Kaplan's Functional and Surgical Anatomy of the Hand

J.B. Lippincott Company

Philadelphia

London   Mexico City   New York
St. Louis   Sao Paulo   Sydney

Third Edition

Kaplan's Functional and Surgical Anatomy of the Hand

Morton Spinner, M.D.

Clinical Professor of Orthopaedic Surgery
Albert Einstein College of Medicine
New York, New York

With 10 Contributors

Sponsoring Editor: Richard Winters
Manuscript Editors: Kristen Frasch,
                    Carol M. Kosik
Indexer: Ruth Elwell
Art Director: Maria S. Karkucinski
Designer: Arlene Putterman
Production Supervisor: J. Corey Gray
Production Assistant: Barney Fernandes
Compositor: Ruttle, Shaw & Wetherill, Inc.
Printer/Binder: Halliday Lithograph

The author and publisher have exerted every effort to ensure that drug selection and dosage set forth in this text are in accord with current recommendations and practice at the time of publication. However, in view of ongoing research, changes in government regulations, and the constant flow of information relating to drug therapy and drug reactions, the reader is urged to check the package insert for each drug for any change in indications and dosage and for added warnings and precautions. This is particularly important when the recommended agent is a new or infrequently employed drug.

3rd Edition

1 3 5 6 4 2

Library of Congress Cataloging in Publication Data
Kaplan, Emanuel B.
   Kaplan's Functional and surgical anatomy of the hand.
   Bibliography: p.
   Includes index.
   1. Hand—Anatomy. 2. Anatomy, Surgical and topographical. I. Spinner, Morton. II. Title. III. Title: Functional and surgical anatomy of the hand. [DNLM: 1. Hand. WE 830 K17f]
   QM548.K3 1984   611'.97   83-11257
   ISBN 0-397-50583-3

iv

"Qu'ils n'oublient jamais que sans anatomie
il n'y a point de physiologie, point de chirurgie, point de médecine."
J. CRUVEILHIER
Anatomie descriptive, 1834

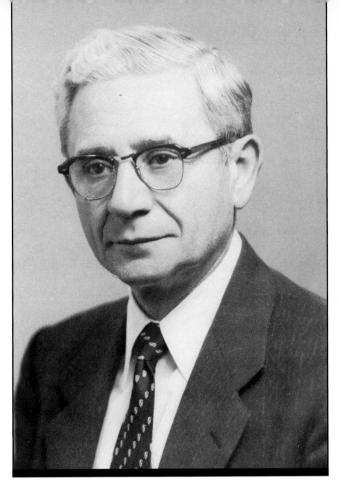

(1894–1980)   Circa 1952

Dedicated to the memory of
EMANUEL B. KAPLAN, M.D.
scholar, anatomist, teacher, clinician
by the editor and contributors

Contributors

JAMES M. HUNTER, M.D.
Professor of Orthopaedic Surgery
Jefferson Medical College of the Thomas Jefferson University
Chief, Hand Surgery Service
Department of Orthopaedics
Thomas Jefferson University Hospital

LEE MILFORD, M.D.
Clinical Professor of Orthopaedic Surgery
University of Tennessee Center for the Health Sciences
Active Staff, Campbell Clinic; Sterling Bunnell Lectureship, 1974
Past President, American Society for Surgery of the Hand, 1974
Consultant in Hand Surgery, Baptist Memorial Hospital,
U.S. Public Health Service, LeBonheur Children's Hospital,
and City of Memphis Hospital, Memphis, Tennessee

MARTIN A. POSNER, M.D.
Associate Clinical Professor Orthopaedic Surgery
Mount Sinai School of Medicine
Chief of Hand Services
Hospital for Joint Diseases Orthopaedic Institute
Mount Sinai Hospital
Lenox Hill Hospital

DANIEL C. RIORDAN, M.D.
Clinical Professor, Orthopaedic Surgery
Tulane University School of Medicine
New Orleans, Louisiana

ROBERT J. SCHULTZ, M.D.
Professor and Chairman
Department of Orthopaedic Surgery
New York Medical College
Director, Sylvester J. Carter Hand Service
New York Medical College

RICHARD J. SMITH, M.D.
Clinical Professor, Orthopaedic Surgery
Harvard Medical School
Chief, Hand Surgery Service
Department of Orthopaedic Surgery
Massachusetts General Hospital
Boston, Massachusetts

ALFRED B. SWANSON, M.D., F.A.C.S.
Professor of Surgery, Michigan State University
    Lansing, Michigan
Chief, Orthopaedic and Hand Surgery Training Program
Blodgett-Butterworth Hospitals
Chief, Orthopaedic and Hand Surgery Research
Blodgett Memorial Medical Center

GENEVIEVE DE GROOT SWANSON, M.D.
Assistant Clinical Professor of Surgery
Michigan State University, Lansing, Michigan
Coordinator, Orthopaedic and Hand Surgery Research
Blodgett Memorial Medical Center

JULIO TALEISNIK, M.D.
Assistant Clinical Professor of Surgery (Orthopaedics)
University of California, Irvine

E. F. SHAW WILGIS, M.D., F.A.C.S.
Assistant Professor of Plastic Surgery at Johns Hopkins Hospital
Assistant Professor of Orthopaedic Surgery at Johns Hopkins Hospital
Director, Division of Hand Surgery, Union Memorial Hospital

Preface

It had long been Dr. Kaplan's intention to revise his text on *Functional and Surgical Anatomy of the Hand*, and several years ago he asked me to assist him in a new edition. When Dr. Kaplan's health failed in 1980, it became apparent that the revision would not be completed within his lifetime. After Dr. Kaplan's death, some of his close scientific friends and students were brought together to complete the work.

It is amazing that Dr. Kaplan, a teacher, a linguist, a research anatomist, and a classical scholar, could have achieved so much in the area of hand surgery. No one person today could hope to attain such mastery over so many aspects of this specialty. For this reason, I am indebted to James M. Hunter of Philadelphia, Lee W. Milford of The Campbell Clinic, Martin A. Posner of The Hospital for Joint Disease, New York, Daniel C. Riordan of New Orleans, Robert J. Schultz of New York Medical College, Richard J. Smith of Massachusetts General Hospital, Julio Taleisnik of California, Alfred and Genevieve Swanson of Grand Rapids, and E. F. Shaw Wilgis of Baltimore for joining me in the revision of Dr. Kaplan's text. All of these contributors were taught by Dr. Kaplan during the past 25 years. All of us share a common bond having been influenced, early on, by this unique man.

Anatomy has not changed since the previous edition of this book was published in 1965. For the most part, changing terminology and attempts to achieve international conformity have necessitated the updating of the text. Dr. Kaplan had strong foreign scientific ties, especially with the French and English. Therefore, the *Terminology for Hand Surgery*, published by the International Federation of Societies for Surgery of the Hand (1970), and the fourth edition of the *Nomina Anatomica* (1975) have been used.

New information about the stability of the wrist and the proximal interphalangeal joint has been included. Recently reported details of the circulation of the flexor tendons and sheath have been added. Redundancies in presentations have been corrected.

Additional illustrations appear in many chapters for increased clarity and understanding of anatomic details. The chapter on surface anatomy has a completely new set of line drawings, which closely follow the description in the text, and will make Dr. Kaplan's classic "cardinal line" observations clearer to all readers. I am grateful to Hugh Thomas, a medical illustrator from New York, for these new drawings. The earlier drawings of C. Kellner and R. Demarest, used in previous editions, have been preserved with only minor changes.

In my work as the editor of this new edition of *Functional and Surgical Anatomy of the Hand,* I have learned a great deal and, again, have been amazed by the depth of Emanuel Kaplan's knowledge. "There is no surgery without anatomy.—It is anatomy, that is all," Dr. Kaplan taught us. One should not read this text to learn how to do a particular operation—rather, one should read it to learn the details of the structures of the hand and their functions. This is the fundamental knowledge one needs to perform whatever surgical procedure is required.

MORTON SPINNER

Acknowledgments

I have been helped in a warm and generous manner by Dr. Irwin Cohen of Manhasset, N.Y. in editing portions of the text. I have used the facilities of the medical library of the New York Academy of Medicine and am indebted to Mrs. Ada Gams, research librarian, for her prompt and tireless expertise.

Several of the contributors wish to express their gratitude to their associates for their assistance. Dr. Julio Taleisnik specifically thanks Dr. R. H. Gelberman and his collaborators, Drs. W. H. Akeson, T. D. Bauman, M. Baumgaertner, J. Menon and J. S. Panagis for the material updating the extraosseous and intraosseous arterial anatomy of the carpal bones.

Dr. James M. Hunter expresses his thanks to his associates, Dr. E. Marshall Johnson, chairman of the Department of Anatomy, Jefferson Medical College, Philadelphia, and Drs. Robert Merkin and Howard Caplan. His numerous hand fellows from 1974 to 1982 helped in the injection techniques and dissections done in the Anatomy Laboratory and Orthopedic Hand Surgery Laboratory. Drs. Scott Jaeger, Naotsune Miyagi, Takeshi Matsui, Michinobu Maeda, and Naoyuki Ochiai are so recognized.

Both Mrs. Virginia Kaplan, Dr. Kaplan's wife, and Mrs. Edith Kaufman, my secretary, assembled Dr. Kaplan's bibliography. Stuart Freeman, medical editor at J.B. Lippincott, and his associates, Richard Winters and Kristen Frasch, have been most cooperative and of great assistance throughout the production of this edition. Special thanks to Maria Karkucinski, art director, for her sincere kindness, understanding, and enormous contributions.

My family, however, provided the greatest contribution to the final product. Jeffrey, my oldest son, relieved me of many household chores that would otherwise have occupied my time. Robert, who has a classics background, advised me frequently as to the appropriate Latin and Greek syntaxes in the text. Steven, my youngest, lost one cheering fan during many of his running races but still encouraged my commitment.

Lastly, I owe my eternal gratitude to my wife, Paula, for her aesthetic eye and loving heart throughout this long period of social hibernation.

M. S.

Preface to the Second Edition

The first edition of this book has been out of print for several years. The favorable acceptance of the first edition and the numerous requests for more information on details of anatomy and function of the hand have prompted the author to add material personally obtained since the publication of the first edition, and also gathered from some of the numerous contributions by anatomists and clinicians who have observed the hand. The author considered it to be important to retain the fundamental parts of the first edition with minor corrections in the text and illustrations. The nomenclature has been changed in accordance with the recommendation of the *Nomina Anatomica Parisiensia*, but some of the familiar names have been retained. The author believes that it is useful, for the sake of simplicity and the elimination of confusion, to retain well-established terms. The periodic changes in anatomic nomenclature which are made by international committees are important and justified, but take time to enter into the clinical literature. Thus, they may at first be confusing to the average clinician. However, there is a tendency among clinicians to introduce new anatomic names not found in the accepted terminology. These new names are usually unnecessary and cause confusion exceeding the permissible level for utility. Unless a new function or a new structure, which had no name previously, is described, such additions are seldom justified.

Changes of nomenclature based on imaginative conceptions are also confusing. Therefore, it should not surprise the reader if some recently introduced, fancied terminology is not to be found in this text.

Further investigations into the details of morphology and function of the hand are imperative because there are still many unanswered questions which beset the hand surgeon and the hand physiologist. Combined efforts by teams of clinicians, anatomists, and kinesiologists will in the future add material for immediate clinical application. These combined efforts will also remove the difficulties often encountered by the hand surgeon in his attempts to wade through complicated mathematical and similar functional explanations. The electromyographic studies of the last few years have already added some valuable material to the functional comprehension of the hand. These will be considered in the light of morphologic studies.

It is hoped that the new edition will continue to be of help to the surgeon who is interested in restoration and preservation of function of the hand. It is also hoped that the new edition will be of help to the anatomist who is interested in special aspects of structure and function of the human hand.

EMANUEL B. KAPLAN

Introduction
to the First Edition

The literature abounds in descriptions of structure and function of the hand. It would appear that the available descriptions are sufficient and that no additional information is required. This impression is erased when the hand surgeon and the hand anatomist are confronted with special problems.

Following World Wars I and II, valuable and instructive studies were made and published. They were based on the abundant material offered by the destructive power of modern weapons applied to the bones and the soft tissues of the upper extremity. The analysis of this material required so much time and attention that observations made by early investigators were not always consulted. Generally, the early anatomists and physiologists understood very well the function of the hand and possessed amazing knowledge of structural detail. Albinus, Winslow, Cloquet and, even earlier, Columbus, Fallopius and many others understand the action of the extensor digitorum communis, the lumbricals and the interrosei, as well as the flexors of the fingers. In the nineteenth century, Gruber, Thompson and others made the most extensive studies of nerve variations, the full importance of which was appreciated only recently. The information obtained by the great anatomists of the eighteenth and the nineteenth centuries, which is not known generally, could be used profitably at present. In 1867, Duchenne, of Boulogne (France), described completely and comprehensively, in a way probably not surpassed by any other observer, the normal and the abnormal functions of the hand. He also placed his description in a proper historical perspective. But his work was overlooked, and much labor was spent, and is being spent, by other investigators who were not, and are not, aware of the observations made by him. The extensive new material and the surgical and the neurologic experiences accumulated since Duchenne's original publication require further study and more precision in the description of the structure of the hand and understanding of the intricacies of its mechanism.

Stimulated by early acquaintance with the work of classical anatomists and by personal experiences in the surgery of the hand, the author collected useful material in the anatomic laboratory over a period of years. Personal studies were made of anatomic structures, and electric stimulation was applied to the muscles of the hand directly during surgical procedures and indirectly. Electric stimulation of muscles of the rhesus monkey also was produced under appropriate conditions. Several gorilla, chimpanzee, rhesus monkey and baboon hands were dissected. Studies were made by the author on the fasciae of the hand, the embryology of the hand, the tendinous apparatus of the fingers and the surgical approaches. Correlation of structure and function was investigated.

There is a general tendency to curtail progressively the time allotted to the teaching of anatomy in the medical schools, but the need for anatomy is greater than ever. It is essential in surgery, where an adequate knowledge of structure could have eliminated inadequate operations performed in the past and those still being performed. Its need in the study of locomotion, rehabilitation, neurologic interpretation and internal medicine, in spite of important strides in biochemistry, biophysics and so forth, should be obvious even to the ignorant.

In the particular instance of the hand, it was considered that the student, the anatomist and the surgeon needed a unified text with descriptions combining structural detail with precise function. Such unification is of practical importance, especially if combined with principles of surgical anatomy. The surgical anatomy should include the description of approaches to various parts, points of repair, possible errors, illustrative procedures and orientation in case of variations.

To obtain all possible facts and to make this book useful, it was necessary to resort to other fields. In the embryologic development of the hand, some comparative anatomic studies were added to bring out such or other detail for understanding of function or structure. Multiple dissections of human hands were necessary to show the most frequent patterns. It was necessary to consider the variations which occur in the hands and to place them in definite groups to grasp their significance and to help the surgeon to meet these variations with comprehension. Comparative anatomic studies were of great help, as they revealed functional relationships of certain structures, offering opportunities equal to planned experiments, because preservation or elimination of structures with known function in different species frequently permits deductions as to the actual significance of variations in the human hand.

The anatomic structures in this book are described from the viewpoint only of function and surgery. Conventional descriptive patterns of anatomy are not followed. Pathology, diagnostic methods and detailed surgical technics are not given, except to clarify an illustration.

The description of anatomic structures in textbooks does not mention the age of the subject. It considers a hypothetical man of average age. The hands of an old person, a child or an adult between 25 and 35 years of age present obvious differences.

With age, some of the finer structures of the fingers and the motor apparatus, especially round the joints, undergo changes that produce limitations of use similar to limitation produced by injury. The fine adjusting mechanism between the flexor and the extensor apparatus is disturbed easily by the slightest injury and loses some of its function at any age, except in the very young. Interference with the adjusting mechanism induced by aging or by inflammatory or metabolic processes is not dissimilar to postoperative fibrosis. Therefore, it is essential to indicate, when possible, at least the difference due to age.

The function and the anatomy of the hand cannot be separated from the function of the forearm or the arm. The limitations of this study to the hand are arbitrary.

References to comparative anatomy are made only to explain function or to understand structure. The author does not contemplate adding material to the discussion of man's relation to other zoologic groups.

It is impossible to separate function of the hand from the central nervous system, but this represents a special field, somewhat outside the immediate need of the surgeon and the functional anatomist, for whom this book is intended primarily.

It was not intended to create an encyclopedia of the hand. This will explain the absence of emphasis on certain subjects which were not studied especially as, for instance, the lymphatic circulation.

The book is illustrated profusely. A few illustrations were obtained from the collections of the Department of Anatomy of the College of Physicians and Surgeons (Columbia University), and their source has been indicated. Aside from these, all the illustrations are original. They were drawn from multiple dissections made by the author and are being published now for the first time.

An attempt has been made to eliminate any misconceptions, and proper credit has been given to the original investigators.

The history of human civilization is replete with special studies of the hand. The expressions, the activities and the configuration of the hand were a constant source of inquiry and inspiration not only to scientists but also to artists, philosophers, men of religion and mystics. In the enormous literature of the past and the present on the subject of the hand, the most curious information can be found alongside rational descriptions. *The Structure, Uses and Abuses of the Hand*, written by William A. Alcott, M.D., and published by the Massachusetts Sabbath School Society of Boston in 1856, may serve as an example. It contains curious advice intermixed with elementary anatomic facts. Although not directly related to our subject, it is of interest to quote one of the many statements in this small book:

Among the parts of the human system to which the hand should *seldom if ever be applied*, except, *perhaps*, to wash them, are the hair, ears, nose, the hollow of the shoulder, knee and hip, the toes and soles of the feet.

This was "sound" advice by a physician and was given not very long ago. Obviously, the advice was not given for the enlightenment of other physicians. The reference is mentioned as an illustration of approach to the study of the hand. It certainly cannot be compared with a famous book, written also in the nineteenth century but many years earlier by the brilliant Charles Bell, *The Hand, Its Mechanism and Vital Endowments as Evincing Design.*

Contrary to custom, the author is not adding a historical survey on the subject of functional and surgical anatomy. Such a study would be profitable and would place the information which we now possess in proper relationship to the scientific acquisitions of the past, but it would be out of bounds in a practical book on surgical and functional anatomy. However, it may be of interest to mention that this subject was treated with great perspicacity even in the beginning of our era. Galen (A.D. 131-201) devoted a large part of *De usu partium* to the subject of the anatomy and the physiology of the hand. In Daremberg's French translation, eighty-seven pages of very important, in every sense up-to-date, material are devoted to the hand.

As mentioned previously, no contribution is made to the interrelation of the mechanics of the hand to the motor and the sensory systems of the central nervous apparatus. The more remote subjects of psychological and psychiatric influences on the hand are not touched upon. However, this field is of great interest.

The *Essai sur la psychologie de la main,* written by N. Vashide and published in 1909, deserves special interest as an attempt to unify function with complexities of "motor image" from the lofty viewpoints of philosophy and psychology.

Attempts to describe firmly established changes in the configuration and the surface creases of the hands of normal and abnormal individuals were made in a book, *The Hand in Psychological Diagnosis,* by Charlotte Wolff, which was published recently. This type of research requires greater amplification. Special training, not possessed by the average surgeon, is the necessary attribute for such studies. These studies could be of great value in the chapters on function of the hand, and in the future they may transcend the morphologic description and the contemporary approach to the immediate mechanisms of hand function.

Congenital deformities are not included in the description because, in contrast with variations which belong to the domain of the anatomist, the congenital deformities fall into the classification of malformations or, perhaps, embryologic arrest. Their surgical management presents special problems that require an individual approach, depending on the type of deformity, age and other factors.

A complete survey of the subject was made in Denmark recently by A. Birch-Jensen. Recently, O'Rahilly, of Wayne University, published a most interesting study on the morphologic patterns in limb deformities and duplications. A. Barsky made an enlightening study of the surgical problems connected with deformities of the hand.

With due apologies for the many omissions, it is hoped that *Functional and Surgical Anatomy of the Hand* will be of help to the orthopedic, the plastic and the general surgeons and to all who are interested in the restoration of function of the hand, also to the anatomist interested in certain aspects of structure and function of the human hand.

E. B. K.

Contents

**Part Three
Surgical
Anatomy**

Part One
The Hand as an Organ

1
The Hand as an Organ

Emanuel B. Kaplan
Morton Spinner

The hand is an important functioning organ requiring rest and performing the greatest part of activities, including locomotion, if need be. The function of the entire upper extremity is to position the hand in space. The arm and forearm position the hand so that we can perform essential tasks. In all its spatial locations the hand not only grasps and releases various objects but transports them as well. Moreover, through the hand, as through sight and hearing, we form a conception of the outside world. It is truly the extension of our brain into the surrounding world; it is the mirror of our innermost response to the outside world.

The function of the hand can be analyzed best when divided into component parts. Although this is somewhat artificial, it permits a better insight into the activity of the hand as a unit. In order to understand the function of the human hand, it is very helpful to compare it with the function of the hands of the anthropoid apes. For different reasons in the past, and even sometimes in the present, observers suspected fundamental anatomic differences between human and anthropoid hands. Actual observations on the action of those hands and on their anatomic structures show that the differences are not very great and at times are indistinguishable.

The most characteristic features of the human hand are the comparative length of the thumb and the almost constant presence of a flexor pollicis longus, which permits great flexibility in the use of the thumb in conjunction with the rest of the hand. The longer thumb of

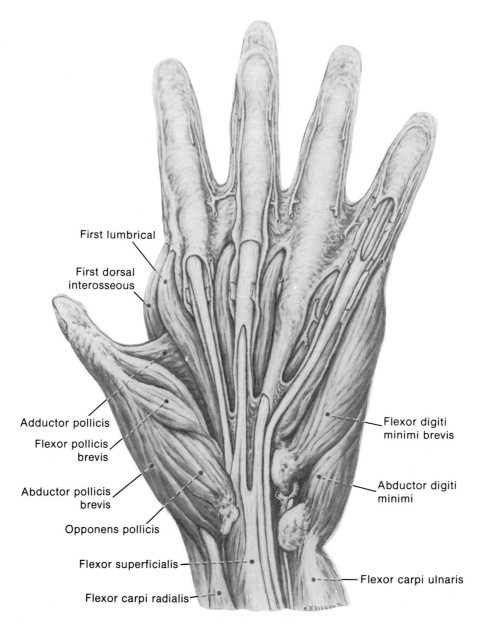

First lumbrical

First dorsal
interosseous

Adductor pollicis

Flexor pollicis
brevis

Abductor pollicis
brevis

Opponens pollicis

Flexor superficialis

Flexor carpi radialis

Flexor digiti
minimi brevis

Abductor digiti
minimi

Flexor carpi ulnaris

FIG. 1–1 The left hand of a gorilla showing the flexor tendons. The thenar eminence reveals a strongly developed abductor brevis, flexor brevis, and opponens. The pisiform is very large and has a special form as can be seen in Figure 1-6. The tendon of the flexor carpi ulnaris is inserted into the entire length of the elongated pisiform on its proximal side, and the abductor of the little finger arises from the entire length of the distal pisiform. (Specimen from the Museum of the Department of Anatomy, College of Physicians and Surgeons, Columbia University, New York, NY)

humans permits better opposition, mostly because of its length and the help of the flexor pollicis longus, which introduces an element of stability. The thenar muscles of the gorilla and of the chimpanzee are almost identical to the thenar muscles of the human hand. The gorilla has good opposition when occasion arises; the other apes have it to a lesser extent. Their ability to seek out and grasp insects is amazing; they actually perform this action by using some opposition between the thumb and the index and middle fingers.

The two distal phalanges of each finger of the anthropoid hand are kept in flexion, permitting the ulnar side of the thumb to touch the radial side of either the distal or the middle phalanx of the index finger. The different groups of the baboon *(Papio)* can fully extend all the phalanges of the fingers and are thus able to touch the volar aspect of the index and especially the middle finger in a manner very similar to human opposition. Slow-motion movie observations made by the author showed distinctly the almost humanlike opposition exhibited by the baboon hand in a rapid grasping of small objects. The gorilla and the orangutan do not have any comparable opposition, but it is not because of the configuration of the metacarpocarpal joint of the thumb (see Figs. 1–1 and 1–2). A valuable study on the subject of power and precision grasp in primates was made by Napier. The nerve supply to these muscles is very similar to the human nerve supply, as attested by many observers (Figs. 1–1 and 1–3).

The hand can be divided artificially into three functional units: the thumb, the index and middle fingers, and the ring and little fingers (Fig. 1–4). The most important actions are performed between the thumb and the index and middle fingers. The ring finger and the little finger form a supporting auxiliary. With the development of fine action, the index finger tends to become more and more independent of the middle finger and the ring and little fingers. This is reflected not only in outward independence but also in separation of the muscle bellies of the index finger from the rest of the flexor profundus and superficialis in many human hands. The thumb forms a separate unit with

FIG. 1–2 The skeleton of an adult human hand, a chimpanzee hand, and a gorilla hand. The pisiform in the gorilla and in the chimpanzee is elongated and somewhat larger than the triquetrum. The most obvious feature is the comparative reduction in the size of the trapezium and the thumb in the anthropoid hand.

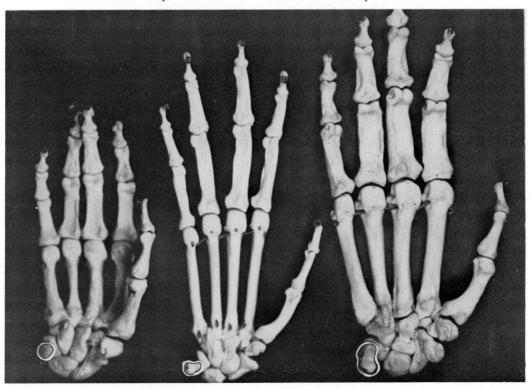

MAN   CHIMPANZEE   GORILLA

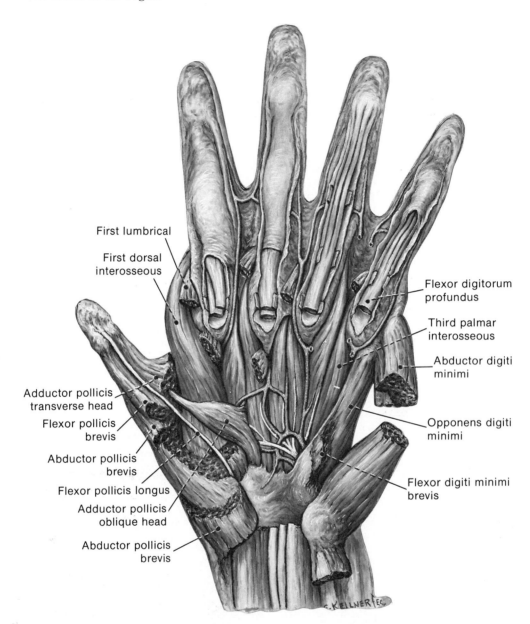

First lumbrical

First dorsal
interosseous

Adductor pollicis
transverse head

Flexor pollicis
brevis

Abductor pollicis
brevis

Flexor pollicis longus

Adductor pollicis
oblique head

Abductor pollicis
brevis

Flexor digitorum
profundus

Third palmar
interosseous

Abductor digiti
minimi

Opponens digiti
minimi

Flexor digiti minimi
brevis

FIG. 1–3 Gorilla's left hand. Further dissection reveals an attenuated flexor pollicis longus tendon in its usual location. The abductor, the flexor brevis, and the opponens of the thumb are seen along with a very small portion of the oblique head of the adductor of the thumb. There are two heads of the transverse portion of the adductor: one originated from the crest of the second metacarpal, the other from the crest of the third metacarpal. The possibility of such origin in the human hand should not be overlooked. The nerve supply to the intrinsic muscles of the hand is not unlike the human nerve supply. (Specimen from the Museum of the Department of Anatomy, College of Physicians and Surgeons, Columbia University New York, NY)

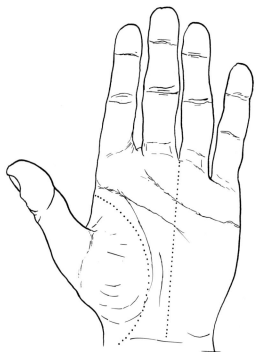

FIG. 1–4 Three functional areas of a hand: the thenar and the thumb; the index and the middle fingers; the ring and the little fingers.

distal crease, which starts at the ulnar border of the palm of the hand and runs radially toward the ulnar side of the index finger, not reaching the web space between the index and middle fingers, is creased mostly when the middle, ring, and little fingers are flexed. An uncreased space remains between the free radial end of this crease and the radial border of the palm of the hand. For flexion of all four fingers, the creasing occurs in the proximal crease of the palm of the hand, which starts from the radial border of the palm of the hand and runs proximally toward, but not reaching, the ulnar border of the palm of the hand. There is an independent area for flexion of the index finger that occurs mostly between the second web space and the junction of the proximal palmar and thenar creases of the hand. The folds that occur when the index finger is flexed do not leave permanent creases in the skin similar to the distal, middle, and thenar creases of the palm, but they are visible when the index is flexed independently (Fig. 1–5).

FIG. 1–5 The left hand, showing the functional creases that appear on flexion of the index finger, the direction of which corresponds to the interspace between the distal crease of the palm and the thenar crease. The long axis of the index finger in flexion corresponds to this interspace. The flexion creases of the index finger run across this space. The broken line indicates the direction of the finger singly flexed.

actual separation of the flexor pollicis longus, low in the forearm, and at the origin of this muscle, from the other long flexor muscles of the hand. The separation of the thumb into an independent unit involves the bones of the wrist as well; actually, both phalanges of the thumb, together with the metacarpal, the trapezium, and the scaphoid bones form a relatively independent functioning unit.

The second functional unit consists of the index and the middle fingers. This is separated into a unit because the most important usages of the hand occur between the thumb as one unit and the index and middle fingers as the other. The index finger occupies a unique position. If one examines the creases of the hand, one sees immediately that the middle finger belongs partly to the third group, which is the supporting group of the hand, and that the index finger occupies an independent position between this supporting group and the thumb. Examining the creases of the palm of the hand, one sees that the

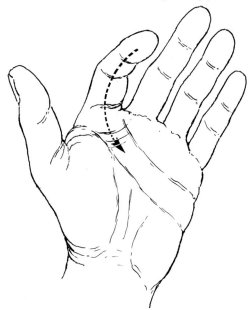

DEFINITION OF MOTIONS OF THE THUMB, THE FINGERS, AND THE WRIST

THE THUMB

The thumb is capable of producing flexion both at the interphalangeal and metacarpophalangeal joints. There is also flexion of the metacarpocarpal joint between the first metacarpal and the trapezium. Motion of abduction and adduction occurs from and to the second metacarpal and takes place in the joint between the metacarpal and the trapezium. There is extension of the distal phalanx in the interphalangeal joint, extension at the metacarpophalangeal joint, and extension at the metacarpocarpal joint. In addition, the thumb is capable of producing opposition. This very specialized motion consists of rotation of the volar surface of the thumb so that from its normal position of rest, perpendicular to the transverse plane of the hand, it is able to face the volar surface of all the fingers after pulling out completely (abduction) from the surface of the palm. Thus, it produces a rotatory motion from the normal 90° of rest to 180° parallel with the transverse plane of the hand.

The joint between the proximal end of the metacarpal and the distal end of the trapezium is a saddle joint; the proximal end of the metacarpal rides in this saddle. Opposition of the thumb is possible because laxity of the capsule of this joint permits not only flexion and extension, and abduction and adduction, but actually some rotatory motion that is combined with the other movements. All these motions are obviously possible because of the activity of the thenar muscles of the thumb, the extensor pollicis longus, and the auxiliary muscles around the thumb, as will be described in Chapter 7. Opposition of the tip of the thumb to the other fingers, especially to the ring and little fingers, is due equally to a varying degree of abduction–adduction that occurs at the metacarpophalangeal joint of the thumb. This important feature was brought out by Duchenne, who explained the important action of the abductor brevis of the thumb.

The activity of the thumb can be divided into abduction occurring at the metacarpocarpal joint, consisting of retraction of the thumb from the second metacarpal, and adduction of the thumb, which also takes place in the metacarpocarpal joint and consists of a motion toward the second metacarpal. Abduction is enhanced by additional abduction at the metacarpophalangeal joint by the abductor brevis; adduction is produced mostly by the adductor of the thumb.

Although it is easy to perceive flexion and extension of the distal and proximal phalanges of the thumb, it is somewhat more difficult to analyze flexion and extension of the metacarpal. Extension at the metacarpophalangeal joint consists of a posterior motion of the metacarpal from the position of rest, and flexion consists of a volar motion of the metacarpal, also from the position of rest. Both motions can be combined with flexion–adduction when the thumb is sliding actively over the surface of the palm and flexion–abduction with the thumb moving away from the palm. The opposite motions are extension–abduction and extension–adduction. Opposition will consist of actual abduction–flexion and rotation of the first metacarpal at the metacarpocarpal joint, aided by flexion and abduction at the metacarpophalangeal joint and extension of the distal phalanx. All these motions are activated by certain muscles, which will be described in detail in the section on the thumb (Chapters 3 and 7).

FINGERS

Each finger of the hand is capable of flexion and extension at the distal interphalangeal joint, at the proximal interphalangeal joint, and at the metacarpophalangeal joint. The latter joint is also capable of abduction and adduction, as well as circumduction, at the metacarpophalangeal joint, thus demonstrating the diarthrodial, multiaxial metacarpophalangeal joint. Each finger is capable of adduction and abduction in relation to its long axis. The middle finger of the hand is chosen as the axis finger; therefore, all motion occurring toward this finger is called adduction, while movement away from this finger is abduction.

WRIST

The function of the fingers of the hand cannot be considered apart from the function of the wrist. Flexion, or volar flexion, of the wrist consists of a motion approximating the volar surface of the forearm and the palmar surface of the hand. Extension, or dorsiflexion, consists of approximation toward each other of the dorsal surface of the forearm and the dorsal surface of the hand. Ulnar deviation is a medial inclination of the hand toward the ulnar side of the forearm, and radial deviation is a radial inclination toward the radial side of the forearm. Circumduction occurs in all of these directions when the moving wrist forms the apex of a cone and the tip of the middle finger describes a circumference.

POSITIONS OF THE HAND

Normally, the inactive hand is at rest with all the constituent parts at rest. This can be changed to the functional position, which is the transition stage from rest to activity.

Position of rest
The position of rest frequently is confused with the functional position of the hand; actually, these two positions differ.

In the position of rest, the hand is dorsiflexed only very slightly, perhaps not more than about 10° to 15° with very slight ulnar deviation; the fingers are flexed at the two interphalangeal and metacarpophalangeal joints, the index finger least and the little finger the most. The position of rest is assumed when the hand is resting on a horizontal surface. When the hand is hanging down, the dorsiflexion of the wrist disappears completely or almost so. The thumb

is abducted slightly, and the pulp of the thumb is either directed to or touches the radial aspect of the distal interphalangeal joint of the index finger.

Functional position
The functional position of the hand is slightly different. In this position, the wrist is much more dorsiflexed, the metacarpophalangeal joints are extended and abducted, the distal and the middle interphalangeal joints are flexed slightly, the thumb is abducted strongly and extended slightly at the carpometacarpal joint, the first metacarpal is rotated so that its radio-ulnar plane is perpendicular to the radio-ulnar plane of the other metacarpals, the metacarpophalangeal joint of the thumb is extended slightly, and the distal phalanx of the thumb is flexed slightly. The functional position permits rapid movement to the various positions of activity.

Pinch positions
In modern usage we are concerned with four types of pinch positions:

1. The *closed round pinch* position permits picking up objects with the index finger or the middle finger and the thumb. The first metacarpal rotates, carrying with it the proximal and the distal phalanges of the thumb so that its pulp touches the pulp of the index finger or the middle finger, the proximal phalanx and the distal phalanx of the thumb are flexed slightly, and the first metacarpal is abducted and flexed slightly at the metacarpophalangeal joint. The index finger is flexed at the metacarpophalangeal joint and also at the proximal and the distal interphalangeal joints. The wrist is dorsiflexed moderately.
2. The *chuck pinch* position is a variant of the closed round pinch in which the distal pulp of the opposed thumb meets the distal pulps of the index and middle fingers when the latter are in contiguity.
3. The *closed elongated pinch* position is a further modification of the closed round

pinch. In this position the thumb and the index finger or the middle finger assume the position of an elongated pincers as in the act of threading a needle. Obviously, under these circumstances the distal phalanges of the index finger or the middle finger and the thumb are extended instead of being flexed.

4. *Key pinch* exists when the thumb is capable only of intimate adduction to the second metacarpal. This latter position has particular relevance in restoration of function following spinal cord injury.

FIG. 1–6 Model of an adult gorilla hand, showing the position of the thumb. Although short, the gorilla thumb has a resting position similar to that of the human thumb. (Specimen from the Museum of the Department of Anatomy, College of Physicians and Surgeons, Columbia University, New York, NY)

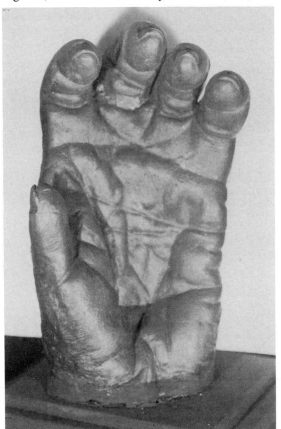

Observations in primates

Observations made by the author on the activity of the hands of a small, young gorilla and a large, young gorilla at the Bronx Zoological Garden showed a wide range of motion of fingers and thumb.

Furthermore, considerable strength of adduction of the thumb was noted by the author when his hand was grasped between the thumb and the second metacarpal of the gorilla. The position of rest of the hand of the gorilla is very similar to that of the human hand, except for the slight extension at the metacarpophalangeal joints, exaggerated flexion of the proximal interphalangeal joint, and strong volar flexion of the wrist. Figure 1–6 is a model of a gorilla hand at rest.

The hand of the chimpanzee is very similar to the hand of the gorilla; however, the thumb is much smaller and comparatively shorter and weaker (Fig. 1–2). While the gorilla appears to use the thumb constantly, the thumb of the chimpanzee gives the impression of being in the way. The fingers of the chimpanzee (a young female), also observed in the Bronx Zoological Garden, appeared to be very agile. The action was very delicate, gentle, controlled, and reasoned. It is well known that the chimpanzee is able to perform a multitude of manual acts resembling human acts, despite suppression of opposition of the thumb, which is substituted by adduction.

The importance of the thumb in the activity of the hand cannot be overestimated, but even in its absence or substitution, it permits a considerable range of useful adaptation. The observation of rehabilitated, intelligent men who have lost parts of their hands proves how much can be regained by compensatory function of the remaining parts. Preservation of function in even seemingly hopeless situations may allow the application of newer and more sophisticated reconstructive and rehabilitative techniques. Restoration of function in these salvaged parts is essential. The task of the surgeon is to preserve this function, even in seemingly hopeless mutilations, because the demands and the responses connected with the activity of the central nervous system produce extraordinary results of rehabilitation.

The gorilla very seldom shows the presence of the flexor pollicis longus; the chimpanzee and the orangutan generally do not possess a flexor pollicis longus. This causes absence of flexion of the distal phalanx, but in actual opposition of the thumb to the fingers, flexion of the distal phalanx of the thumb is not entirely necessary because in opposition, the distal phalanx of the thumb is extended. The flexor pollicis longus acts in this instance as a stabilizer of the distal phalanx. The functional mechanism of opposition is so arranged that the thenar muscles, which are responsible for opposition simultaneously produce extension of the distal phalanx, as will be demonstrated in Chapters 3 and 7. This action of the thenar muscles producing extension of the distal phalanx of the thumb in opposition, even when there is a simultaneous paralysis of the extensor pollicis longus, puzzles the uninitiated.

The extension of the distal phalanx is not caused by the passive stretch of the extensor pollicis longus. The author has found, and it is recognized, that in paralysis of the thenar muscles, when the thumb is brought passively into opposition, the distal phalanx flexes; if the extensor pollicis longus would produce stretch extension of the distal phalanx, the distal phalanx would extend. It was further noted that in cases of traumatic division of the tendon of the extensor pollicis longus over the first metacarpal or in a more proximal location, active opposition of the thumb is accompanied by extension of the distal phalanx.

In the position of pinch for grasping small objects between the index finger and the thumb, the presence of the flexor pollicis longus is very important because without it the half of the pincers formed by the thumb loses the power to hold the distal phalanx of the thumb against the distal phalanx of the index finger.

Inasmuch as the anthropoid apes in their natural activity seldom require the finer pinch, the anthropoid hand seldom requires fine opposition unless specialized activity is required; thus, the Tarsius spectrum, according to authorities and observations during dissections by the author, exhibits a very strong flexor pollicis longus muscle and tendon in the hand. This flexor pollicis longus serves to hold firmly onto branches with the additional help of specialized digital suction pads. In the gibbon, the flexor pollicis longus is apparently attenuated completely, and the thumb is very small and appears to be a hindrance in the brachiating acrobatic activity of locomotion.

The flexor pollicis longus' development is more a function of specialization than of intelligence. The presence of the flexor hallucis longus in the foot of most of the anthropoids and its sophisticated development are well adapted to the survival needs of the anthropoid foot, in contradistinction to the less specialized requirements of the anthropoid hand.

Except under those extraordinary circumstances where both upper extremities are absent (*i.e.*, phocomelia caused by maternal ingestion of thalidomide), the highly developed flexor hallucis longus in the case of the anthropoid foot serves a special function not usually observed in man.

FUNDAMENTAL FUNCTIONS OF THE HAND

To cover the entire range of activity of the human hand, several fundamental functions are required. When opening the hand:

1. Independent flexion of the metacarpophalangeal joints of the fingers
2. Abduction of the fingers
3. Corresponding extension of the middle and the distal phalanges
4. Extension of the metacarpocarpal joint of the thumb
5. Extension of the metacarpophalangeal joint of the thumb

6. Extension of the distal phalanx of the thumb
7. Abduction of the thumb

The motor and the tendinous apparatus for these functions are interconnected into a synchronous system of controlled retention and rapid action with strong tendons for stabilization of the wrist.

When closing the hand, the following functions are required:

1. Independent flexion of the metacarpophalangeal joints
2. Separate flexion of the distal and the middle phalanges
3. Adduction of the fingers
4. Adduction of the thumb
5. Flexion of the distal and proximal phalanges of the thumb
6. Flexion of the metacarpocarpal joint of the thumb
7. Opposition of the thumb

These functions require power more than speed; therefore, the tendinous apparatus is more separated, rounder, and retained in special tunnels, but the power is controlled. For precision, small muscular bodies are called to function. These are short, specialized tendinous arrangements that convert the entire system into a harmonious unit. They are closely knit by fibers and bands of a marvelous retinacular apparatus involving the dorsal and volar aspects of the hand.

The opening and the closing of the hand, as well as the action of the fine adjusting mechanism of the small muscles of the hand, are coordinated with the action of the wrist and consist of slight volar flexion with slight ulnar deviation for opening the hand; dorsiflexion for closing the hand; ulnar deviation for abducting the thumb; and radial deviation for abducting the little finger. All of these motions may occur in either supination or pronation of the forearm.

FUNCTIONAL LENGTH OF TENDONS

The motor units responsible for the activation of the hand are represented by a specialized muscular apparatus that although divided into individual muscles, work in synchrony.

For normal action, a contracting muscle exhibits a comparatively fixed measure of functional length. The term *functional length* means the length through the entire range of motion between the extremes. For instance, the entire functional length of the extensor carpi radialis longus from complete flexion to complete extension of the wrist is about 4 cm for the average hand (measured by the author in fresh cadavers and during surgical procedures). Each tendon involved with movement of the fingers and wrist has a significant average length, and this permits successful application of the principles of transplantation of a tendon of a given functional length for a motion requiring approximately the same functional length. The following figures listed below are averages for the total functional length of the motor units of the hand and the wrist in the normal adult.

TOTAL FUNCTIONAL LENGTH OF THE EXTENSORS OF THE WRIST

Extensor carpi radialis longus, 4 cm (extension–flexion)
  Extensor carpi radialis brevis, 3.5 cm to 4 cm (extension–flexion)
  Extensor carpi ulnaris, 2.5 cm to 3 cm (extension–flexion)

TOTAL FUNCTIONAL LENGTH OF THE FLEXORS OF THE WRIST

Flexor carpi radialis, 5 cm (flexion–extension)
  Flexor carpi ulnaris, 3 to 3.5 cm (flexion–extension)

TOTAL FUNCTIONAL LENGTH OF RADIO-ULNAR DEVIATIONS OF THE WRIST

Flexor carpi radialis, 0.75 cm to 1 cm
  Flexor carpi ulnaris, 1 cm
  Extensor carpi radialis longus, 1.5 cm to 2 cm
  Extensor carpi radialis brevis, 1.5 cm to 2 cm
  Extensor carpi ulnaris, 2.5 cm to 3 cm

Abductor pollicis longus, 1.5 cm to 2 cm
Extensor pollicis brevis, 1 cm to 1.5 cm
Extensor pollicis longus, 1 cm

FUNCTIONAL LENGTH OF THE BRACHIO-RADIALIS AND THE PRONATOR TERES

The total functional lengths of the brachioradialis and the pronator teres are given because these two muscles can be effectively used in muscle transplantations to restore the functions of the fingers: brachioradialis, 3.5 cm to 4 cm (flexion–extension); pronator teres, 2.5 cm to 3 cm (flexion–extension, pronation–supination).

TOTAL FUNCTIONAL LENGTH OF THE MOTORS OF THE THUMB

Flexor pollicis longus, 5.5 cm to 6 cm at the wrist
Extensor pollicis longus, 5.5 cm to 6 cm at the wrist
Extensor pollicis brevis, 3 cm at the wrist
Abductor pollicis longus, 3 cm at the wrist
Adductor pollicis, 1.5 cm to 2 cm at metacarpophalangeal joint
Abductor pollicis brevis, 0.5 cm to 1 cm at metacarpophalangeal joint
Flexor pollicis brevis, 1 cm at metacarpophalangeal joint
Flexor pollicis brevis, 1 cm at carpometacarpal joint

TOTAL FUNCTIONAL LENGTH OF THE MOTORS OF THE FINGERS

The investigation of the functional length of the motor units of the fingers was observed during surgery under local anesthesia; some of the measurements were made on fresh cadavers, and some measurements were made on a specially constructed model. Although the exact length of motion of each tendon is obviously important, the measurements were carried out for the purpose of determining ratios between the functional lengths of various tendons. The measurements were taken at the wrist joint and at the metacarpophalangeal joint with the wrist in a neutral position.

FLEXOR PROFUNDUS

Index—at the wrist, 3 cm; at the metacarpophalangeal joint, about 2.75 cm
Middle finger—at the wrist joint, 4 cm; at the metacarpophalangeal joint, 3.5 cm
Ring finger—at the wrist joint, 4.5 cm; at the metacarpophalangeal joint, 4 cm
Little finger—at the wrist joint, 3.5 cm; at the metacarpophalangeal joint, 3 cm

FLEXOR DIGITORUM SUPERFICIALIS

This tendon gave approximately 0.5 cm to 0.75 cm less functional length than the corresponding flexor profundus for each finger.

EXTENSOR DIGITORUM COMMUNIS

Index finger—at the wrist, 3 cm; at the metacarpophalangeal joint, 3 cm
Middle finger—at the wrist joint, 4 cm; at the metacarpophalangeal joint, 3.5 cm
Ring finger—at the wrist joint, 4 cm; at the metacarpophalangeal joint, 3.5 cm
Little finger—at the wrist joint, 3 cm; at the metacarpophalangeal joint, 2.5 cm
Extensor indicis—slightly shorter than the corresponding extensor communis tendon
Extensor digiti minimi—slightly longer than the corresponding extensor communis tendon

INTEROSSEI

It is very difficult to measure the functional length of these muscles. It varies from finger to finger from approximately 1.25 cm to about 2.25 cm at the metacarpophalangeal joint for the function of simultaneous flexion and extension of the phalanges. The functional length for lateral deviation is approximately 0.5 cm.

LUMBRICALES

The functional length of the lumbrical muscles is surprisingly great. The length of the lumbrical muscle itself varies in the fingers, and the contraction of the muscle may reach about 3.5 cm to

4.5 cm in the middle finger, with correspondingly less length for the other fingers.

The figures given above for the motor units of the thumb, the wrist, and the fingers may vary considerably. In order to establish standards, it will be necessary to measure a larger number of hands of persons in different occupations and especially, in different age groups. It may be correctly assumed that the lumbrical muscles of a violinist or a pianist will have greater lengths of function than the lumbrical muscles of a laborer who uses his hands only for heavy work. The functional length of the tendons of older people is more restricted than that of the tendons of young people or children. The absence of some tendons and the existence of supernumerary tendons may have a definite influence on the function of other tendons.

Boyes has shown the functional length of a muscle or its amplitude may vary in accordance with its relation to the function of joints, crossed by the corresponding muscle and its tendon. This is an important consideration in surgical transfers and substitutions of tendons to restore a lost function, because freeing of a muscle often alters its functional length.

Another important consideration in the kinesiology of muscles is the power of each individual unit. Weber, Fick, von Lanz, and Wachsmuth have correlated muscle cross-sectional area and its strength.

Contributions by Brand and co-workers have recently correlated the relative tension and potential excursion for each of the muscles of the forearm and hand. Precise studies of this type have significant clinical applications.

PRINCIPLE OF COORDINATED ACTION

For normal activity of all the components of the hand, normal function and structure of the moving parts are required. It is obvious that the muscular activity must also be normal. To understand the role of a single muscle, it is necessary to recognize that the muscles work in multiple groups and participate conjointly and synchronously in even the simplest motion.

When a specific action is ascribed to an individual muscle, it means only that there is an active dominance of this muscle over all other muscles that participate in the movement. For instance, in case of direct flexion of the elbow without supination or pronation, all the flexors, including the brachialis, the biceps humeri, the pronator teres, the brachioradialis and secondarily, the supinator, the triceps brachii, the anconeus, and others act as a unit. The dominant muscles in this action are the brachialis and the brachioradialis; the fixation muscles are the active balancing pronator teres and supinator, biceps, and pronator quadratus. The character of predominance of muscle action plays an important role in the interpretation of action of individual muscles and the principle of predominance of action always must be remembered in the interpretation of muscular activity. The usual textbook classification of muscles into separate groups should be interpreted with reservations because this classification does not give a true image of the actual muscular dynamics; it reflects only a limited movement which may vary considerably under specific conditions.

The early anatomists based their definition of muscular activity on the analysis, observed in the cadaver, of motion of muscles stretched between origin and insertion. Such descriptions as noted in the works of Albinus and Winslow are precise and admirable. The modern interpretation of muscle action required the participation of clinicians. These observations were initiated by Duchenne, who was probably the first and the greatest observer and interpreter of muscular action. His studies were based on precise observations of the living subject, normal and abnormal. Although he described in great detail the response of individual muscles to electrical stimulation, he established the important principle that physiologic function of muscles requires participation of other muscles: assistants (synergists), antagonists, fixation muscles, and so on.

In the *Physiology of Motion*, Duchenne states:

Under the name of impulsive muscular associations I understand the synergistic muscular contractions designed to produce any voluntary motion changing the position in any manner in any part of the body. The electrophysiologic experiments and the clinical observations, which I described, threw much light on the study of each of the impulsive muscular associations. They showed that the partial muscular contractions (of each muscle separately) are not a normal thing. These partial muscular contractions are only produced artificially by means of local faradization, or under certain pathological circumstances; that they are always responsible for distortions, as for instance the distortion of the scapula or downward subluxation of the head of the humerus in voluntary elevation of the arm in individuals whose serratus anterior is paralyzed.

If it is considered that muscular functions of the extremities often require the combination of many simultaneous movements which in themselves are a resultant of complex forces, it may be understood how complicated are the impulsive muscular associations which participate in these functions.

In conclusion, every voluntary motion which is executed with precision must be moderated by antagonists, and if this motion is performed in a joint mobile in all directions (arthrodial or enarthrosis), a synergistic collateral contraction of muscles which produce lateral motions must prevent its lateral deviation.

These quotations emphasize the importance of integrated muscular activity in production of any motion. The principle of the dominance of certain muscles in integrated participation with other muscles in a given motion will be considered further under the section on the mechanism of the hand (Chap. 7). A simple concept for better understanding of these mechanisms will be discussed. In the analysis of motion of the various elements of the hand, the normal balance of the hand at rest must also be taken into consideration. The balance is created by the tonic stretch of the antagonistic muscles. The extensors, for instance, are in tonic balance against the flexors. If this principle is not appreciated, errors in interpretation are likely. Although this will be dealt with specifically in the description of the functions of the wrist, the fingers, and the thumb, the following two examples illustrate this principle:

1. At rest, the index finger is kept in slight flexion in all its joints because of a tonic balance between the long flexors, the extensors, and the interossei and the lumbricals. Should the flexor tendons be divided, the index finger immediately assumes a new position. The tonic force of the extensor tendons is counterbalanced by the lumbricals and the interossei. The metacarpophalangeal joint remains in slight flexion, but the distal and the proximal interphalangeal joints are no longer flexed because they are not counterbalanced by the long flexors and therefore extend under the action of the extensor tendons, the lumbrical, and either one or two interossei.

2. In some cases of paralysis of the flexor pollicis longus muscle, tension persists in the muscle. If the thumb is completely hyperextended by the activity of the extensor pollicis longus and then released, the tip of the distal phalanx exhibits a slight degree of flexion at the interphalangeal joint. This slight flexion is obviously not caused by the action of the paralyzed flexor pollicis longus but by the intrinsic tension contributed by the fibrous elements of the tendon–muscle unit.

Modern electromyographic methods emphasize the complexity of the problem of muscle action, and studies using these methods yield varied interpretations of the action of the so-called synergists, antagonists, and stabilizers. More extensive and refined electromyographic studies combined with progressive improvement of instrumentation will provide more definite data; electromyographic studies without further investigation of stimuli controlled by the central nervous system will not suffice. Although pertinent data established by electromyography were useful in normal kinesiology and clinical application, these studies must be combined with other clinical methods of investigation before motion of various parts of the body can be interpreted intelligently.

SKELETON OF THE HAND

The skeleton of the hand consists of the lower end of the forearm articulated with the carpus.

The carpus is articulated with the metacarpals, and the metacarpals are articulated with the phalanges. The carpus and the metacarpals represent an anterior longitudinal and transverse concavity that houses all the important structures responsible for flexion of the fingers of all the interphalangeal and the metacarpophalangeal joints and for extension of the two distal phalanges. It contains the greatest part of the important nerve supply and blood supply of the hand. The concavity of the carpus and the metacarpals results from the configuration of the osseous parts and from the ligamentous apparatus and is maintained and controlled by the intrinsic muscles of the hand. Each of the phalanges has transverse and longitudinal volar concavities adapted to the transmission of the tendinous apparatus controlling flexion of the digits.

TABLE 1–1.
Comparative Nomenclatures for the Bones of the Carpus

Nomina Anatomica Tokyo	International Federation of Societies for Surgery of the Hand	Others
Os scaphoideum	Scaphoid bone	Scaphoid
Os lunatum	Lunate bone	Semilunar
Os triquetrum	Triquetrum	Triangular; cuneiform; pyramidal bone
Os pisiforme	Pisiform bone	Same
Os trapezium	Trapezium	Multangular major, Greater multangular
Os trapezoideum	Trapezoid	Multangular minor, Lesser multangular
Os capitatum	Capitate	Os magnum
Os hamatum	Hamate	Unciform

Excluding the variations that occasionally occur, the carpus consists of eight bones, described in two rows. The distal row contains the trapezium, trapezoid, capitate, and hamate. The proximal row consists of the scaphoid, lunate, triquetrum, and pisiform (nomenclature according to the *Nomina Anatomica Tokyo*; see also Table 1–1). The metacarpal bones are described as the first, corresponding to the thumb; the second, to the index; the third, to the middle finger; the fourth, to the ring finger; and the fifth, to the little finger. There are three phalanges to each finger, but the thumb has only two phalanges. Fortunately, the majority of writers have now adopted the names of proximal, middle, and distal phalanges, which create less confusion.

The description of the osseous structures of the hand relates to an adult hand in which ossification is completed, and each phalanx, metacarpal, and carpal bone consists of osseous tissue throughout. The hand of an infant, a child, or a young adult differs because many parts of the hand skeleton are incompletely ossified. Acquaintance with the sequence of ossification and the status of the growing bones is of importance in surgical anatomy and aids in interpreting functional disabilities of a growing hand (see Table 1–2). The ossification centers in the lower end of the radius, the ulna, the carpal bones, the metacarpals, and the phalanges appear in a regular sequence (Fig. 1–7). The date of the appearance of the centers and their maturation generally occurs earlier in girls than in boys.

It is established that at birth, the metaphyses of the radius, ulna, metacarpals, and all the phalanges are normally present. They appear during the first five months of prenatal development in the following order: radius, ulna, distal phalanges, metacarpals, proximal phalanges, and middle phalanges (see Table 1–2).

FIG. 1–7 The individual carpals and epiphyses in the hand shown are numbered in the approximate order in which their ossification begins: 1, capitate; 2, hamate; 3, distal epiphysis of the radius; 4, epiphysis of the proximal phalanx of the middle finger;* 5, epiphysis of the proximal phalanx of the index finger;* 6, epiphysis of the proximal phalanx of the ring finger;* 7, epiphysis of the second metacarpal; 8, epiphysis of the distal phalanx of the thumb; 9, epiphysis of the third metacarpal; 10, epiphysis of the fourth metacarpal; 11, epiphysis of the proximal phalanx of the little digit; 12, epiphysis of the middle phalanx of the middle finger; 13, epiphysis of the middle phalanx of the ring finger; 14, epiphysis of the fifth metacarpal; 15, epiphysis of the middle phalanx of the index finger; 16, triquetrum; 17, epiphysis of the distal phalanx of the middle finger; 18, epiphysis of the distal phalanx of the ring finger; 19, epiphysis of the first metacarpal; 20, epiphysis of the proximal phalanx of the thumb;* 21, epiphysis of the distal phalanx of the little finger; 22, epiphysis of the distal phalanx of the index finger; 23, epiphysis of the middle phalanx of the index finger;* 23, epiphysis of the middle phalanx of the little finger;* 24, lunate;* 25, trapezium;* 26, trapezoid;* 27, scaphoid;* 28, distal epiphysis of the ulna; 29, pisiform; 30, sesamoid of the adductor pollicis (the sesamoid of flexor pollicis brevis is visible through the head of the first metacarpal, just below the numeral 2 on the epiphysis of the proximal phalanx of the thumb). (Greulich WW, Pyle SI: Radiographic Atlas of Skeletal Development of the Hand and Wrist, 1959)

*Irregularities in the order of appearance are most apt to occur in those centers indicated by asterisks.

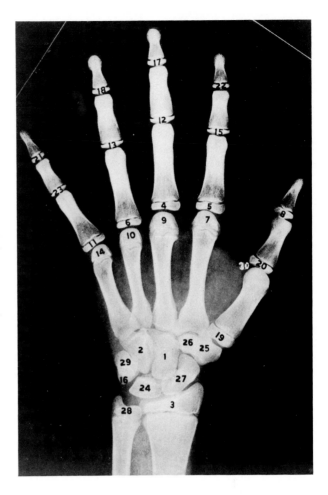

TABLE 1–2.

Appearance of Ossification Centers in Their Normal Sequence and Dates of Complete Ossification and Fusion According to W. Greulich and S. I. Pyle

	Sex	First Appearance (mos.)	Adult Status (yrs.)
1. Capitate	Male	Birth–3	17–18
	Female	Birth–3	15–16
2. Hamate	Male	3	14–15
	Female	3	12–13
3. Distal epiphysis of radius	Male	12–15	18–19
	Female	9–15	17–18
4. Basal epiphysis of proximal phalanx middle finger	Male	15–18	15–17
	Female	9–12	14–16
5. Basal epiphysis of proximal phalanx index finger	Male	15–18	16–17
	Female	9–13	14–15

(Continued)

TABLE 9–2. *(continued)*
**Appearance of Ossification Centers in Their Normal Sequence and Dates of Complete
Ossification and Fusion According to W. Greulich and S. I. Pyle**

	Sex	First Appearance (mos.)	Adult Status (yrs.)
6. Basal epiphysis of proximal phalanx ring finger	Male Female	15–18 9–12	16–17 14–15
7. Capital epiphysis metacarpal index finger	Male Female	15–20 9–13	16–17 15
8. Basal epiphysis of distal phalanx of thumb	Male Female	15–18 12–15	15–15½ 13–13½
9. Capital epiphysis of middle metacarpal	Male Female	15–20 9–13	16–17 15
10. Capital epiphysis of ring metacarpal	Male Female	15–20 9–12	16–17 14–15
11. Basal epiphysis of proximal phalanx little finger	Male Female	18–24 15–18	16–17 14–15
12. Basal epiphysis of middle phalanx middle finger	Male Female	18–24 15–18	16–17 14–15
13. Basal epiphysis of middle phalanx ring finger	Male Female	18–24 15–18	17 15
14. Capital epiphysis of metacarpal of little finger	Male Female	24–30 15–17	16–17 14–15
15. Basal epiphysis of middle phalanx of index finger	Male Female	24–32 15–18	16–17 14–15
16. Triquetrum	Male Female	24–36 18–25	15–16 15–16
17. Basal epiphysis of distal phalanx middle finger	Male Female	18–24 18–24	
18. Basal epiphysis of distal phalanx ring finger	Male Female	18–24 18–24	
19. Basal epiphysis of first metacarpal	Male Female	24–32 18–22	
20. Basal epiphysis of proximal phalanx of thumb	Male Female	24–32 18–22	
21. Basal epiphysis of distal phalanx little finger	Male Female	36–42 18–24	

(Continued)

TABLE 1–2. *(continued)*
Appearance of Ossification Centers in Their Normal Sequence and Dates of Complete Ossification and Fusion According to W. Greulich and S. I. Pyle

	Sex	*First Appearance (mos.)*	*Adult Status (yrs.)*
22. Basal epiphysis of distal phalanx of index finger	Male	36–42	
	Female	24–30	
23. Basal epiphysis of middle phalanx of little finger	Male	42–48	
	Female	24–32	
24. Lunate	Male	32–42	
	Female	30–36	
25. Trapezium	Male	3½–5 yrs	
	Female	36–50	
26. Trapezoid	Male	5–6 yrs	
	Female	3½–4 yrs, 2 mo	
27. Scaphoid	Male	5–6 yrs, 4 mo	
	Female	3½–4 yrs, 4 mo	
28. Distal epiphysis of ulna	Male	5 yrs, 3 mos–6–10 yrs	
	Female	5½–6¾ yrs	
29. Pisiform	Male		17–18
	Female		16–17
30. Sesamoid of adductor pollicis	Male		12–13
	Female		11

Part Two
Structure and Function

2
The Fingers

Osseous and Ligamentous Structures

Martin A. Posner
Emanuel B. Kaplan

The fingers comprise the second, third, fourth, and fifth digits of the hand. This numerical description may be a source of confusion because there are four fingers and five digits—numerically, the second finger is the third digit. It is therefore preferable to use names for the fingers: the index, middle, ring, and little. Referring to the middle finger as the long finger is not acceptable because in some congenital or pathologic conditions this finger is not necessarily the longest (Fig. 2–1).

PHALANGES AND METACARPALS

Each digit normally consists of three phalanges and one corresponding metacarpal. The phalanges are named the *proximal*, the *middle*, and the *distal*. Each phalanx consists of a shaft with a proximal base and a distal head. The proximal and the middle phalanges are somewhat similar in appearance, while the dis-

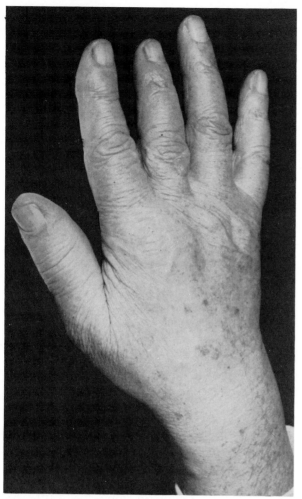

FIG. 2–1 Photograph showing that the middle finger is not always the longest finger.

tal phalanx differs from them considerably. The proximal phalanx of each finger is longer than the middle, and the middle is longer than the distal. The metacarpal of each finger is usually longer than its corresponding proximal phalanx. The longest finger normally is the middle finger, the next is the ring finger, and the shortest is the little finger. The index finger may be either equal to, longer, or shorter than the ring finger. Functionally, the difference in length between the index and ring fingers is of no particular importance.

The proximal phalanx of the middle finger is the longest of the proximal phalanges; the proxi-mal phalanges of the ring and index fingers are approximately equal, and the proximal phalanx of the little finger is the shortest. The middle phalanx of the middle finger is the longest of the middle phalanges, followed in decreasing length by the middle phalanges of the ring, index, and little fingers. The lengths of the distal phalanges differ slightly with the distal phalanx of the middle finger being 1 mm to 2 mm longer than the others. The widths of the phalanges are smaller than the lengths. A possible exception is the distal phalanx of the index finger, which may be the widest of the distal phalanges (except for that of the thumb, which is not considered in this discussion).

The relative lengths of the metacarpals vary. In the majority of hands the metacarpal of the middle finger appears to be the longest of the metacarpals, although the index metacarpal may actually be slightly longer. The metacarpal of the ring finger is usually shorter than the metacarpal of the index finger, and the fifth metacarpal is the shortest. Not infrequently, the metacarpals of the ring and little fingers are much shorter than those of the other fingers, imparting a peculiar asymmetry to the hand.

PROXIMAL PHALANGES

The shaft of the proximal phalanx has a volar concavity in length and width. A ridge along each side of the volar aspect separates this face of the bone from the lateral aspects of the phalanx. The lateral ridges are slightly uneven and do not run to the distal end of the phalanx. The ridges become somewhat wider and inter-rupt approximately at the junction of the distal third with the proximal two thirds, where fre-quently a nutrient foramen is present; the ridges then continue distally to the articular line. Prox-imally, the ridges continue toward the base, where they end in a tubercle for insertion of the collateral ligaments of the metacarpophalangeal joint. The lateral ridges or crests of the phalanx represent the area of insertion of the flexor tendon sheaths. The concavity volarly on the shaft accommodates the flexor tendons. In addition to the nutrient foramina already mentioned, there are other foramina at the junction of the shaft with the head of the phalanx that are usually very small. The dorsal aspect of the shaft is smooth and convex throughout its length and width and is somewhat semioval in transverse section.

The base of the proximal phalanx is wider than the shaft. On its dorsal aspect, there is a slight ridge from side to side separating the dorsal aspect from the proximal articulating end. This ridge serves as a crest for insertion of the capsule of the metacarpophalangeal joint. The midpoint of this ridge is frequently roughened for insertion of a volar slip of the tendon of the extensor digitorum communis, or it represents a reinforcement of insertion of the capsule connected with the midband of the extensor digitorum. Each lateral end of this ridge and the corresponding area of the lateral side of the phalanx show a rough elevation for insertion of the lateral tendon of the interossei. The volar aspect of the base shows a depression between the two tubercles for the collateral ligaments of the metacarpophalangeal joint. This depression accommodates the flexor tendons. Multiple small nutrient foramina are present on the volar aspect of the base. The articular end is smooth, concave in all directions, somewhat oval in configuration, and smaller than the corresponding head of the metacarpal.

The head of the proximal phalanx resembles the distal end of the femur with its two condyles and intercondylar space. The two small condyles of the head of the phalanx are located on the sides of the phalanx with a slight intercondylar depression; the articular surface is more extended toward the volar surface of the phalanx. The entire articular line is more prominent than is the rest of the head and the shaft and has a small tubercule over the middorsal intercondylar line. The lateral sides of the head have circular, depressed areas corresponding to the circumference of each condyle, for insertion of the collateral ligaments of the proximal interphalangeal joint.

The important ratio of the thicknesses of the shaft, head, and base of the proximal phalanges appears to be constant and approximately equals 1:1.3:2. This anteroposterior or volardorsal thickness must be considered when fixation wires are introduced through the long areas of the phalanges. The wire must have a very small diameter because the thickness of the shaft may vary. Normally, it rarely exceeds 8 mm at the thinnest part of the phalanx of the middle finger, and 6 mm in the phalanx of the little finger. This ratio also applies to the middle phalanges which are thinner than the proximal phalanges and have average shaft thicknesses of 4 mm to 5 mm for the middle finger and 3 mm to 4 mm for the little finger. The thickness of the shaft of the distal phalanx is only 2 mm to 3 mm; therefore, the introduction of a fixation wire through the length of the phalanges requires wires less than 1 mm in diameter. Skill and caution must be used to avoid injury to the flexor tendons or the dorsal tendinous apparatus.

MIDDLE PHALANGES

The middle phalanx is shorter than the proximal, although the length ratio can vary in the same individual and even in the same hand. In a fairly large series of hands, it appeared to vary between 2:1 and 1.3:1 regardless of the finger.

Although the general appearance of the middle phalanx is similar to the general appearance of the proximal phalanx, there are distinct differences between the two. The volar aspect of the middle phalanx shaft is not as concave as is the volar aspect of the proximal phalanx. The lateral crests are also thicker, rougher, and wider, occupying mostly the midpart of the shaft. The very minute nutrient foramina are visible on the volar aspect immediately proximal to the articular line of the head. The dorsal aspect of the shaft is somewhat narrower proximal to the head and widens toward the base; it is convex, smooth, and more nearly round than is the dorsal aspect of the proximal phalanx. The configuration of the head is very similar to the head of the proximal phalanx.

The base of the middle phalanx is wider than the shaft. The dorsal aspect shows a transverse ridge separating the base from the articular end. The midpoint of the transverse ridge on the dorsum is strongly elevated into a tubercle for insertion of the midband of the extensor digitorum communis tendon. A prominent tubercle terminates the ridge on each laterovolar aspect of the base for insertion of the collateral ligaments. A prominent volar tubercle is located at the midpoint of the base immediately distal to the articular end. Multiple nutrient foramina are distal to the tubercle. The articular end of the base represents a double concave depression for the two condyles of the head of the proximal phalanx; they are separated by a dorsovolar articular crest corresponding to the intercondylar depression of the head of the proximal phalanx. This crest extends toward the dorsal tubercle of the base dorsally and volarly toward the volar tubercle.

The volar tubercle of the base of the middle phalanx, articulating with the prominent part of the head of the proximal phalanx, forms a volar elevation in relation to the volar shafts of these two phalanges and providing certain mechanical advantages for the function of the flexor tendons. The arrangement of the nutrient foramina in protected areas under tendon insertions is functionally important because by this means the movement of the flexor tendons does not interfere with the blood supply.

DISTAL PHALANGES

The distal phalanges differ in contour from the proximal and middle phalanges. The lengths of these bones, with the exception of that of the thumb, are almost the same for all of the fingers. The distal phalanx of the middle finger may sometimes be 1 mm to 2 mm longer than the others. The widths of the phalanges differ very little except for that of the little finger, which is more slender. The base of the distal phalanx is similar to the base of the middle phalanx, with the width of the base equal to the width of the head of the middle phalanx. The foreshortened shaft is much narrower than the middle phalanx and ends in a roughened crescent that is wider than the distal part of the shaft. On the dorsal aspect, the crescent is 1 mm to 1.5 mm wide; on the volar aspect, the crescent is 3 mm to 4 mm. The base has a few minute nutrient foramina over its volar aspect, and there is a volar tubercle for the joint capsule. There are two lateral tubercles for the collateral ligaments of the distal interphalangeal joint and a posterior dorsal tubercle for the main insertion of the dorsal apparatus. The average length ratios of the middle phalanx to the distal phalanx with the middle phalanx taken as a unit are as follows: index, 1:0.6 to 1:0.9; middle, 1:0.6 to 1:0.7; ring, 1:0.6 to 1:0.7; little, 1:1 to 1:0.8.

METACARPALS

The second, third, fourth, and fifth metacarpals function as the basal intermediaries between the fingers and the carpus. For this reason, these metacarpals are described separately from the first metacarpal, which represents, together with the other structures of the thumb, a functionally separate unit. In discussions of the comparative lengths of the metacarpals, it is sometimes incorrectly stated that the third metacarpal is the longest. The second metacarpal is usually as long as the third, measured from the dorsal aspect, and may be even longer when measured from the volar aspect. The head of the third metacarpal frequently stands out most prominently when all the metacarpophalangeal joints are strongly flexed, however, the prominence of the head of the third metacarpal is not caused by greater length but by its more distal position in relation to the articular line between the metacarpals and the distal row of the carpal bones. Although the second metacarpal is recessed more proximally than the other metacarpals, it actually is usually the longest. The fourth metacarpal is shorter than is the third, and the fifth metacarpal is the shortest if the metacarpal of the thumb is not considered.

The relative lengths of the metacarpals, if the corresponding proximal phalanx is taken as a unit, are as follows: index, 1:1.6 to 1:2.4; middle, 1:1.4+; ring, 1:1.3 to 1:1.5; little, 1:1.7. If the ratios of all these structures are combined and expressed in terms of the distal phalanx as a unit, the relationships in length can be expressed approximately (see Table 2–1).

TABLE 2–1.
Ratios of the Bones of the Fingers

	Distal Phalanx	Middle Phalanx	Proximal Phalanx	Metacarpal
Index	1	1.1–1.4	1.8–2.0	3.2–4.3
Middle	1	1.3–1.8	2.2–2.7	3.0–3.9
Ring	1	1.3–1.7	2.0–2.8	3.0–3.6
Little	1	1.0–1.2	1.6–2.2	2.7–3.9

FIG. 2–2 With the hand in neutral position, a line drawn through the axis of the middle finger and continued through the wrist shows that the lunate bone is on the ulnar side of this line. The forked appearance of the base of the second metacarpal and the styloid process on the radial side of the third metacarpal are constant characteristics of these two bones.

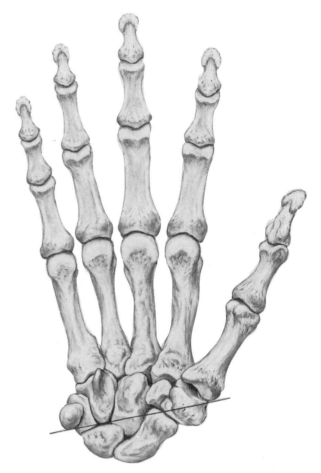

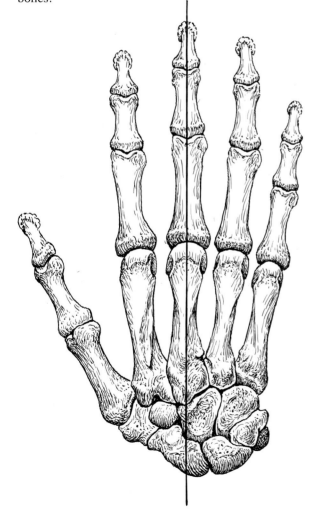

FIG. 2–3 Volar aspect of the skeleton of a human hand. The scaphoid bone is proximal to a line drawn from the proximal edge of the pisiform bone to the proximal tip of the crest of the trapezium. The hook of the hamate bone corresponds exactly to the articular line between the bases of the fourth and the fifth metacarpals.

Each metacarpal shows distinct characteristics in shape and size that make individual recognition easy, especially, for surgeons who rely on these characteristic structures for recognition through operative incisions.

Second metacarpal
The second metacarpal (Figs. 2–2 and 2–3) has a forked base quite different from those of the other metacarpals. The fork is open toward the carpus for articulation with the trapezoid; of its two divisions, the ulnar division is the longer

and articulates with the styloid process of the base of the third metacarpal. The shorter part of the fork is on the radial side and articulates with the trapezium. The space between the two divisions of the fork articulates with the trapezoid. The dorsal aspect of the radial division of the fork serves as an area for insertion of the extensor carpi radialis longus tendon. The apex of the fork which is located distally, presents a depression that is frequently pierced by one or several nutrient arteries arising from the dorsal carpal arch. The ulnar side of the base, which articulates with the styloid process of the third metacarpal, has a small roughened area just distal to the articular facet for insertion of a powerful interosseous ligament that holds together the bases of the second and third metacarpals.

The shaft of the second metacarpal has a flat, triangular dorsal surface immediately proximal to the head. This dorsal surface is limited by lateral ridges that converge toward the dorsum, approximately at the junction of the distal two thirds with the proximal third, to form a single ridge running proximally and ending at the apex of the forked base. The volar surface of the shaft is smoother and more nearly round but becomes more irregular as it approaches the base and the head of the metacarpal. The rough surface near the base is pierced by several small channels for the nutrient vessels.

The head of the second metacarpal is large and irregular, with a smooth convex area that extends further in the volar dorsal direction than in the lateral. An elevated ridge surrounds the articular smooth area. The articular surface descends much more over the volar aspect than over the dorsal aspect. There is a small depression just proximal to the articular surface over the dorsal aspect for insertion of the capsule of the metacarpophalangeal joint. Deep furrows on each side of the articular head proximal to the smooth surface allow for passage of the tendons of the interosseous muscles. On the anterolateral aspect is a tubercle for insertion of the collateral ligaments of the metacarpophalangeal joint.

Third metacarpal

The base of the third metacarpal presents a constant styloid process of the radial side that articulates with the ulnar half of the fork of the base of the second metacarpal and with the capitate bone, or occasionally with a very limited portion of the trapezoid. The relationship of the bases of the second and third metacarpals may vary. When the styloid process of the third metacarpal is shorter, the ulnar part of the fork of the second metacarpal may articulate with a small portion of the capitate bone; the base of the third metacarpal articulates with the greatest part of the distal aspect of the capitate bone. On the radial side of the base just distal to the articulating smooth surface for the second metacarpal base, there is a rough area for insertion of the strong intermetacarpal interosseous ligament. On the ulnar side of the base of the third metacarpal (Fig. 2–4A), there is a double facet for articulation with a similar double facet of the radial side of the base of the fourth metacarpal. The rough area between the two facets, also distal and proximal to them, serves as an insertion area for a strong interosseous intermetacarpal ligament.

On the rough dorsal and volar surfaces of the base, there are several small foramina for the nutrient vessels. The volar surface presents a longitudinal crest extending from just below the metacarpal neck through the entire length of the metacarpal; it joins the crest of the capitate bone for the origin of the adductor muscle of the thumb. The nutrient foramina do not follow a definite pattern, but the nutrient foramina are generally around the bases of the metacarpals and at the junction of the head with the shaft, which is usually located on the volar surface immediately proximal to the circumferential crest of the articular surface. Nutrient foramina on the shaft are inconstant, but when present are on the radial side of the metacarpal.

The shaft of the third metacarpal shows a somewhat flat and triangular dorsal surface. The two lateral ridges of the triangle converge toward the proximal third of the surface and

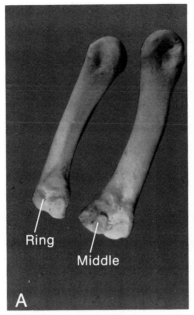
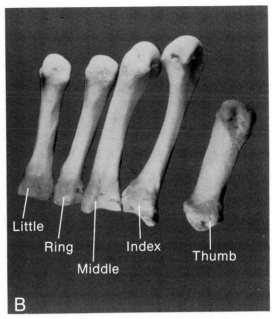

FIG. 2–4 A, Ring and middle fingers (left hand) turned to show the ulnar side of the middle metacarpal and the radial side of the ring metacarpal. **B**, Volar aspect of the metacarpals of the left hand.

form a rough ridge descending toward the base. The triangular area is covered by the tendon of the extensor digitorum communis (Fig. 2–4B). The area lateral to the lateral ridges is the space of origin of the second and third dorsal interossei.

It appears that the metacarpal receives most of its arterial supply from the nutrient arteries at the base and the head, and there is frequently no blood supply from a nutrient artery to the shaft.

The head of the third metacarpal is very similar to the head of the second (Figs. 2–4B and 2–5A). It represents a spheroidal, irregular articular surface. The anteroposterior is round, smooth, and convex and is flatter on each side where a groove for the tendons of the interosseous muscles is present. The articular surface extends much more volarly than dorsally and permits more flexion of the proximal phalanx than extension. Each volar side of the articular surface has a prominent tubercle for

insertion of the collateral ligaments of the metacarpophalangeal joint.

Fourth metacarpal

The fourth metacarpal shows great similarity to the third as far as the head and shaft are concerned, but the base shows distinct differences. The articulating surface of the base has a proximal elevation, dividing its surface into a radial and an ulnar part. The radial part is articulated with the ulnar third of the metacarpal articulating aspect of the capitate bone; the ulnar half of the metacarpal articulates with the radial half of the hamate bone. The articular base of this metacarpal thus projects proximally unlike the forked base of the second metacarpal. The radial side of the base has two small articular facets for articulation with the ulnar side of the third metacarpal (Fig. 2–4A). The roughened area between the two facets serves for insertion of the interosseous intermetacarpal ligament. The ulnar side of the base has a single facet for ar-

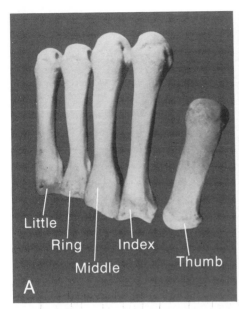 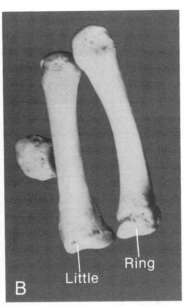

FIG. 2–5   A, Dorsal aspect of the metacarpals of the left hand. **B**, Left ring and little fingers turned to show the ulnar side of the ring finger and the radial side of the little finger.

ticulation with the fifth metacarpal (Fig. 2–5*B*).

Fifth metacarpal

The fifth metacarpal, except for the base, has many similarities to the fourth. The articulating surface corresponding to the ulnar division of the hamate bone actually resembles the shallow saddle configuration of the base of the first metacarpal. The articular surface of the base of the fifth metacarpal is convex in the volardorsal direction and concave in the radioulnar axis. The radial side of the base of the fifth metacarpal has one facet for articulation with the fourth base. The ulnar base has no articular facet but serves for origin of the abductor digiti minimi muscle.

Relationship of the metacarpals to other structures of the hand and wrist

The detailed description of the line of articulation of the metacarpals with the carpal bones is useful because recognition of the characteristics of each bone aids the surgeon in orienting himself in this region (Fig. 2–6). Recognition of the actual localization of the nutrient foramina,

mostly around the bases and heads of the metacarpals, dictates more conservative surgical management of these regions than in dealing with the circulation in the region of the shafts (Fig. 2–7). The arrangement of the joints of each metacarpal with the carpus and between the bases of the metacarpals demonstrates the reason for immobility of the second and third metacarpals and the mobility of the fourth and especially the fifth metacarpals.

INTERPHALANGEAL, METACARPOPHALANGEAL, AND DISTAL INTERPHALANGEAL JOINTS AND LIGAMENTS

The osseous structures and surfaces of the contiguous phalanges, metacarpals, and carpals were described in the preceding section. The capsule of each joint and the ligaments reinforcing the capsule function together as a remark-

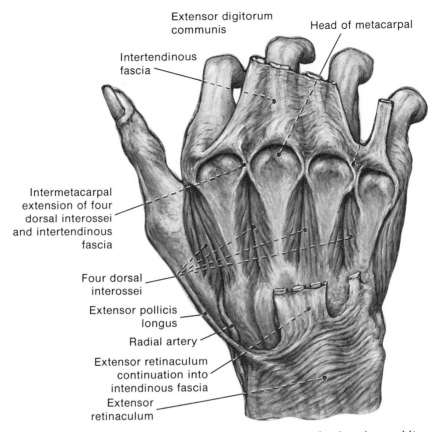

Extensor digitorum communis

Head of metacarpal

Intertendinous fascia

Intermetacarpal extension of four dorsal interossei and intertendinous fascia

Four dorsal interossei

Extensor pollicis longus

Radial artery

Extensor retinaculum continuation into intendinous fascia

Extensor retinaculum

FIG. 2–6 Relationship of all the extensor tendons to the dorsal carpal ligament, to the interosseous muscles, and to the heads of the metacarpals. The fascial sheet of the intertendinous fascia goes around the radial aspect of the second metacarpal and dips between the second and the third heads, then separately between the middle and the ring head, then between the head of the ring and fifth metacarpal, then around the fifth metacarpal head. These fibers are directed toward the dorsal aspect of the deep transverse intermetacarpal ligament. Distal to the distal border of the transverse intermetacarpal ligament, the fibers are directed obliquely toward the tunnels of the flexor tendons. Fibers of the dorsal carpal ligament continue into the intertendinous fascia, uniting all of the extensor tendons. Thus, in this region there are two important anchorages of the extensor apparatus with the retinaculae of the wrist and the hand. The functional excursion of the extensor tendon is somewhat limited by the functioning length of the extensor digitorum communis tendon, and also by the connection of the intertendinous fascia with the extensor retinaculum.

ably efficient unit (Fig. 2–6), particularly in children and young adults whose joints are not affected by any form of arthritis. Although the range of joint motion varies in individuals, the motion is smooth, continuous, and powerful. With prolonged use or excessive demand, the configuration of the joints may change. The round, spherical surfaces become irregular; the ligaments become retracted or stretched, their shiny, fibrous pattern is altered, and they become thicker.

Because the ordinary dissection material used in initial anatomic instruction in medical schools is generally from debilitated, old people, medical students encounter their first discrepancies when they compare idealized atlas illustra-

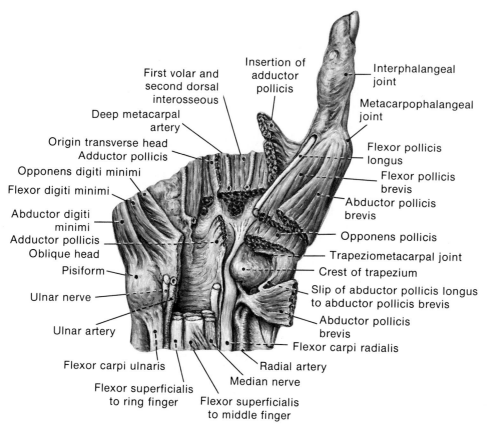

First volar and
second dorsal
interosseous

Insertion of
adductor
pollicis

Interphalangeal
joint

Metacarpophalangeal
joint

Deep metacarpal
artery

Origin transverse head
Adductor pollicis

Opponens digiti minimi

Flexor digiti minimi

Abductor digiti
minimi

Adductor pollicis
Oblique head

Pisiform

Ulnar nerve

Ulnar artery

Flexor carpi ulnaris

Flexor superficialis
to ring finger

Flexor superficialis
to middle finger

Median nerve

Radial artery

Flexor carpi radialis

Abductor pollicis
brevis

Slip of abductor pollicis longus
to abductor pollicis brevis

Crest of trapezium

Trapeziometacarpal joint

Opponens pollicis

Abductor pollicis
brevis

Flexor pollicis
brevis

Flexor pollicis
longus

FIG. 2–7   Relationship of the muscles of the thenar eminence to the deeper structures of the wrist. The volar carpal ligament is completely removed; the roof of the tunnel for the flexor carpi radialis is removed; part of the adductor brevis muscle is excised. The origin of the muscle is shown. The origin of the flexor brevis and the opponens of the thumb is removed. The adductor of the thumb transected near its insertion, with removal of a large segment of the muscle, shows the insertion of the tendon of the flexor carpi radialis into the base of the third metacarpal. The origin of the adductor from the crest of the third metacarpal and from the carpus is demonstrated. A few small, deep common digital arteries are shown. Part of the muscles from the proximal part of the intermetacarpal spaces was removed to show the metacarpal origin of the adductor muscle and the bases of the second and third and a very small part of the fourth metacarpals. The origins of the flexor brevis pollicis and the opponens pollicis are removed to show the trapezium with its crest, underneath which passes the flexor carpi radialis tendon. Distal and radial to the trapezium, a fissure leading into the metacarpophalangeal joint is indicated. The flexor carpi radialis covers the capsule of the carpal joints. It completely covers the trapezoid bone. The abductor brevis is separated from the trapezium, showing its partial origin on the scaphoid bone. The scaphoid bone is covered by the tendon of the flexor carpi radialis. The muscle is separated from the capsule covering the trapezionavicular joint. The ulnar artery and nerve are located volar to the carpal ligament. All the tendons and the median nerve pass dorsal to the volar carpal ligament.

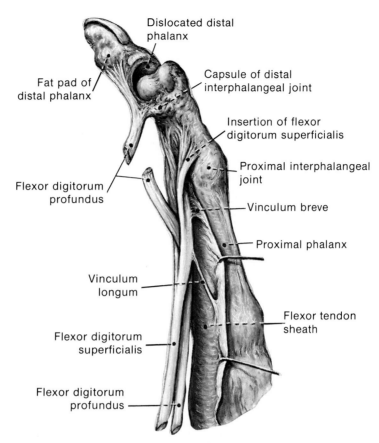

Dislocated distal
phalanx

Capsule of distal
interphalangeal joint

Fat pad of
distal phalanx

Insertion of flexor
digitorum superficialis

Proximal interphalangeal
joint

Flexor digitorum
profundus

Vinculum breve

Proximal phalanx

Vinculum
longum

Flexor tendon
sheath

Flexor digitorum
superficialis

Flexor digitorum
profundus

FIG. 2–8   Distal phalanx disarticulated to show the relationship of the insetion of
the tendon of the flexor profundus into the base of the distal phalanx and into the fat
pad and capsule of the distal interphalangeal joint. The twist of the flexor sublimis
slip and also the long and short vincula are demonstrated.

tions with their dissections. It is important to
remember that ligaments vary with age.

DISTAL INTERPHALANGEAL JOINTS

The distal interphalangeal joint bears two
important insertions, that of the flexor profundus on its volar aspect and that of the extensor
apparatus on its dorsal aspect. Injuries to the
joint or to either of the tendons produce characteristic deformities that can seriously impair
function of the digit. The problem of injuries to
this joint and the mechanism will be discussed
later.

The distal joint is formed (Fig. 2–8) by the
junction of the base of the distal phalanx with
the head of the middle phalanx. The head of the
middle phalanx has a bicondylar smooth surface
with an intercondylar depression, and the base
of the distal phalanx has a corresponding concave surface with an anteroposterior elevated
ridge that fits into the intercondylar valley. The
smooth surface of the head covered with hyaline
cartilage extends dorsally for a considerable
distance, reflecting the passive hyperextension
possible at the joint. Volarly, the articular surface permits flexion to almost 90° but this is less
than that of the head of the proximal phalanx,
where there is greater flexion. The condyles of
the head of the middle phalanx are asymmetri-
cal in width, anteroposterior length, and projection. The difference in projection of the two

condyles results in deviation of the long axis of the distal phalanx from that of the middle phalanx. This is true of each of the fingers except the middle finger, in which the long axis of both phalanges are the same. The adjacent fingers deviate toward the central digit with the distal phalanx of the index finger inclined ulnad and the distal phalanges of the ring and little fingers inclined radially.

The articular surface of the base of the distal phalanx is less extensive than that of the head of the middle phalanx. It consists of concave radial and ulnar condyles that are asymmetric corresponding to the differences between the condyles of the head of the middle phalanx.

The intercondylar ridge of the distal phalanx extends dorsally and ends in a rough, elevated tubercle that is more prominent than the flat volar surface. The resulting fit of this articulation is such that in addition to flexion and extension, some degree of rotation also takes place, which facilitates optimal positioning of the finger tips in prehension.

The base of the distal phalanx and the head of the middle phalanx are held together by a capsule attached to the crest, which surrounds the cartilaginous surface and separates it from the shaft of the phalanx. The capsule is reinforced laterally by thick collateral ligaments that are inserted into the sides of the head of the middle phalanx and run in a distal and volar direction for insertion into the laterovolar tubercle of the base of the distal phalanx. Accessory collateral ligaments are more volar and extend from the sides of the phalangeal head to the sides of the palmar plate. The palmar plate provides for volar stability and serves as a floor for the flexor profundus tendon. This plate blends distally into the nonarticular surface of the base of the distal phalanx and intermixes its fibers with the terminal fibers of insertion of the flexor profundus tendon. Proximally, the plate is

FIG. 2–9   Dorsal apparatus of the middle finger of the right hand, completely removed from the finger, is shown from the volar aspect. The division of the tendon into a fanlike structure of the extensor digitorum communis tendon and the intimate connection of the central part of the extensor communis with the capsule of the joint are demonstrated. The open capsule, separated from the proximal interphalangeal joint, is shown. The so-called triangular ligament over the middle phalanx is demonstrated. At the proximal interphalangeal joint, the intimate connection of the lateral bands with the capsule is indicated.

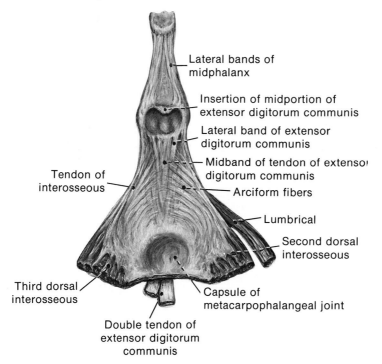

Lateral bands of midphalanx

Insertion of midportion of extensor digitorum communis

Lateral band of extensor digitorum communis

Midband of tendon of extensor digitorum communis

Tendon of interosseous

Arciform fibers

Lumbrical

Second dorsal interosseous

Third dorsal interosseous

Capsule of metacarpophalangeal joint

Double tendon of extensor digitorum communis

attached to the neck of the middle phalanx, but there are no "check-rein" ligaments, so that hyperextension of the joint is permitted.

The fibrous tunnel of the flexor tendons also participates in the formation of the tendinocapsuloligamentous unit of the distal interphalangeal joint. The fibrous tunnel adheres to the palmar plate and adds its fibers to the reinforcement of this plate. The insertion of the flexor profundus tendon in this proximity adds to the complexity of this joint. Before its insertion into the base of the distal phalanx, the flexor profundus tendon fans out over the entire width of the joint and very frequently divides longitudinally into two terminal tendons instead of one. The divided or fanned-out tendon is inserted into the entire width of the distal base, blending with the distal fibers of the palmar plate of the joint and the periosteum and also sending some fibrous extensions into the fat pad of the finger tip (Fig. 2–8).

Over the joint itself, the flexor profundus tendon is completely free and glides smoothly within its protective fibrous tunnel. It is connected for blood supply with the palmar plate through nonrestricting short vincula tendinum. Immediately under the palmar plate, numerous small foramina for vessels are found over the volar base of the distal phalanx and proximal to the articular head of the middle phalanx. The foramina permit passage of multiple nutrient arteries and are probably more important than the conventional nutrient artery that enters the shaft of the middle phalanx.

The dorsum of the joint has no reinforcing ligament, but the terminal part of the extensor apparatus of the finger serves as a reinforcement firmly adhering to the capsule from the dorsal edge of one lateral collateral to the dorsal edge of the opposite lateral collateral ligament. The adherence of the extensor apparatus is wide, and the insertion of the tendinous part of the extensor apparatus is made over a wide area, not only into the dorsal tubercle of the base of the distal phalanx. The insertion of the extensor apparatus extends distally to the root of the nail. The fibers of the extensor blend totally into capsular fibers and the periosteum (Figs. 2–9, 2–10, and 2–11).

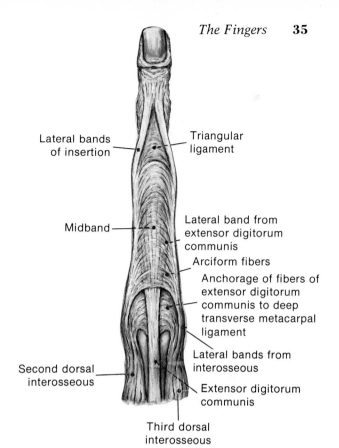

FIG. 2–10 Dorsal view of a finger. The interossei are inserted into the lateral bases of the proximal phalanx and into the interosseous expansion. The tendon of the extensor digitorum passes over the metacarpophalangeal joint and is then incorporated in the expansion of the interossei. The fibers of the dorsal expansion are arciform, running from the lateral bands of the interossei toward the extensor digitorum tendon. The tendon of the extensor digitorum fans out from a narrow band over the metacarpophalangeal joint, becoming wider as it runs distally in the expansion toward the proximal interphalangeal joint where it covers almost entirely the distal part of the proximal phalanx. The most collateral parts of the extensor digitorum join the lateral bands of the interossei. This union of the fibers of the extensor digitorum tendon and the lateral bands of the interossei is more volar than the dorsal aponeurosis, which runs over the tendon of the extensor digitorum. The central part of the fanlike expansion of the extensor digitorum communis stops at the base of the middle phalanx. The dorsal expansion over the area of insertion of the central portion of the extensor digitorum does not continue beyond this area; instead, a thin, resistant membrane is found between the lateral bands, which continue their course toward the distal phalanx. The insertion of the reunited lateral bands into the base of the distal phalanx occurs over a wide ridge, completely covering the dorsal aspect of the distal interphalangeal joint. The distal part of the insertion is covered by the root of the nail.

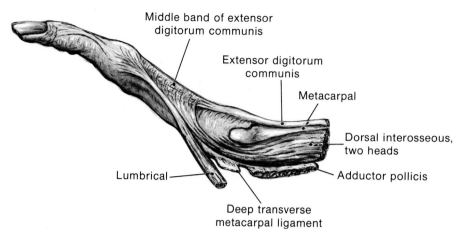

Middle band of extensor
digitorum communis

Extensor digitorum
communis

Metacarpal

Dorsal interosseous,
two heads

Adductor pollicis

Lumbrical

Deep transverse
metacarpal ligament

FIG. 2—11   Middle finger of the right hand, showing important areas of anchorage of the dorsal apparatus to the metacarpophalangeal and interphalangeal joints. A sheath extends volar from the extensor digitorum tendon and blends into the collateral ligaments of the capsule of the metacarpophalangeal joint and into the deep transverse metacarpal ligament. Distal to the transverse intermetacarpal ligament the same extension is anchored by oblique fibers to the tunnel of the flexor tendons. Then, the extensor apparatus recedes to its dorsal component, which is loosely connected with the periosteum of the dorsum of the proximal phalanx. Further distally, the apparatus extends volar to the proximal interphalangeal joint, where it forms the second anchorage. The fibers of connection are oblique, permitting distal and proximal motion over the proximal interphalangeal joint. Then, the apparatus again recedes to the dorsum of the middle phalanx, where it is separated from the periosteum by loose areolar tissue. Over the distal interphalangeal joint, a third anchorage occurs between the apparatus and the distal interphalangeal joint and the distal part of the tunnel of the flexor profundus. (Note that the origin of the adductor pollicis is approximately in the same plane as the plane of the deep transverse metacarpal ligament.)

The volar or palmar plate and the dorsal capsule of the joint reinforced by the terminal tendon of the extensor apparatus each display an intra-articular thickening. The dorsal capsular thickening protrudes into the dorsal part of the joint between the base of the distal and the head of the proximal phalanx; the volar thickening fills the space between the volar part of the distal phalanx and the head of the middle phalanx. The interior of the joint is covered with a thin synovial membrane that, at times protrudes in the form of small diverticuli between the fibers of the lateral collateral ligaments and the volar plate.

Investigation of the relationship of the extensor apparatus and the tunnel of the flexor tendons performed on unembalmed cadavers (and microscopically on fetal material) disclosed that the two are intricately connected by fibers running somewhat parallel with the direction of the lateral collateral ligaments between the edges of the extensor apparatus and the tunnel of the flexor tendon. These fibers are more superficial than are the lateral collateral ligaments and they serve as an anchorage for the extensor apparatus to the flexor area of the finger in the region of the distal interphalangeal joint, without interfering with the activity of the terminal part of the flexor profundus tendon.

The skin around the distal interphalangeal joint is fixed to the deeper structures, particularly around the nail and finger tip. Along the sides of the joint the skin is attached to Cleland's ligaments, which at the distal level become continuous with the lateral interosseous ligaments (extending from the lateral tubercles of the phalangeal base to the lateral aspects of the ungual tuberosity). The fixation of the skin frequently results in lesions with dislocation of the joint.

PROXIMAL INTERPHALANGEAL JOINT

Proximal interphalangeal joints differ from the distal interphalangeal joints in the connections between the ligaments and the extensor and flexor systems. The osseous articular ends entering into the anatomic combination of this joint are similar to those of the distal interphalangeal joint. Except for a slight variation in size, there are no differences in the proximal interphalangeal joints of the four fingers; however, there is no asymmetry of the condyles of the proximal phalanx or compared to the middle phalanges of the index, ring, and little fingers. The symmetry of the condyles of the proximal phalanx maintains the longitudinal axis of the proximal interphalangeal joint.

Structure

The capsule of the joint consists of two collateral ligaments on the medial and ulnar sides of the joint, a volar or palmar plate volarly, and thinner ligaments above the collateral ligaments and between the collateral ligaments and volar plate (the accessory collateral ligaments). Dorsally, the capsule is actually the extensor mechanism, which overties the synovial membrane.

The lateral collateral ligaments are strong, thick bands stretched between the lateral circular depressions on each side of the head of the proximal phalanx and the laterovolar tubercle of the base of the middle phalanx.

This ligament is inserted firmly into the volar base of the middle phalanx, but mainly at the lateral margin, where it is confluent with the fibers of the collateral ligament. There is no significant fibrous attachment of the volar plate to the area of the volar tubercle of the median ridge of the middle phalanx. This tubercle is inserted covered with cartilage. In the central

portion of the base of the middle phalanx the volar plate is loosely attached to the periosteum. The resulting configuration of this distal portion of the plate is that of a meniscus with a recess between it and the volar articular facet of the middle phalanx. This anatomic arrangement permits the plate to retract from the base at the middle phalax when the joint is flexed.

Just dorsal to the lateral margin of the volar plate at the intercondylar recess of the proximal phalanx is a distinct aperature that permits access of a branch of each digital artery supplying the midline viniculum. Proximally, the volar plate is firmly anchored to the bone just inside the second annular (A_2) pulley and confluent with the origin of the first cruciate (C_1) pulley. This proximal attachment has a swallow-tail configuration that provides easy access for branches of the digital arteries to reach the tendon sheath (Fig. 2–12). In extension, the thickest part of the volar plate is in contact with the phalangeal condyles. The thickness of the plate averages 1.5 mm. and there is a constant ratio of 1:3 between volar plate thickness and condylar radius, which increases the moment arm of the superficialis by 25%. The volar plate thus enlarges the articular cavity, permitting the head of the proximal phalanx to remain in contact with a cartilaginous surface in flexion. The cartilaginous plate covers more than half of the joint's volar surface and then thins out into a fibrous membrane that covers the rest of the volar surface of the joint. In flexion of the joint, the fibrous membrane folds, permitting the volar cartilaginous plate to approximate the volar surface of the shaft of the proximal phalanx without compression; in extension, the fibrous membrane stretches. Thus, the cartilaginous plate permits normal excursion of the head of the proximal interphalangeal joint. The volar plate also serves as the floor of the tunnel for the flexor tendons of the finger. By its attachment to the base of the middle phalanx, the volar plate protects the action of the flexor tendons. Although instability of the proximal interphalangeal joint is mainly a function of the collateral ligament and volar plate, the contrac-

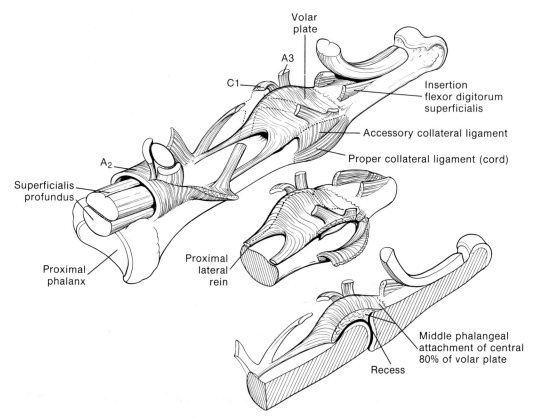

Volar
plate

A3

C1

Insertion
flexor digitorum
superficialis

Accessory collateral ligament

Proper collateral ligament (cord)

A₂

Superficialis
profundus

Proximal
phalanx

Proximal
lateral
rein

Middle phalangeal
attachment of central
80% of volar plate

Recess

FIG. 2–12 Diagrammatic representation of the proximal interphalangeal joint detailing the relationships of the volar plate to the components of the flexor sheath.

tion of the extensor or flexor apparatus of the finger greatly enhances it. With the two motors completely relaxed, a light lateral motion of the interphalageal joints can be produced passively with ease.

The dorsal aspect of the proximal interphalangeal joint has a complex arrangement of fibers reinforcing the capsule. The integrity of this arrangement contributes to the smooth working of the joint. The slightest disturbance of one of the elements of the articular unit produces deformities that indirectly affect the distal interphalangeal and the metacarpophalangeal joints and restrict their motion.

The complexity observed in this region results from the connections of the extensor apparatus with the capsule and the collateral ligaments. A study of the joint in adult and fetal

hands showed that the extensor digitorum, which fans out over this joint, has a central portion–the midband–and the lateral portions called the *lateral bands*. The central portion or midband adheres to the capsule of the joint and cannot be separated from it. The midband with the capsule is firmly inserted into the dorsal tubercle of the base of the middle phalanx and into the entire ridge of the base of the middle phalanx on each side of the dorsal tubercle. The lateral bands continue the insertion of the midband to the laterovolar tubercles until they intermingle with the most dorsal parts of the collateral ligaments, which are inserted into the laterovolar tubercles of the base of the middle phalanx.

The most lateral parts of the extensor apparatus are thick because they represent a

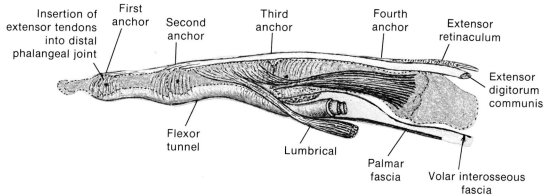

FIG. 2–13 Diagrammatic drawing of the anchorages of the extensor apparatus. Anchorage 1 connects the extensor apparatus to the distal interphalangeal joint. Anchorage 2 connects the dorsal apparatus to the proximal interphalangeal joint. Anchorage 3 connects the dorsal apparatus with the metacarpophalangeal joint. Anchorage 4 loosely connects the dorsal carpal ligament with the intertendinous fascia of the extensor digitorum communis. The palmar fascia adheres to the tunnel of the flexor tendons. The flexor tendon tunnel is separated artificially from the plate of the metacarpophalangeal joint. The interosseous fascia continues into the plate at the deep transverse intermetacarpal ligament. The lumbrical muscle is retracted superficial to the palmar fascia to illustrate the connection of the palmar fascia with the tunnel of the flexor tendon.

combined structure, consisting of the lateral parts of the communis tendon and the continuation of the interosseous tendon on the ulnar side of the finger and the interosseous and the lumbrical tendon on the radial side of the finger. The insertion of the fanned-out lateral parts of the extensor digitorum communis that adhere to the capsule is deeper; the more superficial part of the thickened lateral bands continues toward the distal part of the middle phalanx for terminal insertion into the base of the distal phalanx. According to the investigations of the author, there is no phase in the fetal development of the finger in which a separate tendon for the interosseous or the lumbrical can be traced beyond its junction with the extensor apparatus. Therefore, apparently the extensor apparatus is a functional unit and the various bands and fibers are the result of functional demands by the muscles and not differentiated, preformed tendons or tendinous slips.

The dorsal aponeurosis has a definite connection with the capsule of the joint through the midportion of the extensor communis, through its fanning-out lateral fibers and through the lateral, thick bands that transmit the action of the interossei and the lumbricals. In addition to all of these fibers, the dorsal apparatus is connected with the flexor tunnel in the form of a second anchorage of the extensor apparatus to the flexor surface of the finger. The anchorage consists of long fibers that emanate from the lateral bands, pass distally over the joint, and run toward the flexor tunnel (Figs. 2–13, 2–14, and 2–17) in a direction generally parallel with the lateral collateral ligaments.

The intra-articular surface is covered with a synovial membrane that stops at the edge of the hyaline cartilage, covering the head of the proximal phalanx and the base of the middle phalanx.

Function

The proximal interphalangeal joints are important in the control of extension and flexion of the entire finger. In extension of the joint, the dorsal expansion must remain properly centered to avoid displacement in relation to the transverse

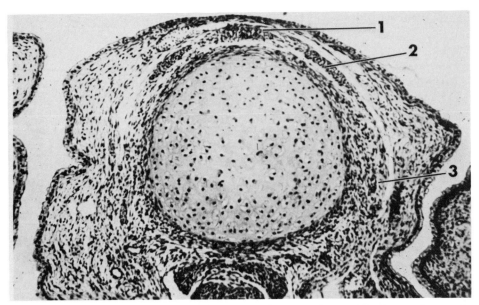

FIG. 2–14 Section through the proximal phalanx of the middle finger of an early fetus, showing the condensation of the extensor apparatus over the dorsum of the phalanx into three bands. The expansion of this apparatus runs around the phalanx toward the tunnel of the flexor tendons. (1) Midband of extensor tendon; (2) lateral band; (3) lateral band extends to level of the flexor tendon tunnel.

axis of the joint and the longitudinal axis of the finger. In flexion, the dorsal expansion must maintain its central position without displacement volar to the transverse axis of the joint.

This problem apparently was of interest to anatomists in the past. As early as 1742, Weitbrecht described retinacular ligaments that held the dorsal expansion over the proximal interphalangeal joints connecting the lateral bands of the extensor expansion over the middle phalanx with the lateral sides of the flexor tendon's tunnel. He also described cutaneous ligaments connecting the extensor expansion with the skin (see Fig. 6–26).

The retinacular ligaments have evoked much interest in recent years. A number of anatomists and surgeons specializing in hand reconstruction contributed to the study of the morphology and function of these retinacular fibers. The complicated mechanism of action of the interphalangeal and metacarpophalangeal joints in their simultaneous participation results

primarily from the actions of the extensor digitorum, the flexor superficialis, and the flexor profundus, together with the lumbrical and interosseous muscles. The functional length of each of these muscles, the power, and the sequence of their contributions in a given movement was never studied completely. The characteristics of insertions of these muscles make the problem of proper mechanics of action even more complicated. As shown by Haines, Landsmeer, Stack, and before them by Hanck, Montant and Baumann, Sunderland and later by Sunderland, Valentin, Littler, Riordan, Tubiana and others, there is no doubt that the retinacular ligaments play a role in the dynamics of finger action. However, a full comprehension of this role will be possible only after the mechanics of the action of all the participating muscles, with their differences of power, length, sequence, and degree of participation have been established completely.

In embryologic studies of the extensor

expansion over the proximal interphalangeal joint, the author found fibers connecting the lateral bands with the flexor tendon's fibrous sheath at an early stage of development. This was confirmed in a study on the developmental anatomy of the extensor expansion (O'Rahilly). In the same study, deeper attachment between the lateral bands and the border of the proximal phalanx could not be observed. There have been varying descriptions of the extensor apparatus over the proximal interphalangeal joints in relation to the retinacular arrangement. This will be discussed further in relation to function of the intrinsic and extrinsic muscles of the hand.

METACARPOPHALANGEAL JOINT

The metacarpophalangeal joint is formed by the irregularly spheroidal head of the metacarpal and the broad concave base of the proximal phalanx. It is not a hinge or ginglymoid joint like the interphalangeal joints, but a multiaxial condyloid joint permitting flexion, extension, abduction, adduction, and to a slight degree, circumduction. The most extensive movements are flexion and extension. The joint consists of a capsule, two collateral ligaments, two accessory ligaments, and a glenoidal ligament or volar plate. The capsule is somewhat loose and is attached to the elevated crest surrounding the smooth, articular surface of the head of the metacarpal and the ridge similarly separating the articular concave base from the shaft of the proximal phalanx. The laxity of the capsule permits the motions of the proximal phalanx and even a minimal amount of distraction and a very minimal range of rotation.

The lateral collateral ligament, situated on the radial and ulnar sides of each joint, is a very thick (1.5 mm to 3 mm) band, 4 mm to 8 mm wide, with an average length of about 12 mm to 14 mm. Reinforcing the capsule, this ligament is taut in flexion and more relaxed in extension; however, its tightness in flexion still permits some abduction and adduction. Although it contributes to stability to a certain extent, the actual stability of the fingers at the metacar-

pophalangeal joint is provided by the contraction of the intrinsic muscles and the tautness of the flexor tendons and the extensor apparatus. The collateral ligament arises in a special depression of the lateral subcapital area of the metacarpal, then runs distally toward the base of the proximal phalanx and fans out widely from the lateral tubercle of the base to the accessory ligament, which runs toward the volar plate. (Figs. 2–15 and 2–16). On the dorsal border, the collateral ligament blends with the dorsal capsule of the metacarpophalangeal joint. The accessory portion of the ligament is firmly united to the volar plate. The plate is fibrocartilaginous and is firmly inserted into the volar base of the proximal phalanx. Proximally, it thins out into a flexible membranous ligament that is attached to a line on the volar side of the metacarpophalangeal neck immediately proximal to the cartilage-covered head of the metacarpal.

The volar plate on the volar aspect of the metacarpal with the two accessory ligaments on the sides enlarges the cavity of the metacarpophalangeal joint, permitting the head of the metacarpal to remain in the articular cavity when the proximal phalanx is in full flexion. The head of the metacarpal is covered with cartilage over about three fourths of its spherical dorsovolar surface.

The volar plate appears very early in the fetal development of the hand. It forms, apparently, a continuous structure with the accessory ligaments. At this stage of development, the volar plates are not connected between the metacarpals (Fig. 2–18); with further development, the volar plates become connected from the index finger to the little finger, forming the deep transverse intermetacarpal ligament, which appears at this stage of development (Figs. 2–19 and 2–20). While the dorsal surface of the volar plate is in contact with the head of the metacarpal, the volar surface of this ligament is in contact with the flexor tendons, which pass from the proximal part of the hand into the fingers. Each pair of the long flexors (superficialis and profundus) is surrounded by the vaginal ligament, which is actually a tunnel, adherent to the

(Text continues on page 44.)

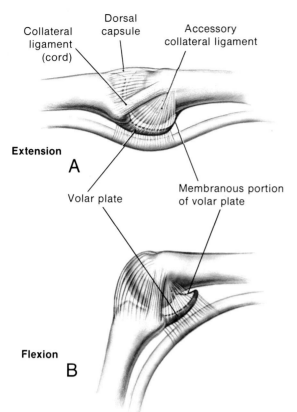

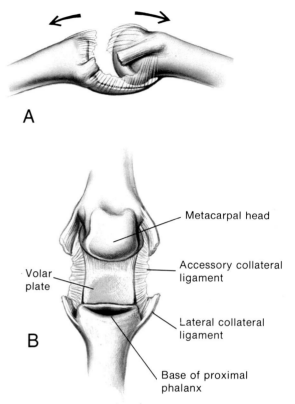

FIG. 2–15 Metacarpophalangeal joint. Note the relationships of the collateral ligaments, volar plate, and dorsal capsule in extension (**A**) and flexion (**B**).

FIG. 2–16 Metacarpophalangeal joint with dorsal capsule remove and lateral and accessory ligaments divided.

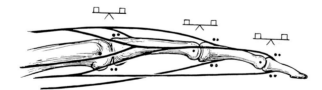

FIG. 2–17 Balance of forces over the joints of the finger. Single dots represent the axes flexion-extension of each joint. Double dots represent the areas of action of the corresponding tendons at each joint. At the metacarpophalangeal joint, the balance is between the extensor tendon on the dorsum and the interosseous lumbrical component at the volar aspect. At the proximal joint, the insertion of the extensor apparatus into the dorsum of the middle phalanx is balanced against the flexor sublimis. At the distal joint, the insertion of the extensor apparatus is balanced against the flexor profundus. (From Kaplan E.B.: Anatomy, injuries and treatment of the extensor apparatus of the hand and the digits. Clin Orthop 13:24, 1959.)

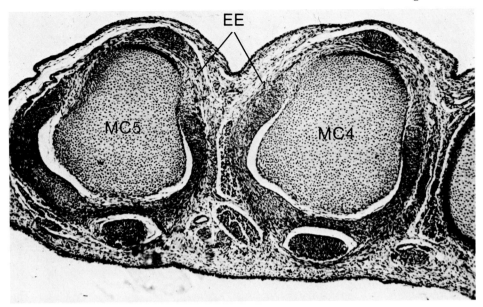

FIG. 2—18 Section of an early fetal hand through the metacarpal heads. The extensor expansion (EE) runs toward the side of the capsule; the deep intermetacarpal ligament is not evident as yet, and the midpalmar aponeurosis is practically absent.

FIG. 2—19 Section of the hand of a 4-month-old fetus through the metacarpal head at the level of the deep transverse metacarpal ligament (**A**). The deep transverse metacarpal ligament is dorsal to the lumbrical canal at the bottom of the illustration. The fibers of the dorsal apparatus do not penetrate the transverse intermetacarpal ligament. The transverse intermetacarpal ligament shows its direct continuation into the anterior plate of the metacarpophalangeal joint (**B**), which separates the joint from the long flexors.

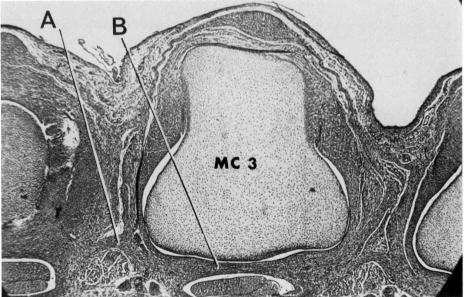

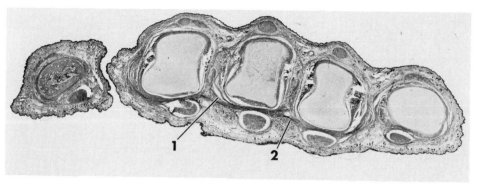

FIG. 2–20   Transverse section through the metacarpal heads of the left hand of a 5-month-old fetus. The fibers surrounding the metacarpal heads and connected with the expansion of the tendons of the extensor digitorum contribute to the formation of the deep transverse intermetacarpal ligament. These fibers do not penetrate the deep transverse metacarpal ligament. The deep transverse metacarpal ligament continues directly into the volar plate of the metacarpophalangeal joint. There is no indication of the pretendinous bands of the midpalmar fascia, which are seen more clearly in transverse sections of the adult hand. The section runs through the distal phalanx of the thumb, showing the extensor brevis together with the extensor longus, prolonged into the distal phalanx. (1) Fibers of extensor expansion; (2) deep transverse metacarpal ligament.

volar plate and completely surrounding the flexor tendons. It is formed by circular fibers (Fig. 2–21). The accessory volar ligament sometimes shows in its depth the presence of a small sesamoid (Fig. 2–23).

The deep transverse metacarpal ligament begins to appear, approximately, toward the end of the third month of fetal development (Fig. 2–18). In the adult (Figs. 2–21 and 2–23), it is continuous with the volar plates and extends

between the metacarpals and the bases of the proximal phalanges in the second, third, and fourth web spaces (Fig. 2–24). It continues to the palm of the hand, becomes thinner, and blends with the anterior fascia that covers the interossei muscles. In the interdigital spaces its sharp distal edge is about 10 mm proximal to the *interdigital skin* fold. The space between the fold and the distal edge of the ligament is filled with areolar fatty tissue. The width of the ligament in

FIG. 2–21   **A,** Transverse section of the hand through the heads of the metacarpals of the second, third, fourth, and fifth fingers. **B** and **C,** The hoods over the metacarpophalangeal joint were dissected out to show the separation of the hood from the metacarpal heads. The skin of the palm of the hand was dissected to show the pretendinous bands of the midpalmar fascia and the transverse, superficial metacarpal ligament. The hood extends to the lateral collateral ligaments and to the deep transverse metacarpal ligament without perforating the deep transverse metacarpal ligament. Four tunnels of the flexors and their relationship with the lumbricals and the neurovascular bundles are indicated. ▶

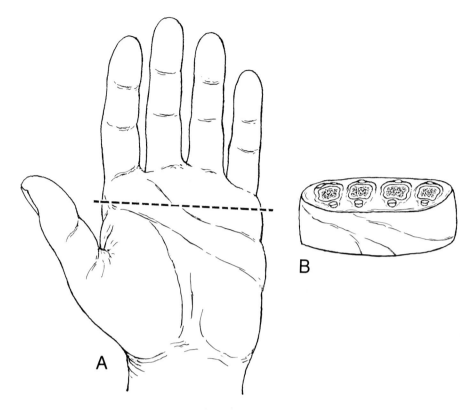

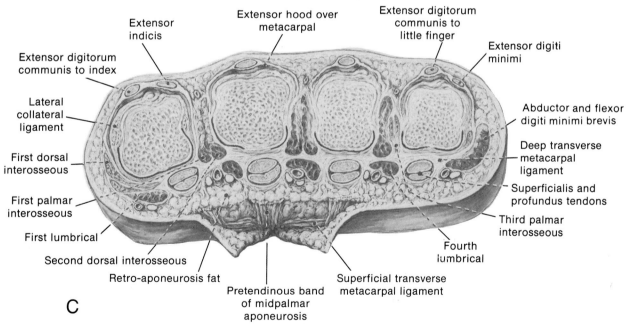

Extensor
indicis

Extensor hood over
metacarpal

Extensor digitorum
communis to
little finger

Extensor digiti
minimi

Extensor digitorum
communis to index

Lateral
collateral
ligament

First dorsal
interosseous

First palmar
interosseous

First lumbrical

Second dorsal interosseous

Retro-aponeurosis fat

Pretendinous band
of midpalmar
aponeurosis

Superficial transverse
metacarpal ligament

Fourth
lumbrical

Abductor and flexor
digiti minimi brevis

Deep transverse
metacarpal
ligament

Superficialis and
profundus tendons

Third palmar
interosseous

C

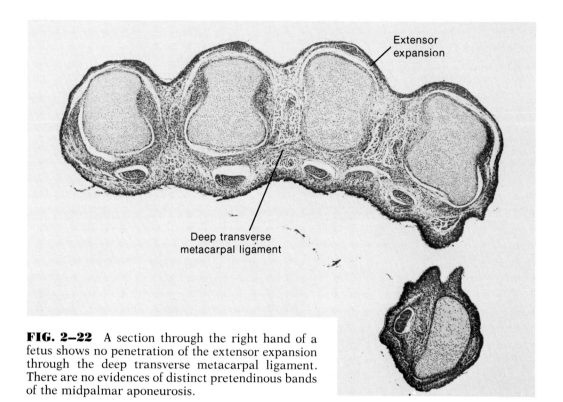

Extensor
expansion

Deep transverse
metacarpal ligament

FIG. 2–22 A section through the right hand of a fetus shows no penetration of the extensor expansion through the deep transverse metacarpal ligament. There are no evidences of distinct pretendinous bands of the midpalmar aponeurosis.

each intermetacarpal space equals the width between the corresponding metacarpals. The height of the ligament varies from 9 mm to 12 mm. Volar to the transverse metacarpal ligaments are the lumbrical muscles, with the beginning of their tendinous parts, and the neurovascular bundle. Dorsal to ligaments pass the tendons of the interosseous muscles (Fig. 2–23).

In direct relation to the collateral ligaments lie the tendons of the interosseous muscles. Although further consideration of these muscles will be given in the chapter on hand muscles, it may be mentioned now that the tendons of the interossei are located in a depression on each side of the metacarpal neck and head and are covered with a part of the extension hood that forms a complete tunnel for these tendons and prevents dislocation from this position. This anatomic detail, important from a functional viewpoint, refutes the assertion of some observers that under certain circumstances the

interossei, which are flexors of the metacarpophalangeal joint, may displace dorsally and become extensors. The authors have never seen such a dorsal displacement and doubts its possibility.

The relationship of the extensor digitorum communis to the metacarpophalangeal joint deserves a detailed description in view of its importance to the function of the finger. The extensor digitorum or the combined extensor digitorum and the proprius of the index and little fingers runs in the form of tendons to the head of the metacarpal. On arriving at the heads, the tendons expand into a wider structure. The tendon itself begins to fan out and is joined and covered by an aponeurotic extension of the tendon of the interosseous, which is located on each side of the finger. The aponeurotic extension is sometimes double and appears to enclose the tendon of the extensor digitorum (Fig. 2–10).

If the tendon of the extensor communis is lifted and retracted distally as in Figure 2–6, it

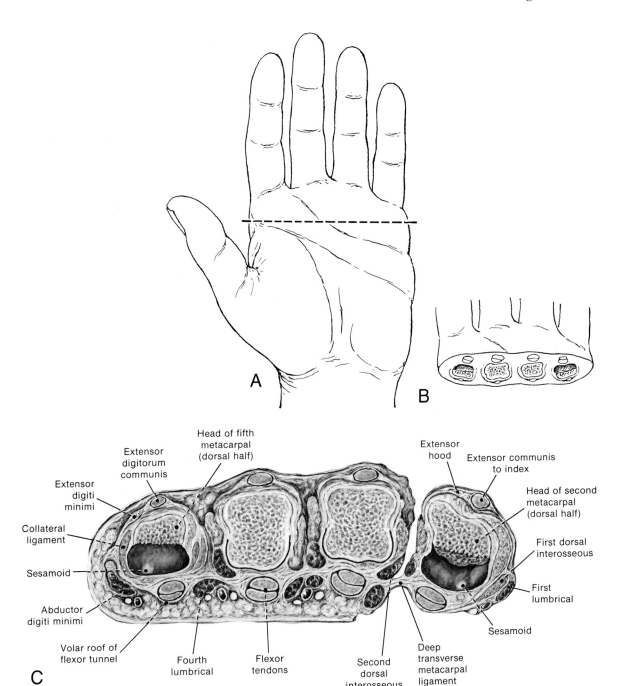

FIG. 2–23 **A** and **B**, Cross-section showing in direct view the structures through the metacarpal heads. **C**, The volar half of metacarpal heads 2 and 5 are removed to show the depth of the joint. The interossei muscles between the second and the third metacarpals are removed to show the relation of the extensor hood to the capsule and the collateral ligament of the joint. It shows the thickness of the deep transverse metacarpal ligament and its distance from the dorsal and volar surfaces of the hand. As can be seen, the fibers of the dorsal apparatus do not penetrate through the deep transverse metacarpal ligament.

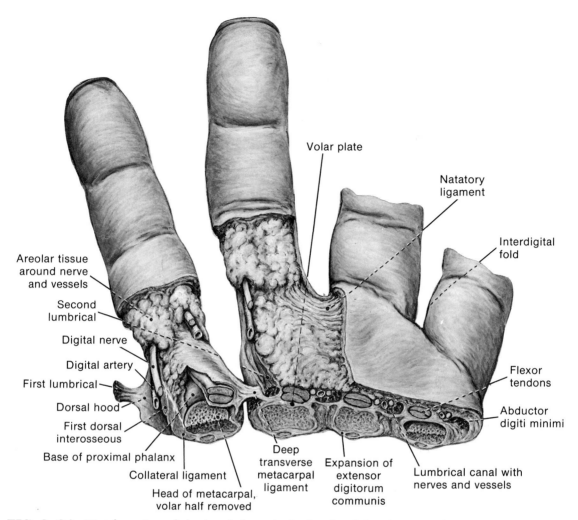

FIG. 2–24 Distal section of the hand through the heads of the metacarpals to indicate the location of the deep transverse metacarpal ligament in relation to the interdigital fold, also to show the relationship of this ligament to the joint line of the metacarpophalangeal joint. The interdigital or natatory ligament is shown with its continuation into the dense subcutaneous fat of the palm and the subcutaneous tunnel that surrounds and covers the digital nerve and artery. Note that there is a continuation of the dorsal expansion over the metacarpal head toward the deep transverse metacarpal ligament between the metacarpal heads and toward the collateral ligament of the metacarpophalangeal joint on the radial side of the index finger and the ulnar side of the little finger. The volar half of the head of the fifth metacarpal and the volar half of the head of the index finger metacarpal are removed to show the depth of the metacarpophalangeal joint.

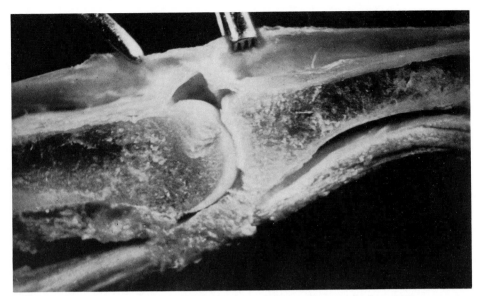

FIG. 2–25 Sagittal section of a metacarpophalangeal joint of a finger. The extensor digitorum tendon is lifted up to show the connection of the extensor digitorum tendon to the capsule of the joint.

can be separated from the capsule of the metacarpophalangeal joint, but the sides of the expansion dip in between the metacarpal heads. The separation of the expansion and the tendon from the capsule of the metacarpophalangeal joint can be seen clearly in Figure 2–9, which represents the complete dorsal apparatus of the finger separated from the head of the metacarpal, the metacarpophalangeal joint, the proximal phalanx, the proximal interphalangeal joint, the middle phalanx, and the distal interphalangeal joint with the distal phalanx.

In contrast with the proximal and distal interphalangeal joints, in which the tendons adhere intimately to the posterior capsule, the extensor apparatus shows only a depression for the head of the metacarpal and the metacarpophalangeal joint; however, loose connections between the palmar surface of the extensor apparatus and the dorsal aspect of the capsule are almost always present and at times may assume the aspect of fibrous slips (Fig. 2–25). In a previous study, the author found the presence of such slips in about 38.5% of a series of 140 fingers. If the dorsal apparatus is completely divided and separated across the dorsum of the proximal phalanx, and the extensor tendon is

completely divided over the metacarpal, and traction is applied to the distal end of the divided extensor digitorum tendon on the metacarpal, the proximal phalanx will hyperextend. If in addition to the division of the extensor apparatus and the extensor digitorum tendon the lateral connections are also completely divided so that the extensor expansion and the extensor tendon are completely disconnected from all attachments, traction applied to the distal end of the extensor tendon will again produce hyperextension of the proximal phalanx. Of course, no action will be transmitted to the two distal phalanges.

This experiment indicates that in most of the hands a connection exists between the capsule of the metacarpophalangeal joint and the extensor tendon; however, if the experiment by traction is repeated forcibly a number of times, the connection between the tendon and the capsule can be disrupted. Apparently, the connection between the capsule of the joint and the extensor tendon plays a double role: it reinforces the to-and-fro action of the extensor expansion over the metacarpophalangeal joint, and it stabilizes the midband of the extensor over the center of the joint. In rheumatoid arthritis, the almost con-

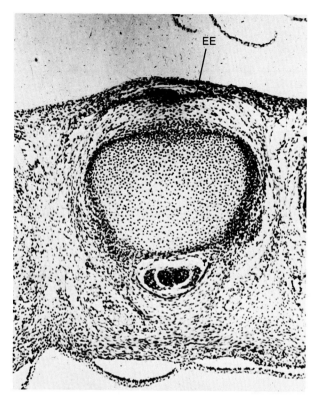

FIG. 2–26 Section through the base of the proximal phalanx of the middle finger of a 40-mm fetus. Distal to the deep transverse intermetacarpal ligament, the extensor expansion (EE) surrounds the phalanx in this area. The direction of the fibers around the phalanx is clearly seen.

stant presence of synovitis produces a disruption of the connecting fibers between the extensor tendon and the capsule and thus facilitates the sliding of the extensor tendon to the side with a corresponding drift of the fingers.

Complete sections through the metacarpophalangeal joints in the adult and in fetal hands show that the extensor expansion extends over the metacarpophalangeal joint and its lateral aspects, covering the lateral collateral ligaments, finally reaching the volar plate with its flexor tendons tunnel. Figures 2–18, 2–19, 2–25, 2–26, and 2–27 show the development of this structure in fetal hands. In the adult hand (Fig. 2–3), the dorsal aponeurotic expansion can be seen radiating toward the anterior aspect of the

fingers. There is, at times, adhesion of the expansion even to the lateral collateral ligament (Figs. 2–21 and 2–23). Thus, in this area another anchorage is established, connecting the extensor apparatus to the flexor surface similar to the anchorages over the distal and proximal interphalangeal joints.

FIG. 2–27 Section through the metacarpophalangeal joint of a 5-month-old fetus showing the connection of the extensor tendon (ET) with the capsule of the dorsum of the metacarpophalangeal joint over the base of the proximal phalanx. The expansion of the tendon of the extensor digitorum communis runs along the lateral aspect of the metacarpophalangeal joint with oblique connections with the collateral ligamentous apparatus (CL). Several layers over the dorsum of the joint indicate that motion of flexion and extension is possible.

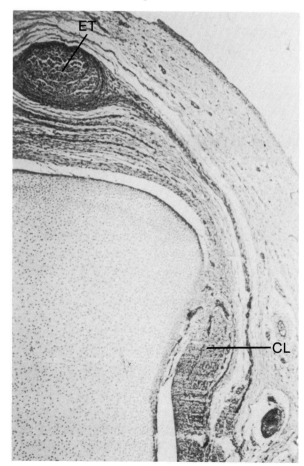

Lymph, Blood, and Nerve Supplies of Interphalangeal and Metacarpophalangeal Joints

Robert J. Schultz
Emanuel B. Kaplan

The blood supply of the interphalangeal joints is derived from branches of the proper digital arteries of the fingers. These branches arise proximal to the interphalangeal joint, enter the joint in the midlateral plane, and supply the capsule and synovium. The metacarpophalangeal joints are supplied by branches of the common and proper digital arteries, which arise from the palmar arterial arches. Arterial branches from the dorsal arterial arches supply the dorsal aspect of the metacarpophalangeal and sometimes the dorsal aspect of the proximal interphalangeal joints. The venous drainage from the small joints of the fingers passes directly into the superficial dorsal veins of the fingers and the superficial palmar veins. There appear to be no veins accompanying the proper digital arteries.

The anatomy of the lymphatic drainage from the joints of the fingers was presented in an excellent comprehensive study by Sappey. According to his study, osseous tissue is probably completely devoid of lymphatic drainage. He felt that the synovial membrane has no lymph vessels, with most of the lymph drainage occurring from the periarticular structures. Newer studies, however, have demonstrated that the synovial membrane contains two plexuses of lymphatics: a deep layer and a superficial layer. One layer is found directly under the endothelium and the other layer is found in the subsynovial tissues. The lymph vessels drain directly into larger trunks that accompany the proper digital arteries. The lymph vessels of the metacarpophalangeal joints drain directly into lymph trunks accompanying the palmar arterial arches or the superficial dorsal collectors.

The nerve supply to the finger joints has been studied by many authors. Head noted that proprioception in joint movement remains intact despite nerve laceration if the tendons have not been lacerated. He felt that deep sensibility was provided by the motor nerves that pass into the joint with the tendons and blood vessels. Stoppford's contribution was related to stereognosis. He felt that the afferent articular impulses were provided by the nerves in relation to their cutaneous distribution.

Schultz and Krishnamurthy have recently studied the innervation of the small joints of the fingers using gross anatomic dissections and microscopic cross-sections. They noted that the proximal interphalangeal joints are innervated by articular branches that arise from the proper digital nerves (Fig. 2–28) on the radial and ulnar sides of the digit proximal to the proximal interphalangeal joint, pass in a dorsolateral direction, and enter the joint in the midlateral plane, bifurcating just before entering the joint. They are accompanied by an articular arterial branch arising from the proper digital artery. The artery and nerve enter the joint capsule through a common portal and then pass to the synovium. The point of entry of the nerve lies between the lateral bands and the attachment of the fibrous sheath to bone. In the capsule, the nerve fibers are found predominantly in a lateral and palmar location. No articular branches enter the capsule from the nerves passing dorsal to the joint. These nerves remain dorsal to the extensor mechanism.

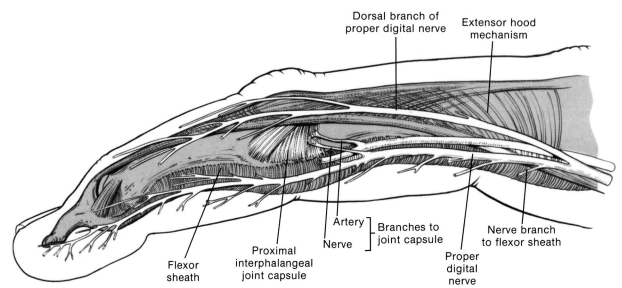

FIG. 2–28 Diagramatic representation of the innervation to the proximal interphalangeal joint. Note the dorsolateral course adopted by the articular nerve and artery after their origins from the palmar proper digital nerve and artery. Note also the bifurcation of the nerve prior to entering the joint.

The Muscles and the Tendon Systems of the Fingers

Emanuel B. Kaplan
James M. Hunter

The muscles of the fingers are described separately from the muscles of the thumb and the wrist, which are discussed separately in Chapters 3 and 4. The real meaning of the relationship of the muscles and the frequent variations that occur in the hand as a whole become much clearer when seen in the light of comparative anatomic and embryologic studies.

In the analysis of the muscular system it is preferable to eliminate the frequently used term of *anomaly* for muscles that have an origin or insertion differing from accepted descriptions. It is more in line with the findings of comparative anatomy and embryology to classify all the differences as variations.

The anomalous structures fall into a different group produced by external causes: disease, exposure to radiation, or other damaging influences, either during development or in later stages. The so-called cases of developmental arrest probably also fall into the group of changes produced by abnormal chemical or physical agents.

The comparative anatomic investigations of Humphry help explain a number of variations encountered in the hand. In more modern and more nearly complete studies, Strauss and Haines advanced the understanding of the development of the musculature. LeDouble and Testut collected a large series of muscular variations and correlated them wih the findings of others. A discussion of these investigators follows.

The upper-limb girdle develops in the same way as the ribs and costal cartilages in the transverse intermuscular septum of the ventral muscles in the plane of the middle or internal oblique stratum. Essentially, they derive from the middle stratum and may be considered as serially homologous with the muscles passing from septum to septum or from rib to rib in front and behind them. It has also been shown that the external stratum of the external oblique muscle is prolonged on the limbs as a more or less complete funnel; therefore, the muscles are derivatives of the two outer strata of the ventral muscles, and they contribute largely to the muscular basis of the limbs. The muscle tissue of the limbs in the primitive form is segmented into transverse planes corresponding to the axial, cartilaginous, or osseous segments, thus resembling the disposition of the muscles in the trunk; but in the trunk, the muscle fibers, particularly the superficial fibers, are often not confined to their particular segments. The muscles of any division of a limb usually consist of three layers: the fibers of the segment itself, or the "intrinsic fibers"—of these the proximal series pass from the girdle to the first segment of the limb; the fibers derived from the distal segment, or the "extrinsic fibers"; more superficial fibers derived from the ventral muscles, or the superficial "ventral appendicular fibers." The components of these three layers are blended together in a variety of ways, making it almost impossible to define to which layer they belong.

THE PRONATOFLEXOR AND SUPINATOEXTENSOR MASSES

In vertebrates, the muscles located on the flexor surface of the forearm are segregated in an anatomic system described by Humphry and called the *pronatoflexor mass*. The extensor surface was segregated into a supinatoextensor mass.

The *pronatoflexor mass*, which is undifferentiated in its area of origin at the medial epicondyle of the humerus and the corresponding parts of the ulna and radius, divides distally into separate units and distinct sections. The degree of development and differentiation varies according to the zoologic group and is subordinated to the variable functions of the forearm and the hand; thus, in certain reptiles and amphibians in which the movements of the hand are not differentiated, the muscular mass is entirely undivided. In the higher vertebrates, the functions of the hand become more nearly perfect, the needs become more multiple, and the muscles that are to accomplish those movements become more divided and more individualized. In man, out of this pronatoflexor mass we find two common flexors completely separated: an individualized flexor for the thumb and also a separate pronator. The entire mass divides into two layers: a deep layer that forms the deep flexors and the pronator quadratus and a superficial layer that divides into distinct sectors, an ulnar sector that forms the flexor carpi ulnaris, a radial sector that forms the pronator teres and the flexor carpi radialis, and an intermediary sector that forms the flexor digitorum sublimis and the palmaris longus.

In the intermediate sector, the palmaris longus expands into the palmar fascia, where it blends with the fibers of the flexor carpi ulnaris. The flexor digitorum sublimis is a more important muscle because it absorbs a great part of the flexor carpi ulnaris and of the palmaris longus, which has a tendency to disappear.

The elements of the carpometacarpals, the metacarpophalangeals, and the phalangeals follow the quadrate pronator in uniting or retaining their union with the flexor profundus; however, advancing distally, they often separate and attach themselves to the sides of the phalanges, forming the lumbricals from their lateral parts and the retinacula from their middle parts. The phalangeal fibers are probably included in the latter but occasionally remain separate and often disappear. The lumbricals are found chiefly on the deep surface of the angles between the tendons of the flexor profundus. In the cases of the thumb and little finger, their elements remain in part or wholly on the metacarpals and form the short flexors. For this reason, the lumbricals are not usually present on the tendons of these digits, or only one is present, lying on the radial side of the tendon to the little finger. More rarely, there is one on the ulnar side of the tendon to the little finger. In some animals, the lumbricals pass from both sides of the several tendons of the flexor profundus to both sides of the fingers with one on the ulnar side of the flexor profundus to the thumb, and one on the radial side of the little finger, making eight lumbricals. In mammals, these are usually combined into four lumbricals.

To put it another way, the lumbricals and the retinacula may be regarded as parts of the common flexor mass, which instead of becoming segmented into metacarpophalangeals and phalangeals, retain their connection with the flexor tendons and are separated with them from the metacarpus and the carpus. However, they are not detached from the phalanges to which they pass accordingly from the flexor tendon.

Their connection with the extensor tendons in man and some mammals is a reminder of the blending of antagonistic muscles into a common sheath, which is one of the features of a primitive limb.

The flexor profundus does not only absorb or retain annexed to it these various elements of the deep stratum of the pronator flexor mass, in most animals above the salamander, the flexor profundus also retains its connection with the terminal middle portion of each digital division of the superficial stratum or superficial flexor and passes on to the terminal phalanx, while the lateral portions of the superficial flexor tendons, by disconnecting themselves from the middle terminal portion, stop at a preceding phalanx. In this way, the deep flexor perforates the superficial flexor, which splits, allowing the flexor to pass.

Tendons of this type, passing along the digit, ordinarily divide into three parts when approaching a joint. Of these, the lateral parts are attached to the phalanx immediately on the distal side of the joint; the middle part runs to the next joint, where a similar process is repeated. This is best seen in the digits of birds and reptiles where there are more than two phalanges. It is also exemplified in the usual arrangement of the tendons of the superficial and deep flexors of the digits; these are considered as segments of one flexor prolongation on the digit.

This flexor prolongation first detaches the lumbricals to the first phalanx from its sides, then continues to run. In a similar manner, it detaches the slips of the flexor superficialis to the middle phalanx, repeats the same process according to the number of phalanges and finally reaches the distal phalanx.

The *supinatoextensor mass* leads to the development of the extensor muscles of the forearm. The division of the superficial stratum of this mass into three sectors (radial, middle, and ulnar) is more distinct than in the pronatoflexor masses. Owing to the convexity of the elbow, they are more often cut off from the continuity of the muscles of the humerus than are the pronatoflexor masses.

Traced downward, the middle sector commonly extends on the digits forming the extensor digitorum communis. Sometimes, the radial sector reaches no farther than the lower end of the radius. In mammals, only a segment of it is inserted into the inner edge of the radius, constituting the brachioradialis. This may extend to the inner edge of the thumb or may spread over the palmar surface of the forearm. Other segments passing close to the carpus form the extensor carpi radialis; the ulnar sector (the extensor carpi ulnaris) is inserted into the other side of the metacarpus. The abductor digiti minimi is segmented from the lower end of this sector and represents a continuation of the extensor carpi ulnaris to the ulnar side of the hand. The abductor pollicis is a continuation of the more or less segmented radial section on the thumb. This shows that the three sectors of the superficial sheath of the supinatoextensor mass may be imperfectly segmented from the others, and each may be extended on the digits, or partly or wholly arrested at the more proximal points.

The deep layers of the supinatoextensor masses generally correspond to the deep pronatoflexor masses. The outer mass represents the supinator; lower down it forms the abductor pollicis longus. Still more distal, it runs in one or two portions on the pollex, forming the extensor pollicis brevis. Still more distal, it extends to the index or other fingers, forming an extensor profundus. It is evident that the muscles called extensors of the pollex, the index, and others are really derivatives of the extensor profundus. In the same way as the elements of the deep flexor stratum, the elements of the extensor stratum are usually continued further distally on the phalanges than are the elements of the superficial stratum.

In mammals, the greater part of the superficial stratum is inserted into the middle phalanx. The deeper stratum, arising from the radius and the ulna, and the still deeper stratum interossei are continued to the distal phalanges. When tendons of the superficial extensors are continued distally with prolongations of the deep stratum to the terminal phalanges, they are usually derived from the marginal parts of the digital tendons; the middle part of each tendon is inserted into the more proximal phalanx. When the tendons of the superficial extensor reach to the terminal phalanges without sagittal prolongations of the deep stratum, it is nevertheless the marginal parts of the tendon that reach the phalanges.

The disposition is reversed for the flexor tendons. The flexor tendons show that the deeper and more prolonged tendon occupies the middle position and continues its course distally to the terminal phalanx, while the superficial tendon is inserted into one or usually both margins of a more proximal phalanx. When the superficial and deep flexors are fused into one and that one subdivides to supply the several phalanges, the middle part is usually more prolonged and never receives any marginal additions from the deeper stratum.

In higher animals in which the metacarpals admit little movement to and from one another, the interossei change their transverse direction to a course more parallel with the digits, and they extend on the phalanges and sometimes blend with the extensor tendon. In the simple limbs of some of the lower animals, the interossei are mere bands passing between the metacarpals, drawing the digits together, and antagonizing the abductors of the marginal digits.

The muscles that show differentiation of the pronatoflexor or supinatoextensor group of Humphry may therefore show, in man, multiple variations, the significance of which can be grasped or interpreted from the viewpoint of the anatomist and especially the surgeon. How to interpret an additional muscle, whether to call it an atavistic reversal to the original, or whether to interpret an absent muscle as a developmental arrest is of little interest to the surgeon who must suspect what the additional or absent muscle represents anatomically and what function is connected with the structure.

The muscles that move the fingers are represented by two groups: the long extrinsic muscles originating in the forearm, and the short intrinsic muscles, originating in the hand.

LONG EXTRINSIC MUSCLES

The long extrinsic muscles are located on the volar and the dorsal aspects of the forearm and the hand. The muscles originating from the volar surface of the forearm are flexors; the muscles originating from the dorsal aspect of the forearm are extensors.

LONG FLEXORS

The two long flexors are the flexor digitorum profundus and the flexor digitorum sublimis.

The *flexor digitorum profundus* originates in the forearm from the proximal two thirds of the volar and medial surfaces of the ulna, extending to an area just below the coronoid process of the ulna, near the fibers of insertion of the brachialis. The fibers of the flexor profundus extend toward the medial side of the ulna, where the muscle is in contact with the fibers of the supinator, situated more radially. On the medial side, more proximally, the muscle originates

from the septum, which separates the flexor profundus from the flexor carpi ulnaris and occasionally from the radius, slightly distal to the bicipital tuberosity on the edge of the medial border of the radius. The origin also extends to the ulnar half of the interosseous membrane. The origin of the flexor profundus runs alongside the origin of the flexor pollicis longus, which is located on the radial side of the interosseous membrane, where both muscles contiguously descend almost to the origin of the pronator quadratus.

The muscular belly, which is formed by fibers running a straight distal course, finally divides into four muscular bundles in the distal third of the forearm. The most radial bundle is more widely separated and runs toward the index finger. The bundle to the little finger is sometimes separated from the bundles to the third and the fourth (middle and ring) fingers. A flattened tendon soon appears following each bundle. The fleshy fibers descend on the dorsal surface of these tendons much more distally than on the volar surface, reaching the proximal edge of the osteofibrous tunnel of the wrist (Fig. 2–29). The division between the tendon to the ring and little fingers sometimes occurs within the osteofibrous tunnel of the wrist. The relation of these tendons to the tendons of the superficialis through the wrist tunnel and in the palm of the hand will be described with the tendons of the flexor superficialis.

The *flexor digitorum superficialis* is superficial to the flexor digitorum profundus. It is a large, flat, fleshy muscle that originates in the forearm from the medial epicondyle of the humerus in common with the other epicondylar muscles. The fibers arise from the anterior and medial surfaces of the epicondyle, from the medial collateral ligament of the elbow, and from the medial aspect of the coronoid process medial to the origin of the pronator teres and medial to the insertion of the tendon of the brachialis with which the flexor sublimis forms intimate connections. From here, the line of origin runs an oblique course along the oblique line of the radius—a line separating the radius into an anterosuperior supinator surface and an

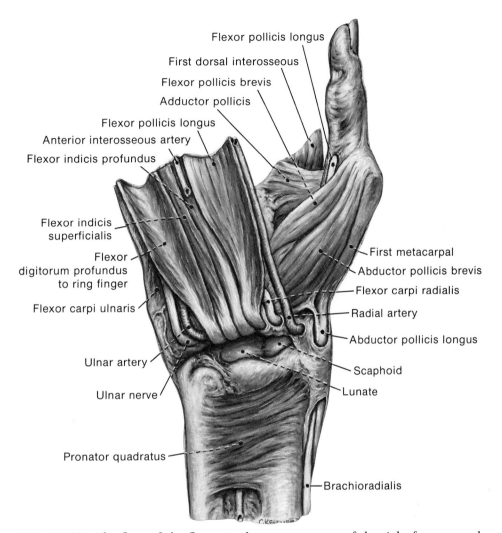

Flexor pollicis longus
First dorsal interosseous
Flexor pollicis brevis
Adductor pollicis
Flexor pollicis longus
Anterior interosseous artery
Flexor indicis profundus
Flexor indicis superficialis
Flexor digitorum profundus to ring finger
Flexor carpi ulnaris
Ulnar artery
Ulnar nerve
Pronator quadratus

First metacarpal
Abductor pollicis brevis
Flexor carpi radialis
Radial artery
Abductor pollicis longus
Scaphoid
Lunate
Brachioradialis

FIG. 2—29 The floor of the flexor tendon compartment of the right forearm and thumb. All the long flexors of the fingers were retracted distally to show the relation of the brachioradialis insertion, which actually forms a floor for the tunnel through which the tendons of the abductor pollicis longus and the extensor pollicis brevis pass. The additional insertion of the abductor pollicis longus into the abductor pollicis brevis is shown in this specimen. The retraction of the tendons exposes the radiocarpal joint.

anterior-inferior surface for the flexor pollicis longus. The line is about 6 cm to 8 cm long, running from the bicipital tuberosity to the anterior border of the radius.

The origin of the flexor digitorum superficialis thus has two heads, one ulnar and the other radial with fibrous band stretching between the two heads. The median nerve and the ulnar artery pass under this band to continue their course over the more deeply situated flexor profundus muscle. Following the origin, a large, flat muscular belly descends distally, completely covering the flexor profundus muscle (Fig. 2–29). The ulnar border is straight, and in the lowermost part of the forearm it deflects toward the radial side, thus uncovering the most ulnar part

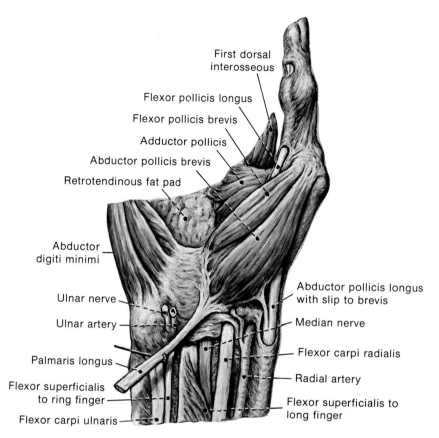

First dorsal
interosseous

Flexor pollicis longus

Flexor pollicis brevis

Adductor pollicis

Abductor pollicis brevis

Retrotendinous fat pad

Abductor
digiti minimi

Ulnar nerve

Ulnar artery

Palmaris longus

Flexor superficialis
to ring finger

Flexor carpi ulnaris

Abductor pollicis longus
with slip to brevis

Median nerve

Flexor carpi radialis

Radial artery

Flexor superficialis to
long finger

FIG. 2–30 Flexor tendons of the distal right forearm and thumb. The palmaris longus is partially inserted into the abductor pollicis brevis. The flexor carpi ulnaris is continuous through the pisiform with the abductor digiti minimi, and the fat pad of the midpalmar space is seen ulnar to the abductor pollicis.

of the pronator quadratus. The radial border of the muscle is oblique toward the ulnar border of the forearm and leaves the lower half of the flexor pollicis longus muscle exposed.

Slightly distal to the middle of the forearm, the muscle belly is divided into four parts or bundles: two bundles are located more superficially and run toward the middle and the ring fingers; the other two bundles are situated deeper for the index and little fingers. The muscle fibers to the index finger are usually bipenniform. The fibers to the middle finger are unipenniform on the radial side of the tendon. The muscle fibers descend distally toward the transverse carpal ligament.

The special disposition of the fleshy fibers of the middle finger form an interesting relation to the median nerve. The median nerve normally emerges on the radial side of the fleshy fibers of the middle finger, which cross the median nerve obliquely in a distal and ulnar direction (Fig. 2–30). This relation of the median nerve to the flexor superficialis in the distal part of the forearm may be compared with the relation of the median nerve in the proximal part of the forearm. The fibrous band of origin of the flexor superficialis crosses the median nerve in a distal and radial direction.

The tendons of the flexor superficialis reach the osteofibrous tunnel of the wrist together with the tendons of the flexor profundus. They enter the tunnel and usually retain a constant relation between themselves (Fig. 2–31). Enclosed in the synovial bursa in layers, the flexor superficialis to the middle finger—the strongest and most cylindrical—lies most superficially, alongside the flexor superficialis tendon of the ring finger, which is located on the ulnar side of the tendon superficialis to the middle finger. The tendon of the flexor superficialis to the little finger is most ulnar and at the wrist may be quite variable and can be absent or cordlike in appearance. There is always some connection to the little finger through the mesotendon system.

Variations should be noted clinically because a variety of flexion contractures of the little finger are related to shortening of the superficialis tendon system. Dissections show continuations of the synovial bursae into the palm and into the finger associated with long continuing vinculum in the finger (see Fig. 2–33). This complexity is at times correctible by tenotomy of the superficialis in the forearm or palm.

The tendon of the flexor superficialis to the index finger is found deeper and toward the tendon of the flexor superficialis of the middle finger. In the same horizontal plane with the flexor indicis superficialis, the four tendons of the flexor profundus are found. It must be mentioned that the flexor superficialis to the index finger has a tendency to shift completely under the tendon of the flexor superficialis of the middle finger; in this case, the tendon of the flexor profundus to the index finger lies immediately dorsal to the median nerve.

The tendons of the fingers

After the tendons emerge from the carpal tunnel into the palm of the hand, the superficialis and the profundus form a regular two-layer arrangement, with the superficialis occupying a superficial position and the profundus running deeper to the superficialis. The tendons diverge from the carpal tunnel radially toward the fingers. In passing in the proximal palm of the hand, the flexor profundus tendons give origin to the lumbrical muscles. It must be noted that although the lumbrical muscles originate from

the tendons of the flexor profundus, they cover the tendons of the flexor superficialis for more than half of the diameter of the superficialis tendon and sometimes conceal the superficialis completely.

Further distally, the tendons of the flexors enter the fibrous sheaths over the distal ends of the metacarpals just proximal to the metacarpophalangeal joints. The two tendons still run in the same orders: the superficialis is the superficial and the profundus is the deep (Fig. 2–21). After the tendons cross the metacarpophalangeal joint, their diameters and dispositions begin to change. The flexor profundus begins to penetrate into the flexor superficialis, which flattens out (Figs. 2–32 and 2–33). The perforation occurs through a considerable length of the superficialis tendon.

A longitudinal line appears in the middle of the tendon of the flexor superficialis at varying points in the vicinity of the metacarpophalangeal joint on the volar surface of the tendon. Approximately over the middle of the proximal phalanx, the longitudinal line over the volar surface of the tendons of the flexor sublimis becomes deeper and splits into two halves to let the tendon of the flexor profundus run through to the surface. Each half of the sublimis tendon first covers the corresponding half of the penetrating flexor profundus, then the superficialis turns around so that the anterior surface of each half becomes lateral in relation to the flexor profundus. Each half then runs posterior to the flexor profundus and emerges on the other side of the flexor profundus. In this passage, posterior to the flexor profundus, the halves cross each other. Each lateral half of the flexor sublimis, which changed from an anterior position to a lateral and then a posterior after crossing, lies in contact with the flexor profundus on its opposite side. Thus, one half of the flexor superficialis that before the penetration of the flexor profundus was, let us say for illustration, on the radial side of the flexor profundus will change its surface in contact with the profundus tendon to a posterior and then an ulnar position, producing a complete twist.

Only about half of the fibers of each half of the superficialis tendon cross posteriorly to the

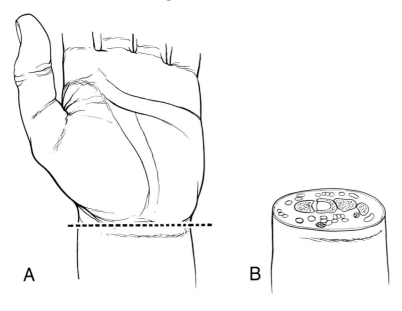

A

B

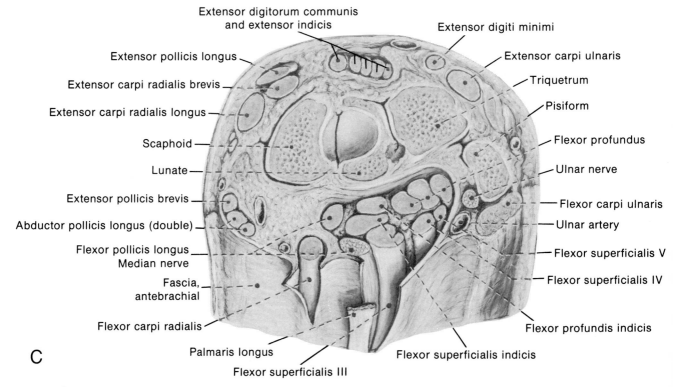

Extensor digitorum communis
and extensor indicis

Extensor digiti minimi

Extensor pollicis longus

Extensor carpi ulnaris

Extensor carpi radialis brevis

Triquetrum

Extensor carpi radialis longus

Pisiform

Scaphoid

Flexor profundus

Lunate

Ulnar nerve

Extensor pollicis brevis

Flexor carpi ulnaris

Abductor pollicis longus (double)

Ulnar artery

Flexor pollicis longus
Median nerve

Flexor superficialis V

Fascia,
antebrachial

Flexor superficialis IV

Flexor carpi radialis

Flexor profundis indicis

C

Palmaris longus

Flexor superficialis indicis

Flexor superficialis III

FIG. 2–31 **A** and **B**, Transverse section through the left wrist to demonstrate the relationship of tendons and bones at the wrist joint. The proximal segment was dissected, the volar skin was removed, and the palmaris longus tendon was freed from its sheath. The antebrachial fascia that encloses the median nerve and the flexor tendons and the proximal part of the carpal tunnel was opened longitudinally. The separate tunnel for the flexor carpi radialis was partially opened. Separate from the carpal tunnel, between the flexor carpi ulnaris and the transverse carpal ligament, a separate tunnel for the ulnar artery and nerve is found. It is known in the French nomenclature as the *tunnel of Guyon*.

flexor profundus; the other half continue on the same side of the tendon and insert into the lateral crest of the volar surface of the middle phalanx where they unite intimately with the crossed fibers of the other side as far distal as the neck of the proximal phalanx. Over the proximal phalanx the posterior crossing of the superficialis tendon forms a plate that can be separated from the periosteum of the phalanx and lifted up until stopped by the insertion of the ends of the superficialis tendon into the volar crests of the middle phalanx (Figs. 2–32 to 2–34).

The opening of the superficialis tendon serves as a tunnel for the passage of the flexor profundus tendon on its proximal half over the proximal phalanx. The distal half of the opening is narrowed by the passage of a constant mesotendon from the floor of the flexor tendons sheath, or rather periosteum, to the tendon of the flexor profundus. Vincula tendinum firmly connect the slips of the bifurcation of the flexor superficialis with the floor of the tunnel. Some of these vincula are slender and long; some of them are very much broader (Fig. 2–33).

The Chiasma Tendinum of Camper. The fibers of the flexor superficialis, which are noted distal to the perforation, form a pattern so similar to the chiasma opticum that it was called *chiasma tendinum* by Peter Camper, who described it and illustrated it in his *Demonstrationum Anatomico-Pathologicarum*, published in 1760 (Fig. 2–35). It is curious to note that a similar and very beautiful illustration of the chiasma was given by Bernard Siegfried Albinus in his *Historia, Musculorum Hominis* in 1774, but this intersection was not called chiasma tendinum. Camper was probably the first to call it chiasma tendinum, but he refers to the description of this structure by Albinus. Albinus gives the following names to the different parts of this apparatus: *tendo sublimis truncatus,* for the undivided sublimis tendon; *caudae duae, in quas sublimis tendo se findit,* for the division of the tendon in two parts; *pars quam emittunt, quaque cohaerent inter se,* the underlying decussation under the tendon profundus; *extrema caudarum ultra*

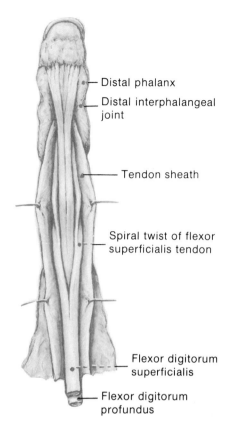

Distal phalanx

Distal interphalangeal joint

Tendon sheath

Spiral twist of flexor superficialis tendon

Flexor digitorum superficialis

Flexor digitorum profundus

FIG. 2–32 The flexor tendon tunnel is opened to show the flexor superficialis and the flexor profundus tendons *in situ.* Note division of the flexor profundus into two flat tendons as it crosses the distal interphalangeal volar plate to insert on the distal phalanx. Perforation of the flexor superficialis and the twist of the lateral slips of insertion of the superficialis are demonstrated.

partem illam, qua cohaerent inter se, the distal end of the decussation; *pars illa qua adjacentem tendineum Profundi contidunt,* the adjacent lateral divisions of the sublimis in contact with the tendon of the profundus; and *ultima caudarum extrema, inserta ossi secunda,* the insertion of the sublimis into the middle phalanx.

The division of the sublimis tendon into these component parts is seldom described and may be of importance in helping to overcome failures in tendon surgery in the regions of the finger also so aptly called "no-man's land."

(Text continues on page 64.)

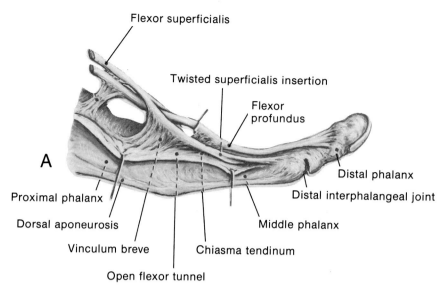

A

Flexor superficialis
Twisted superficialis insertion
Flexor profundus
Distal phalanx
Distal interphalangeal joint
Middle phalanx
Chiasma tendinum
Proximal phalanx
Dorsal aponeurosis
Vinculum breve
Open flexor tunnel

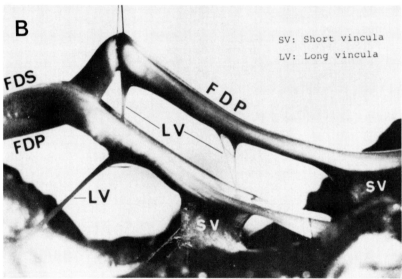

B

SV: Short vincula
LV: Long vincula

FDS
FDP
FDP
LV
LV
SV
SV

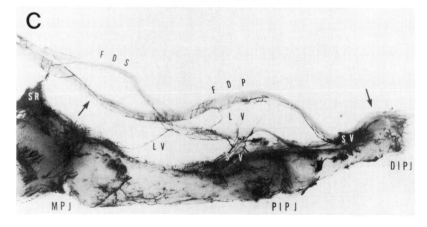

C

FDS
FDP
SR
LV
LV
SV
SV
MPJ
PIPJ
DIPJ

◀ **FIG. 2–33 A,** Details of insertion of the flexor superficialis and the profundus tendons into the phalanges of a finger. The flexor tendon tunnel is completely open. The joint line of the distal interphalangeal joint is indicated. The perforation of the flexor superficialis by the profundus over the proximal phalanx lets the tendon of the flexor profundus pass through. The twist of the slips of the insertion of the flexor superficialis is indicated. The vincula tendinum are firmly connected with the bifurcation of the flexor superficialis at the floor of the tunnel. Another vinculum connects the flexor profundus with the floor. The insertion of the tendon of the flexor profundus into the distal phalanx occurs not only into the volar base but extends beyond the base and into the fat pad of the distal phalanx. **B,** The lateral view of the flexor digitorum profundus and the flexor digitorum superficialis. The typical anatomy of the long and short vincula is seen. **C,** Vascular supply to vinculum and tendon. Injection-prepared specimen (Matsui). Arrows show crossover zones of the intrinsic blood of the flexor digitorum profundus.

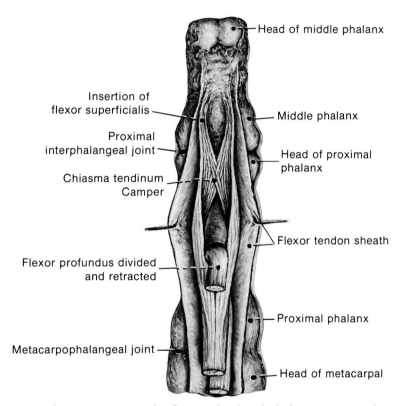

Head of middle phalanx

Insertion of flexor superficialis

Middle phalanx

Proximal interphalangeal joint

Head of proximal phalanx

Chiasma tendinum Camper

Flexor tendon sheath

Flexor profundus divided and retracted

Proximal phalanx

Metacarpophalangeal joint

Head of metacarpal

FIG. 2–34 Flexor apparatus of a finger. The distal phalanx is removed, together with the distal part of the flexor profundus. The proximal part of the flexor profundus is retracted proximally. The perforation of the flexor superficialis tendon by the tendon of the flexor profundus occurs over the volar surface of the proximal phalanx. The two lateral slips of the flexor sublimis tendon rotate completely. Part of those fibers cross to the other side of the phalanx and continue into the middle phalanx where they insert into the lateral volar crest of the middle phalanx. The other part of the rotated slip continues on the same side and inserts on the corresponding side of the phalanx into the crest of the middle phalanx. The intersection of fibers, which is similar to the intersection of the neurofibers of the chiasma opticum of the second cranial nerve, is called the *chiasma tendinum of Camper.* The chiasma tendinum forms a plate underneath the flexor profundus and can be lifted off the periosteum and the capsule of the proximal interphalangeal joint. The distal ends of the slips of the flexor superficialis usually stop a few millimeters proximal to the neck of the middle phalanx.

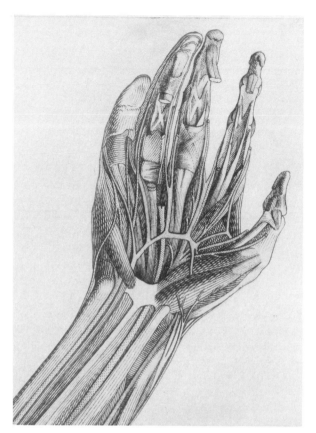

FIG. 2–35 Demonstration of the chiasma tendinum of Camper. (From Camper P: Demonstrationum Anatomico-Pathologicarum, Liber Primus, Continens Brachii Humani Fabricam et Morbos, 1760)

Albinus' nomenclature is quoted to show how precise and detailed were the anatomic descriptions of the anatomists of this period.

Considerable independent motion is possible between the flexor superficialis and the flexor profundus. The perforation of the superficialis serves the purpose of a most efficient pulley. The vincula normally permit sufficient motion; however, the vincula may restrict motion even in the absence of adhesions between the tendons of the superficialis and profundus, especially if fibrosis occurs in the vincula between the distal

part of the perforation and the profundus tendon.

After emerging from the sublimis tendon, the distal end of the profundus tendon spreads out over the distal interphalangeal joint, occupying a wide line over the area of insertion into the distal phalanx. Frequently, the tendon is divided into two divergent bands with a longitudinal separation between them. The division of the flexor profundus tendon frequently begins just distal to the passage of the tendon through the perforation in the sublimis and is maintained until insertion takes place into the distal phalanx. The area of insertion does not stop at the base itself, but extends more distally for about one third of the phalangeal height. The tendon is intimately connected with the capsule of the distal interphalangeal joint.

It may be of interest to note that exactly the same disposition of the flexor profundus tendons was observed in the hands of the gorilla and the chimpanzee, which the author had occasion to dissect. The insertion of the profundus, the chiasma tendinum, and the splitting of the superficialis tendon were exactly similar (Fig. 1–3).

The comparison of the human hand with the skeletons of hands of the gorilla and the chimpanzee shows great similarity in the configuration of the phalanges (Fig. 1–2). The other bones show differences that cannot be considered too great. The general pattern of these hands is amazingly similar. The difference can be detected mostly in the enormous size of the pisiform bone, which is much more elongated and massive than is the human pisiform. The configurations of the navicular bones are somewhat different; however, the triquetral bones of the gorilla and the human are very similar. It is obvious that similar bones are usually connected with a similarity of muscles that take origin from these bones. That fact is observed in the arrangement and in the variation of the muscles with some eliminated and some added, as seen in the human hand.

Anatomy of Flexor Tendons— Pulley, Vincular, Synovia, and Vascular Structures

James M. Hunter

THE RETINACULAR AND SHEATH SYSTEMS

Advances in reconstructive hand surgery emphasize improved functional results and refinements of old and new techniques in tendon surgery. The sheath or digital theca should be studied in minute detail because the vascular and synovial fluid concepts of tendon nutrition cannot be understood without understanding the reinforcing ligamentous systems that produce order and efficiency for tendon gliding.

THE RETINACULAR SYSTEM

The retinacular system of the digit is a series of connecting reinforcing fibers lined by a thin layer of synovium. Its function is to hold the flexor tendons close to the bone and the volar joint plate surfaces, thereby producing the maximum mechanical advantage for joint flexion. Retinacula also function as pulleys in other locations in the body. For example, the illustration of Andreas Vesalius in his *De Humane Corporis Fabrica 1543*, Figure 2–36, shows the bowstringing effect of the extensor hallucis longus when the ankle retinaculum is absent. Forces act to extend the ankle joint rather than the great toe. Clinically, by preservation and reconstruction of pulley retinaculum systems is critical to maximim restoration of digital function.

Each digit has five annular ligaments (Fig. 2–37): A_2 and A_4 arise exclusively from bone and are broad and rigidly fixed to the outer volar edge of the proximal and middle phalanx; A_1, A_3, and A_5 arise from bone and volar joint plate. These ligaments adjust with movement, holding the flexor tendon close to the joint. They are narrower than are A_2 and A_4. A_1 is a thick pulley, but A_3 and A_5 often are thin with filmy, circumferential fibers. The three cruciform pulleys C_1, C_2, and C_3 serve as reinforcing extensions of the annular pulleys along with a C_0 or variable fiber between A_1 and A_2. The cruciates prevent herniation of the sheath during extension and flexion of the finger. C_1 is the most discrete and well formed. Figure 2–37A shows the crossing fibers beyond A_2; C_2 at times seems absent, but in these instances it is probably incorporated into the proximal tapered rim of A_4. The annulae and cruciates are best observed in the index and middle fingers, because they are designed to withstand hard gripping forces. This system is less distinct and more variable in the ring and little fingers.

The retinacular system of the finger is supported by two other biomechanical designs. The first is an additional retinacular system proximal to the A_1 pulley at the metacarpophalangeal joint. The A_1 pulley forces are in part relieved by a preannulus, a complex made up of the peritendinous band of the palmar aponeurosis (Figs. 2–11 and 2–13) connected to the deep transverse metacarpal ligaments. The preannulus system of the palm leads the flexor tendon directly to A_1. If A_1 has been divided (*i.e.*, in the surgical treatment of trigger finger), this preretinalculum may represent an important factor in preventing mechanical bowing and lateral drift of the flexor tendon.

The second support system to the retinaculum of the finger is the flexor digitorum superficialis. Before its penetration by the profundus, the tension of the superficialis acts as a buttress against the profundus tendon and pro-

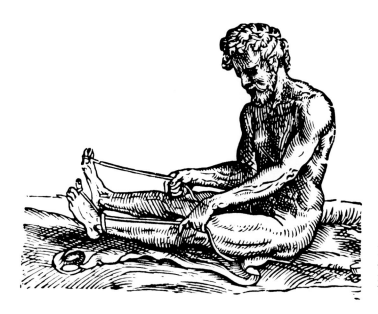

FIG. 2–36 Bowstringing effect of the extensor hallucis longus when the ankle retinaculum is absent. (From Andreas Vesalius: De Humane Corporis Fabrica, 1543)

FIG. 2–37 **A** and **B**, Pulley system of the digit.

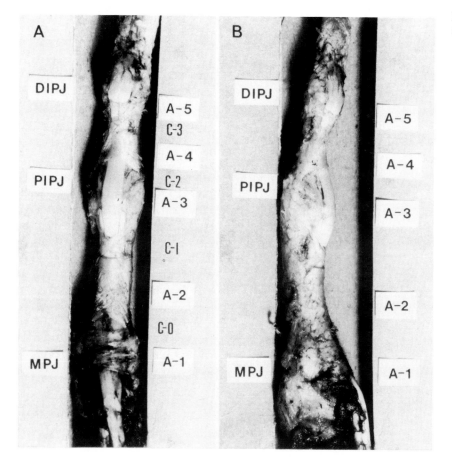

duces a more even distribution of force against the A_2 retinaculum; however, this double tendon system, beautifully arranged for good mechanics, appears to be poorly arranged from the nutritional standpoint. Some typical problems observed at this location will be discussed further under Intrinsic Vascularization.

The fibrous sheath system at the proximal interphalangeal joint level deserves special consideration. A well-formed C_1 system can be studied in the middle finger (Figure 2–37A). The oblique fibers of C_1 may be single in lateral fingers and thin and filmy in the little finger. Consistently, however, they are part of a fibrous pulley system at the proximal interphalangeal joint that adjusts during flexion and extension of the finger. This system includes C_1, A_3, and C_2. The oblique fibers of C_1 anchor to the bone at the distal edge of A_2; crossing obliquely over the flexor tendons, the fibers course into the capsular ligamentous complex of the volar lateral surface of the joint (Figs. 2–38A and B). A_3 is the center of the sling, and as the fibers leave their lateral location they cross obliquely proximal to the distal edge and over the flexor tendon again to anchor into bone at the proximal edge of A_4. The lateral retinacular ligament, described by Landsmere, seems to blend with the retinacular sling fibers at the proximal interphalangeal joint apex. Assuming that in the clinical situation all annulars are found intact, a loss of C_1 and C_2 represents only a small change in flexion efficiency.

However, following an injury where major pulley reconstruction is required, the proximal interphalangeal joint flexor retinacular sling offers a functional model worthy of careful study. Figure 2–38C shows the A_2, C_1, A_3, and C_2 complex in relief. The tissues are edematous and thickened owing to chronic synovitis from a rupture of the flexor digitorum profundus tendon 4 months earlier. The thin sheath has been excised at the edges of the retinaculum to outline the shrouds of the proximal interphalangeal sling system. The importance of effective pulley control at the proximal interphalangeal joint has been emphasized by laboratory studies indicat-

ing that the proximal interphalangeal joint has the largest vertical arc of motion of all finger joints and is the most important joint in bringing the finger in contact with the distal palmar crease.

FINGER RETINACULUM LABORATORY STUDY

A laboratory pulley experiment further emphasizes the significance of the normal retinacular digital system and the importance of placement of reconstructed pulleys at key biomechanical locations. In this experiment with fresh cadaver fingers, the metacarpal is secured with screws to a work board. The flexor and extensor tendons are given equal tension with wire sutures, and all excursions remain constant. In Figure 2–39A, the retinacular system of the middle finger is normal and undisturbed; a full range of motion is seen at the proximal interphalangeal and distal interphalangeal joints, and the palm and fingertips touch. In Figure 2–39B all pulleys have been removed except for A_2 over the proximal phalanx; the proximal interphalangeal flexion arc is significantly reduced, and nearly all of the distal interphalangeal joint flexion is lost. In Figure 2–39C, all pulleys are removed; the prepucial fold and the vincula restrain the tendon, producing proximal interphalangeal flexion; however, metacarpophalangeal motion is reduced and distal interphalangeal motion is totally absent.

For comparison, a nearly perfect pulley reconstruction is accomplished using copper wire. This is not possible in clinical practice, but it is applicable to this study. Three key sites of pulley placement produce full proximal interphalangeal joint motion, a more than normal flexion of the metacarpophalangeal joint, and nearly full flexion of the distal interphalangeal joint. This combination permits a complete closure of the fingertip to the palm (Fig. 2–39D). Finally, to emphasize the importance of controlled proximal interphalangeal joint flexion, the copper wire placement is shifted from the A_3 position at the apex of the proximal interphalangeal joint to the proximal

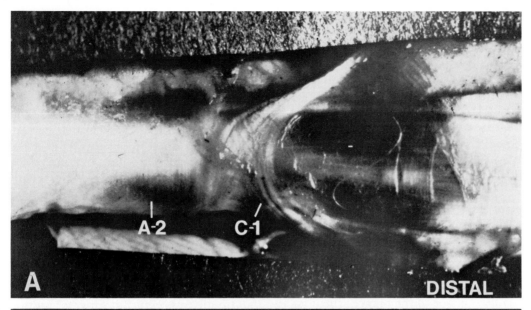

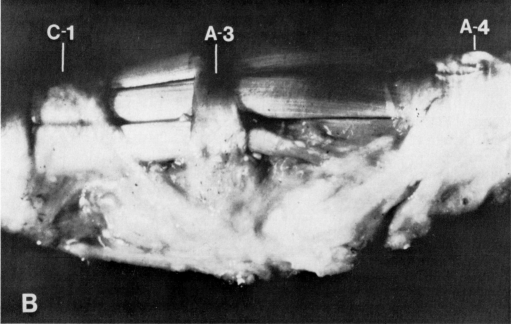

FIG. 2–38   Pulley system at the proximal interphalangeal level. Note the A$_2$, C$_1$, A$_3$, and C$_2$ components of the sheath system. **A** and **B**, Dissection specimens; **C**, from an operative case of a 4-month-old flexor digitorum profundus rupture. ▶

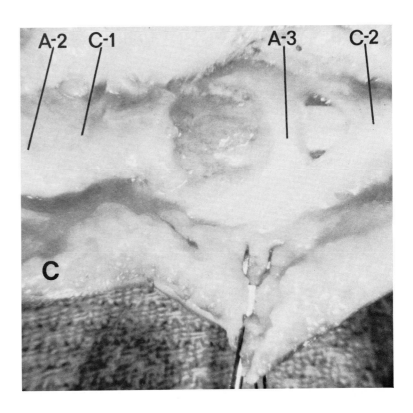

A₄ position just distal to the proximal interphalangeal joint (Fig. 2–39E). The proximal interphalangeal joint motion arc increases, but the metacarpophalangeal joint and distal interphalangeal joint ranges of motion are reduced.

The results, as shown in Figures 2–39D and 2–39E, can be applied to the clinical practice of pulley reconstruction. Under constant excursion of the tendon, if a pulley is reconstructed near a particular joint, there is essentially no gain in flexion exhibited at that joint. Instead, and most important, the other two joints gain significantly owing to their increased relative mechanical advantage. Hence, adding a pulley near or over the proximal interphalangeal joint will increase flexion at both the distal interphalangeal and metacarpophalangeal joints. One would presume that the annular pulley system is functionally exact, but in fact it is not because every factor means something to total function. For

example, when the cruciate retinacula are removed, or when a two-tendon system is replaced by one tendon as in a tendon grafting procedure, slack develops in the gliding tendon system and total function is reduced.

To emphasize this point in the laboratory, we performed an experiment to reconstruct a five-pulley system of over 100% efficiency. Reconstruction of a pulley at the head of the metacarpal rather than proximal to the head of the metacarpal brought the tendon closer to the metacarpophalangeal joint than it would naturally be. Almost all of the increases in efficiency—2% at the metacarpophalangeal joint, 5% at the proximal interphalangeal joint, 21% at the distal interphalangeal joint—occurred at the two distal joints. This principle of overworking one joint to gain at the other two could be helpful in improving hand rehabilitation after tendon reconstructive surgery.

(Text continues on page 72.)

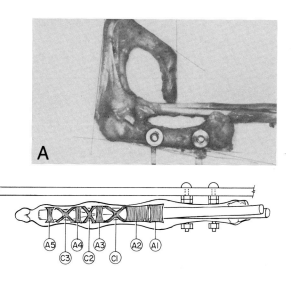

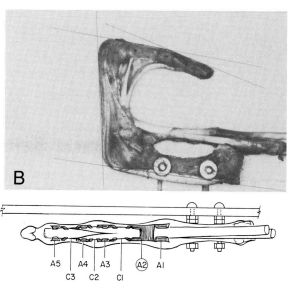

FIG. 2–39 An anatomic experiment of the relationship of pulley system injury and its effect on flexion of the digit. **A**, Normal retinacular system; note full range of motion. **B**, All pulleys removed except for A_2. There is significant reduction of proximal interphalangeal motion and nearly all distal interphalangeal motion. **C**, All pulleys are released; there is reduced flexion of the proximal interphalangeal through the intact vinculum. Metacarpophalangeal joint motion is also reduced significantly; distal interphalangeal joint motion is absent. **D**, Three sites of pulley reconstruction demonstrate nearly complete flexion arc of the digit. **E**, Leaving no pulley near or over the proximal interphalangeal joint results in decreased flexion at the distal interphalangeal joint. ▶

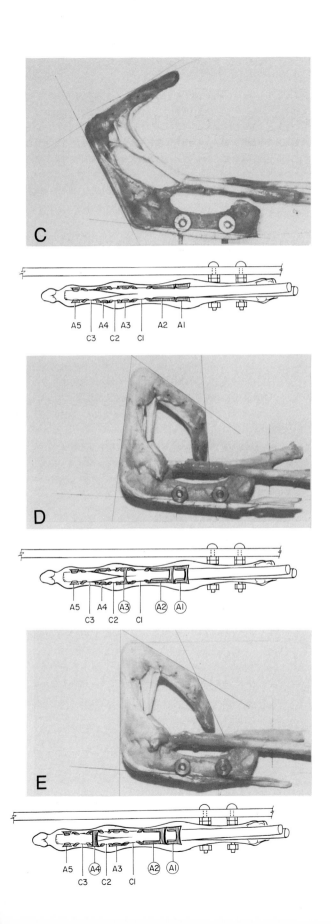

C

A5　A4　A3　　A2　A1
　C3　C2　　C1

D

A5　A4　(A3)　(A2)　(A1)
　C3　C2　　C1

E

A5　(A4)　A3　　(A2)　(A1)
　C3　C2　　C1

THE DIGITAL SHEATH

The digital synovial sheaths are contained in the tunnel of the flexor tendons. Under the slightest pressure, the synovial sheaths distend in places where they are not compressed and become bulbous; they very seldom present the cylindrical, regular appearance seen in anatomic illustrations. Inside the digital sheaths, the tendons are not attached by a continuous mesotendon to the synovial wall; instead, there are separate synovial bands, the vincula tendinum brevia and longa. There are usually two types of vinculum brevia. One vinculum is found at the insertion of the flexor profundus tendon into the distal phalanx. It is triangular and unites the dorsal surface of the tendon with the synovial wall. The other short vinculum is quadrilateral and runs between the synovial wall of the proximal phalanx and the two tendons. The long vinculum is represented also by two types. One group unites the two tendons near the midline; the other group unites the superficialis tendon with the periphery of the synovial wall (Figs. 2–8 and 2–33).

Each tendon has its own separate synovial investment. The vincula carry blood vessels and nerves, which probably run in the walls of the small arteries. The radial synovial bursa has a wide, interrupted synovial fold that connects the tendon in the thumb with the synovial wall. The blood and nerve supply of the ulnar synovial sac is provided through the interspaces on the radial, extrasynovial side of the sac. The synovial membrane between the tendons and the walls of the osteofibrous tunnels and the wall of the sac has several folds that permit free motion of the tendons. In addition to all the synovial sacs on the volar surface, another small sac covers the tendon of the flexor carpi radialis in its passage under the crest of the multangulum major. This synovial covering extends for 1.5 cm to 2 cm between the scaphotrapezial and trapezio-metacarpal joints of the thumb. The synovial sheaths of the flexor tendons and their extensions are discussed with the synovial sheaths of the hand (Figs. 2–41 and 2–43). Studies of intrinsic vascularization have augmented our knowledge of the digital sheaths.

When the digital fibrous tendon sheath is viewed from the dorsal aspect (*i.e.*, the side where it is contiguous to the tendon), the pulley is lifted so that the annular and cruciate portions can be clearly seen (Fig. 2–40*A*). This is an un-

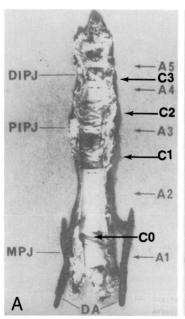
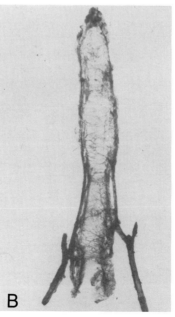

FIG. 2–40   A, The digital fibrous tendon sheath viewed from its dorsal aspect. **B**, The tendon sheath receives its blood supply from the proper digital artery by multiple fine blood vessels.

usual view of the retinacular system of the finger, and the anatomy is particularly clear, in this middle finger presentation. Note A_5, C_0 (variable fiber) between A_1 and A_2, and C_1, C_2, and C_3. Of special interest is the grooved impression that runs longitudinally against the five retinacula of the digit. The smooth grooving of the under or dorsal side of the flexor retinaculum corresponds to the close tolerance of the flexor tendon system and part of the synovial fluid propulsion plan, which keeps the tendon collagen moistened and soft for pressure gliding. The course of the proper digital artery is closely related to the tendon sheath (Fig. 2–40B) and the retinacula and outer sheath receives its nutrition from multiple fine blood vessels that layer off the digital arteries as they pass from proximal to distal.

The interior of the sheath is lined by synovium. Fine arteries enter the synovium separately from the digital arteries. The deep synovium and the floor of the sheath receive arteries from the four transverse communicating arteries. The vincula carry the synovium to the dorsum of the flexor tendons with arteries from the transverse communicating arteries (Fig. 2–41).

THE PARATENON SYSTEM (PALM)

The flexor superficialis and profundus tendons, from their musculotendinous origin to the level of the proximal portion of the flexor digital sheath, have a uniform intratendinous vascular pattern. This was described in 1975 by Caplan, Hunter, and Merklin in the *Symposium on Tendon Surgery*. Edwards, Brockis, and Smith have also confirmed these observations. The basic unit of tendon vascularization, the fascicle, consists of collagen bundles and their investing connective tissue, the endotenon. Within the interfascicular connective tissue, in a uniform cross-sectional distribution, is found the basic vascular unit—a single arteriole and one or two venules. This system is oriented longitudinally, paralleling the longitudinal course of the tendon fascicles; however, there are frequent cross connections between the intratendinous vessels and

between the segmental vessels of the surrounding paratenon. This system ends at the point where the palmar vessel branches on the volar surface of the flexor digitorum superficialis (FDS) and profundus (FDP) tendons with their investing mesotenon become intratendinous, forming the prepucial fold (Mayer). Anatomically, this occurs at the base of the proximal phalanx under the proximal A_1 retinaculum.

VASCULAR ANATOMY OF FLEXOR TENDONS

The vascularization of flexor tendons has come under considerable scrutiny in recent years because of advances in hand surgery and the need for more predictable results after tendon repair and reconstructive surgery. Successful procedures are now performed that were, in the past, considered theoretical or technically questionable: surgeons now routinely perform tenorrhaphy of flexor tendons in "no-man's land," the palm, and the forearm, as well as reconstructive procedures such as grafting of tendons in one and two stages, implantation of tendon prostheses, complex pulley reconstruction, and replantation of digits in hands by microsurgical techniques. These advances have provoked investigation about how the flexor tendon system derives basic nutrition and how its nutritional state changes with injury and repair. Detailed investigation of the intrinsic microcirculation of the human flexor tendons is of utmost importance because the healing of vascularized tissues is governed by its blood supply.

Leo Mayer pointed out the segmental sources of the extrinsic vasculature: musculotendinous junction as a continuation of the perimyseal vessels, paratenon vessels, plical and vincular vessels (mesotenon) in sheathed areas, and tendinosseous junction as a continuation of the periosteal vessels. Mayer stated that within the tendon "vessels travel in the hilum of the tendon, in the epitenon, and in the connective tissue septa between the tendon bundles (the endotenon)" and that these vessels "anastomose freely by transverse and oblique branches." Ed-

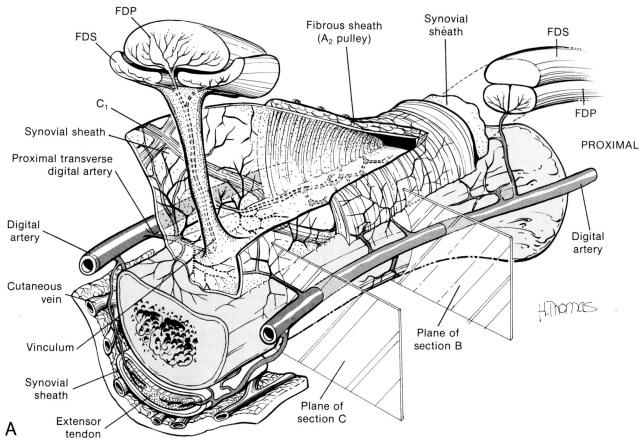

FIG. 2–41   A, Diagrammatic three-dimensional representation of the central communicating arterial system of the finger at the proximal interphalangeal level. Note the proximal transverse artery supplying the flexor tendons, flexor sheath, and the synovial bed of the tendons. **B**, Cross-section at the level of the A_2 pulley; the flexor tendon is segmental through the vincula. The retinaculum has a separate blood supply from the digital artery. **C**, Cross-section at the C_1 level. The synovial sheath blood supply is supplied by the transverse digital artery to the vinculum.

wards further defined the intrinsic pattern as simple and uniform throughout the tendon. Each tendon fascicle is surrounded by endotenon carrying a series of longitudinally oriented vascular bundles (an arteriole and two larger venules). These vessels are fed from surface vessels by transversely oriented vessels of the same size that thread their way around and between the fascicles and link the longitudinal system into a uniform plexus. All vessels and capillary loops are interfascicular, and none penetrate into the collagen bundles.

Brockis and Smith confirmed this interfascicular pattern in human flexor tendons and made an additional observation peculiar to the flexor digitorum profundus in the area of the proximal and distal interphalangeal joints. At these points, the longitudinal system is "upset by an artistic grouping of peculiar vertical loops originating from the dorsal channel or the vincula longae and breve." Peacock showed that in dogs the longitudinal circulation through intrinsic vessels was nonexistent for distances greater than one third the length of isolated tendons.

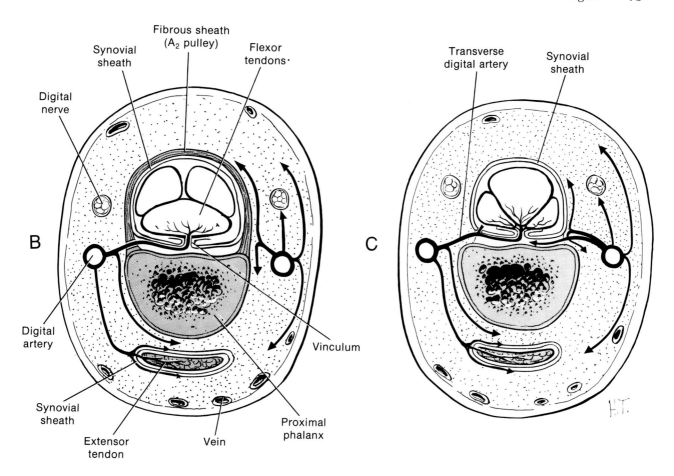

Young and Weeks, studying monkeys, concluded that within the digital sheath the flexor digitorum profundus at the proximal end of the sheath was less well perfused than distally; the distal portion of the flexor digitorum profundus was perfused by the vinculum breve; the proximal portion was perfused by the palmar vessels; and the vinculum longa alone could not maintain normal levels of perfusion.

Clearly, there has been a continuing effort to study the vascularity of flexor tendons and to relate this knowledge to a better understanding of the reaction of flexor tendon tissues to injury in the processes of healing. The sections that follow augment the work of these authors and should broaden our base of thought for further study of this fascinating subject.

BLOOD SUPPLY TO THE FLEXOR TENDON SUPERFICIALIS AND PROFUNDUS MUSCLE

The blood supply to the flexor superficialis and the profundus was studied in detail by Salmon and Dor. These studies disclosed that the arterial circulation of the muscular body of the superficialis is assured by the artery of the median nerve, by a large artery branch of the ulnar for the epicondylar muscles, and by the branches of the ulnar artery supplying the medial segment of the belly. The radial artery supplies a narrow strip of the muscle on the lateral side of the muscular body. The flexor profundus is supplied principally by the ulnar artery, by the anterior interosseous, or by a branch from the common trunk of the interossei. The artery accompanies the muscular branch of the median nerve, which supplies this muscle. The artery of the epicondylar muscles supplies a great part of the proximal belly of the muscle. Important anastomoses are established between the arteries in the substance of the flexor superficialis and separately in the substance of the profundus. The authors considered the possibility of arterial territorial divisions with the blood supply deriving from definite arteries for specific muscular bundles for the index, middle, ring, and little fingers.

A number of important investigations on the blood supply of the tendons appeared in recent years in the American and foreign literatures. In connection with the blood supply of the tendinous parts of the flexors, it is necessary to repeat and emphasize the description of the blood vessels found in the region of the phalanges and the interphalangeal and metacarpophalangeal joints. The blood supply to the tendons is derived from the peritendinous vascular network (Potenza, Gambier, Asvazadurian, Venturini Mittelmeier), and apparently there is no significant difference between the extensor and flexor tendons. The investigations were carried out mostly in relation to tendon healing in various animals; however, observations in tendons in various periods of healing in the human hand showed patterns identical to those seen in animals in the forearm and arm.

BLOOD SUPPLY TO FLEXOR TENDONS IN THE FINGERS

More than 60 upper extremities (from fresh cadavers or traumatically amputated specimens) were used, with ages ranging from 11 to 88 years. After the vascular system was flushed with physiological saline solution, each specimen was injected with diluted India ink-latex solution through both radial and ulnar arteries by means of hand syringes and manual pressure, until clean fluid exited from the venous system. The injection was a five- to ten-fold dilution with physiological saline solution of a 2:1 mixture of an amorphous carbon suspension. The carbon particles were in an alkaline suspension and were less than $0.1\ \mu$ in diameter (the diameter of

a red blood cell is $7.5\ \mu$). By maintaining alkaline solutions of latex, clumping of carbon particles was not a problem. A concern about small carbon particles passing through the blood vessels or capillary walls did not materialize in our specimens; neither did we observe any interaction between the injected material and the vessel wall.

The specimens were fixed with 10% formalin. After dissection, they were dehydrated with methyl alcohol and placed in a solution of tricresyl phosphate and tributyl phosphate (11:2) to make them transparent, as described by Caplan and associates.

In some specimens, the tissues were returned to 10% formalin by reversing the steps of the clearing procedure. This was done to reduce the hardness of the tendons, which were then cut into approximately 5-mm sections and returned to the clearing solution. This permitted the study of tendon cross-sections at the various levels of the profundus tendon, so that the location of the intrinsic tendon vessels could be ascertained. Photographs of these cleared specimens were taken by tansillumination.

The normal vascular anatomy of the flexor tendons will be discussed by using the flexor digitorum profundus tendon as a model. The vascular pattern for the superficialis tendon can be observed in the illustrations, and the segmental distribution will be emphasized as well. The paratenon gives a predictable vascular pattern to the flexor tendons in the forearm and palm. The synovial reflection or sheath begins in the distal third of the palm, and it is here that tendon nutrition is affected by a combination of vascular and synovial fluid diffusion. This system seems to be uniquely specific to support the strenuous demands of grip and gliding through a lifetime. The earlier discussions of the synovial sheath emphasized the importance of the retinaculum and the specific fine vascular support given by the digital artery to this portion of the sheath so that synovial fluid can be exchanged and distributed over the tendon surfaces (Fig. 2–41). The second part of the synovium is on the floor of the sheath over the phalanges. Vascular distribution here is also

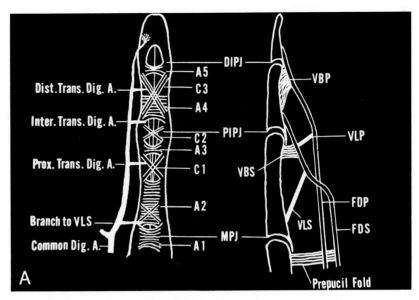

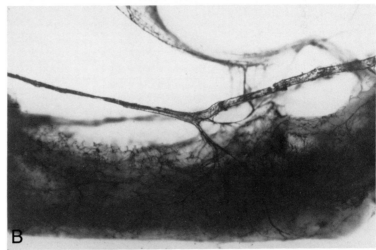

FIG. 2–42 **A**, The vascular supply to the flexor tendons is by four transverse communicating branches of the digital arteries. VLS is vinculum longus superficialis; VBP is vinculum breve profundus; VLP is vinculum longus profundus; VBS is vinculum breve superficialis. **B**, Note the communicating vessels at the proximal interphalangeal level.

arterial, principally through the direct communication of four transverse branches of the digital arteries (Fig. 2–42A). These communicating arteries send branches to bone as nutrient arteries, and to the volar joint capsule, dorsal synovium, and vincula. Figure 2–42B shows the direct communicating arteries at the proximal interphalangeal joint and superficialis short vinculum level. This level is the source of the central segment of the arterial system within the tendon.

The overall view of the intrinsic vascularity of the profundus tendon can best be reviewed in a unique injection study, permitting a composite view of the longitudinal vascular arrangement in cross-section. A fourth-decade specimen was chosen, and the injected finger, after being photographed, was subjected to a chemical softening process that permitted 34 serial cross-sections to be arranged as cleared specimens and stained specimens side by side (Fig. 2–43). This study gives a two-dimensional view of the intrin-

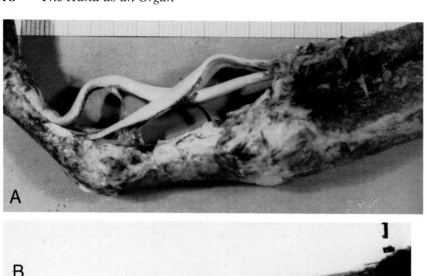

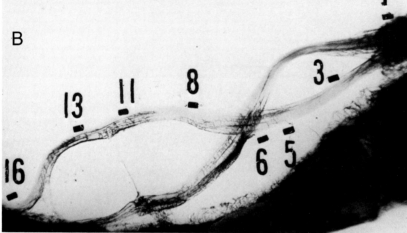

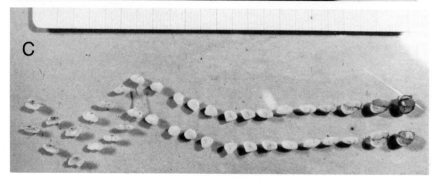

FIG. 2–43 **A,** Injected right long finger of a 42-year-old woman. The dissection of the soft tissues and sheath is completed. This flexor digitorum profundus (FDP) has middle and mixed types of long vinculum. **B,** This is the key illustration for Figures 2-44 through 2-49. This slide has been prepared from 2–43A, after being cleared for translumination photography. Double cross-section (cleared and histologic stain) will be seen at levels 1, 3, 6, 8, 11, and 16. Level 1 is the prepucial fold level; 3, a watershed zone; 6, a mixed VLP connection; 8, between two long vincula; 11, at the VLP distal; 16, at the VPB level. (Note that dark irregular patches may represent artifact of histologic preparation.) The author believes the irregular spaces represent nutrient channels within the tendon substance. Fine fingers of synovium can be seen entering the tendon from the dorsal surface. **C,** Cut into 34 cross-sections (5 mm thick), these will be divided into two groups by adjacent section: 17 cross-sections are clear specimens; 17 cross-sections are histologic specimens stained with hematoxylin and eosin H & E. Slides were studied at various levels of the FDP tendon with a microscope.

sic vascular nutrition of the flexor tendon. The vascularity of the tendon can be studied from the prepucial fold of the palm, where there is arterial venous flow from the paratenon through the changeover to a segmental vascular distribution within the sheath. The quadrants and surfaces of the tendon show clearly that the vascular channels project in a loop fashion over the intertendinous spaces. The dorsolateral quadrants are in surface contact with the synovial surface of the fibro-osseous system. There is a close relationship for fluid flow and diffusion because the shape of the tendon conforms to the shape of the sheath (Fig. 2–46) and the shape of the flexor digitorum profundus conforms to the contour of the split surfaces of the enveloping flexor digitorum superficialis tendon. This study presents a vascular anatomic basis to aid in the evaluation of clinical results after flexor tendon injury and repair.

The longitudinal blood vessels, which are evenly distributed throughout the tendon in the palmar region, are supplied from the synovial reflection at the entrance to the flexor tendon sheath (Fig. 2–44). These longitudinal blood vessels run close to the periphery of the tendon and

FIG. 2–44 **A** and **B**, The proximal end of digital sheath VDP and VDS. The epitenonlike tissue is thick, continuous synovium of the prepucial fold, is layered against the tendon tissue, and is very vascular. (Note that the vessels are located in the intrafascicular connective tissue, not in the tendon fascicles. The vessels are distributed relatively evenly in cross-section.)

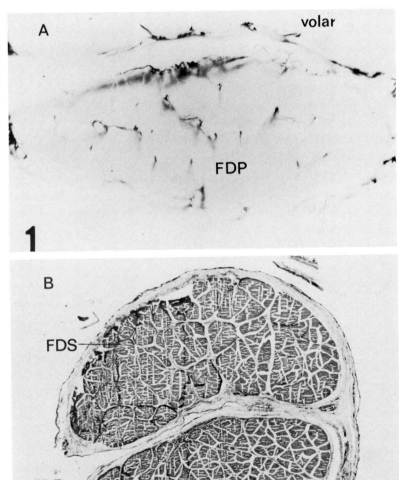

gradually decrease in number until at the proximal phalanx they are situated centrally or on the volar side, and are essentially absent on the dorsal side (Fig. 2–45). Distal to the proximal phalanx down to the attachment of the short vinculum, the tendons are supplied by blood vessels from the long and short vincula. In this area, blood vessels run longitudinally along the dorsal side of the tendon (Fig. 2–46). There are essentially no blood vessels along the volar side. At the proximal phalanx there is a crossover of the intertendinous vessels, with the vessels running longitudinally and decreasing in number forming the distal-end capillary loops (Fig. 2–45). These blood vessels are located centrally or volarly proximal to the crossover and arranged dorsally distal to the proximal phalanx. The blood vessels in the area extending from the beginning of the fibrous tendon sheath of the flexor digitorum profundus tendon to the attachment of the short vinculum represent two distinct systems of blood vessels: a proximal system running from the palm in the periphery and supplied by the synovial reflexion, and a distal digital system originating from the long and short vincula (Figs. 2–44 through 2–49).

At the bony attachment of the flexor digitorum profundus tendon, blood vessels run from the volar epitenon proximally and from the short vinculum distally through the tendon, so that a crossover of these blood vessel systems occurs in the vicinity of the distal interphalangeal joint (Figs. 2–47 and 2–49).

Anastomotic rami connect blood vessel systems that run longitudinally in the intertendinous plane almost parallel with one another.

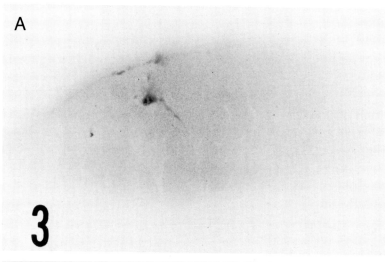

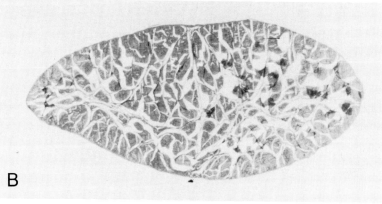

FIG. 2–45 A and **B**, This level is distal to Level 1 and close to the watershed zone. Distribution of vessels is biased to the volar half of the flexor digitorum profundus. At this level, the dorsal half is avascular.

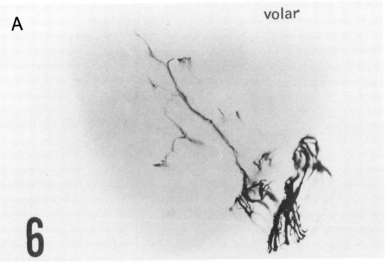

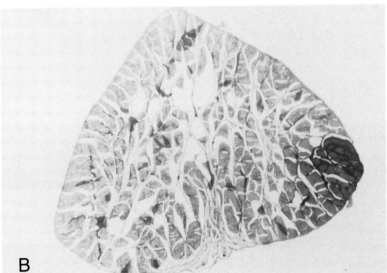

FIG. 2–46 **A** and **B**, This level is distal to the watershed zone and insertion of mixed type of vincula (VLP) dorsally. The intrinsic synovium and blood vessels are located dorsally between two longitudinal halves of the FDP. Triangular shape of the flexor digitorum profundus was due to two slips of the flexor digitorum superficialis compressing the tendon proximal to the chiasm of Camper.

The vascular loopings are seen in the tendon and in its dorsal lateral borders (Fig. 2–50*A*). In the anteroposterior view of the flexor digitorum profundus tendon, large, dorsally located central blood vessels run longitudinally in its midportion (Fig. 2–50*B*). The branches and vascular looping progress laterally from the central dorsal vessel. Throughout the length of the tendon, the volar surfaces generally remain avascular. The distribution of the intrinsic blood vessels in the profundus tendon vary in all the fingers of the same hand, depending on the vincular variation and the age of the individual. Before looking at the vascular changes in each decade of life, the anatomy of the vincular system within the finger should be reviewed with respect to its variations in different fingers.

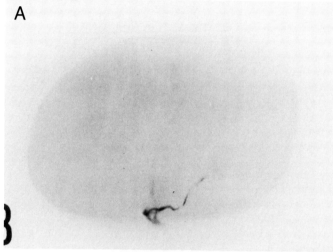

A

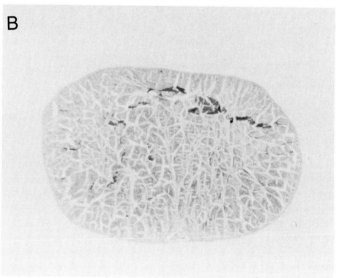

B

FIG. 2–47 **A** and **B**, The zone of decreased vascularity between two types of VLP, the centrally located dorsal synovium and blood supply branches into the substance of the tendon.

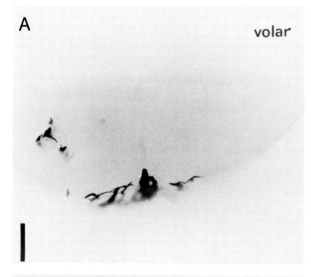

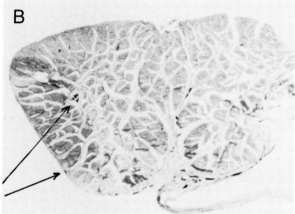

FIG. 2–48 A and **B**, Cross-section at the distal VLP longitudinal synovium; intrinsic vessels are recognized entering the central portion on the dorsal half of the FDP. The volar quadrant is avascular, and dorsally the synovium and vessels extend to the lateral borders of the tendon. Note the capillary looping (*arrow*).

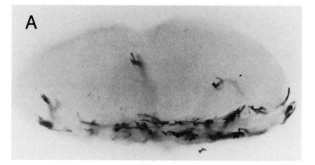

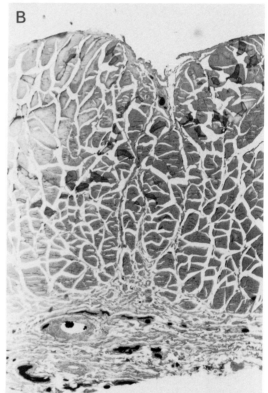

FIG. 2–49 A and **B**, Cross-section at the proximal level of the distal phalanx, VBP dorsal connective tissue of the VBP contains many blood vessels. The vascular bed likely represents arteries and veins at this distal location.

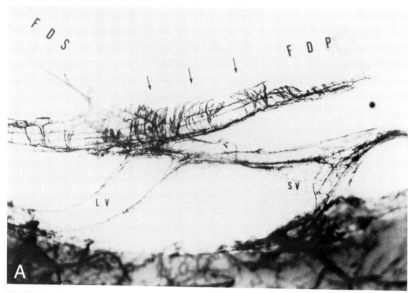

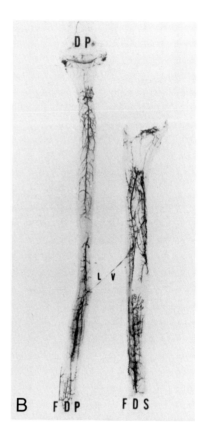

FIG. 2–50 **A,** Vascular loopings are noted in the dorsolateral aspect of the flexor tendon. The blood vessels pass longitudinally in the intertendinous planes. **B,** Anteroposterior view of injected specimen. The FDP tendon has large central blood vessels running longitudinally.

THE VINCULAR SYSTEM IN THE DIGITAL SHEATHS

In the digital canal, both flexor tendons have two kinds of vincula, the short and long vincula, which are folds of the mesotendon. The short vinculum of the superficialis tendon arises from the membranous part of the volar plate of the proximal interphalangeal joint and is attached to the superficialis decussation. This short vinculum contains many arterial vessels, which arise mainly from the proximal transverse digital artery (Figs. 2–42 and 2–52). The short vinculum of the profundus tendon is a thin triangular-shaped mesotendon arising along the distal two-thirds of the middle phalanx. The arterial supply to this vinculum is primarily from both the interphalangeal and distal transverse digital arteries. These two short vincula were consistently found in all dissected fingers (Figs. 2–52, 2–53, and 2–54).

In our study, the long vincula, which have been considered to be the major channels of the segmental blood supply to the flexor tendons in the digital canal, were found to be of various types and to differ from each other in the four fingers studied. Ochiai classified three patterns of distribution of the long vinculum of the superficialis tendon and five of the long vinculum of the profundus tendon.

The long vinculum of the superficialis tendon arises from the transverse communicating artery at the radial or ulnar side of the base of the proximal phalanx and attaches to one of two slips of the superficialis just proximal to the decussation. These two long vincula are classified as the radial and ulnar type respectively. The radial and ulnar types were found in approximately equal distribution in 130 fingers studied. Twenty-five percent of these fingers had both radial and ulnar types. No long vinculum was found in one third of fingers, and was principally absent in the long and ring fingers.

The five types of distribution of the long vinculum to the profundus tendon are designated as the distal, middle, mixed, proximal, and absent. The distal type arose at the level of the insertion of the superficialis tendon and attached to the profundus tendon directly. Its blood supply came mainly from the interphalangeal transverse digital artery. This type was very rare and was found in only five percent of the fingers studied.

The middle type bridged between the profundus and the decussation of the superficialis tendon as the direct continuation of the short vinculum of the superficialis. Its blood supply came from the proximal transverse digital ar-

tery. This type was the most common and was found in approximately 75 percent of the fingers studied (Fig. 2–51A).

The proximal type arose from the synovial membrane between the two slips of the superficialis and attached to the profundus where it passed through the superficialis. Its arterial supply came from the long vinculum of the superficialis tendon (Fig. 2–52).

The mixed type had the same relationship to the two tendons as the proximal type, but in this type there was no long vinculum of the superficialis. Its blood supply came from the short vinculum of the superficialis indirectly through

FIG. 2–51 A 10-hour-old middle finger with middle-type long vinculum to the profundus (VLP). **A,** Large arrow shows crossover in FDP tendon. Three small arrows show avascular volar surface of profundus tendon. **B,** Enlarged details at the metacarpophalangeal joint level. Note the dense arrangement of vessels in the synovial fold level proximal to the proximal joint of the finger. The changeover from volar to dorsal vessel arrangement occurs at the arrow.

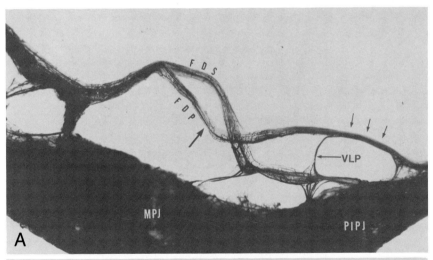

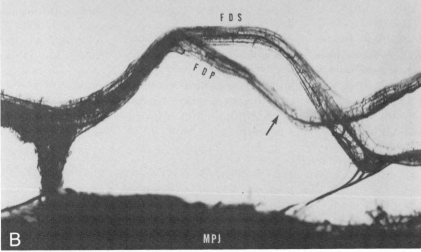

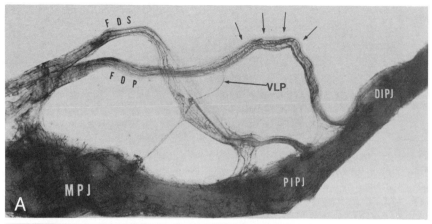

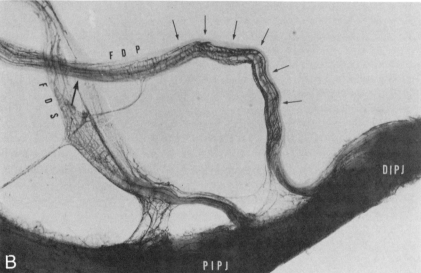

FIG. 2–52 A 26-year-old middle finger with proximal-type long vinculum (VLP) to the profundus. **A**, Small arrows indicate an avascular volar aspect of the profundus tendon. **B**, Large details of A and the vascular arrangement of the chiasm of Camper. The large arrow shows the crossover of longitudinal blood vessels in the profundus tendon.

the synovial membrane between the two slips of the superficialis. This type was found in 20 of the 130 fingers studied. The ring finger presented with this pattern in most instances.

No long vinculum of the profundus was found in six percent of fingers studied, principally in the long and ring fingers. Multiple vincula were occasionally seen, especially in the middle type of the long vinculum of the profundus.

In the index finger, the most common combination was the middle-type long vinculum of the profundus and the radial-type long vinculum of the superficialis. The second most common combination was the middle-type long vinculum of the profundus and both the radial- and ulnar-types long vincula of the superficialis. If one looks only to the long vinculum of the superficialis tendon, the radial type and the combined radial and ulnar types are found most of the time.

In the long finger, a dominant pattern was not found. A combination of the middle-type long vinculum of the profundus and the radial-type long vinculum of the superficialis (Fig. 2–51) or a combination of both middle and proximal types of long vinculum of the profundus and the radial and ulnar type long vincula of the superficialis was found most frequently. Absence of the long vincula of both the profundus and superficialis was noted in 10% of long fingers studied.

In the ring finger, the mixed-type long vinculum to the profundus was found in almost half of the ring fingers studied. In 18 of 30 fingers studied, a long vinculum of the superficialis was not found. The combination of the middle and mixed-type long vinculum of the profundus and the absent-type long vinculum of the superficialis, or a combination of the mixed-type long vinculum of the profundus and the absent-type long vinculum of the superficialis tendon, was the pattern most frequently found.

In the little finger, the combination of the middle-type long vinculum of the profundus and ulnar-type long vinculum of the superficialis was most commonly found. A combination of the middle- and proximal-type long vincula of the profundus and ulnar-type long vinculum of the superficialis, and a combination of the middle-type long vinculum of the profundus and the radial- and ulnar-type long vincula of the superficialis was also observed. In this finger, almost all long vincula of the superficialis originated from the ulnar side of the finger and 70% of the ulnar types of the long vincula consisted of the broad mesotendon, which was fused to the short vinculum of the superficialis.

The special combination of the absent type of both the profundus and superficialis was found in three fingers. However, this combination was not found in either the index or in the little finger.

CLINICAL CORRELATION

The absence of the long vinculum of the superficialis in 36% of long fingers and 60% of ring fingers studied is of particular interest. In the index finger, only three were absent and in the little finger only two were absent. When one looks at the rupture of the distal flexor profundus insertion, one would suspect that there is some correlation between the absence of this vinculum and the fact that some patients also have a total absence of the long vinculum of the flexor digitorum profundus. These vincula are known to act as check ligaments in various respects. The superficialis was mentioned earlier as a reinforcing portion of the pulley system.

Another example of a problem that a clinician could relate to this anatomical data is that of flexion contracture of the fifth finger, a very common congenital anomaly. I have observed that the long vinculum of the superficialis are quite commonly connected on the ulnar side of the fifth finger by a long, broad mesotendinous system. This system can produce a mesotendon type of connection from the middle phalanx across the proximal phalanx into the palm and, at times, through the ulnar bursa system into the distal forearm. Because this is the only finger in which this particular type of broad mesotendinous vinculum occurs, one cannot avoid the probable correlation of this anatomical pattern. The surgeon would do well to keep this in mind when managing this difficult problem in children.

FLEXOR TENDON VASCULAR CHANGE WITH AGE

The results of tendon repair following flexor tendon injury vary. The intrinsic pattern of blood distribution by level in the finger has been shown to be segmental, suggesting that portions of a tendon may be rendered avascular following injury. The volume distribution of intrinsic tendon blood flow varies with age, but the patterns remain essentially the same through the decades of life.

In newborns the intrinsic blood vessels show even distribution and dense arrangements and are well developed in the vincula. A crossover of longitudinally oriented blood vessels occurs at the proximal phalanx level. The volar surface remains essentially avascular between the proximal phalanx and the short vinculum (Fig. 2–51).

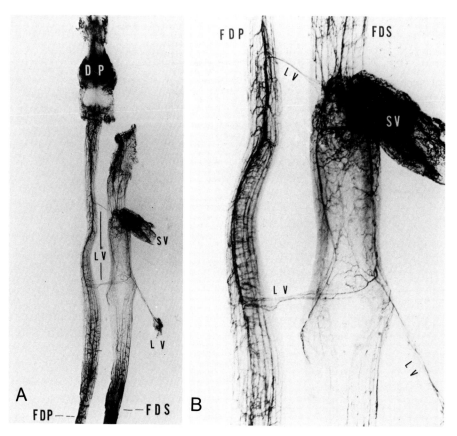

FIG. 2–53 A 21-year-old index finger. **A**, Anteroposterior view of flexor digitorum profundus and superficialis tendons. **B**, Details of tendons at the level of the long and short vincula. DP is distal phalanx; SV is short vincula; LV is long vincula.

These latter features are consistent with blood vessel arrangements in old and young hands. Specifically, in young hands of the second and third decades (Fig. 2–52), the basic arrangement of vessels is seen. From the proximal phalanx to the attachment of the short vinculum, the tendon is rich in blood vessels supplied from the long and short vincula; typically, no volar blood vessels are observed.

In the anteroposterior view of the tendons, large well-developed blood vessels are prominent in the middle of the tendon from the attachment of the short vinculum to a point near the more proximal long vinculum. More proximally, a number of longitudinal blood vessels connect with one another by anastomatic rami (Fig. 2–53). The chiasma tendinum of Camper forms a gliding plate for the flexor profundus. The blood vessels are richly supplied from the anastomosis along the volar surface of the middle phalanx (Fig. 2–53B) between distal and proximal long vincula.

In later decades (as seen in Fig. 2–54; the sixth decade), the longitudinal blood vessels after leaving the synovial reflections in the palm become dorsally located as they enter the fibrous sheath. The vessels diminish in number and at the flexor superficialis bifurcation become almost nonexistent in some cases. Between the bifurcation and the bone insertion, the profundus tendon is supplied by blood vessels from the long vincula through the short vincula of the flexor superficialis (Fig. 2–54). The volar segment of the profundus tendon is essentially

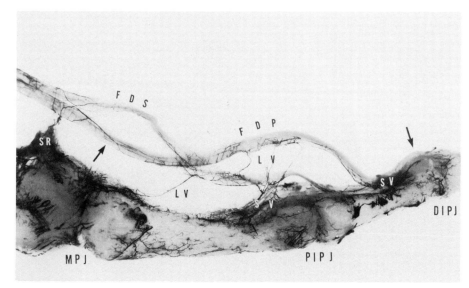

FIG. 2–54 A 52-year-old ring finger. Arrows indicate sites of crossover of intratendinous longitudinal blood vessels of the profundus tendon. (SR is synovial reflection). (From Matsui T, Merklin RJ, Hunter JM: A microvascular study of the human flexor tendons in the digital fibrous sheath. J Jap Orthop Assoc 53: 307–320, 1979)

avascular in the later decades, suggesting a fluid nutritional dependence from the sheath with the gliding dispersion of synovial fluid along the surface of the flexor retinaculum. These anastomatic features of a reduced intrinsic vascular flow in the later decades as compared to a profuse intrinsic vascular flow in the young decades tends to correlate with the clinical observation that the reduced quality and predictability of flexor tendon healing often varies with age.

FLEXOR TENDON VASCULAR CHANGES FOLLOWING INJURY

Movement of the hand is produced by muscle contraction and tendon gliding. In this environment, synovial fluid propulsion and blood flow are arranged to support tendon integrity for function and stress. Following tendon injury, vascular and synovial fluid channels are disturbed, and the biologic response to injury is depressed. As the vascular anatomy of the synovium and tendon within the sheath is segmental, injury at specific levels on the tendon

may be critical to tendon healing. This is emphasized in a fresh-cadaver experiment prepared in our laboratory by Dr. Matsui. Before injection of the vascular system, injury was simulated by a series of delicate operations during which fine copper wires were selectively tied around vinculae or tendons. Specimens were then routinely prepared for transillumination photographic study. From a series of 30 experiments, two hands from the early and late decades of life were selected to correlate injury with anatomic variations and age. The first hand (Fig. 2–55A and B) shows vascular characteristics of the late decades of life. Blood vessels are sparse in the periosteal synovial bed and in the typical dorsal tendon arrangement, suggesting a balance toward synovial fluid nutrition and away from vascular flow nutrition in the tendon. In the second hand (Fig. 2–56A and B) the illustration by comparison shows vascular characteristics of the early decades of life; the blood vessels are profuse in the periosteal synovial bed and the intratendinous connective tissues.

The first hand (Fig. 2–55A and B) is a 54-

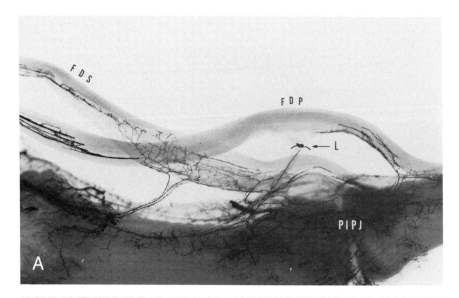

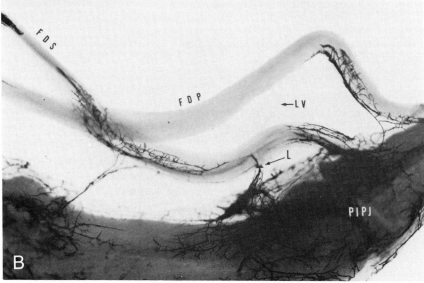

FIG. 2–55 A, Ligation injury (L) in a 54-year-old middle finger to the vinculum longus profundus. Note the avascular segment of the profundus. **B**, Ligation injury (L) in a 54-year-old index finger to a short vinculum superficialis resulted in an extensive injury to the FDP.

year-old specimen. In Fig. 2–55*A*, a middle-finger ligation (L) of the long vinculum profundus produced an avascular segment of the profundus tendon. In Figure 2–55*B*, an index-finger ligation (L) of the short vinculum superficialis resulted in a more extensive avascular segment of the profundus tendon. The long vinculum

profundus is more proximal in this finger and obviously depends on blood flow from the short vinculum superficialis. Segmental blood supply to the more proximal portion of the superficialis tendon is through the presence of the long vinculum superficialis. In other specimens not shown, the tendon of the superficialis was li-

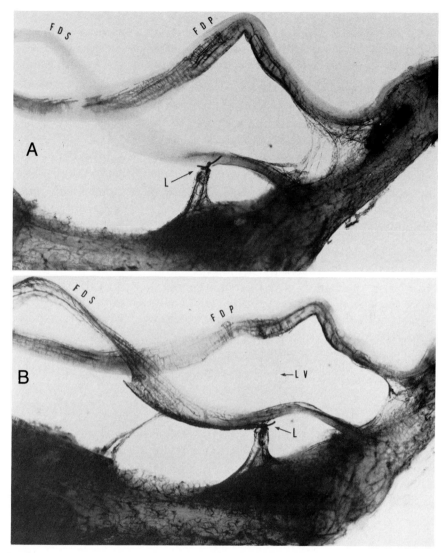

FIG. 2–56 **A**, Ligation (L) of the short vinculum in a 26-year-old middle finger produced an avascular flexor digitorum superficialis. **B**, Ligation (L) in a 26-year-old index finger of the short vinculum failed to produce any abnormality of the flexor digitorum profundus or superficialis despite no flow through the long vinculum (LV).

gated at the level of the chiasm of Camper and the long vinculum superficialis with no effect on the profundus blood flow. In addition to the clinical significance of injury that damages the superficialis synovial bed the clinician is reminded that resection of the superficialis tendon at the level of the short vinculum may seriously compromise vascular flow to the pro-

fundus tendon and initiate scar contracture of the proximal interphalangeal joint.

The second specimen (Fig. 2–56A and B) is 26 years of age, the earlier decade of life. A middle-finger ligation (L) of the short superficialis vinculum rendered the superficialis almost avascular; the long vinculum superficialis and long vinculum profundus were both absent in this instance. In the index finger, by comparison, a complete vascular pattern remains in the superficialis despite ligation (L) injury to the short vinculum. There is no flow through the long vinculum with minimal if any change probably caused by the extensive long longitudinal vascular arrangement.

Figure 2–56*A* shows an interesting variation of the vascular flexor tendon anatomy observed in approximately 10% to 15% of middle and ring fingers of 80 specimens reviewed. There is no long vinculum proximal to the short vinculum of this profundus tendon. Long intravasicular vascular channels originate from a broad, short vinculum profundus and from the proximal palmar synovial fold (the preputial fold of Mayer). Ligation injury of the profundus tendon distally or proximally would likely render a large segment of this tendon avascular. Interestingly, this vascular arrangement shows that although segmental at the proximal phalanx level, long interfascicular vascular flows are possible. This correlates and supports the probability of a similar type of vascular nutri-tion in the long tendon grafts gliding within the pseudosheaths formed by a gliding stage-I tendon implant.

In summary the surgeon should bear in mind that the absence of or the location of the vincula will vary with the finger studied and that these factors will vary with age. Application of these basic facts helps to explain the unpredictable results of flexor tendon repair following tendon injury in the digital sheath. The surgeon should consider that after injury and repair a failed result may be explained on an anatomic basis and not necessarily on faulty surgical technique or how quickly surgery was carried out after injury. In this day and age, some patients and their legal counsel think they know more about treatment and expected results than does the surgeon. The truths of anatomy can add the strength to forcefully explain to the patient why a result may be predictably less than expected and that after a judicious delay, reconstructive tendon surgery and hand therapy can again return good hand function.

Extrinsic Muscles of the Fingers

Emanuel B. Kaplan
James M. Hunter

LONG EXTENSOR MUSCLES

The three long extensors of the fingers are the extensor digitorum communis, the extensor proprius of the index, and the extensor proprius of the little finger. The origin of these muscles is different; the terminal insertion is similar. Phylogenetically the muscles derive from the supinatoextensor group of Humphry. The investigation of Strauss on the phylogeny of the human forearm extensors, among other ideas, brought a better understanding of the variations of these muscles.

The extensor muscles are represented by three basic groups in tetrapods: the brachioantebrachial, the antebrachiomanual, and the manual. The first originates from the elbow matrix; the other two, from the wrist matrix. The brachioantebrachial group has three divisions: the humeroradial, represented in mammals by the extensors carpi radiales longus and brevis, the supinator, and probably the brachioradialis; the humerodorsal, represented by the extensor digitorum communis; the humeroulnar, forming the extensor carpi ulnaris and the extensor digiti minimi. The antebrachiomanual group becomes the abductor pollicis longus with secondary development of the extensor pollicis brevis and primary development of the extensor profundus reduced to the extensor pollicis longus and the extensor proprius indicis. The muscles of the brachioantebrachial and the antebrachiomanual group exhibit distal phylogenetic migration and replace the third basic manual group.

The extensor digitorum communis

The most superficial muscle of the extensor group, the extensor digitorum communis originates from the lateral epicondyle of the humerus and from a small area posterior to the radial notch of the ulna. The origin from the humeral epicondyle occurs in common with the other muscles the extensor carpi radialis brevis and the extensor digiti minimi. Some of the fibers of origin come from the antebrachial fascia, which covers these muscles. The ulnar origin intermingles with the ulnar fibers of the supinator through a fibrous reinforcement of the insertion. The muscular belly begins slightly proximal to the origin and consists of a flat muscle running in a distal direction between the extensor carpi radialis brevis on the radial side and the extensor digiti minimi and the extensor carpi ulnaris on the ulnar side. The muscular belly covers the supinator in the upper third of the forearm.

Approximately in the lower third of the forearm, the muscle splits in four tendons, which separate and proceed toward the dorsal carpal ligament of the wrist accompanied by the tendon of the extensor indicis proprius. On reaching the posterior aspect of the lower end of the radius, the tendons of the extensor communis, covered with a synovial bursa, engage under the dorsal carpal ligament in a special smooth, bony groove between Lister's tubercle on the radial side and a shallow canal for the extensor digiti minimi on the ulnar side. Lister's tubercle is a very important point of reference because immediately under it on the ulnar side lies the tendon of the extensor pollicis longus, immediately ulnar to it is the tendon of the extensor digitorum communis, and immediately radial to it is the tendon of extensors carpi radialis brevis and longus (Fig. 2–57; *see also Fig. 3–14*).

On emerging from under the dorsal carpal ligaments the extensor tendons diverge radially toward the fingers. The fascia that covers the dorsal carpal ligament extends onto the synovial bursa and fuses with the intertendinous fascia. This loose fascial fusion forms a definite anchorage that restrains the extensor tendons from overstretching in a distal direction when the fingers are completely flexed; it appears to contribute to the system of dorsal anchorages, which was described over the distal and the proximal interphalangeal joints and also over the metacarpophalangeal joints as anchorages 1, 2, and 3. This last anchorage will thus form anchorage 4 (Figs. 2–6 and 2–13). Over the carpus the tendons run over the lunate and the capitate bones, diverging on the ulnar side toward the triquetral and on the radial side toward the scaphoid (Fig. 2–31). Over the metacarpal shafts the tendons spread out from the radial side of the fifth metacarpal to the ulnar side of the second metacarpal. They repose on the posterior interosseous fascia enclosed in the intertendinous fascia and covered by the supratendinous fascia *(see Fig. 2–63)*.

Extensor digiti minimi
The extensor digiti minimi originates from the posterior aspect of the radial epicondyle of the humerus from a common tendon for the epicondylar muscles, medial to the origin of the extensor communis, radial to the origin of the extensor carpi ulnaris, and posterior to the supinator. The origin of the muscle adheres to the antebrachial fascia. The muscle belly is long and narrow and runs distally until it joins the ulnar side of a tendon over the radiocarpal articulation. It then engages under the extensor retinaculum; crossing the hamate bone posteriorly, it runs toward the base of the fifth metacarpal in its own synovial sheath.

Over the dorsum of the hand, the extensor digiti minimi is represented by a double tendon running from the wrist to the point of insertion. The tendon from the extensor digitorum usually is absent and is represented by a small extension in the form of a junctura. Only in rare cases is there a separate tendon from the extensor digitorum, and then it usually runs as a third tendon to the little finger. In a recent study (Schenck), it was found that even in the presence of more than two tendons of the little finger the

extensor digitorum may still be represented by a single short extension from the extensor digitorum of the ring finger near its metacarpophalangeal area to the extensor digiti minimi near the metacarpophalangeal joint of the little finger.

Extensor indicis
The extensor indicis originates at a point deep in relation to the extensor digitorum communis from the distal third of the ulna, distal to the origin of the extensor pollicis longus, from the corresponding area of the interosseous membrane, and from the septum separating these two muscles. The muscular fibers run distally and join a tendon just proximal to the proximal edge of the dorsal carpal ligament. The tendon runs anterior to the extensor digitorum tendons in the same synovial sheath and then to the ulnar side of the extensor communis to the index finger. Over the metacarpals all of the extensor tendons run toward their corresponding fingers. The pattern and the number of the tendons to the fingers is never constant. The most varied combinations occur and may differ even in the hands of the same individual. The tendon of the extensor indicis proprius is almost constantly on the ulnar side of the extensor communis tendon to the index. The extensor to the little finger is almost constantly on the ulnar side of the tendon of the extensor communis to the little finger (Fig. 2–57; *see also Fig. 6–16*).

The extensor indicis and the extensor digiti minimi have comparatively independent origin; however, the extensor digitorum, which is independent of the muscles mentioned, binds the action of the index, middle, ring, and little fingers into a common unit. Some independence of the common extensor tendon to the index finger has been observed in instances in which the extensor indicis proprius has been used for transfer. The extensors of the index and little fingers permit an almost complete independence of motion; however, the middle and ring fingers are so bound by the common origin of the different parts of the extensor digitorum that independent motion of these fingers is limited considerably. Generally, the limitation of exten-

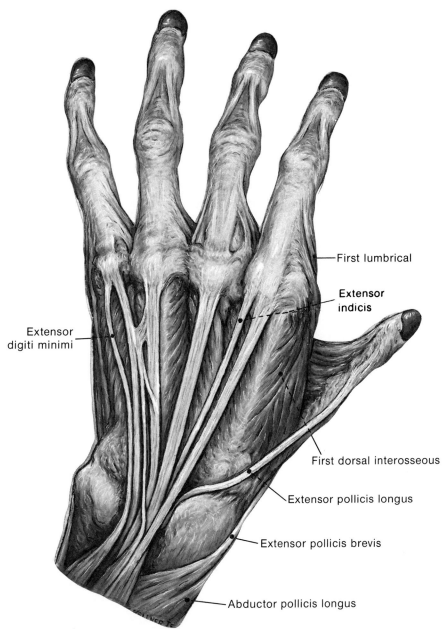

First lumbrical

**Extensor
indicis**

Extensor
digiti minimi

First dorsal interosseous

Extensor pollicis longus

Extensor pollicis brevis

Abductor pollicis longus

FIG. 2—57 The left hand of a gorilla. The extensor tendons to the fingers, showing
an independent extensor indicis, a strong and independent extensor digitorum
communis tendon to the index and the middle fingers. The extensors to the ring and
the little fingers exhibit a complicated pattern with a distinct extensor minimi to the
little finger. The lumbrical muscles are inserted into the radial side of the extensor
apparatus of each finger. Were it not for the short thumb, it would be difficult to
differentiate this hand from a human specimen. (Specimen from the Museum of the
Department of Anatomy, College of Physicians and Surgeons, Columbia University,
New York, NY)

sion of the ring finger while the others are flexed does not interfere with the usual activities of the hand, but there are instances in which limitation of extension of the ring finger becomes annoying. It happens sometimes in musicians, especially pianists, and causes them great mental distress.

The tendons of the extensor digitorum are connected by short oblique slips running in a distal direction, usually from the medius to the index and ring fingers and from the ring to the little finger. In the last case, as mentioned before, it may represent the only extensor digitorum tendon to the little finger. The slips between the various tendons of the extensor digitorum are usually found in the distal part of the dorsum of the hand proximal to the metacarpophalangeal joints. The slip is known as the *junctura tendinum*, or according to the Nomina Anatomica Parisiensia, as the *connexus intertendineus*.

The intertendinous slips were considered to be responsible for restriction of individual extension of the ring finger; however, attempts to correct the restriction of individual movement of the ring finger by surgical division of the juncturae did not increase the individual movement of the ring finger because the restriction is caused by the interconnection in the common muscular mass of the extensor digitorum at its origin. This can be proved easily by electric stimulation of the various parts of the extensor digitorum (Fig. 2–58).

Extensor tendon variation

The variations of the tendons of the three extensors may assume different forms. The following is a résumé based on literature and personal observations.

The extensor digitorum may exhibit an absent tendon or a very attenuated tendon to the little finger. Five tendons may be observed instead of four, the increase dependent on a double index, middle, ring, or little finger. Six tendons are sometimes observed by a double tendon to two fingers simultaneously or a triple tendon to the middle finger. Eight tendons may be observed by a doubling of each tendon. Ten and eleven tendons also were observed. A complete unseparated extensor sheet was observed

running from the carpus to almost the base of the proximal phalanges. This variation is often seen with congenital anomalies of the digits (*e.g.,* adactylia and acheiria).

An extensor proprius to the middle finger was observed with a tendon located under the extensor digitorum with a separate muscular body parallel with the body of the extensor indicis proprius. The extensor proprius to the little finger may be absent or fused with the extensor communis to the little finger or with the extensor carpi ulnaris; or it may be double or may send a tendinous slip to the ring finger.

The extensor indicis may be absent or diminished in size or become double with insertion into the index only, or the index and the middle fingers, or the index and the extensor pollicis longus. The extensor may even change its origin to the carpal bones or the dorsal carpal ligament.

For comparison with the extensor tendons of the human hand, the dorsal aspect of the hand of a gorilla is presented (Fig. 2–57). The arrangement of the tendons in the gorilla differs little from the variants of a human hand. Perhaps, it may be noted that the tendons to the middle and the index fingers are almost completely isolated. This may be a confirmation of the observation of Strauss, who found an advanced isolation of the individual tendons of the extensor communis in all the higher primates except the gibbon. Strauss believed that the overdevelopment of the flexors has probably been a most important factor in limiting the evolution of the extensor musculature in anthropoids. In the anthropoids, the extensors as a whole are not as developed as in man. Although the extensor muscles in man are still subordinate in action to the flexor muscles, they are more differentiated than are the extensors of the anthropoids.

While the number and the form of the extensor tendons vary greatly over the metacarpal shafts, their behavior over the metacarpophalangeal joint and their course toward the terminal insertion become constant. As mentioned before, the tendons of the extensor indicis proprius and the tendon of the extensor digiti minimi join their corresponding extensor com-

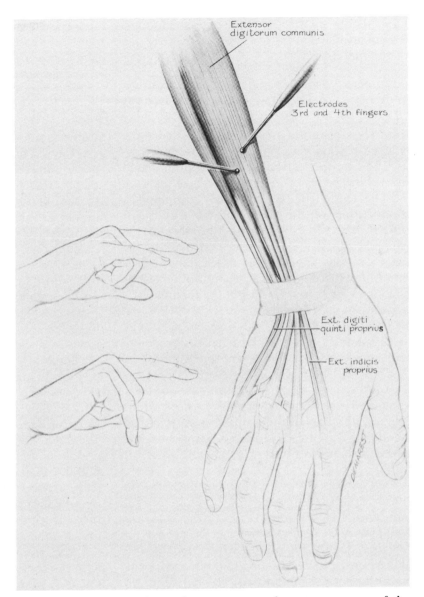

FIG. 2—58 When stimulated with an electric current, the common mass of the extensor digitorum produces extension of four digits that is not increased by section of the juncturae tendinum. Extension of the index and the little fingers is possible when the flexors of the ring and middle fingers are flexing these two fingers. Extension of the ring finger at the metacarpophalangeal joint when the little and middle fingers are flexed but the index is extended is practically impossible even under strong electric stimulation although the juncturae are completely divided.

munis tendon on the ulnar side of the communis and form one tendon over the dorsum of the metacarpal head.

DORSAL APPARATUS OF THE FINGER

From the dorsum of the metacarpal head, the extensor tendon participates in a design involving the capsule of the metacarpophalangeal joint, the tendons of insertion of the interossei, and the tendon of the lumbrical muscle. The organization of the fibers of the apparatus located over the dorsum and the sides of the proximal phalanx and over the proximal and the distal interphalangeal joint has a definite pattern. Many investigations of the minutiae of this fibrous apparatus were made because the mechanism of action of extension and flexion of the constituent elements of a finger could not be well explained. Some of the parts of the dorsal apparatus were described as continuations of the tendons of the interossei, some others as prolongations of the lumbrical tendon. Apparently, the arrangement of the various fibers of the dorsal apparatus is a response to functional demands and therefore appears late in the development of the small muscles of the hand.

Serial sections of fetal hands studied by the author failed to show definite tendons for the interossei and the lumbricals (Figs. 2–14 and 2–59). Areas of condensation of cells occur in the evolving dorsal apparatus, which include the long extensor corresponding to the lateral bands of the apparatus and to the dorsum, but the entire dorsal apparatus forms initially a continuum with the flexor tunnel, retaining oblique connections in later development only at the distal and the proximal interphalangeal and the metacarpophalangeal joints (Figs. 2–18 and 2–20). It is very difficult, if not impossible, to separate the description of the terminal insertion of the extensor communis from the other parts because the insertion actually represents a functioning unit with an intimate interconnection between all the component parts.

The dorsum of the finger (Fig. 2–10), which was isolated from all other fingers with all the phalanges in extension, shows the fibers of the dorsal apparatus from the metacarpophalangeal joint to the distal phalanx and the nail. The tendon of the extensor digitorum communis runs over the metacarpophalangeal joint. Fibers from the sides of the proximal part of the tendon run toward the lateral ligaments of the metacarpophalangeal joints and transfix the tendons of the interosseous muscles, which are attached to the lateral tubercles of the proximal phalanx in a tunnel so that the interossei cannot luxate dorsally even in strong hyperextension of the metacarpophalangeal joint. A short distance more distally the extensor communis tendon penetrates into a dorsal membrane. This membrane exhibits a more or less pronounced, semilunar edge crossing the extensor tendon. Parallel with this edge arciform fibers are observed running in the substance of the membrane from one side of the finger to the other until these fibers reach the area of the proximal interphalangeal joint. The sides of the membrane are represented by thickened bands running distally toward the sides of the proximal interphalangeal joint. These bands turn toward the dorsum of the middle phalanx and unite near the head of the middle phalanx. Continuing their course they form a wide, ribbonlike structure that inserts into the base of the distal phalanx, not only into the dorsal tubercle but along an elevated ridge, limiting the articular base of the distal phalanx.

The lateral bands are in direct continuation with the parts of the tendons of the interosseous muscles, which insert into the dorsal apparatus. Normally, on the radial side of each finger the tendon of the lumbrical muscle is also inserted slightly distal to the insertion of the interosseous. The illustration (Fig. 2–10) does not show the insertion of the lumbrical because normally this insertion cannot be seen directly from the dorsal aspect of the finger.

The tendon of the extensor communis can be seen through the membrane as a fanning-out structure that shows a tendency toward condensation of its fibers into a midportion and two lateral portions. The lateral divergent fibers run toward the lateral bands of the dorsal aponeurotic membrane. The midband stops at the base of the middle phalanx where it is inserted.

A lateral incision of the dorsal apparatus of the finger with the dorsal aponeurosis retracted from the phalanges shows the strong insertion of the midband into the base of the middle phalanx. The undersurface of the apparatus shows one lateral band, the midband, and the arciform fibers between the midband and the lateral band, which is longitudinally incised. The loose connection of the extensor tendon with the capsule of the metacarpophalangeal joint is also visualized. The incision over the side of the metacarpophalangeal joint emphasizes the intimate connection of the dorsal apparatus with the interossei and the tunnel of the flexor tendons (Figs. 2–60, 2–61, and 2–62).

A better study of the dorsal aponeurosis can be made on removal of the entire apparatus from the finger. The dorsal apparatus shows the relation of the interossei, which actually fuse into the lateral sides of the dorsal membrane. The arrangement of the arciform fibers permits some independent motion between the peripheral lateral band and the midportion of the extensor communis (Fig. 2–61).

The volar aspect of the removed apparatus shows the gradual convergence of the arciform fibers toward the midband and the lateral collateral ligament. The intra-articular space of the proximal interphalangeal joint shows how the midband contributes to the formation of the posterior wall for this joint and ends in the fibrous or fibrocartilaginous intra-articular protrusion. The metacarpophalangeal joint is completely separated from the dorsal membrane because the dorsal membranous apparatus contributes to the formation of the dorsal capsule. Figure 2–9 shows the lateral prolongations of the apparatus after they were separated from the collateral ligaments.

The dorsal apparatus spreads out between the metacarpophalangeal joints to form a tunnel for the tendons of the interossei and becomes attached to the deep transverse intermetacarpal

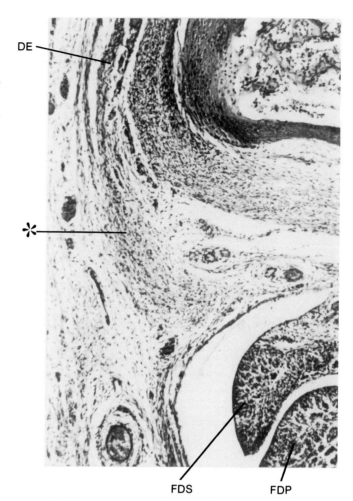

FIG. 2–59 Large magnification of a section of a finger near the proximal interphalangeal joint in a 5-month-old premature infant. The fibers of the dorsal expansion (DE) running parallel with the capsule of the joint, outside of the capsule, are directed and intimately connected by the transverse retinacular ligament of Landsmeer (✻) with the dorsolateral aspect of the tunnel which encloses the flexor superficialis (FDS) and the profundus (FDP) tendons.

ligament (Fig. 2–21). As was mentioned previously, the dorsal apparatus acquires oblique attachments in the region of the proximal and distal interphalangeal joints with the flexor tunnel and the articular plate of the joints. These attachments permit a limited dorsal shift of the entire apparatus. A limited volar shift is also

(Text continues on page 102.)

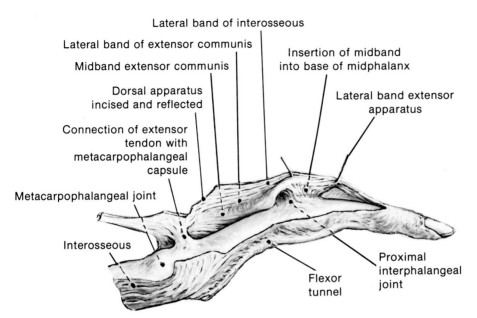

Lateral band of interosseous

Lateral band of extensor communis

Midband extensor communis

Insertion of midband into base of midphalanx

Dorsal apparatus incised and reflected

Lateral band extensor apparatus

Connection of extensor tendon with metacarpophalangeal capsule

Metacarpophalangeal joint

Interosseous

Proximal interphalangeal joint

Flexor tunnel

FIG. 2–60   Ring finger of the right hand, ulnar aspect. Dorsal apparatus incised longitudinally from the metacarpophalangeal joint to the distal interphalangeal joint. The extensor digitorum communis and the dorsal apparatus are reflected, showing the connection of the tendon with the base of the proximal phalanx. Insertion of the tendon of the extensor digitorum communis into the base of the middle phalanx is shown.

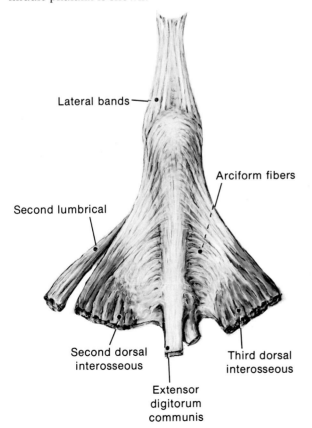

Lateral bands

Arciform fibers

Second lumbrical

Second dorsal interosseous

Third dorsal interosseous

Extensor digitorum communis

FIG. 2–61   Dorsal apparatus of a third finger completely removed from the phalanges and from the metacarpophalangeal joint. Dorsal aspect. Over the metacarpophalangeal joint the interosseous muscles show the connection with the lateral bases of the proximal phalanx and also the insertion of these muscles into the lateral bands of the dorsal aponeurosis. The fibers from the interossei toward the extensor tendon are first horizontal; they gradually change their course to more and more oblique fibers. The underlying tendon of the extensor digitorum communis shows the fanning out of the deep fibers, with their termination in the lateral bands. The tendon of the extensor communis does not actually divide into three separate bands; rather, it is a continuous fanlike structure with thin interruptions, with a more or less condensed central portion and spread-out lateral bands. The tendon actually spreads out over the entire dorsal capsule of the proximal interphalangeal joint.

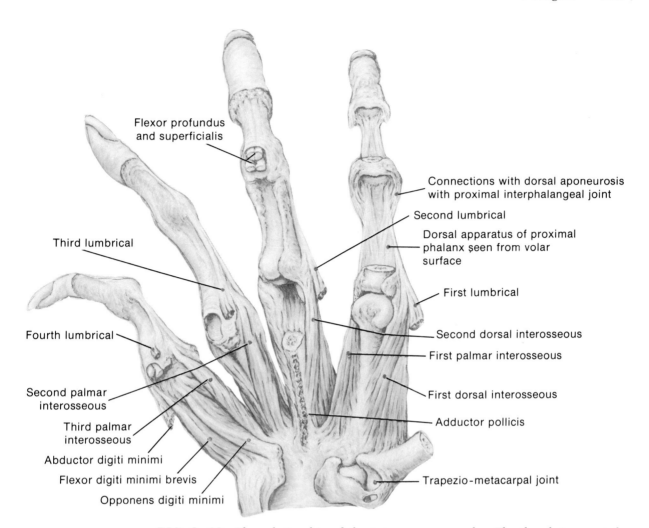

Flexor profundus
and superficialis

Connections with dorsal aponeurosis
with proximal interphalangeal joint

Second lumbrical

Dorsal apparatus of proximal
phalanx şeen from volar
surface

Third lumbrical

First lumbrical

Fourth lumbrical

Second dorsal interosseous

First palmar interosseous

Second palmar
interosseous

First dorsal interosseous

Third palmar
interosseous

Adductor pollicis

Abductor digiti minimi

Flexor digiti minimi brevis

Trapezio-metacarpal joint

Opponens digiti minimi

FIG. 2–62 The relationship of the interosseous muscles. The thumb is resected
through the first metacarpal, the metacarpophalangeal joint is opened, and the
proximal and middle phalanges of the index finger are removed almost entirely,
leaving the bases of these phalanges only, to show the intimate connection of the
dorsal apparatus to the distal, middle, and proximal phalanges and the metacarpophalangeal joint. The first dorsal interosseous is shown in its entirety, as are the
second, the third, and the fourth dorsal interossei. The head of the third metacarpal is
removed to show the relationship of the interossei to the metacarpophalangeal joint.
The ring and little fingers were dislocated at their bases at the metacarpocarpal joint
and rotated toward the ulnar side to demonstrate their radial aspects. The ring finger
shows the origin and the insertion of the second palmar interosseous; the little finger
shows the insertion of the third volar interosseous. A double insertion of the volar
interosseous into the base of the proximal phalanx and into the dorsal aponeurosis in
the ring finger and a single insertion into the dorsal aponeurosis of the little finger are
shown.

possible but is maintained in balance by the integrity of the dorsal apparatus over the proximal interphalangeal joint from one lateral to the other lateral side of the structures just proximal to the joint. These structures are mostly the fanned-out fibers of the tendon of the extensor digitorum communis obliquely connected with the lateral collateral ligaments of the proximal interphalangeal joint. An abnormal volar shift is also prevented by the membrane between the lateral bands over the dorsum of the middle phalanx, the triangular ligament (Fig. 2–10).

INTRINSIC MUSCLES

The intrinsic muscles of the fingers form four distinct and important groups: the dorsal and the palmar interossei, the lumbricals, and the muscles of the hypothenar and the thenar eminences. (The thenar muscles will be dealt with separately.)

Infrequently, the dorsum of the hand shows a few muscular bundles ending in short tendons inserted into the second and the third, or even into the fourth finger or into the corresponding interossei. The muscular fibers are located dorsal to the tendons of the extensor communis. These muscular fibers originate from the bones of the carpus or the metacarpals. The muscle is probably similar to the extensor brevis of the foot and was called *extensor digitorum brevis manus.*

We believe that this muscle was first described by Albinus in 1734 as a short extensor in the hand. LeDouble made a study of this muscle in a monograph published in 1895. The frequency, as reported by many anatomists, varied greatly. According to Caldwell, Anson and Wright (1943), the variation was seen in some 3% of the population. In the authors' experience, this muscle was encountered occasionally. The possible existence of this muscle must be remembered in surgery of the dorsum of the hand. When the existence of this muscle is unknown, it may lead to an erroneous diagnosis and may be taken for a dorsal ganglion, a tumor of the dorsum, or even a hematoma after injury.

The extensor digitorum brevis manus muscle represents a homologue of the extensor brevis of the foot (extensor digitorum brevis). It originates from the carpal bones, usually in the region of the scaphoid and the lunate or the metacarpal bases in this region, and inserts into the tendons of the extensor digitorum near the metacarpophalangeal joints of the middle, ring, or other fingers.

INTEROSSEOUS MUSCLES

The interosseous muscles are located between the metacarpal shafts and are described as the dorsal and the palmar interossei according to their relation to the axis of the hand and their relative position to the palmar and the dorsal aspect of the intermetacarpal spaces (Figs. 2–62 and 2–63).

Most of the anatomists consider that there are three palmar interosseous muscles and four dorsal. The characteristics of the palmar interosseous is the location of its origin on the metacarpal in relation to the axis. The axis of the hand passes longitudinally through the middle metacarpal and finger. The palmar interosseous originates by a single belly from the palmar two thirds of the metacarpal shaft facing the axis of the hand. The insertion of the palmar interosseous is on the proximal phalanx corresponding to the metacarpal origin; therefore, the palmar interosseous is an adductor toward the axis of the middle finger.

The dorsal interosseous originates by means of two muscular bellies from the adjacent metacarpals. The larger belly arises from the entire anterolateral surface of the metacarpal that faces away from the axis of the middle finger. The smaller belly is attached to the remaining anterolateral third of the shaft of the metacarpal that faces the axis of the middle finger (Fig. 2–64). The insertion of the muscle takes place on the proximal phalanx of the side of the larger origin of the muscle. The dorsal interosseous is an abductor of the fingers away from the axis of the middle finger.

When the palmar surface of the hand is completely denuded of all structures including

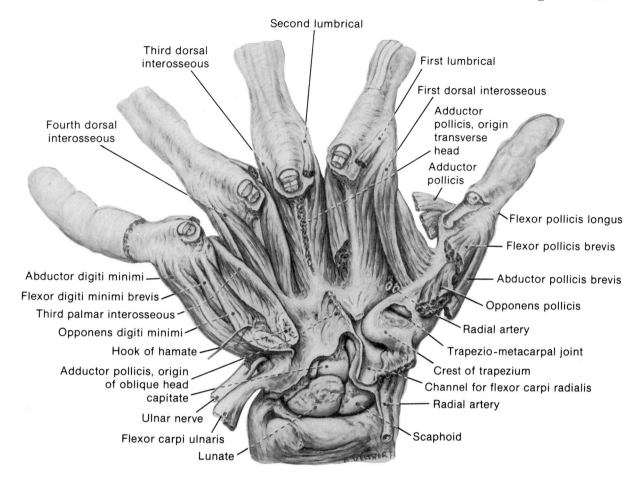

Second lumbrical

Third dorsal interosseous

First lumbrical

First dorsal interosseous

Adductor pollicis, origin transverse head

Adductor pollicis

Fourth dorsal interosseous

Flexor pollicis longus

Flexor pollicis brevis

Abductor pollicis brevis

Abductor digiti minimi

Flexor digiti minimi brevis

Third palmar interosseous

Opponens digiti minimi

Hook of hamate

Adductor pollicis, origin of oblique head

capitate

Ulnar nerve

Flexor carpi ulnaris

Lunate

Opponens pollicis

Radial artery

Trapezio-metacarpal joint

Crest of trapezium

Channel for flexor carpi radialis

Radial artery

Scaphoid

FIG. 2–63 Normal relationship of the interossei and other deep structures of the hand. The metacarpocarpal joint of the thumb is opened, the tunnel for the flexor carpi radialis is uncovered, and the origin of the oblique fibers of the adductor pollicis shows its intimate connection with the tunnel of the flexor carpi radialis. The radiocarpal capsule was opened; the hook of the hamate bone was divided and reflected to the ulnar side to demonstrate clearly the origin of the third volar interosseous and of the flexor brevis and opponens to the little finger.

the anterior interosseous fascia, the palmar and the dorsal interossei are exposed and can be seen from this side of the hand (Fig. 2–63). When the dorsum of the hand is similarly denuded of all structures, only the dorsal interossei can be seen (Fig. 2–6) from the dorsal side of the hand.

Palmar interosseous muscles
There are three palmar interosseous muscles, although this is not generally accepted. The small muscular belly usually connected with the

flexor pollicis brevis is considered by some anatomists to be the additional palmar interosseous muscle. For comparative anatomic reasons, perhaps this is justified; however, it is simpler and more practical to admit the presence of three palmar interossei. They are numbered from the radial to the ulnar side of the hand (Fig. 2–64). The first is between the second and the third metacarpals with insertion into the base of the ulnar side of the proximal phalanx of the index. The second is found be-

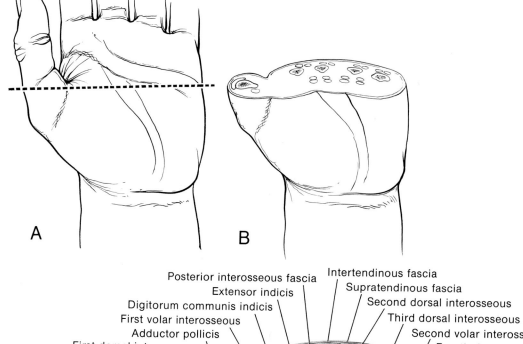

A

B

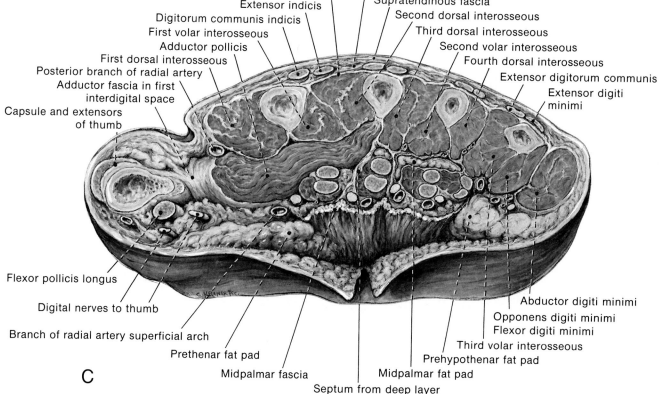

Posterior interosseous fascia
Extensor indicis
Digitorum communis indicis
First volar interosseous
Adductor pollicis
First dorsal interosseous
Posterior branch of radial artery
Adductor fascia in first
  interdigital space
Capsule and extensors
  of thumb

Intertendinous fascia
Supratendinous fascia
Second dorsal interosseous
Third dorsal interosseous
Second volar interosseous
Fourth dorsal interosseous
Extensor digitorum communis
Extensor digiti
  minimi

Flexor pollicis longus

Digital nerves to thumb

Branch of radial artery superficial arch

Prethenar fat pad

Midpalmar fascia

Septum from deep layer
to third metacarpal

Midpalmar fat pad

Third volar interosseous
Prehypothenar fat pad

Abductor digiti minimi
Opponens digiti minimi
Flexor digiti minimi

C

FIG. 2–64 A, B, and **C**, Section of the left hand passing through the middle of the second, the third, the fourth, and the fifth metacarpals and obliquely through the proximal phalanx of the thumb. The relationship of the palmar aponeurosis to the subcutaneous fat is shown. The midpalmar fat pad is also indicated. The septum from the deep layer to the crest of the third metacarpal comes from the ulnar bursa (see Fig. 6-6.)

tween the third and the fourth metacarpals with insertion into the base of the radial side of the proximal phalanx of the ring finger. The third palmar interosseous is located between the fourth and the fifth metacarpals with insertion into the base of the radial side of the proximal phalanx of the little finger.

The insertions of the palmar interossei have been described in detail. Although the descriptions are generally similar, slight discrepancies are noted in the description of the manner of attachment of the palmar interossei into the base of the proximal phalanx and into the dorsal apparatus. Some anatomists found that the palmar interosseous is mostly attached to the dorsal apparatus and has no insertion or very insignificant insertion into the anterolateral base of the proximal phalanx. Salisbury asks the following question: "It has been shown that the lumbricales are on the side of the interossei with the greater insertion into the proximal phalanges. May this not be accepted as evidence that the lumbricales do assist in interphalangeal extension, being more highly developed where the dorsal interossei are unable to act on the extensor apparatus?"

In view of Salisbury's findings in the investigations of the interosseous muscles, his question has a certain implication. He came to the conclusion based on a study of 30 hands, that the palmar interossei are inserted, with few exceptions, wholly into the extensor expansions and that the first dorsal inserts wholly into the lateral base of the proximal phalanx. He also found that the other three dorsal interossei have a variable insertion, more frequently into both the extensor apparatus and the base of the proximal phalanx. Salisbury's question creates an impression that he suspects that the lumbricals act in substitution for the absent part of the insertion of the dorsal interosseous into the dorsal expansion. This may be true in some cases but should not be taken to mean that the lumbricals function in substitution for the absent or the weak insertion of the dorsal interosseous into the dorsal apparatus. In the author's experience, hands were found in which the lumbricals coex-

isted with very strong insertions of the dorsal interosseous into the dorsal apparatus.

It is necessary to consider that the study of insertions of small muscles in general, and of the interossei in particular, is beset with difficulties. The material obtained is usually preserved and represents mostly an advanced age group with frequent arthritic changes of the smaller joints. For precise information, investigations must be supplemented by serial sections of a larger number of normal hands and by sections of fetal hands. In large series, the variations of insertions are so persistent that it is difficult to state whether a distinction between the two should be made at all. Even in the case of the insertion of the first dorsal interosseous, which is generally described as having only one insertion into the lateral tubercle of the base of the proximal phalanx, it is found not infrequently that the insertion extends prominently into the dorsal apparatus.

Function is the essential factor. It does not necessarily depend on the variation of insertions or the number of muscle bellies; it may be connected also with the variations of nerve supply. It is probably true that additional muscle variations, or a more efficient nerve, or a more elastic and efficient ligamentous apparatus make the difference between subjects with great dexterity and others who have clumsy and inept fingers, but the relation between anatomic perfection and efficiency of function is obviously not a constant factor. It is not of very great importance whether an interosseous muscle on one side has a perfect double or single insertion if the interosseous on the other side of the finger has an insertion that contributes to the function of the finger producing what the interossei normally do together, or with the assistance of the lumbrical.

The insertions of the palmar interosseous are similar to the insertions of the dorsal interosseous with the exception that the palmar interosseous does not always possess the insertion into the lateral tubercle of the base of the proximal phalanx but instead inserts almost exclusively into the dorsal apparatus by a round, fairly long tendon. The tendon expands and contributes to the fibers of the dorsal apparatus which are connected with the midband of the extensor digitorum communis tendon and also to the lateral bands of the dorsal apparatus; however, it must be emphasized that an insertion into the lateral tubercle of the base of the proximal phalanx is frequently found.

Dorsal Interosseous Muscles.
There are four dorsal interosseous muscles. The first is located between the first and second metacarpals and is inserted into the radial side of the metacarpophalangeal component of the index finger. The second is inserted into the radial side of the metacarpophalangeal region of the middle finger. The third is inserted into the ulnar side of the metacarpophalangeal area of the same finger. The fourth is attached to the ulnar side of the metacarpophalangeal region of the ring finger (Figs. 2–62 and 2–64).

The tendon of the interosseous is formed by fusion of the tendinous structures of the muscle bellies of the dorsal interosseous. On its approach to the metacarpophalangeal joint it assumes its connections with the capsule, the extensor digitorum tendon, and the dorsal apparatus. These connections, variously described in their detail, have a bearing on the function of the entire finger. The tendon divides into two heads: One head is round and is inserted into the base of the proximal phalanx, normally volar to the axis of the dorsovolar extension-flexion of the metacarpophalangeal joint. The axis of extension and flexion passes transversely through the head of the metacarpal in a radioulnar direction. The other head of the tendon is flatter and approaches the dorsal apparatus with a slight twist to join the apparatus (Fig. 2–11).

The part of the interosseous tendon that is inserted into the lateral base of the proximal phalanx is connected loosely with the collateral ligaments, although at times it may adhere to the capsule. Usually, it is contained in its place by the expansion of the extensor apparatus, which surrounds the metacarpophalangeal joint on each side and turns volad to join the intermetacarpal deep transverse ligament (Lig. metacarpeum transversum profundum, NAP) and the fibrocartilaginous plate of the volar aspect of the metacarpophalangeal joint (Figs. 2–19 and 2–23).

The extensor apparatus usually does not unite with the tendon of the interosseous inserted into the phalanx, so a certain amount of motion of the tendon of the interosseous is possible without transmission to the dorsal apparatus. At times, both are firmly united; however, whether united or free, the tendon of the interosseous apparently does not normally shift dorsally to the axis of extension-flexion of the metacarpophalangeal joint and therefore normally never becomes an extensor of the proximal phalanx at the metacarpophalangeal joint.

The insertions of each of the dorsal interossei are variable. It was stated previously by several investigators that the first dorsal interosseous does not, as a rule, insert into the dorsal aponeurosis and that the only insertion of the first dorsal interosseous is confined only to the lateral tubercle of the base of the proximal phalanx of the index finger. In the previous edition of this book, it was stated that the first dorsal interosseous may not have any insertion into the dorsal apparatus. It was since found that the first dorsal interosseous almost constantly inserts into the dorsal apparatus, although in certain instances the extension of the second distal phalanges by the first dorsal interosseous may not be as strong as the extension of these two phalanges by the first lumbrical.

Faradic or sinusoidal stimulation of the exposed first dorsal interosseous during surgical procedures always produces a more or less intense extension of the two distal phalanges of the index. The dorsal apparatus in this case still retains the usual relationship with the radial side of the metacarpophalangeal joint; retention of the tendon of the first dorsal interosseous prevents the possibility of its shifting dorsally (Figs. 2–21 and 2–23). The second dorsal interosseous has the typical double insertion. The third dorsal may sometimes show an attenuated insertion into the dorsal apparatus. The fourth dorsal usually has a typical double insertion.

Variations Among the Interossei

The variations affecting the interossei can be understood in the light of comparative anatomy as outlined before. The palmar interossei may have a double origin with two tendons, each tendon inserted into a corresponding finger, or one or all palmar interossei may be absent. The dorsal interossei may have an extended origin from the bases of the metacarpals and even of the carpal bones. The second dorsal interosseous may be inserted into the ulnar side of the base of the second metacarpal—similar to the insertions of the interossei in the foot. The axis of the hand is then considered as running through the second digit, instead of the middle. They may have a reduced number of bellies of origin.

The Blood and the Nerve Supply of the Interossei

The distribution of the blood supply of the interossei was investigated by Salmon and Dor. Vascularization is abundant and derives from the deep palmar arch and from the common digital (metacarpal) arteries of the superficial palmer arch. The dorsal arch does not appear to contribute to the pattern of vessels supplying the dorsal interossei.

The innervation of all the interossei comes from the deep branch of the ulnar nerve, which is covered on its volar surface by the deep interosseous fascia. Rauber also described an occasional additional innervation of dorsal interossei muscles by the posterior interosseous branch of the radial nerve after it supplies the dorsal aspect of the carpal bones. It must be mentioned that rarely the entire nerve supply to the intrinsic muscles of the hand may derive from the median nerve through an anastomotic branch with the ulnar nerve over the flexor profundus in the proximal part of the forearm. This anastomosis will be described later in the text.

MUSCLES OF THE HYPOTHENAR EMINENCE

The hypothenar eminence is a separate group of three muscles involved with the activity of the little finger. The name is derived from the Greek word *thenar*, which means palm of the hand. The function of the muscles of the hypothenar eminence affects not only the little finger but the entire hand, as will be described later in the text. A fourth muscle not directly connected with the function of the hand or the little finger sometimes is described with the hypothenar eminence as the palmaris brevis. This muscle is represented by an accumulation of a variable number of muscular fibers in the cutaneous structures of the hand and will be described with the fascia of the hand. The three muscles of the hypothenar eminence are the abductor digiti minimi, the flexor digiti minimi brevis and the opponens digiti minimi (Figs. 2–30 and 2–65).

The *abductor digiti minimi* originates chiefly from the distal part of the pisiform bone, from the pisiform hamate ligament, and from a part of the volar carpal ligament in the immediate vicinity of the pisiform bone. The muscle almost constantly has two bellies separated from origin to insertion. The fibers of origin are in almost direct continuation with the tendon of the flexor carpi ulnaris, intermingling freely (Fig. 2–30); however, the contraction of the flexor carpi ulnaris does not produce simultaneous abduction of the little finger. The contraction of the abductor brevis, on the other hand, does not produce flexion of the wrist but pulls the pisiform in a distal direction with simultaneous contraction of the palmaris brevis. The muscle continues its course toward the base of the proximal phalanx, forming a double tendon of which one is inserted into the lateral tubercle (ulnar) of the proximal phalanx and the other into the dorsal apparatus. This double insertion is similar to the insertion of a dorsal interosseous. The muscle is also similar in function. This may be verified on the cadaver by traction applied to the abductor digiti minimi and also by direct stimulation of the abductor digiti minimi in the living.

The *flexor digiti minimi brevis* originates from the volar carpal ligament, the hook of the hamate bone of which it occupies the anterior and the ulnar side, and from the pisiform-

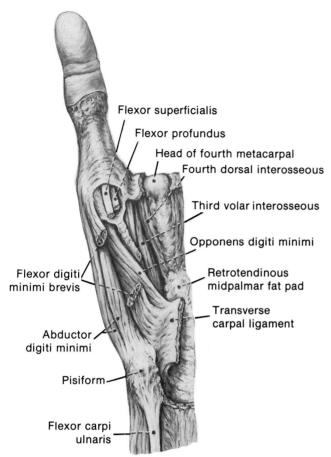

Flexor superficialis

Flexor profundus

Head of fourth metacarpal

Fourth dorsal interosseous

Third volar interosseous

Opponens digiti minimi

Retrotendinous
midpalmar fat pad

Transverse
carpal ligament

Flexor digiti
minimi brevis

Abductor
digiti minimi

Pisiform

Flexor carpi
ulnaris

FIG. 2—65   Fifth finger of the right hand. Relation of
the hypothenar muscles to the transverse ligament,
the pisiform bone, and the flexor carpi ulnaris. The
abductor digiti minimi has a double origin and is in
direct continuation with the flexor carpi ulnaris. Part
of the flexor digiti minimi brevis is excised to show the
opponens. Part of the flexor brevis originates from the
pisiform–hamate ligament.

hamate ligament. The muscle is covered partly
by the abductor. A small interval separates the
muscle from the abductor digiti minimi for
passage of the deep palmar branches of the
ulnar artery and the ulnar nerve (Fig. 2–63).
The muscle almost completely covers the muscle belly of the opponens. The insertion of the
flexor takes place volar to the phalangeal insertion of the abductor on the anterior part of the
lateral tubercle (ulnar) of the base of the proximal phalanx.

The *opponens digiti minimi* is a small muscle completely covered by the flexor brevis. It
originates from the hook of the hamate bone,
medial to the origin of the flexor brevis, and
from the ligament uniting the hook of the
hamate and the pisiform bone. A few fibers
originate from the undersurface of the volar
carpal ligament. The fibers of the muscle run
distally toward the fifth metacarpal and are
inserted by short, tendinous slips into the whole
length of the ulnar side of the shaft of the
metacarpal. The deep branches of the ulnar
artery and nerves pass through the fibers of the
muscle. On its radial side, it is in close contact
with the third palmar interosseous muscle.

The Variations Affecting the Hypothenar Muscle

The abductor digiti minimi may be absent or
fused with the flexor brevis, or it may extend its
origin over the entire pisiform bone; it may have
a single belly instead of a double. In the author's
experience, the double belly is more frequent;
others believe it to be less frequent. Very infrequently, an additional muscle originating from
the distal part of the forearm and running a
superficial course to the abductor digiti minimi
with fused insertions may be observed. The
origin of this additional muscle may be the flexor
carpi ulnaris or the flexor carpi radialis or the
palmaris longus. These variations are important
to keep in mind because they may cause confusion in surgical approaches to the anterior
aspect of the wrist.

The flexor brevis may fuse completely with
the abductor digiti minimi or may be absent; it
may send an additional extension into the metacarpal shaft between the opponens and the
palmar interosseous. Frequently, the opponens is
fused with the flexor brevis or with the abductor;
generally, it varies very little.

The blood supply of the muscles of the
hypothenar muscle is abundant and comes from
branches of the deep branch of the ulnar artery
and from the common digital. The arteries enter
the muscle from the deeper surface nearer the
origin of the three muscles.

The nerves to the hypothenar muscles all come from the ulnar nerve *(see Fig. 5–16)*. The abductor muscle is supplied by the deep branch before the deep branch penetrates between the abductor and the flexor; the branch enters the muscle on its ulnar side. The flexor brevis is supplied by a branch from the deep branch and enters the muscle near its origin on the deep aspect of the muscle. The opponens is supplied by one or two branches from the same deep branch and receives the nerves on its volar aspect. The palmaris brevis is usually supplied by a superficial branch of the ulnar nerve before the emergence of the digital nerve for the ulnar aspect of the little finger.

LUMBRICAL MUSCLES

There are four lumbrical muscles. They are located on the radial side of the flexor tendons and are inserted on the radial side of the dorsal apparatus (Fig. 2–66); their function is important. Sometimes, the muscles may be absent, and in this case the interossei substitute for their action. They are found in many mammals and are very evident in the anthropoids (Fig. 1–1); the muscles are quite variable.

The origin of these muscles normally occurs from the tendon of the flexor profundus in the palm of the hand. The first and the second lumbricals originate from the radial side of the flexor profundus of the index finger and from the flexor profundus tendon of the middle finger, respectively. The third arises from the contiguous third and fourth flexor tendons, and the fourth from the contiguous fourth and fifth flexor profundus tendons. The lumbricals are numbered from the radial to the ulnar side of the hand. The lumbrical to the index is the first and to the little finger, the fourth. The first and the second lumbricals are unipenniform; the third and the fourth are bipenniform. At times there seems to be a blending of the lumbrical muscle fibers of the middle, ring, and little fingers so that the three lumbrical muscles seem to be tripenniform in origin. This lumbrical complex, indicating the tendons to the ulnar side of the palm can present complex functional problems after injury. The fibers thicken in adhesions, and the connective tissues can blend the lumbrical mass into one, producing a form of functional quadregia and imbalance.

The lumbrical muscles usually arise from the radial and volar surface of the flexor profundus tendon. The extent of origin is surprisingly long. The average length of origin of the first lumbrical on the flexor profundus of the index finger is about 3 cm and reaches the level of the crest of the multangulum major. The length of origin of the second lumbrical on the tendon of the flexor profundus is about 4 cm. The third lumbrical runs for about 4 cm on the radial side of the flexor profundus of the ring finger and for about 2 cm on the ulnar side of the flexor profundus of the medius. The fourth lumbrical may run for about 3 cm to 3.5 cm on the radial side of the flexor profundus of the little finger and for approximately 1 cm to 1.5 cm on the ulnar side of the profundus tendon of the ring finger. The proximal end of the lumbrical origin forms a fine, elongated, pointed, muscle belly that reaches the transverse level of the distal end of the pisiform bone for the middle, ring, and little fingers when the fingers are extended. When the fingers are flexed, the proximal ends of the origin of the lumbricals are pulled into the carpal canal and may reach the level of the distal end of the radius.

The muscle fibers run with the flexor tendons toward the radial side of the fingers. In the palm of the hand, the lumbricals may completely cover the tendons of the flexor superficialis (Fig. 2–64). As soon as the flexor tendons enter their respective tunnels, the lumbricals diverge radially and repose on the deep transverse intermetacarpal ligament in company with the digital nerves and vessels; however, the first lumbrical has no intermetacarpal ligament on which to rest. It remains in contact with the radial side of the metacarpophalangeal joint and maintains the relationship with the vessel and the nerve (Figs. 2–21 and 2–24).

In transverse sections of the hand through the heads of the metacarpals, the tendons of the

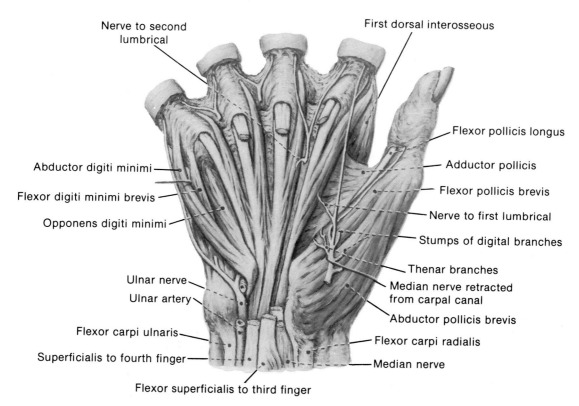

FIG. 2–66   The usual arrangement of the lumbrical muscles with the fingers extended. The area of origin of the first lumbrical is about 3 cm long and extends almost to the distal point of the crest of the multangulum major. The origin of the second lumbrical is about 4 cm long. The third lumbrical occupies about 4 cm in length of the flexor profundus to the ring finger and about 2 cm on the ulnar side of the flexor profundus tendon in the middle finger. The lumbrical of the little finger extends for about 3.5 cm on the radial side of the profundus of the fifth finger and about 1.5 cm on the ulnar side of the profundus of the ring finger. Flexion of the fingers pulls the fleshy fibers of the lumbrical muscles deep into the carpal canal and may reach as far proximal as the distal end of the radius. The fleshy fibers of the flexor superficialis muscle to the third finger descend on the tendon more distally than on any other flexor tendon of the hand. The median nerve was divided at the wrist, and the distal segment was pulled out from the carpal canal. The common digital branches to the index and the middle finger and to the middle and the ring finger were excised.

flexors are found in separate compartments formed by the volar plate of the metacarpophalangeal joint posteriorly and the vaginal ligaments of the flexor tunnel anteriorly and on the sides. The lumbricals with their vessels and nerves are placed between the flexor tunnels in compartments bound by the transverse intermetacarpal ligament dorsally and by the palmar subcutaneous fat pad and the natatory ligament volarly (Figs. 2–23, 2–24, and 2–66).

While passing through the special compartment, the lumbrical still consists of its muscle body. Only when it reaches the level of the base of the proximal phalanx does it begin to form a tendon that flattens out and joins the radial side of the extensor apparatus. Its fibers of continuation run distally from the fibers of the lateral bands of the dorsal apparatus, but not separately, as far as the head of the proximal phalanx (Fig. 2–11). The angle of approach of the lumbrical from the flexor tendon to the dorsal apparatus is about 30°. The tendon lies distinctly volar to the transverse axis of rotation of the metacarpophalangeal joint. It cannot slip dorsally because of its intimate connection with the flexor tendon. Normally, therefore, it cannot become an extensor of the metacarpophalangeal joint. It must be emphasized again that no splitting into separate tendons of the fibers of the lateral parts of the dorsal apparatus could be observed in the fetal material investigated by the author. The tendinous part of the lumbrical muscle varies in length. In the material examined by the author, the free part of the tendon from the muscle belly to the insertion was found to be approximately 15 mm for the index finger, 8 mm for the middle finger, 4 mm for the ring finger, and only about 2 mm to 3 mm for the little finger.

The total length of the lumbrical may reach or exceed 90 mm to 95 mm for the index finger, about 80 mm to 85 mm for the middle finger, 70 mm to 72 mm for the ring finger and 50 mm to 60 mm for the little finger. It may be expected that a muscular belly having a length of about 80 mm to 85 mm with a diameter of 8 mm to 10 mm as some of the lumbricals have, may develop considerable traction strength. The lumbrical muscles should not be regarded as trivial in their functional role. Their variational absence may cause an observable impediment in the function of the hand.

Variation in the lumbricals

The most important variations observed in the lumbricals were well reported in the past. The surgeon is interested mostly in the possible variations and their relative occurrence rather than in the precise frequency of the variations. The most frequent variation, as observed by the author and reported by others, concerns the third lumbrical, which forms a double tendon—one for the ulnar side of the middle finger and one for the radial side of the ring finger. In another variation, the third lumbrical may have an insertion into the ulnar side of the middle finger only. The lumbricals may be very attenuated or even absent—especially the third and the fourth. A few rare variations have been observed

by the author. A long tendon originated from the deep surface of the origin of the flexor sublimis in the forearm and passed through the carpal canal, forming the first lumbrical distal to the carpal canal with typical insertion into the dorsal apparatus of the index finger. A long tendinous structure was seen originating from the flexor or indicis profundus, forming an independent lumbrical for the index finger. A similar structure was found originating in the forearm from the flexor pollicis longus and from an accessory pollicis longus and then proceeding distally, ending as a lumbrical to the index finger. The absence of the first and the second lumbricals has been reported in the literature.

All known variations should be kept in mind in dealing with interpretation of afflictions, injuries, and surgical treatment of hands. The significance of the variations may be made clear by referring to the analalysis of Humphry and more modern investigators.

Blood supply to the lumbricals

The abundant blood supply that the lumbricals receive indicates that when they are present their function, is apparently important. According to Salmon and Dor, the blood supply reaches the muscular bellies from their volar and dorsal aspect.

Each muscle is supplied on its deep or dorsal aspect with a lumbrical artery, a branch of the deep volar arch. The branch runs distally and volarly. It is about 20 mm to 30 mm long and divides into an ascending and descending branch entering the first and the second lumbricals at about the middle of the muscle; the branch for the third and the fourth lumbricals enters the muscle more distally. At times, the arteries enter the muscle more superficially, winding around their radial side. Sometimes, an additional branch is derived from the volar interosseous artery of the forearm. The volar aspect of the muscle is supplied by small branches of the digital arteries from the superficial arterial arch.

Nerve supply

The standard description of the nerves supplying

the lumbricals shows that the first and the second lumbricals are supplied by the branches of the median nerve; the third and the fourth, by the branches of the ulnar nerve; however, the nerve supply is variable and will be considered in the chapter on the general nerve supply of the hand. The nerves usually enter the muscles at about the middle third of the muscle on the radial side for lumbricals 1 and 2 and from the deep dorsal side for lumbricals 3 and 4.

The role of the lumbricals, which will be considered further in the section on motors and mechanism of action of the fingers, is of great importance. Inasmuch as the lumbricals constitute a connection between the flexor and extensor mechanism of the fingers, they obviously have a moderating and controlling action on the two motors.

Studies of this action have been made from various angles. Electromyographic and histologic investigations are being constantly carried on. In a recent study on the proprio-

ceptive innervation of the lumbricals, valuable information was obtained (Rabischong). The complexity of this innervation and the different types of proprioceptive receptors in the lumbrical muscles were found to be far more abundant than in any other striated muscle. Rabischong considers the lumbricals can be regarded as true tonsiometers supplying minute peripheral stimulations in the flexion-extension antagonistic activity; therefore, it is advisable in surgical procedures to avoid any disturbance of the lumbrical muscles. It is better to avoid using the lumbrical muscles to protect tendon suture lines in tendon surgery in the palm of the hand. Every possible effort should be made not to disturb the lumbricals or their blood and nerve supply. Lumbrical function is so complex that when function is altered after injury, you may find it a good practice to perform a tenotomy of the lumbrical during flexor tendon reconstruction procedures rather than risk restricted tendon motion due to lumbrical imbalance.

3
The Thumb

Emanuel B. Kaplan
Daniel C. Riordan

By its position and function, the thumb differs from the other fingers; it differs as well in structure and the arrangement of the motors and in the configuration and length of the bones. There are notable variations in the length of the thumb from person to person. The thumb is of special interest to the hand surgeon, the physical anthropologist, and the comparative anatomist. The important function of the thumb is its movement in opposition to the index finger, and to the other fingers. Since Duchenne described opposition as a combined movement involving the metacarpocarpal joint, the proximal joint, and the distal interphalangeal joint, various interpretations have been added. Opposition and its relation to the function of the hand will be considered in the section on function. The differences in the abilities of various species to use the thumb has been studied, but more extensive studies are necessary. The relation of thumb function to the presence or absence of the flexor pollicis longus in certain anthropoids and to the ability to fully extend the fingers in certain other species requires further observations.

The bones of the thumb differ from the bones of the other digits in size and in the relation of the proximal phalanx to the carpus. The skeleton of the thumb consists of two rather than three phalanges and one metacarpal. The metacarpal of the thumb was subjected to intensive investigation to determine whether it is a true metacarpal or a proximal phalanx. These investigations are of interest and show a variety of viewpoints not of immediate importance to the surgeon or to the subject of function. It must be noted that the metacarpal of the thumb shows the same characteristic of ossification as the phalanges; all other metacarpal bones develop from a central nucleus for the shaft and the secondary distal epiphysis in the head. The metacarpal of the thumb, like the phalanges, develops from a central nucleus and a secondary proximal epiphysis in the base. The developmental similarity of the first metacarpal to the phalanges does not change the present-day consideration of the first metacarpal as a true metacarpal. It is accepted by many that the thumb is actually deprived of the middle phalanx. Many believe that in triphalangeal thumbs, the additional phalanx represents the missing middle phalanx of the thumb. It should be noted that when the triphalangeal thumb is present, the metacarpal base does not have a saddle joint articulating with a bone shaped like the trapezium. In such triphalangeal thumbs, the metacarpal base is flat and articulates with a carpal bone shaped like the trapezoid rather than like the trapezium. The triphalangeal thumb therefore does not have the ability to circumduct.

The proximal phalanx of the thumb is shorter than the proximal phalanges of the other fingers; it is longer than the middle phalanges of the other fingers. The distal phalanx is longer than the distal phalanges of other fingers by 2 mm to 4 mm. It is also wider and thicker than the distal phalanges of other fingers. The base of the distal phalanx is about 3 mm thicker anteroposteriorly than the thickest base of the distal phalanx of the middle finger. The width of the base is about 1.5 times wider than the widest base of the distal phalanx of the middle finger. The ratio of the lengths of the phalanges and the metacarpals of the thumb, if the distal phalanx is taken as a unit, is as follows: 1 (distal phalanx), 1.1 to 1.6 (proximal phalanx), 1.6 to 2.6 (metacarpal). The thickness of the proximal phalanx of the thumb is approximately equal to the thickness of the proximal phalanx of the index finger—an average of 5 mm to 6 mm. The metacarpal of the thumb is the shortest of all metacarpals except the triphalangeal thumb, in which case it is equivalent in length to the metacarpal of the ring or little finger.

PHALANGES AND METACARPAL

The distal phalanx of the thumb is similar to the distal phalanges of the other fingers (Figs. 2–2 and 2–3). Except for its greater length and width, it differs only slightly. The lateral and the anterolateral tubercles are more accentuated. The volar aspect of the base for insertion of the flexor pollicis longus appears to be more excavated and rougher. The dorsal aspect of the base shows a thick crest just distal to the articular surface that is slightly more elevated in the middle. The crest and the mid-elevation serve as areas of insertion for the extensor pollicis longus. The articular surface is divided by a midcrest into two concave surfaces for articulation with the head of the proximal phalanx.

The proximal phalanx consists of a head, a shaft, and a base. The head is similar to the head of the proximal phalanx of the other fingers. The articulating area is wider and larger, extending slightly more over the volar surface of the shaft with a line of demarcation separating the articular surface from the volar and dorsal surfaces of the shaft. The shaft has no lateral crests, and the borders are more nearly round; very seldom can a nutrient foramen be found on the surface of the shaft. The base of the proximal phalanx has multiple large foramina over the volar surface for nutrient vessels. The lateral tubercles are prominent. The dorsal aspect of the base has a crest separating the shaft from the articular surface. The crest represents the area of insertion of the extensor pollicis brevis. The articular surface of the base differs from the articular surfaces of the bases of other fingers; it is flatter and less excavated in order to accommodate the head of the metacarpal, which is not spheroidal as are the heads of the other metacarpals.

The first metacarpal is the shortest and differs in the configurations of its head and base. The shaft is broader, and its anteroposterior thickness is relatively less pronounced. The average thickness in the midshaft normally varies from 6 mm to 11 mm. The average thickness of the phalanges and metacarpals is emphasized because of the general use of fixation wires through these small bones in surgery and treatment of fractures, which necessitates choosing wires of appropriate diameter.

The head of the first metacarpal is much less spheroidal than the heads of the other metacarpals because it favors hinge-joint action in contrast with the universal-joint action possible in the metacarpophalangeal joints of the other fingers. Apparently this is characteristic not only of the human hand but also of the anthropoid hand (Fig. 1–2). The anterolateral tubercles are prominent. The articular surface is wide and flat and has a quadrilateral appearance; the volar side is slightly larger and extends on the volar surface of the shaft. A slight depression is found in the volar midline between the tubercles of the head (Fig. 2–3). Each tubercle articulates with the corresponding sesamoid.

The base of the metacarpal is most characteristic and differs greatly from all the other metacarpals. There are no articular facets on either side because this metacarpal does not articulate with other metacarpals. The only articular surface is found on the proximal side of the base for articulation with the trapezium. The articulating surface of the metacarpal is convex in the transverse direction and concave in the dorsovolar direction (Fig. 3–1). The articular surface is separated from the shaft by a crestlike ridge that stands out over the circumference of the articular surface. The configuration of the base is significant because it plays an important role in the mechanism of opposition of the thumb; it represents half of the saddle joint that it forms with the corresponding surface of the trapezium.

JOINTS OF THE THUMB

The joints of the thumb present distinct differences when compared with the corresponding joints of the other fingers. The differences are

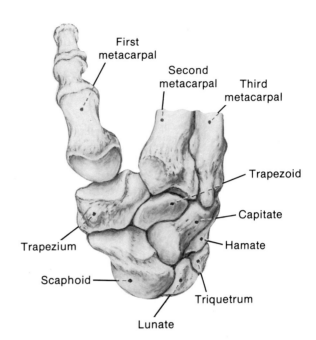

FIG. 3–1 The skeletal column of the thumb. The first metacarpal is flexed showing the saddle joint of the trapeziometacarpal joint, which permits ample rotation for complete opposition.

of general interest but are of special significance to the surgeon because they help to indicate some of the possible failures in surgical treatment around the joints.

INTERPHALANGEAL JOINT

The interphalangeal joint of the thumb is formed by the base of the distal phalanx and the head of the proximal phalanx. It is a massive hinge joint with a strong capsule and ligaments usually permitting only insignificant lateral motion. The capsule is attached to the ridge of the articular surface of the base and to the ridge of the articular surface of the head of the proximal phalanx. The capsule is reinforced by two collateral ligaments and their extensions into the volar fibrocartilaginous plate. The tendon of the flexor pollicis longus passes over the plate to reach its insertion, which occurs over a wide and sometimes deeply excavated surface of the volar surface of the base between two tubercles that are placed over the lateral borders of the volar surface of the base of the phalanx. A sesamoid embedded in the tendon just proximal to the base of the phalanx is occasionally present and should not be mistaken for an avulsion fracture of the flexor pollicis longus insertion into the distal phalanx.

The dorsal base of the distal phalanx just distal to the insertion of the capsule has a slightly elevated ridge for insertion of the extensor pollicis longus alone or with the extensor pollicis brevis, which sometimes passes over its area of normal insertion and proceeds toward the base of the distal phalanx. The dorsal insertion consists of longitudinal fibers continuing from the tendon of the extensor pollicis longus or the combination of the extensor longus and brevis tendons. The single or combined tendon has a well-defined edge on each side of the joint.

On minute dissection and in transverse sections of fetal thumbs, the pattern of the tendon insertion is found to be similar to the insertion patterns of the distal interphalangeal joints of other fingers. Oblique fibers are found uniting the tendon with the collateral ligaments for ultimate connection to the tunnel of the flexor pollicis longus (Fig. 3–2). These fibers are parallel with the direction of the collateral ligaments of the joint and securely anchor the dorsal tendon to the volar apparatus without interfering with the motion of the joint. The tendon of the extensor also adheres to the dorsal part of the capsule of this joint. The lateral collateral ligaments are inserted into the rough lateral depressions on each side of the head of the proximal phalanx and the lateral tubercles of the head. From this area, they run distally and volarly to the lateral tubercles of the base and to the fibrous or fibrocartilaginous plate of the volar aspect of the joint.

METACARPOPHALANGEAL JOINT

The metacarpophalangeal joint is formed by the connection of the metacarpal head and the base

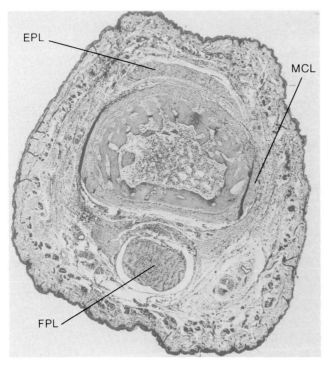

EPL

MCL

FPL

FIG. 3–2 Section through the distal end of the proximal phalanx of the thumb of a premature 5-month fetus. The tendon of the extensor pollicis longus (EPL) with expansion toward the medial collateral ligament (MCL) and toward the tunnel of the flexor pollicis longus (FPL) is demonstrated.

of the proximal phalanx with the addition of the two sesamoid bones, which are constantly present. The lateral sesamoid is usually larger than the medial sesamoid. A capsule unites the osseous elements of the joint. It is inserted into the ridge separating the articular surface of the shaft of the proximal phalanx and the metacarpal. The capsule is thin dorsally and much thicker on the volar surface. The capsule is reinforced on each side by the collateral ligaments, which are inserted into the sides of the head of the metacarpal and run distally and volarly to the base of the proximal phalanx. Each collateral ligament is inserted into the lateral tubercle of the base of the proximal phalanx and into the corresponding sesamoid. The two sesamoids are incorporated into the fibrocartilage or the volar plate of the joint; thus, the collateral ligament and volar plate with the sesamoid actually form a continuous structure (Fig. 3–3). The tunnel of the flexor pollicis longus is intimately connected to the volar plate so that

the tunnel also becomes an integral part of the apparatus, connecting the lateral ligaments and the volar plate with the sesamoids. The volar plate with the sesamoids and the capsule are firmly attached to the volar base of the proximal phalanx and move as a unit with the proximal phalanx in flexion and extension. In flexion, the volar plate moves toward the volar aspect of the shaft of the metacarpal, and in extension it moves away from the volar aspect of the metacarpal.

The metacarpophalangeal joint can be flexed and extended. The range of flexion is usually less than that of the other metacarpophalangeal joints; extension is normally about 180 degrees. A few persons can achieve extreme hyperextension of this joint, whereas others are unable to extend this joint even to 180 degrees; some can flex this joint only to 25 or 30 degrees. The joint can show a certain degree of lateral inclination produced by the pull of the abductor brevis muscle. The role of this angulation in

FIG. 3–3 Section through the metacarpophalangeal joint of a fetal right thumb. The expansion of the fibers from the (EPL) run into the adductor pollicis (AP) on the ulnar side and into the abductor pollicis brevis (APB) on the radial side. The flexor tunnel for the FPL is shown intimately wedged between the radial and the ulnar sesamoids in intimate connection with the short muscles of thumb, which themselves are in intimate connection with the expansion of the tendon of the EPB. The EPL tendon is located nearer the ulnar side of the thumb over the dorsum of the phalanx. The ulnar collateral ligament is seen deep to the extensor expansion. The volar plate (VP) is visualized between the sesamoids.

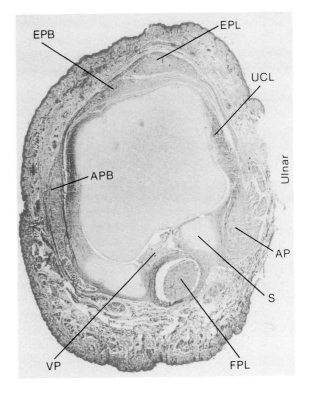

opposition was first analyzed by Duchenne and will be discussed in the section on function. Generally speaking, there is a certain degree of relaxation of the collateral ligaments in extension and a tightening of the collateral ligaments in flexion. In older individuals, the lateral collateral ligaments lose flexibility and show marked restriction of lateral motion.

The dorsum of the joint is in contact with the tendinous apparatus of the long and short extensors of the thumb; the lateral parts of the joint are integrated with the short muscles of the thumb. The specific relationship of these structures to the capsular and ligamentous apparatus of the metacarpophalangeal joint is responsible for the characteristic differences of action between the thumb and the other fingers. These details are described along with the motor of the thumb.

The arrangement of the articular surfaces, the lateral ligaments, and the volar ligament with the sesamoid are important in understanding the movement of this joint. The configuration of the head of the metacarpal is different from that of the other metacarpals: it is somewhat quadrilateral with the dorsal side slightly wider than the volar side. The cartilaginous surface of the head is divided into two units: one articulating with the base of the proximal phalanx and the other, more volar, with the sesamoids.

The ligaments of the thumb reinforce the capsule. The dorsal capsule is thin and is in direct relationship with the tendon of the extensor pollicis longus to which it adheres. The volar side of the joint is covered by a thick glenoid ligament or volar plate that contains the two sesamoids. The plate intimately adheres to the volar base of the proximal phalanx and somewhat more loosely to the neck of the metacarpal. In flexion and extension, the sesamoids remain in contact with the articulating area of the metacarpal head; however, there is a sufficient area of contact between the sesamoid articulations and the corresponding articulations on the volar surface of the metacarpal head to permit the sesamoids to move proximally for contact of the base of the proximal phalanx with the volar part of the metacarpal head in flexion. The collateral ligaments, similar to those in the other metacarpophalangeal joints, consist of two types: one collateral (the cord portion) runs from the lateral side of the metacarpal to the lateral tubercle of the proximal phalanx on each side of the metacarpophalangeal joint, and the other runs more volar to the sesamoids and the volar plate (Figs. 3–4 and 3–5), in a similar manner. The two sesamoids are connected by transverse fibers. A tunnel adherent to the connecting transverse fibers serves for the passage of the tendon of the flexor pollicis longus.

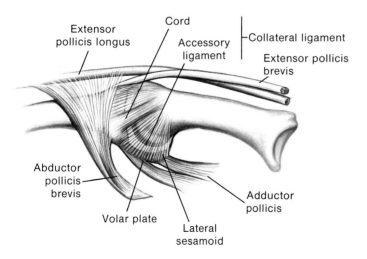

FIG. 3–4 Radial side of the metacarpophalangeal joint of the right thumb. Diagrammatic presentation of details of the joint and intrinsic and extrinsic tendon insertions.

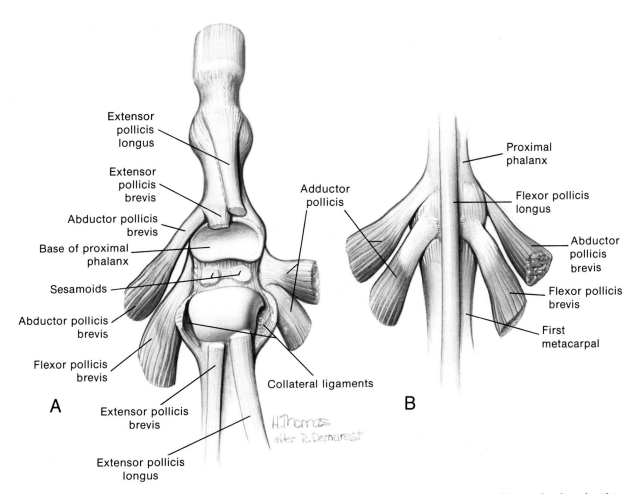

Extensor
pollicis
longus

Extensor
pollicis
brevis

Abductor pollicis
brevis

Base of proximal
phalanx

Sesamoids

Abductor pollicis
brevis

Flexor pollicis
brevis

Adductor
pollicis

Collateral ligaments

A

Extensor pollicis
brevis

Extensor pollicis
longus

H.Thomas
after R.Demarest

Proximal
phalanx

Flexor pollicis
longus

Abductor
pollicis
brevis

Flexor pollicis
brevis

First
metacarpal

B

FIG. 3–5 A, Inner view of the metacarpophalangeal joint of the right thumb. This is a dorsal view of the metacarpal joint of the right thumb in which the dorsal capsule is removed, the lateral ligaments are excised, and only the parts attached to the metacarpal are shown. The accessory ligaments are excised, leaving only a small part under the lateral ligaments. The volar plate with the sesamoids is shown at the bottom of the joint. **B,** Volar view of the metacarpophalangeal joint of the right thumb.

The literature contains little information on the function of the sesamoids. The most common belief is that the sesamoid bones are located near joints to increase the leverage of certain muscles connected with tendons running to these joints, but this general statement may be easily challenged. Although the patella may be considered in this category, it is difficult to see the function of a fabella in the lateral gastrocnemius or of the sesamoids in the abaxial metacarpal bones of certain animals in which they have no particular function, as in the manus of a pig. Intratendinous inclusions may also have varied significance and function, as exemplified by the occasional presence of an ossicle in the popliteus tendon.

The sesamoids are present under all the metacarpophalangeal joints of carnivora. In the

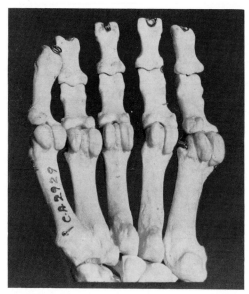

FIG. 3–6 Volar aspect of the forepaw of a North American bear. The first metacarpal is on the left.

it is more to our purpose to inquire what are their anatomical associations in those animals in which their development is carried to a further state of perfection than that seen in Man. When the bones are developed in their dump-bell form, the grip of the dumb-bell forms a pulley groove over which the flexor tendons run, and at the two knobs of bone at either end are the flexor insertions of the short intrinsic muscles. In whatever animal metacarpophalangeal sesamoids are found, they are always present in association with the short intrinsic digital flexors.

Jones concludes with the statement

They are not produced by pressure or hard work, they are not caused by old age, but they are ossicles in the tendons of insertion of a fluctuating group of intrinsic muscles which produce flexion of the metacarpophalangeal joints.

The solution of the problem, as mentioned above, will have to include an explanation of the function of the sesamoids not only in the hand but in all areas where they are present.

The metacarpophalangeal joint of the thumb is of great interest and importance because of its specialized function in opposition. The joint is formed by the base of the first metacarpal and the trapezium bone and it is a saddle joint that permits only a certain form of motion. The articular surface of the base of the first metacarpal has a concave surface in the anteroposterior plane and a convex surface in the lateral direction, with the middle part of the anterior aspect of the articular surface elevated. The trapezium has a reverse arrangement of its articular surface to accommodate the base of the metacarpal. The articular surface is convex in the anteroposterior direction and concave from side to side. The configuration of the articular surfaces is such that only a certain type of movement was once considered possible. The base of the metacarpal, according to Fick, could move only in abduction and adduction or flexion and extension. Fick stated that opposition was a combined motion involving no rotation of the metacarpal around its longitudinal axis but rather a complex of flexion adduction. The reverse motion was called *reposition* and was concerned chiefly with extension. The whole

American bear, two sesamoids are present at each metacarpophalangeal joint (Fig. 3–6). Tendons of the flexors of the toes pass through tunnels confined between each group of two sesamoid bones. The bear carries the weight of his forefoot mostly on the front part of his foot. Do the sesamoids then act as protectors and stabilizers of the flexor tendons in the midline of the joint? In the human thumb, the flexor pollicis longus runs through an area over the metacarpophalangeal joint that functionally sustains more pressure than other areas of the hand.

It is known that in hallux valgus deformities the two sesamoid bones are deflected laterally with the flexor hallucis longus tendon between them, and with rotation of the proximal phalanx, the flexor tendon follows the sesamoids to the lateral side. The abductor and the adductor muscles remain inserted into their corresponding sesamoids, but their function is distorted, whereas the relationship of the flexor hallucis tendon and the sesamoids remains the same. In his *Principle of Anatomy*, the famous anatomist, Jones, stated in reference to sesamoids

motion, according to Fick, was dictated by the arrangement of the articular surfaces. Clinical observations made since Fick's accurate analysis have brought out additional explanations.

CARPOMETACARPAL JOINT

Cornacchia described the mechanism of action occurring in the carpometacarpal joint. He stated that rotation around the longitudinal axis of the metacarpal takes place within a limited range of 15 to 20 degrees, passively or actively, at the termination of flexion of the metacarpal. The rotation, according to this author, is possible because of elasticity of the articular cartilage and because the *capsule of the joint is lax.*

The issue of the capsule's laxity is important. It is obvious that a saddle joint permits limited motion in accordance with the form of contiguous surfaces, but clinicians are also aware that rotation of the metacarpal definitely occurs. Dissection of the carpometacarpal joint reveals the reason for the possibility of rotation. The capsule uniting the base of the metacarpal with

the trapezium is very lax and can be distended easily by injection of a fluid into the joint. On opening the capsule (Fig. 3–7), the extent of the intra-articular space demonstrates that the surfaces are not kept together tightly. Anteriorly it is reinforced by muscular fibers of the thenar muscles and posteriorly by the extensor pollicis longus and brevis; however, all these reinforcements do not significantly restrict the rotation of the metacarpal around its axis on the fixed trapezium.

The carpometacarpal joint of the thumb was generally not described in sufficient detail. With the development of interest in the movement of opposition of the thumb and the disabling fractures of the base of the first metacarpal, interest in the carpometacarpal joint contributed to a number of studies; however, it must be mentioned that Weitbrecht gave a precise description of the joint and its ligaments and a simple but correct interpretation of function in 1742. Duchenne gave a comprehensive functional explanation of opposition of the thumb in relation to the metacarpocarpal joint in 1867, and

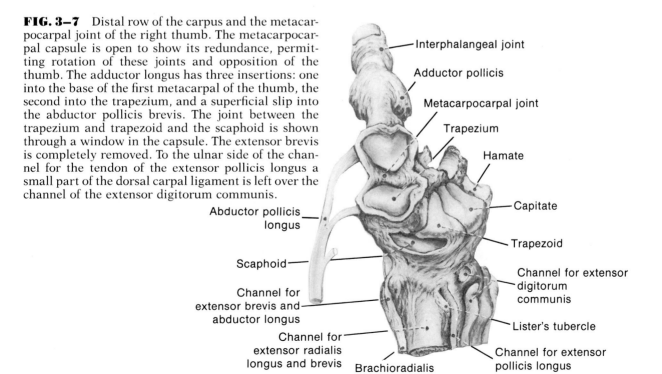

FIG. 3–7 Distal row of the carpus and the metacarpocarpal joint of the right thumb. The metacarpocarpal capsule is open to show its redundance, permitting rotation of these joints and opposition of the thumb. The adductor longus has three insertions: one into the base of the first metacarpal of the thumb, the second into the trapezium, and a superficial slip into the abductor pollicis brevis. The joint between the trapezium and trapezoid and the scaphoid is shown through a window in the capsule. The extensor brevis is completely removed. To the ulnar side of the channel for the tendon of the extensor pollicis longus a small part of the dorsal carpal ligament is left over the channel of the extensor digitorum communis.

Interphalangeal joint

Adductor pollicis

Metacarpocarpal joint

Trapezium

Hamate

Capitate

Trapezoid

Channel for extensor digitorum communis

Lister's tubercle

Channel for extensor pollicis longus

Abductor pollicis longus

Scaphoid

Channel for extensor brevis and abductor longus

Channel for extensor radialis longus and brevis

Brachioradialis

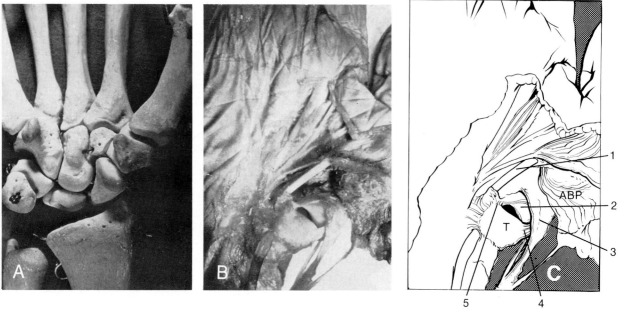

FIG. 3—8   A, Volar view of an articulated right wrist. The first metacarpal on the right shows the articulation of its base with the trapezium. The pointed beak is directed toward the tubercle of the trapezium. The hamate is on the left side of the illustration with the hook of the hamate standing out. **B** and **C**, Right hand. The metacarpocarpal joint is exposed; the capsule of the joint is removed; the abductor pollicis brevis is separated from the joint and is retracted distally. (1) Tendon of FPL; (2) base of the first metacarpal with its beak; (3) the APL inserted into the base of the first metacarpal; (4) lateral ligament; (5) ulnar ligament; (T) trapezium.

FIG. 3—9   A, Right thumb metacarpocarpal joint. Bones of the joint in opposition and flexion. **B**, Same, in abduction, extension, and traction.

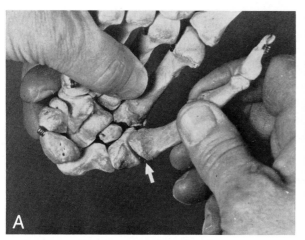
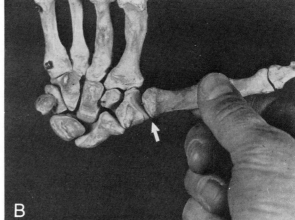

comprehensive studies have been made by several recent investigators (Bunnell, Gedda, Moberg, Stenner, and Napier). Our multiple dissections and observations of fractures of the base and the shaft of the first metacarpal have led to a more precise description of the carpometacarpal joint, confirming the findings of Gedda and Napier.

The following illustrations show the configuration of the first metacarpal and the trapezium, the bony structures constituting the joint. The base of the first metacarpal shows a triangular beak that in neutral position of the thumb is oriented toward the ridge of the trapezium (Fig. 3–8A). The beak of the base of the first metacarpal and the most distal part of the ridge on the tubercle of the trapezium are united by a strong ligament—the ulnar ligament of the carpometacarpal joint (Figs. 3–8B and C). The lateral side of the base of the first metacarpal, immediately proximal to the insertion of the tendon of the abductor pollicis longus, is the site of insertion of a lateral ligament that connects

this area of the metacarpal with the lateral side of the trapezium (Figs. 3–8B and C); thus, the capsule of the carpometacarpal joint is reinforced by a strong ulnar ligament and a lateral ligament. A dorsal reinforcement is found between the dorsal aspect of the base of the first metacarpal and the trapezium, and this reinforcement, or dorsal ligament, is covered by the tendons of the extensor pollicis brevis and longus with their intertendinous fascia.

In flexion and opposition of the thumb, the beak of the base of the first metacarpal fits into the area of the trapezium, corresponding to the most distal part of the tubercle of the trapezium (Fig. 3–9A). In abduction, extension, and traction, the beak of the first metacarpal base is elevated and pulled away from the trapezium (Fig. 3–9B). The ulnar ligament, which unites the tubercle of the trapezium and the beak of the metacarpal base does not permit much retraction (Fig. 3–10) unless the protruding beak is broken off. The ulnar ligament retains the fragment near the trapezium, but the rest of the

FIG. 3–10 A, Metacarpocarpal joint with the right thumb in abduction, extension, and traction with ulnar ligament intact. The beak of the base of the metacarpal remains in the vicinity of the trapezium. **B,** Metacarpocarpal joint in radial rotation of the thumb. Rotation still maintains the relationship of the metacarpal beak and the trapezium in the presence of an intact ulnar ligament.

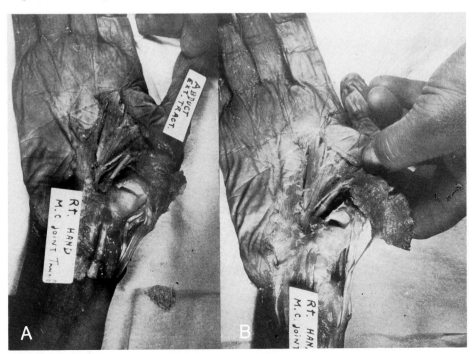

metacarpal base with the metacarpal shaft is retracted posteriorly by the abductor longus and the two extensors of the thumb.

The capsule is attached to the ridge of the base of the first metacarpal, which surrounds the articular surface at a distance of 1.5 mm to 2 mm, contributing to the formation of an intra-articular recess all around the articular surface of the base.

BLOOD AND NERVE SUPPLY

The blood supply of the thumb is derived from branches of the radial artery, the first dorsal metacarpal, and the small branches of the dorsal carpal artery. The nerve supply follows Hilton's law. The nerves supplying the thenar muscles also supply the articular branches to the joint.

MUSCLES OF THE THUMB

The thumb is supplied with long muscles originating from the forearm and with short muscles of the thenar eminence originating from the structures of the wrist and hand. The long muscles are the flexor pollicis longus, the extensor pollicis longus, the extensor pollicis brevis, and the abductor pollicis longus. The short muscles are the abductor pollicis brevis, the flexor pollicis brevis, the opponens pollicis, and the adductor pollicis.

LONG MUSCLES

Flexor pollicis longus

The flexor pollicis longus has a large area of origin from almost the entire middle third of the volar surface of the radius to the ulnar side of the oblique line of insertion of the flexor superficialis and proximal to the insertion of the pronator quadratus. The origin extends over the radial third of the interosseous membrane of the forearm. On its ulnar side and in the same plane is found the flexor digitorum profundus. The flexor pollicis longus is covered by the radial head of the flexor digitorum sublimis, which separates the long flexor of the thumb from the pronator teres.

The muscle frequently receives an additional muscular slip from the coronoid process or from the medial condyle of the humerus, or from both (Fig. 3–11). The additional muscle is known as the *accessory muscle of Gantzer* (Fig. 3–11*A*). When present, it originates in common with the flexor superficialis and runs parallel with the ligament of Weitbrecht (chorda obliqua). In a series of 76 upper extremities examined by Mangini, the accessory head was observed in both forearms in 62% of cases. In most cases, the accessory head originated from the medial epicondyle of the humerus in association with the common origin of the forearm flexors. In 22% the origin was from the coronoid process, in 9% from the intermuscular fascia between the flexor superficialis and the flexor profundus. Occasionally the origin was from the medial epicondyle of the humerus and the coronoid process of the ulna simultaneously. The accessory muscle most frequently presents an independent tendon that runs parallel with the main tendon of the flexor pollicis longus.

A tendinous structure appears high in the muscle mass and gradually becomes round and independent of the muscle fibers on the ulnar side of the muscle. The muscle fibers descend with the tendon on its radial side to the level of the carpus and enter the carpal canal to the radial side of the flexor indicis profundus covered by the tendon of the flexor carpi radialis (Figs. 2–7 and 2–31).

In its course in the lower third of the forearm, the tendon crosses almost perpendicularly the transverse fibers of the pronator quadratus; it is then hidden completely behind the volar carpal ligament and more distally by the flexor brevis of the thumb until it reaches the proximal part of the metacarpophalangeal joint, where it appears in its flexor sheath in its course to its terminus on the volar side of the distal phalanx. In its passage over the volar surface of the metacarpophalangeal joint, the tendon is enclosed in its sheath and firmly wedged between the two sesamoids, which are themselves firmly entrenched in the fibrocartilaginous plate attached to the volar base of the proximal phalanx. The tendon passes somewhat nearer to the medial (ulnar) sesamoid, which is also the smaller and rounder sesamoid (Figs. 3–3 and 3–8).

Variations of the Flexor Pollicis Longus. The variations are of interest to the surgeon because they are not uncommon and may present problems of interpretation in muscular and nerve injuries. In humans, the muscle is completely separate from the flexor profundus digitorum, but phylogenetically, both derive from a common muscle mass, which makes it possible to find a common flexor profundus without division of the flexor pollicis longus into a separate muscle. The flexor pollicis longus may unite with the flexor indicis profundus, which separates from the rest of the profundus group. Not infrequently, an accessory flexor digitorum profundus to the index finger arises from the primary or secondary head of origin of the flexor pollicis longus (Fig. 3–11A and B). Rarely, this variant muscle arises from the distal third of the radius (Fig. 3–11C). Linburg (1979) demonstrated this anomaly in 25% of cadaver limbs, bilaterally in 6%. He reported four cases of probable chronic tenosynovitis caused by this variant.

Different combinations may occur between the flexor pollicis longus and the flexor superficialis and the other muscles because they derive from a common phylogenetic group of the pronatoflexors of Humphry.

The following variations have been reported: (1) more or less complete union of the two flexors—fusion of the different digital portions of the same muscle: termination of a flexor superficialis fleshy portion in the flexor profundus or in the long tendon that joins a tendon of the flexor profundus more distally; independent tendons of the flexor superficialis of the middle, ring, and little fingers united (ring and middle, little and ring); all sublimis tendons fused in the palm; fusion without perforation of the fourth and fifth; (2) absence of the radial origin of the flexor superficialis; (3) radial origin for the flexor profundus with tendons to the index or to the index and the thumb; (4) digastric flexor superficialis; (5) absence of the flexor to the little finger with a replacement from the anterior volar ligament; (6) supernumerary flexors with insertions either into the volar carpal ligament or the palmar aponeurosis; (7) independence of some of the tendons of the flexor profundus of either the index or the little finger; (8) supernumerary lumbricals; (9) fusion with other muscles.

Multiple arrangement normally seen in the anthropoids and monkeys may be observed as variations in humans. Frequently, the flexor pollicis longus is absent in the gorilla and chimpanzee. In the few anthropoid specimens that the author has dissected, no tendon to the distal phalanx was found. A vestige of the tendon, apparently without function and disappearing in the direction of the flexor profundus digitorum, is sometimes found (Fig. 1–3). The distal phalanx of the gorilla and chimpanzee does not show the deep excavation for the insertion of the tendon on the volar surface of its base observed in the distal phalanx of the human hand.

The author has dissected two hands of the same animal of a Tarsius Spectrum and found a separate muscle belly with a long, strong tendon representing the flexor pollicis longus; this has been reported by others.

Interestingly, the feet of the gorilla and the chimpanzee have well-developed flexor hallucis longus muscles. The muscle functions very efficiently and in a manner similar to that of the flexor pollicis longus of the human hand.

Blood and Nerve Supply. The arterial blood supply comes from the radial artery through two or three small branches entering the muscle at the junction of the middle and lower third, and from the anterior interosseous on the ulnar side of the muscle. Normally, the artery of the median nerve is not a source of supply, but this artery may occasionally also supply the muscle. The accessory muscle belly is supplied by a branch of the ulnar artery. No intramuscular anastomoses can be demonstrated by roentgenography. The muscle is innervated by a branch of the anterior interosseous of the

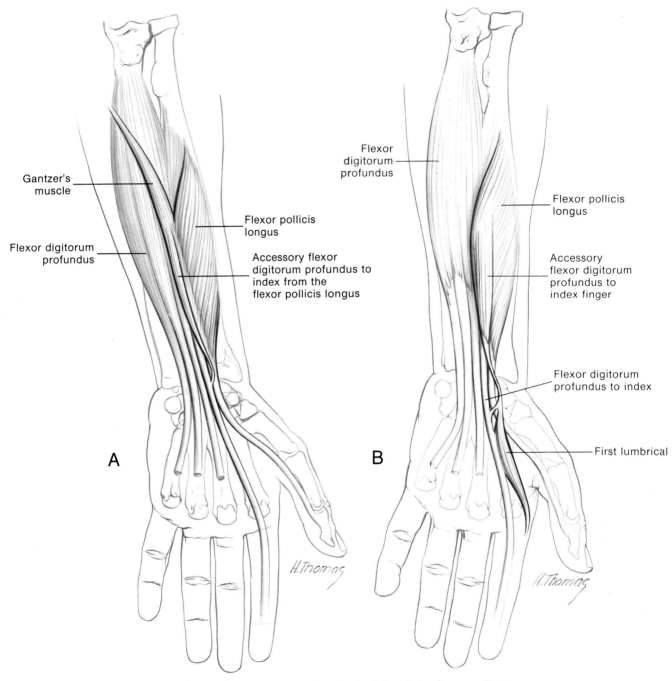

FIG. 3–11 A, Gantzer's muscle, an accessory head of origin of the flexor pollicis longus. This specimen had in addition an accessory flexor digitorum to the index finger, which arose from Gantzer's muscle. **B**, An accessory flexor digitorum profundus to the index finger is seen arising from the proximal portion of the flexor pollicis longus. In this anatomic specimen the anomalous muscle inserted both into the first lumbrical and the flexor digitorum profundus to the index finger. **C**, An accessory flexor digitorum profundus to the index finger arising from the distal radius. (From Dr. Emanuel B. Kaplan's anatomical sketches, circa 1924.)

median nerve. It branches off the anterior interosseous approximately 10 cm distal to the medial epicondyle of the humerus, in the vicinity of the nerve supplying the flexor digitorum profundus.

Extensor pollicis longus

The extensor pollicis longus originates together with the extensor pollicis brevis, the abductor pollicis longus, and the extensor indicis proprius from a common area of the posterior aspect of the mid-forearm. The extensor pollicis longus is located between the abductor pollicis longus and the extensor pollicis brevis, which originate more proximally, and the extensor indicis proprius, which originates more distally.

The extensor pollicis longus comes off the middle third of the posterior aspect of the ulna in a narrow strip extending distally and ulnad to the interosseous membrane and adhering to the intermuscular septum that separates the extensor indicis proprius from the extensor carpi ulnaris. The muscle fibers converge in a bipenniform mode and join a tendon that enters a special groove on the posterior aspect of the radius covered by the dorsal carpal ligament (Fig. 3–12). This tendon crosses the two radial extensors of the wrist from the ulnar to the radial side, finally coursing over the dorsum of the first metacarpal toward the dorsum of the metacarpophalangeal joint and widening over the proximal phalanx (Figs. 3–13 and 3–14). It crosses the interphalangeal joint over the dorsum and reaches its final insertion over the dorsum of the base of the distal phalanx, where it spreads widely (Fig. 3–13).

Extensor pollicis brevis

The extensor pollicis brevis originates from a small area of the ulna just proximal to the extensor pollicis longus and running parallel with and proximal to the origin of the extensor pollicis longus. It comes off the adjacent area of the interosseous membrane and impinges on the middle third of the contiguous part of the dorsal aspect of the radius. The muscle runs in a distal and lateral direction with the tendon of the abductor pollicis longus, which lies more lateral. Both tendons travel toward the posterolateral

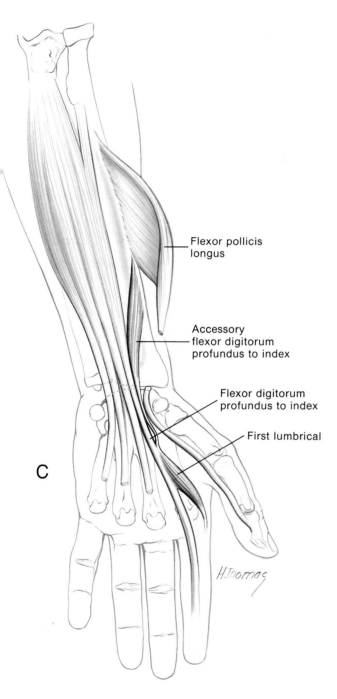

Flexor pollicis longus

Accessory flexor digitorum profundus to index

Flexor digitorum profundus to index

First lumbrical

C

H. Thomas

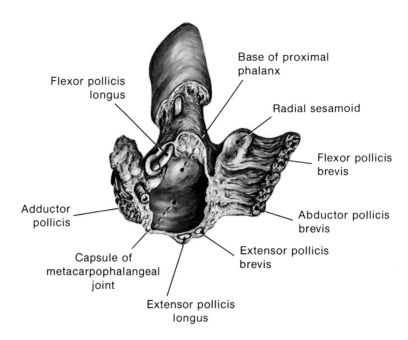

Flexor pollicis longus

Base of proximal phalanx

Radial sesamoid

Flexor pollicis brevis

Abductor pollicis brevis

Extensor pollicis brevis

Adductor pollicis

Capsule of metacarpophalangeal joint

Extensor pollicis longus

FIG. 3–12   The thumb of the right hand disarticulated at the metacarpocarpal joint to show the base of the proximal phalanx. The capsule of the joint was cut longitudinally, and the radial sesamoid was reflected to the radial side of the thumb after separation from the phalanx. The ulnar sesamoid was not dissected out. The flexor brevis is inserted into the radial sesamoid; the abductor brevis is inserted dorsal to the sesamoid and partly into the sesamoid. On the ulnar side the adductor is inserted into the sesamoid. The fibers of the abductor and the adductor are shown on continuation with the aponeurosis, which encloses the extensor pollicus longus and brevis. The tendon of the FPL is shown in its tunnel, which is partly dissected. The tunnel with the flexor tendon is located somewhat nearer to the ulnar sesamoid than to the radial sesamoid.

aspect of the dorsum of the radius where they enter a common groove under the cover of the dorsal carpal ligament. Within this first compartment the extensor pollicis brevis tendon may be separated from the abductor pollicis longus tendon by a fibrous septum so that each tendon has its own compartment. This septum may occasionally be a bony septum forming two completely separate compartments, one for each tendon. (These anatomic variations must be recognized when treating de Quervain's stenosing tenosynovitis.) The tendon continues its course after abandoning the companion tendon of the abductor pollicis longus and runs toward the metacarpophalangeal joint. It crosses the dorsum of this joint almost in the middle and inserts into the dorsal base of the proximal phalanx (Fig. 3–13).

Abductor pollicis longus

The abductor pollicis longus originates in the most proximal location of the common group from the lateroposterior aspect of the ulna, between the origin of the supinator muscle proximally and the extensor pollicis brevis distally. The course of the muscle fibers is very oblique distally and laterally. Additional origin in the same direction takes place from the interosseous membrane and the medial contiguous part of the posterior aspect of the radius just proximal to the origin of the extensor pollicis brevis. The muscle runs together with the muscle belly of the extensor pollicis brevis and crosses the two tendons of the radial extensors in the lower third of the posterolateral aspect of the forearm (Fig. 3–14). The muscular fibers end on a tendon that emerges on the deep part of the muscle. The

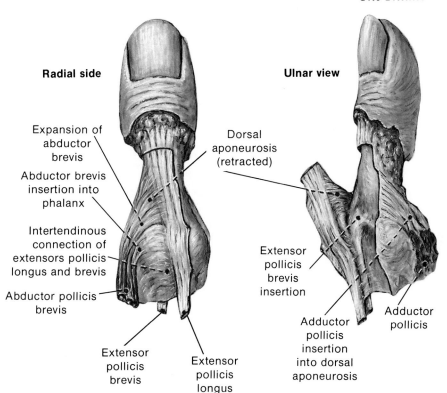

Radial side

Expansion of
abductor
brevis

Abductor brevis
insertion into
phalanx

Intertendinous
connection of
extensors pollicis
longus and brevis

Abductor pollicis
brevis

Extensor
pollicis
brevis

Extensor
pollicis
longus

Ulnar view

Dorsal
aponeurosis
(retracted)

Extensor
pollicis
brevis
insertion

Adductor
pollicis
insertion
into dorsal
aponeurosis

Adductor
pollicis

FIG. 3–13 Disarticulated right thumb at the metacarpophalangeal joint, dorsal and ulnar views. The dorsal aponeurosis is connected with the extensor pollicis longus. The extensor pollicis longus tendon is placed somewhat ulnad. On the radial side of the thumb, the extensor pollicis brevis is concealed by the dorsal aponeurosis and appears to be deeper than the extensor pollicis longus. On the radial side of the thumb, the tendon of the abductor pollicis brevis is extended toward the extensor pollicis longus after its insertion into the radial base of the proximal phalanx. The extension of the abductor pollicis brevis toward the dorsal aponeurosis consists of transverse and oblique arched fibers similar to the arciform fibers of the dorsal aponeurosis of the fingers.

An incision is made through the tendon of the extensor pollicis longus, and the tendon is retracted toward the radial side of the thumb. The ulnar view of the thumb shows the insertion of the extensor pollicis brevis into the base of the proximal phalanx. The tendon of the extensor pollicis longus is shown in its course toward the distal part of the thumb. The deep surface of this tendon shows its connection with the fascia and the capsule over the metacarpophalangeal joint. The arciform fibers connecting the abductor pollicis brevis with the tendon of the extensor pollicis longus are shown from the deep surface. Arciform fibers connecting the adductor pollicis are shown on the ulnar side of the thumb divided by the incision through the dorsal aponeurosis on the ulnar side of the tendon of the extensor pollicis longus.

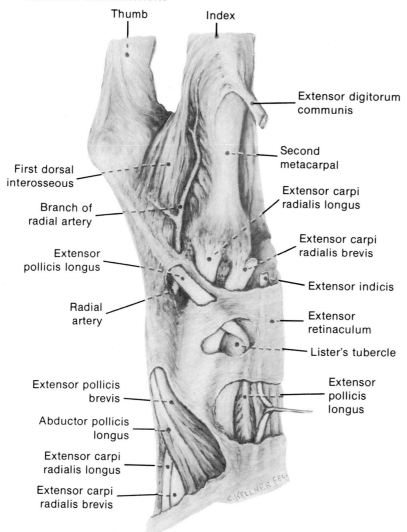

Thumb Index

Extensor digitorum communis

Second metacarpal

First dorsal interosseous

Extensor carpi radialis longus

Branch of radial artery

Extensor carpi radialis brevis

Extensor pollicis longus

Extensor indicis

Radial artery

Extensor retinaculum

Lister's tubercle

Extensor pollicis brevis

Extensor pollicis longus

Abductor pollicis longus

Extensor carpi radialis longus

Extensor carpi radialis brevis

FIG. 3—14 Radial half of the dorsum of the carpus right hand showing the first metacarpal and intercarpal space. Relationship of the important tendons in this region. A window was made into the dorsal carpal ligament of the wrist; another window was cut slightly proximal to it. The following relationship is to be noted: the extensor carpi radialis longus is inserted into the radial base of the second metacarpal, the extensor carpi radialis brevis is inserted into the ulnar base of the second metacarpal, and a short stump for the third metacarpal is shown separated from the third metacarpal. Just proximal to this insertion, a very interesting relationship can be noted: immediately distal to Lister's tubercle, two tendons are found crossing in the form of a letter X. These are invariably the extensor pollicis longus crossing the extensor carpi radialis brevis, which runs underneath the first tendon. A more distal X is formed by the tendon of the extensor pollicis longus with the extensor carpi radialis longus which runs underneath the extensor pollicis longus tendon. Very frequently Lister's tubercle conceals the tendon of the extensor pollicis longus. Just proximal to the Lister's tubercle the extensor pollicis longus becomes fleshy; the bipenniform appearance of the fleshy fibers permits its easy recognition. The anatomic snuff-box is covered with fascia. The radial artery can be seen in the depth. The first dorsal intermetacarpal artery is either a branch of the radial artery directly or of the dorsal carpal radial artery.

tendon, with the accompanying tendon of the extensor pollicis brevis, enters the groove on the lateral aspect of the radius under the cover of the dorsal carpal ligament. Finally, it inserts into the radial side of the base of the first metacarpal, sending a tendinous slip to the abductor pollicis brevis and a deep slip to the trapezium (Fig. 3–7).

Variations of the long extensors
The variations of the long extensor muscles of the thumb can be classified into several groups. In the largest group, the tendons of the long extensors may become double, and this division may progress proximally into the muscle body; in this case, the additional extensor may be considered as an extensor accessorius (Fig. 3–15). The extensor brevis may be completely absent or may not extend beyond the middle of the metacarpal, as is almost always found in the hand of the anthropoid ape (Fig. 2–57). The extensor pollicis brevis may be completely fused with the abductor pollicis longus. Not infrequently, the extensor pollicis longus is reinforced by a supernumerary extensor from the extensor digitorum communis.

The abductor pollicis longus is one of the most variable muscles of the forearm and very frequently represents supernumerary insertions for the first metacarpal, the annular ligament, the thenar muscles, or the trapezium. Complex forms sometimes occur in which there are two tendons for the first metacarpal and one for the trapezium, or there may be three tendons that divide more or less farther proximally, one for the metacarpal, one for the trapezium, and one for the abductor pollicis brevis. The division of the abductor tendon with a slip for the abductor pollicis brevis is so frequent that it may almost be considered normal. In some specimens there are four tendons: three divisions for the first metacarpal and one extending into the first dorsal interosseous. At times, a double abductor longus muscle can be observed, with one inserted in the usual location, forming the ulnar portion, another radial portion having two or three tendons for the first metacarpal, and a

fourth tendon for the opponens. The division into four tendons may assume a variety of insertions, as stated by Tesut: There may be two for the metacarpal, one for the short abductor of the thumb, and one for the short extensor of the thumb. The muscle may be completely absent when fused with the extensor brevis.

There is one other muscle that can be considered a supernumerary extensor longus. It is located between the extensor of the index and the extensor pollicis longus, with a double tendon and insertion into the thumb and index finger. This muscle may completely replace the extensor indicis or the extensor longus of the thumb, or it may coexist with other muscles.

Blood and nerve supply of the long extensors
The abductor longus and the extensor pollicis brevis are supplied by arterial branches from the lateral branch of the dorsal interosseous artery. The arterial branch runs between the abductor pollicis longus and the supinator muscles and supplies the long abductor. The other muscles are supplied by branches of the dorsal interosseous and the dorsal branch of the volar interosseous. The arteries do not enter the muscles with the nerves, but separately, forming more extensive anastomoses in the intermuscular planes than within the muscles. The nerve supply to the abductor and the two extensors is from the deep branch of the radial nerve. A deep division of the deep branch supplies the muscles entering their dorsal surfaces.

SHORT MUSCLES

The short muscles of the thumb are usually described as the muscles of the thenar eminence. The most superficial radial is the abductor pollicis brevis; and the deepest radial is the opponens. The only muscle on the ulnar side is the adductor pollicis, if the additional palmar interosseous is disregarded.

To eliminate confusion it is necessary to repeat that a few anatomists describe in addition to the three known palmar interossei an additional palmar interosseous that according to

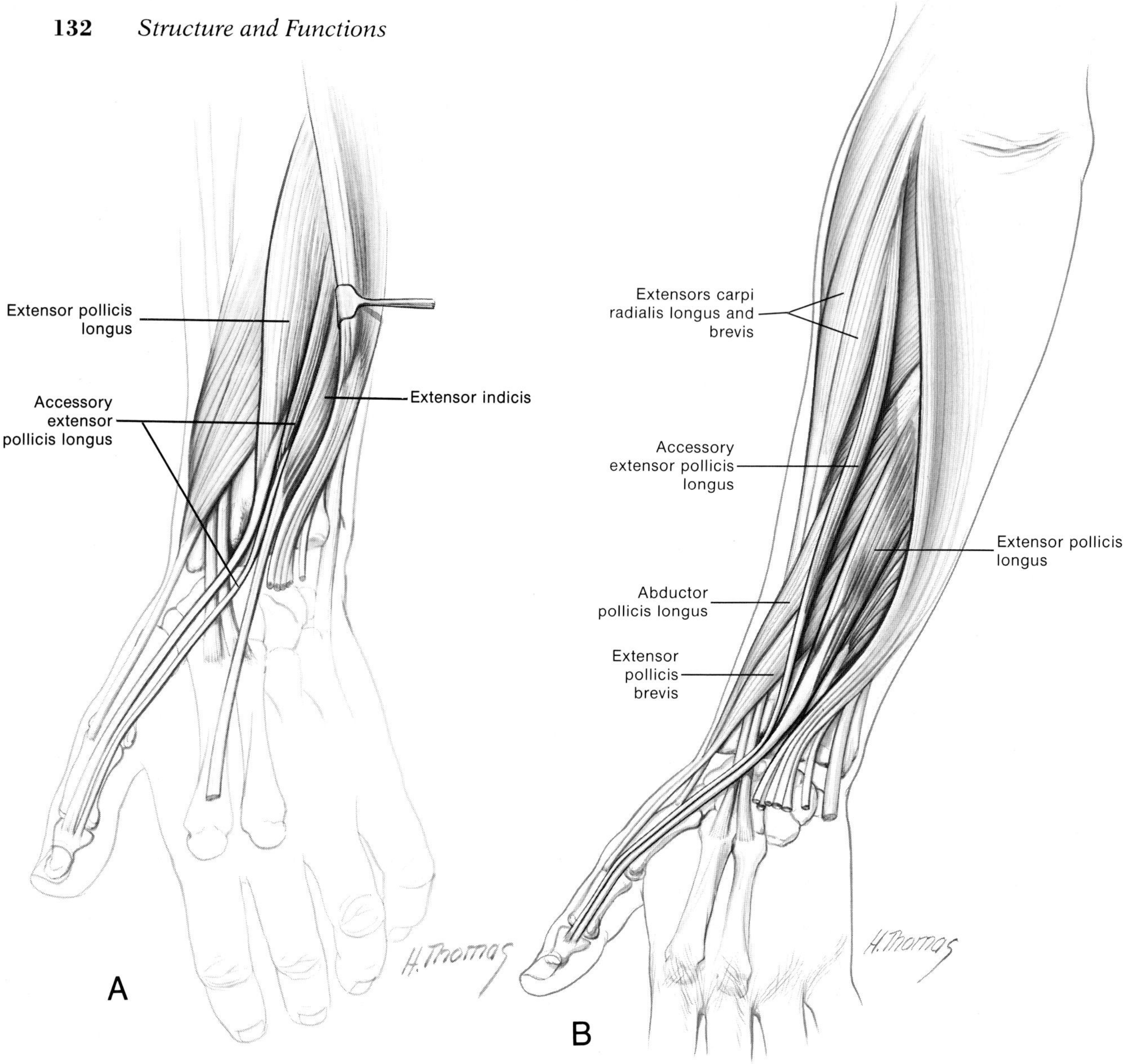

Extensor pollicis longus

Accessory extensor pollicis longus

Extensor indicis

Extensors carpi radialis longus and brevis

Accessory extensor pollicis longus

Extensor pollicis longus

Abductor pollicis longus

Extensor pollicis brevis

A

B

FIG. 3–15 A, Accessory extensor pollicis longus arising from the distal ulna. **B**, Accessory extensor pollicis longus arising from the aponeurosis of the extensor carpi radialis brevis (From Dr. Emanuel B. Kaplan's anatomical sketches, circa 1927.)

their description is located in the first interosseous space. This additional palmar interosseous originates from the anteromedial surface of the first metacarpal and from a small area on the anterior surface of the trapezium. Its few muscular fibers run parallel with the first metacarpal and according to this description, are inserted with the tendon of the adductor pollicis into the ulnar sesamoid. When this muscle exists, it is difficult to separate it from the adductor pollicis into a real muscle unit; however, it is often described as the first palmar interosseous. From practical, clinical, and surgical viewpoints, it is preferable to eliminate it completely; therefore, the muscle that is normally located in the second interosseous space and is inserted into the ulnar side of the index finger is now known universally as the first palmar interosseous.

Abductor pollicis brevis

The abductor pollicis brevis is the most superficial muscle of the thenar eminence. Immediately on removal of the skin and the thin fascia of the eminence, the muscle appears in its entirety with the muscle fibers running from the wrist to the metacarpophalangeal joint. On its posterior border, a few muscle fibers of the opponens emerge from underneath it.

Abductor pollicis brevis

The abductor pollicis brevis is the most superficial muscle of the thenar eminence. Immediately on removal of the skin and the thin fascia of the eminence, the muscle appears in its entirety with the muscle fibers running from the wrist to the metacarpophalangeal joint. On its posterior border, a few muscle fibers of the opponens emerge from underneath it. On its anterior border, other muscular fibers of the flexor pollicis brevis run almost parallel with the fibers of the abductor (Fig. 3–16).

The muscle fibers of the abductor brevis arise from the lateral half and the distal border of the volar carpal ligament (Fig. 3–16), which, in this area covers the crest of the trapezium and the tubercle of the scaphoid bone. The tubercle of the scaphoid bone lies dorsal to the tendon of the flexor carpi radialis (Fig. 2–63), and the volar carpal ligament lies volar to the tendon so that the fibers of the abductor brevis do not originate directly from the scaphoid bone (Fig. 3–16), as is occasionally stated. Frequently, an additional slip from the abductor pollicis longus joins the abductor brevis (Fig. 3–16). The muscular fibers are directed toward the metacarpophalangeal joint, which they cross, becoming transformed into a tendon about 8 mm wide that adheres to the capsule of the lateral aspect of this joint. A few fibers of this tendon join the tendon of the flexor pollicis brevis, which is inserted into the radial sesamoid (Figs. 3–12 and 3–16), and a few other fibers join the dorsal apparatus of the thumb. The muscle may have a line of cleavage

separating each group of fibers into two separate bellies.

Flexor pollicis brevis

The flexor pollicis brevis is located under the abductor brevis and medial to the opponens. The muscle has two heads of origin, one slightly deeper than the other (*see Fig. 7–17*). The origin of the superficial head is from the distal lateral border of the volar carpal ligament and from the anterior surface of the tunnel of the flexor carpi radialis near the insertion of this tendon into the base of the second metacarpal (Figs. 3–16, 3–17, and 3–18) and from the crest of the trapezium, which is covered by the anterior carpal ligament. The origin of the deeper head comes from the anterior surface of the trapezoid to the ulnar side of the tunnel for the tendon of the flexor carpi radialis and the contiguous part of the capitate bone proximal to the insertion of the oblique head of the adductor pollicis (Fig. 3–18), all covered by the volar intercarpal ligaments. The deep head of the flexor brevis seems to continue into the origin of the oblique portion of the adductor pollicis. The two heads, which are located deeper and toward the opponens in the area of origin (*see Fig. 7–17*), become more superficial on reaching the insertion in the region of the metacarpophalangeal joint. The two heads unite and form a trough for the passage of the flexor pollicis longus, which rests on the ulnar side of the flexor brevis. The fibers of the flexor brevis converge toward a tendon near the metacarpophalangeal joint, and adhering to the capsule, which is very thin in this region, reach the lateral sesamoid enmeshed in the volar fibrocartilaginous plate and insert into the lateral sesamoid (Figs. 3–12 and 3–16) and the lateral tubercle of the base of the proximal phalanx. An expansion is sent to the dorsal apparatus of the thumb.

Opponens pollicis

The opponens pollicis originates from immediately under the origin of the abductor brevis, volar to the origin of the flexor brevis from the volar ligament and the ridge of the trapezium, which is covered by the fibers of the

(Text continues on page 136.)

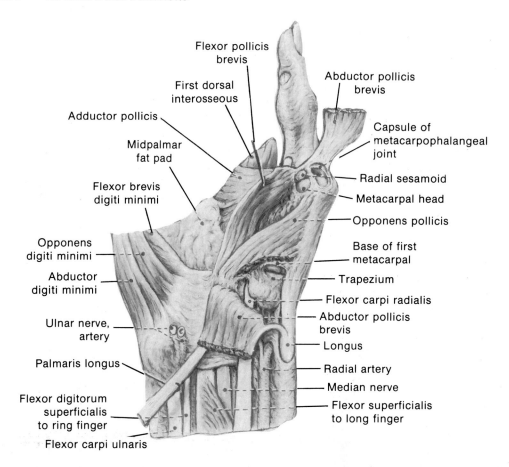

Flexor pollicis
brevis

First dorsal
interosseous

Adductor pollicis

Midpalmar
fat pad

Flexor brevis
digiti minimi

Abductor pollicis
brevis

Capsule of
metacarpophalangeal
joint

Radial sesamoid

Metacarpal head

Opponens pollicis

Opponens
digiti minimi

Abductor
digiti minimi

Ulnar nerve,
artery

Palmaris longus

Flexor digitorum
superficialis
to ring finger

Flexor carpi ulnaris

Base of first
metacarpal

Trapezium

Flexor carpi radialis

Abductor pollicis
brevis

Longus

Radial artery

Median nerve

Flexor superficialis
to long finger

FIG. 3–16 Insertion and origin of the muscles of the thenar eminence of a right hand. The abductor muscle is divided in the middle, the origin is reflected proximally, and the insertion distally. Two windows are cut out in the capsule of the metacarpophalangeal joint to show the insertion of the abductor brevis into the base of the proximal phalanx and into the capsule of the metacarpophalangeal joint. A few fibers are extended to the radial sesamoid. The tendon of insertion of the flexor brevis was divided from the tendon of the abductor brevis and retracted. Its insertion into the sesamoid bone and the capsule was divided.

The origin of the abductor brevis is from the volar carpal ligament, from the tunnel through which passes the tendon of the flexor carpi radialis, from the trapezium and the scaphoid bone. A slip from the abductor pollicis longus into the brevis is shown. The origin of the flexor pollicis brevis, deeper than the abductor, from the volar carpal ligament is indicated. The opponens muscle originates from the volar carpal ligament, radial to the origin of the flexor brevis, also from the trapezium and from the capsule of the carpophalangeal joint of the thumb. A window was cut into the opponens muscle to show the trapeziometacarpal joint and the crest of the trapezium bone. The insertion of the tendon of the abductor longus into the base of the first metacarpal is demonstrated. Distally to the distal end of the volar carpal ligament, all the tendons are removed to demonstrate the deep midpalmar fat pad.

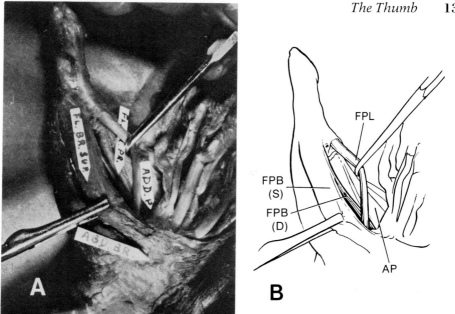

FIG. 3–17 **A** and **B**, Muscles of the left thenar eminence. The origin of the abductor pollicis brevis is indicated. The radial or superficial head of the flexor pollicis brevis (FPB[S]) is held in a forceps and retracted on the left. The tendon of the flexor pollicis longus (FPL) is retracted with a hook to show how the deep or ulnar head of the flexor pollicis brevis (FPB[D]) crosses posterior to the retracted FPL tendon from the adductor pollicis (AP) side to the lateral side of the metacarpophalangeal joint to join the superficial head of the FPB(S).

FIG. 3–18 Wrist of the left hand showing the carpal canal from its distal end with the tendons removed. The fingers are forcibly hyperextended at the metacarpophalangeal joint, and the thumb is strongly hyperextended. This illustration demonstrates the relationship of the origin of the short muscles of the thumb to the tendon of the flexor carpi radialis, to the carpal canal and to the volar carpal ligament. The tendon of the flexor carpi radialis is immediately dorsal to the deep head of the flexor brevis. Immediately radial to the tendon of the flexor carpi radialis is the crest of the trapezium bone. More radial to the tendon of the flexor carpi radialis one can observe the metacarpotrapezial joint of the thumb, reinforced by an oblique ligament.

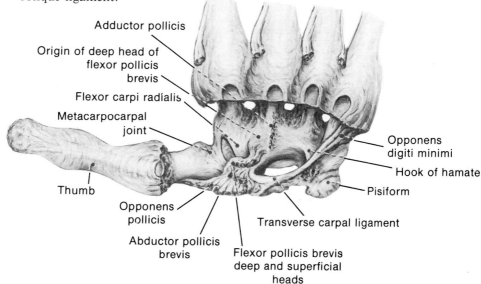

volar carpal ligament, and from the capsule of the carpometacarpal joint of the thumb (*see Fig. 7–17*). The muscle may be formed by two layers of fibers that reunite and insert directly into the lateral aspect of the first metacarpal, running an oblique course radially and distally. The fibers of the muscle near the origin are in immediate contact with the volar surface of the carpometacarpal joint of the thumb (Figs. 2–7 and 3–16).

Adductor pollicis

The adductor pollicis is located on the radial side of the hand and extends from just below the neck of the third metacarpal to the wrist, covering the second dorsal, the first palmar, and the first dorsal interossei and inserting into the ulnar side of the base of the proximal phalanx of the thumb. It is the deepest muscle of the thenar eminence and arises by two heads, the transverse and the oblique. The transverse head originates from the volar crest of the third metacarpal, from the neck of the metacarpal to the base, and from the volar aspect of the base of this metacarpal. The origin impinges on the proximal part of the metacarpophalangeal joint of the middle finger. This head also originates from the ligaments covering the base of the second metacarpal and from the anterior interosseous fascia (Fig. 2–63). The oblique head originates from the ligaments of the carpus, covering the capitate and the trapezoid and the tunnel of the flexor carpi radialis near the insertion of the tendon of the flexor carpi radialis into the base of the proximal phalanx near the origin of the flexor brevis pollicis (Fig. 3–18). A small, tendinous arch is always found either in the oblique or transverse head or between the two heads for the passage of the deep branch of the ulnar nerve and the deep arterial volar arch.

The two heads of the muscle converge toward a short tendon inserted into the ulnar sesamoid, which is intimately united with the fibrocartilaginous anterior plate of the metacarpophalangeal joint. It was mentioned previously that the plate, with the sesamoids, is united firmly with the proximal phalanx and united loosely with the neck of the metacarpal. The entire action of the adductor is thus transmitted to the phalanx. The short tendon of the adductor, besides its insertion into the sesamoid, has two extensions. One extension is inserted into the ulnar lateral tubercle of the proximal phalanx, and the other is attached to the dorsal apparatus of the thumb.

The dorsal apparatus of the thumb is formed by the tendon of the extensor pollicis longus, the extensor pollicis brevis, the expansion of the abductor brevis on the radial side, and the expansion of the adductor on the ulnar side. The tendon of the extensor pollicis longus runs obliquely from under Lister's tubercle on the dorsum of the radius to the thumb (Fig. 3–14). It reaches the ulnar side of the base of the first metacarpal and proceeds distally, covered with a fascia (Fig. 3–19). Running over the ulnar side of the dorsum of the first metacarpal, it crosses the ulnar side of the metacarpophalangeal joint and continues until it reaches the proximal phalanx. It expands over the proximal phalanx and, running toward the base of the distal phalanx, inserts over a wide line. A section through the proximal phalanx (Fig. 3–2) shows the width of this tendon when the extensor brevis does not expand beyond the base of the proximal phalanx.

The tendon of the extensor pollicis brevis (Fig. 3–19) runs on the radial side of the thumb in its own fascial plane. It crosses the metacarpophalangeal joint and reaches the base of the proximal phalanx, where it divides into a superficial and a deep portion (Fig. 3–13). The deep portion is inserted into the proximal phalanx in the middle of its dorsal base; the superficial continues on to the dorsum of the proximal shaft, contributing fibers to the dorsal apparatus of the dorsum on the radial side. The superficial fibers occasionally reach the base of the distal phalanx and are inserted into the base, together with the extensor longus. In these cases, the extensor brevis may act as an extensor of the distal phalanx when the extensor longus is divided completely (Fig. 3–20). A cross-section near the metacarpophalangeal joint through the head of the proximal phalanx may show a double-plane disposition of the terminal part of the extensors brevis and longus, with the brevis

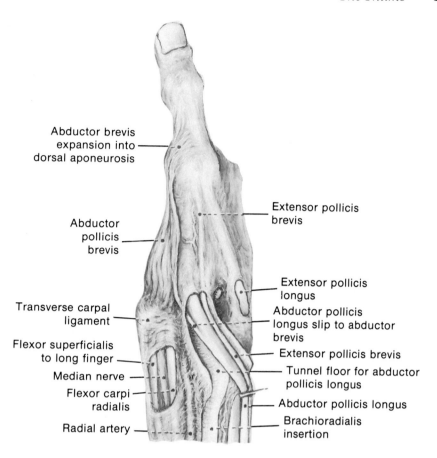

Abductor brevis expansion into dorsal aponeurosis

Abductor pollicis brevis

Extensor pollicis brevis

Extensor pollicis longus

Abductor pollicis longus slip to abductor brevis

Transverse carpal ligament

Extensor pollicis brevis

Tunnel floor for abductor pollicis longus

Flexor superficialis to long finger

Median nerve

Flexor carpi radialis

Abductor pollicis longus

Radial artery

Brachioradialis insertion

FIG. 3–19 Right thumb, radial aspect showing the rarely shown but important relationship of the tendon of insertion of the brachioradialis. The tendon of the brachioradialis ends in a wide fanlike structure, much thinner than the tendon itself, which covers the lower tip of the lateral aspect of the radius forming a floor for the tendons of the abductor longus and the extensor brevis with all their variational subdivisions. In this illustration, the abductor longus with its slip of insertion into the abductor brevis, together with the tendon of the extensor pollicis brevis are retracted dorsad, showing the floor of the tunnel for these tendons. The sheath that forms the dorsal part of the tunnel of passage for these tendons is removed for better exposure.

Volar to the tendon of the brachioradialis, the radial artery is demonstrated. Volar to the artery, one can see the tendon of the flexor carpi radialis, the median nerve, and the flexor sublimis to the middle finger. The most volar structure is the tendon of the palmaris longus. Dorsal to the exposed tendons of the abductor longus and the extensor brevis in the depths of the anatomic snuff-box, the radial artery can be seen, and the dorsal to that a small segment of the tendon of the extensor pollicis longus can be seen through a window in its tendinous sheath. At the metacarpophalangeal joint, the oblique and the transverse fibers emanating from the abductor brevis are clearly shown crossing the dorsum of the extensor pollicis longus, which is seen by transparency.

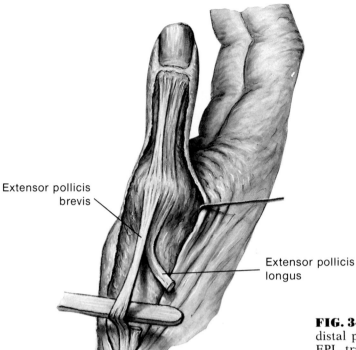

Extensor pollicis
brevis

Extensor pollicis
longus

FIG. 3–20 The EPB can on occasion insert into the distal phalanx. In this instance with division of the EPL, traction on the tendon of the EPB produces complete extension of the distal phalanx of the thumb.

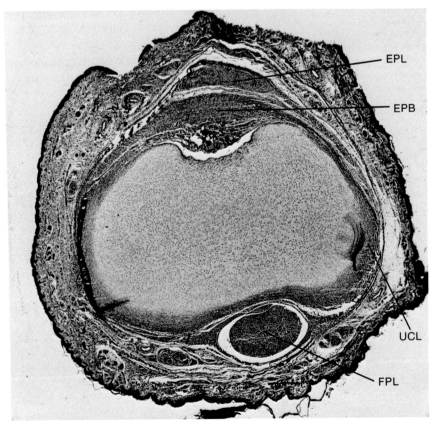

EPL

EPB

UCL

FPL

FIG. 3–21 Metacarpophalangeal joint of a 5-month premature infant. Section through this joint. The EPB is intimately connected with the dorsum of the joint. The EPL is completely separated from the EPB. The expansion of the extensor brevis and longus toward the collateral ligament of the joint shows that it continues to the tunnel of the FPL.

tendon situated deeper (Fig. 3–21). The insertion of the extensor brevis into the distal phalanx is very frequent; a few anatomists maintain that it is the most frequent. In the author's experience, the tendon of the extensor brevis is inserted mostly into the base of the proximal phalanx. The extensor longus tendon usually is wider than the extensor brevis; however, they may occasionally be equal in width; very rarely, the extensor brevis may be slightly wider.

Over the dorsum of the metacarpal the two tendons move independently in their own fascial planes. The extensor brevis has no lateral motion and moves only along its axis longitudinally in extension and flexion; however, the extensor longus, in addition to its motion in the longitudinal direction of flexion and extension can move laterally either to the radial or ulnar side of the metacarpal. The entire range of lateral motion is not more than 10 mm to 12 mm from the extreme ulnar to the extreme radial position; however, this motion is important because it permits adduction and abduction of the thumb. The tendon moves laterally only in its oblique course between the tubercle of Lister on the radius and the metacarpophalangeal joint. Over the dorsum of the metacarpophalangeal joint, the two extensor tendons receive the fibers of expansion of the abductor brevis and occasionally the flexor brevis on the radial side and of the adductor on the ulnar side (Figs. 3–22 and 3–23). These fibers of expansion run directly across the extensors in the proximal part of the dorsal apparatus and in a more oblique course toward the distal part of the thumb. This pattern is very similar to the arrangement of the fibers of expansion of the dorsum of any other finger.

There is some difference of opinion concerning the relationship of the insertion of the abductor brevis to the dorsal expansion of the thumb. Some observers find no extension of the abductor brevis into the dorsal expansion and therefore consider that the abductor brevis does not produce any extension of the distal phalanx of the thumb, while abduction of the thumb is achieved by this muscle.

The author's investigation of the manner of insertion of the abductor brevis on a large number of hands (over 300) combined with observations during surgery for other conditions of Faradic stimulation of the normal abductor brevis showed that there is a constant extension of the abductor brevis into the extensor expansion (Fig. 3–23). Faradic stimulation of the isolated abductor brevis produced abduction of the thumb combined with extension of the distal phalanx and a moderate flexion at the metacarpocarpal joint. The degree of abduction, especially extension of the distal phalanx, varied but was always present. In median nerve paralysis, the abductor brevis, the flexor brevis (superficial head), and the opponens all are involved in loss of opposition; however, the abductor brevis and especially the flexor brevis appeared to be more responsible than is the opponens. Of course, it is well known that stimulation of the flexor brevis produces flexion at the carpometacarpal joint accompanied by rotation because of the special configuration of this saddle joint and the special structure of the ligaments and the capsule, which permit functional rotation of this joint.

The insertion of the adductor pollicis occurs in three areas in the region of the ulnar side of the metacarpophalangeal joint: the ulnar side of the base of the proximal phalanx, the ulnar sesamoid, and the medial, most distal part of the neck of the first metacarpal. The most superficial part of the tendon that goes to the ulnar sesamoid extends toward the expansion with some torsion of its fibers (Fig. 3–23). Faradic stimulation of the adductor produces adduction of the thumb with simultaneous extension of the distal phalanx. (Further consideration of this problem will be treated in the section on the mechanism of opposition.)

The entire combination of the ligamentous and the tendinous structures over the metacarpophalangeal joint shows great similarity to the metacarpophalangeal joint of any other finger. The dorsal apparatus, consisting of the extensor tendons and the expansion of the short muscles, surrounds the metacarpophalangeal joint and reaches the volar plate, which includes the sesamoids of the thumb and the tunnel of the flexor pollicis longus tendon. The dorsal expan-

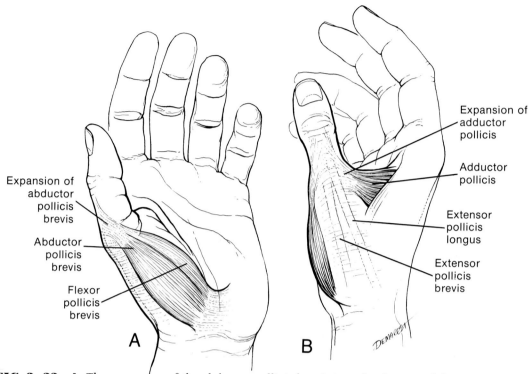

Expansion of
abductor
pollicis
brevis

Abductor
pollicis
brevis

Flexor
pollicis
brevis

A

Expansion of
adductor
pollicis

Adductor
pollicis

Extensor
pollicis
longus

Extensor
pollicis
brevis

B

FIG. 3–22   A, The expansion of the abductor pollicis brevis into the dorsum of the proximal phalanx of the thumb. It forms a dorsal expansion or apparatus with the extensors longus and brevis of the thumb. The flexor pollicis brevis is usually not extended to the dorsal apparatus but it may occasionally join the extension of the abductor brevis. **B,** The connection of the adductor pollicis with the dorsal expansion of the thumb.

sion occasionally adheres to the collateral ligaments; thus, an important anchorage unites the extensor apparatus to the immobile flexor tunnel and slightly mobile volar articular plate. The construction of the dorsal apparatus permits independent extension of the distal phalanx by traction applied separately to three structures: the tendon of the extensor pollicis longus; the tendon of the extensor pollicis brevis, when its insertion reaches the distal phalanx; and the thenar muscles of the thumb (adductor on the ulnar and abductor on the radial side).

Variations of the thenar muscles
The variations of the thenar muscles generally consist of fusion between the different bellies or more distinct separation of the muscles into

double bellies for the abductor or triple bellies for the flexor brevis. The opponens frequently divides into two layers. The opponens is sometimes inseparable from the flexor brevis.

We found that in a gorilla hand the tendon of insertion of the abductor pollicis brevis continued its insertion beyond the radial base of the proximal phalanx into the radial base of the distal phalanx. Functionally, this insertion would act to pull the thumb away from the other fingers, probably to permit greater freedom of action for the fingers of the anthropoid hand. It would not be surprising to occasionally find such a variation in the human hand. The general arrangement of the thenar muscles in the gorilla hand is very similar to that of the human hand (Fig. 1–1).

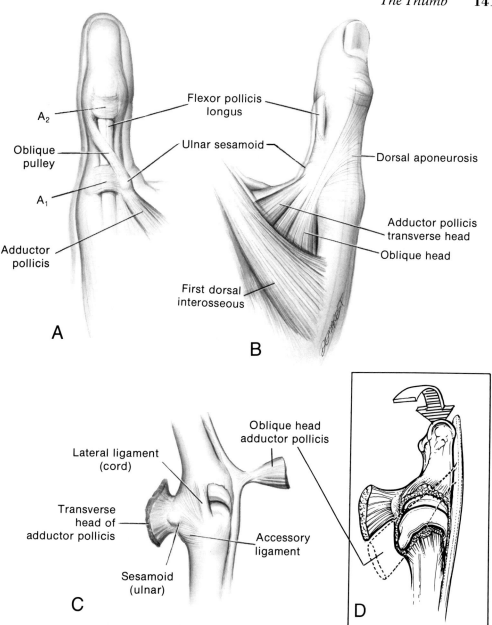

FIG. 3–23 **A**, The volar aspect of the left thumb. **B**, The ulnar side of the left thumb. **C**, The ulnar side of the thumb with the adductor pollicus (transverse head) inserted into the ulnar sesamoid to the metacarpal and to the proximal phalanx. The oblique part of the muscle expanded into the dorsal aponeurosis is lifted to show the collateral ligaments of the metacarpophalangeal joint to the thumb. There is definite torsion of the fibers of the adductor expansion into the dorsal aponeurosis. The capsule of the joint is excised between the EPL tendon and the lateral ligament of the joint. In slow stretching of the capsule, the head of the metacarpal may dislocate through this area. **D**, In acute injuries of the ulnar aspect of this joint, the dorsal capsule and the collateral ligament are torn, and the head dislocates into the area of rupture.

Blood and nerve supply of the thenar muscles

The short abductor derives its blood supply from the superficial volar branch of the radial artery; it is superficial to the nerve. The opponens is supplied by the superficial volar branch of the radial or from the first intermetacarpal, posterior to the nerve entering the opponens. A number of very small arteries coming from the anterior network of the wrist also supply the opponens. The flexor brevis is supplied by the first dorsal metacarpal artery for the superficial head. The artery enters the muscle near its origin, medial to the nerve; the deep head receives its supply from a branch or branches of the deep volar arch. The adductor pollicis is supplied by the branches of the radial artery, the deep arch, and the metacarpal arteries. The nerves of the thenar muscles are classically described as deriving from the median and ulnar nerves. The abductor brevis, the opponens, and the superficial head of the flexor brevis are supplied by the motor branch of the median nerve. The deep head of the flexor brevis and the abductor pollicis are supplied by the ulnar nerve.

Experiences with nerve injuries in World Wars I and II, Korea, and Vietnam proved the existence of numerous variations of the nerve supply to these muscles. These variations must be reckoned with for accurate diagnosis and treatment, and they will be considered in connection with function and the general nerve supply to the hand.

Pollicization

Daniel C. Riordan

Sir Charles Bell, in *The Hand, Its Mechanism and Vital Endowments As Evincing Designs* (1837), stated that "the thumb is called pollex because of its strength and that strength is necessary to the power of the hand, being equal to that of all the fingers." The power of the human hand depends on the length, strength, free lateral motion, and perfect mobility of the thumb.

A child born without a thumb (Fig. 3–24) is socially and physically handicapped to varying degrees, depending on whether the absence is unilateral or bilateral and whether there are associated anomalies that complicate the situation, such as absence of the radius. The absence of one thumb, however, is not an indication for pollicization. If a patient has four normal fingers and a thumb on one hand, and four normal fingers and no thumb on the other hand, I do not believe that any attempt at pollicization should be made. I have seen adults who can dress themselves, button buttons, comb hair, tie ties, feed themselves, and earn a living with bilateral absence of the thumb and four normal fingers. I have seen one such gentleman who admits that there are some things he cannot do, such as hold a large glass with a single hand, but his most embarrassing problem is his inability to shake hands in a normal manner. He states that this is a "right-handed world" and that if the right thumb is absent, efforts should be made to restore it if possible. He insisted that his son, who was also born with no thumbs, should have a thumb made on the right hand, so that he would be able to shake hands when he became an adult.

An absence of a thumb can occur as an isolated anomaly but is usually associated with other congenital anomalies. The radius may be normal, hypoplastic, or completely or partially absent, and such conditions can be unilateral or bilateral. With complete absence of the radius, there is usually complete absence of the thumb, but occasionally in the thrombocytopenia radial aplasia syndrome (Fig. 3–25) a normal thumb is present despite the complete absence of the radius. Hypoplastic or absent thumbs may occur in a number of syndromes, such as Fanconi's (pancytopenia-dysmelia), Holt–Oram, trisotomy 18 with multiple malformations, Rothmund–Thompson, Treacher Collins, the ring-D chromazome abnormality, and the pseudothalidomide or true thalidomide syndromes.

In patients with bilateral absence of the thumb, pollicization of the index finger should be the procedure of choice. The absence of the thumb represents a 40% loss of function in the normal hand whereas loss of the index finger deprives the hand of only 20% of its function. Because it is a "right-handed world," in bilateral absence, pollicization in the right hand should be done first. Most parents will invariably ask for the second thumb to be made after the reconstruction and recovery of the first thumb.

FIG. 3–24 Total absence of the thumb on the left; normal thumb on the right.

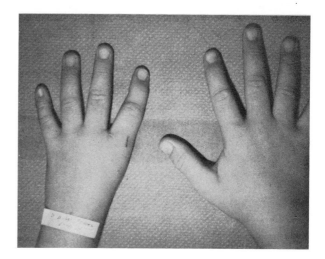

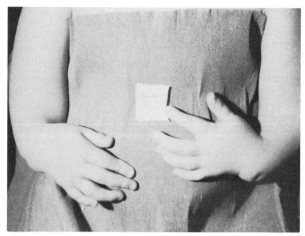

FIG. 3–25 Bilateral absence of the radius with good thumbs in a case with thrombocytopenia (megalokaryocytopenia).

FIG. 3–26 Absence of the thumb in a hand with stiff proximal interphalangeal joints of the index, long ring, and little fingers.

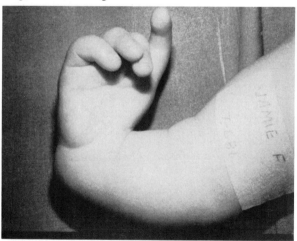

In congenital absence of the thumb, two types of reconstruction are possible. A recession or shortening of the index finger, leaving it in its regular position but increasing the angle between the second and third metacarpals, has been described by Littler and is recommended only when the parents will not accept full pollicization. This operation does provide some prehension, and without full pollicization, it is probably the best that can be done. The present-day concept of transplantation of the index finger with its bone, joints, tendons, and its neurovascular supply was described by Littler in 1953. This was a considerable improvement over the method described by Bunnell in 1944, and further contributions have been made by Iselin in 1955, Ahstrom in 1973, and Buck–Gramcko in 1971.

Although it is surgically possible to transfer any one of the four fingers into the thumb's position, transference of the index finger is favorable because the child would normally use this as the pincher between the index and long fingers and because the long, ring, and little fingers are the power gripping part of the hand. Also, if the index finger is lost there is quick transfer of precision activities to the long finger, with little loss of skill.

In radial aplasia (Fig. 3–26), stiffness of the index and long fingers is quite common, and some feel that this is a detriment to transferring the index finger. If one remembers that the metacarpophalangeal joint is to become the carpometacarpal joint, which usually has a good range of motion, good motion can be provided at the key basal joint of the new thumb, and the relative stiffness of the interphalangeal joints will not interfere significantly with the function of the reconstructed thumb. Fusion can be performed later if necessary, when the positioning of the stiff joints is not adequate.

One occasionally sees a five-fingered hand (Fig. 3–27) or, rarely, a six-fingered hand with no thumb. The most satisfactory way of providing opposition is to pollicize the most radial finger by moving this ray out of the transverse palmar plane of the other digits and transferring the intrinsic muscles as described by Littler. In a six-fingered hand (Fig. 3–28) this usually means that three interosseous muscles can be transferred into the new pseudothenar eminence, which will be even more lifelike in appearance than in the five- or four-fingered hand.

The operation should be performed as early as possible, reducing the time during which the child may develop unsatisfactory habit patterns, as well as an unfavorable body image from the psychological impact of a visible deformity. A child becomes aware of his or her hands and thumbs at about 3 months, and eye-hand coordination and habit patterns of the hand are set between 6 and 24 months. The surgery should be performed between 6 and 12 months, so that the hand can be in the correct position during the formative months.

The operative technique consists of the following six major steps:

1. Planning and mobilization of the skin flaps for adequate thumb web coverage
2. Isolation and identification of the neurovascular bundles of the index finger with great care taken to preserve the dorsal venous network, which is extremely important in the preservation of the digit to be transferred
3. Identification of the long extensors and flexors and the interossei and the detachment of the interossei from the index proximal phalanx so that they may be transferred more distally to reconstruct the thenar and adductor muscles

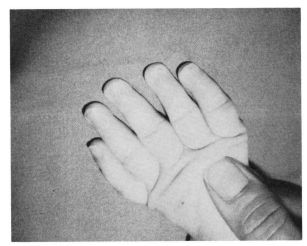

FIG. 3–27 Five-fingered left hand; no thumb is present, and it is replaced by three-jointed finger and a metacarpal with a distal epiphysis.

FIG 3–28 **A**, Six-fingered hand with no thumb. **B**, One month postoperative, the second most radial finger has been pollicized and shows the fullness of the reconstructed thenar eminence with the transferred three interossei. **C**, The infant shows the automatic grasp reflex and thenar eminence fullness of the pollicized finger 1 month following surgery.

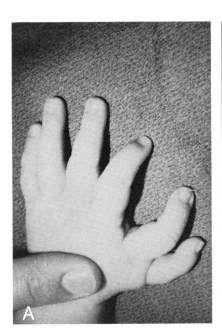
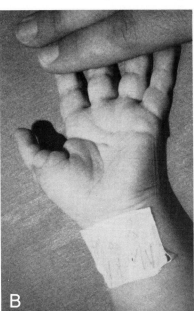
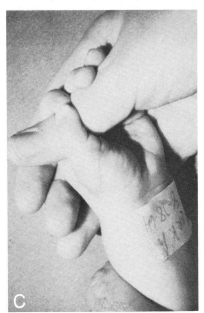

4. Shortening of the finger to the relative length of the thumb by removal of the metacarpal shaft from the epiphyseal plate to the base of the second metacarpal

5. Rotation of the thumb by suturing the cartilaginous metacarpal head anterior or palmar to the base of the stump of the second metacarpal.

6. Attachment of the interossei to the radial and ulnar sides of the transplanted digit, shortening of the extensor tendon, release of the A_1 and A_2 pulleys, rotation of the skin flaps, and closure of the wounds.

The skin incisions are outlined in a manner similar to those described by Buck–Gramckov; however, the dorsal, V-shaped incision on the proximal phalanx and metacarpal head area is not split, and the S-shaped incision is a more deeply curved S shape on the palmar side (Fig. 3–29A, B, and C). The skin flap on the palmar aspect over the metacarpal head is dissected free. The subcutaneous fat is left attached to the finger in order not to disturb the digital vessels and nerves as the finger is being prepared for rotation. In the closure, the palmar flap will become the thumb web, and part of the dorsal, V-shaped flap will become the thenar and dorsoradial side of the reconstructed thumb. Great care must be taken during the dissection to preserve the dorsal veins draining the finger because these veins are as important as is the arterial supply. The deep transverse metacarpal ligament must be sectioned in order to allow the finger to be shortened and rotated, permitting mobility of the entire finger (Fig. 3–29D and E). In some cases, it will be necessary to split the nerve more proximally on the ulnar side of the index finger, and it will occasionally be necessary to tie off the branch of the common digital artery to the radial side of the long finger to allow the free proximal migration of the ulnar digital artery of the index finger. These structures are usually easily seen once the deep transverse metacarpal ligament has been sectioned, and the surgeon can then decide whether the artery to the radial side of the long finger should be sacrificed as the finger is being shortened and rotated.

Both the first dorsal and first palmar interossei are detached from their bony insertions on the base of the proximal phalanx. Taking a small bit of the oblique fibers of their insertion into the extensor mechanism allows for mobilization of these two interossei. Care must be taken in their proximal portion to preserve the nerve and blood supplies. These muscles are stripped subperiosteally from the metacarpal shaft, which then allows cutting of the metacarpal shaft near its base. Care must be taken to leave enough bone for the insertion of the flexor carpi radialis and the extensor carpi radialis longus.

At this stage the extensor digitorum communis and extensor indicis are separated and identified, and the communis is cut at the level of the joint. The junctura between the extensor communis of the index and long fingers is detached, and the extensor indicis is cut about one inch proximally (Fig. 3–29F). These ends are tagged so that they can later be repaired and shortened. The communis will become the new abductor pollicis longus, and the extensor indicis will become the extensor pollicis brevis. A knife is used to cut through the epiphyseal plate, and then the bone's shaft is cut off with a small bone cutter after the base of the metacarpal has been visualized (Fig. 3–29E, insert). This then frees the index finger to be rotated approximately 120 degrees and shortened into its new position of opposition. It is quite important that the second metacarpal head is sutured in front or on the palmar side of the stump of the second metacarpal because this second metacarpal head will now become the new trapezium and should be in front of the transverse plane of the other metacarpals (Fig. 3–29G). This will make the new reconstructed thumb sit in the position of a normal thumb. The second metacarpal head is sutured into position with the head rotated as it would be if the finger were hyperextended, which will help prevent the occasional tendency for marked hyperextension of this new metacarpal and help to tighten this metacarpophalangeal joint. Kirschner wires are not usually necessary, but some nonabsorbable suture should be passed through the cartilaginous head and into the second metacarpal base to hold the metacarpal head in the desired position.

At this point, the tourniquet is usually released and the return of circulation and the viability of the flaps are evaluated. In most cases, inflow of blood will be adequate and sometimes exit of blood may be delayed because of kinking of the venous structures by the shortening of the digit; however, this is usually adequate if care has been taken to preserve the dorsal veins, and the various parts can then be sutured. The first

dorsal interosseous should be advanced as far distally as possible and sutured into the lateral band near the proximal interphalangeal joint of this index finger, which will make this muscle act as the abductor pollicis brevis. On the ulnar side of the thumb, the first palmar interosseous is sutured as far distally as possible on the ulnar side to the lateral band near the proximal interphalangeal joint, and this will function as the adductor of the thumb. The extensor digitorum communis is then sutured to the extensor mechanism over the proximal phalanx,

(Text continues on page 150.)

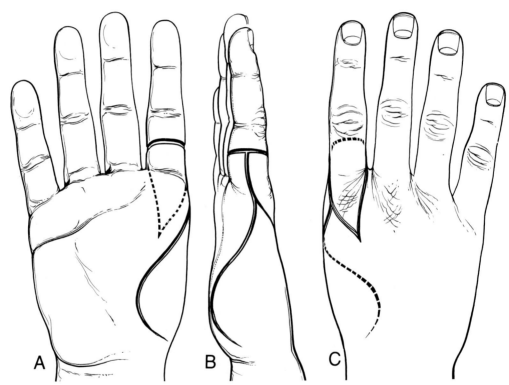

FIG. 3–29 A, **B**, and **C**, Riordan pollicization technique, skin incisions. **D**, Detailed anatomy of the finger to be pollicized. **E**, Section of the deep transverse metacarpal ligament mobilizes the digit. Ligation of the arterial branch to the long finger may be necessary as well as longitudinal splitting of the common digital nerve. **E** (insert), Removal of the shaft of the metacarpal permits rotation and shortening of the finger to be pollicized. **F**, The levels of incision of the extensor digitorum communis, extensor indicis, and interossei are presented. **G**, The second metacarpal head is sutured and hyperextended in front of the base of the stump of the second metacarpal. **H**, The A₁ and A₂ pulleys are opened. **I**, The extensor digitorum communis, extensor indicis and interossei are advanced distally and sutured.

(Continued on next two pages)

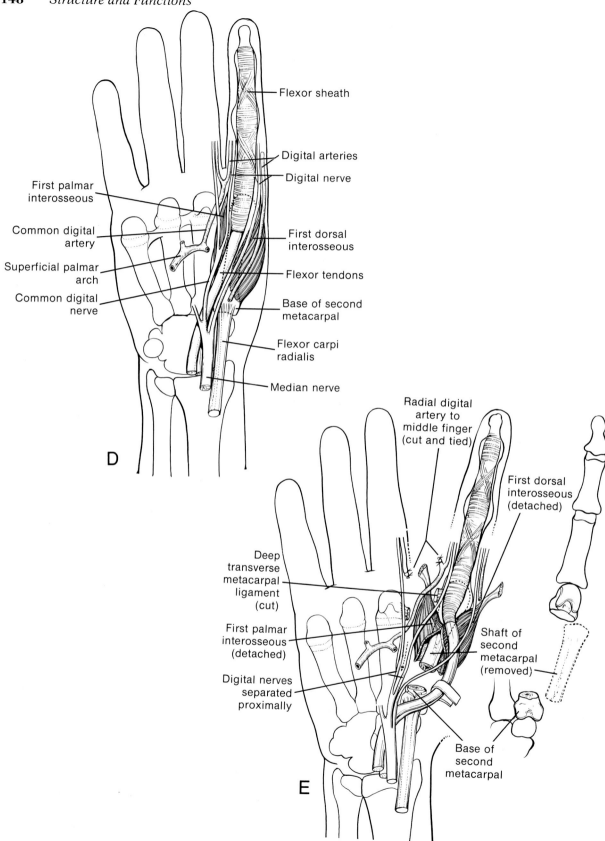

Flexor sheath

Digital arteries

Digital nerve

First palmar interosseous

Common digital artery

Superficial palmar arch

Common digital nerve

First dorsal interosseous

Flexor tendons

Base of second metacarpal

Flexor carpi radialis

Median nerve

D

Radial digital artery to middle finger (cut and tied)

First dorsal interosseous (detached)

Deep transverse metacarpal ligament (cut)

First palmar interosseous (detached)

Digital nerves separated proximally

Shaft of second metacarpal (removed)

Base of second metacarpal

E

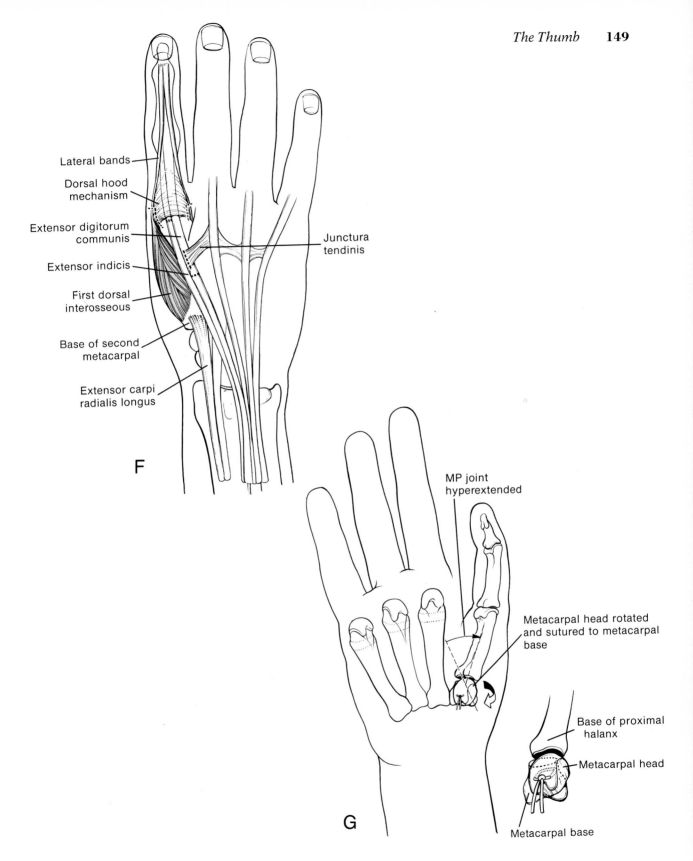

Lateral bands

Dorsal hood mechanism

Extensor digitorum communis

Extensor indicis

First dorsal interosseous

Base of second metacarpal

Extensor carpi radialis longus

Junctura tendinis

F

MP joint hyperextended

Metacarpal head rotated and sutured to metacarpal base

Base of proximal halanx

Metacarpal head

Metacarpal base

G

(Continued)

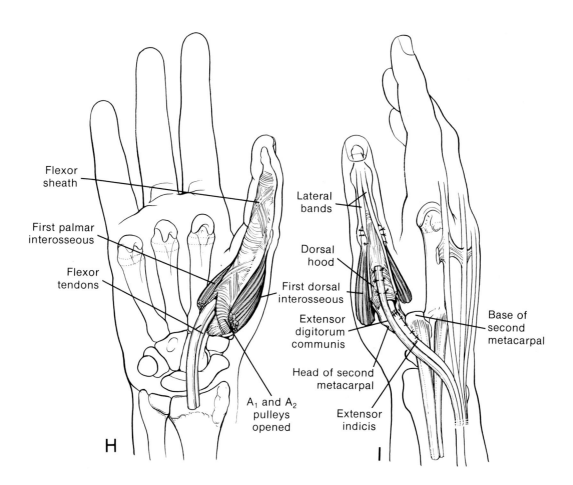

Flexor
sheath

First palmar
interosseous

Flexor
tendons

Lateral
bands

Dorsal
hood

First dorsal
interosseous

Extensor
digitorum
communis

Head of second
metacarpal

Extensor
indicis

A_1 and A_2
pulleys
opened

Base of
second
metacarpal

H   I

and this will act as the abductor pollicis longus; the extensor indicis is overlapped and shortened, depending on the amount of shortening that has taken place, which will vary with the age and size of the child (Fig. 3–29H and I).

At this point, if there is no problem with circulation, the A_1 and A_2 pulleys are visualized and opened, allowing the flexor tendons to bowstring away from the metacarpal head and proximal phalanx, so that the flexors of the finger will approach this at an angle similar to that of the normal flexor pollicis longus of a normal thumb (Fig. 3–29H). The skin flaps are now transferred and closed with fine 6/0 catgut sutures. Care is taken to use small needles, placing the stitches close together and not more than 1 mm to 1.5 mm from the edge of the skin. The sutures should not be pulled tight; if they are too tight, the hand will swell and the sutures will cut through the tissues and cause an increase in scarring. With loose closure of the wounds, drains may not be necessary; however, if a tighter closure is preferred, a small drain connected to a suction apparatus should be used in the most proximal part of the wound.

A pressure bandage should be applied with skill. Some nonadherent, fluffy bandages should be used to apply gentle pressure, but should be loose enough to allow for swelling and expansion of the tissues so that they do not strangulate. Plaster splints are used to immobilize both the elbow and the hand because most children can very easily get out of bandages unless they are carefully applied with the elbow flexed at least 90 degrees. Elevation of the hand should be carried out for a minimum of 48 hours after the

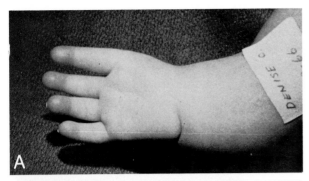

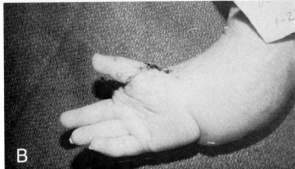

FIG. 3–30 **A**, Six-month-old child postcentralization for absent radius, preoperative for pollicization of index finger. **B**, Three weeks postoperative.

procedure, and the parents should be instructed to keep the hand at chin height at all times, whether the child is vertical or horizontal. This bandage is maintained for 3 weeks uninterruptedly. After 3 weeks, a small bandage is applied to the hand to keep the thumb in opposition for an additional week, although the child at this point is allowed complete mobility (Fig. 3–30). Because children heal more quickly than do adults, the tendons will become quite adherent and the child will have a difficult time getting a satisfactory range of motion if full immobilization is maintained for 6 weeks.

Postdressing training is usually easily done on small children by placing interesting objects in front of them for grasping while occupying the normal hand (or the hand not operated on) so that the child will use the pollicized side. With an older child, two-handed toys or play equipment can be used that will automatically make the child grasp and extend the finger. It usually does not take very long for a child to develop the new habit pattern of using the index finger now transformed to the position of a thumb (Fig. 3–31).

FIG. 3–31 **A**, Preoperative left hand of a 4-year-old without a thumb and stiff proximal interphalangeal joints of the index, long and ring fingers. **B**, Four years after pollicization of the index finger, the pollicized digit is slightly longer than desired. Fingers now fully extend after traction and 4 years of active use as the major hand.

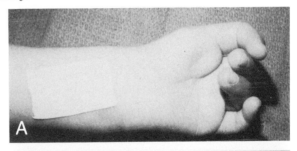

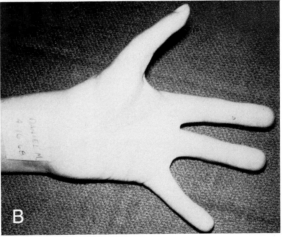

4
The Wrist

Emanuel B. Kaplan
Julio Taleisnik

The wrist is the anatomic bridge uniting the hand with the forearm. For descriptive purposes, its limits can be set between a horizontal plane passing through the distal border of the pronator quadratus muscle proximally and through the carpometacarpal articular line distally. The bony structures enclosed between these limits are represented by the distal end of the radius and the ulna and the eight bones of the carpus.

OSSEOUS STRUCTURES OF THE WRIST

RADIUS

The distal articular surface of the radius is triangular in shape. The apex is directed toward the radial styloid process—a bony prominence that can be felt as the lowermost point of the radius on the lateral aspect of the wrist. The base of the triangle is concave and is part of the ulnar notch for articulation with the head of the ulna. The entire articular surface is biconcave and covered with hyaline cartilage; it is divided into two facets by a smooth, anteroposterior ridge. The lateral facet is triangular for articulation with the scaphoid; the ulnar facet is quadrilateral for articulation with the lunate. The volar margin of the articular surface is a rough, narrow strip not wider than 2 mm to 4 mm in its ulnar half. Radially, it merges with the anterior aspect of the styloid and widens into a small triangular area containing a few vascular foramina—usually two larger ones and a few minute openings. This narrow area with the triangular widening is separated from the volar

153

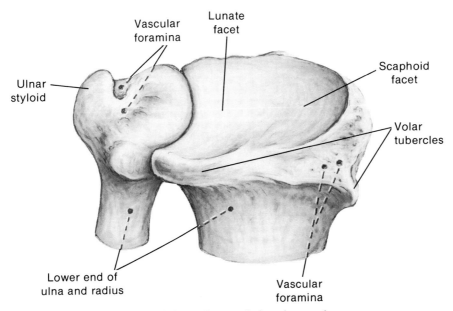

FIG. 4–1 Anterior distal end of the radius and the ulna to demonstrate constant vascular foramina at the base of the styloid process of the ulna and over the anterior ridge of the distal end of the radius (right forearm).

surface of the radius by an elevated ridge that ends in a prominent tubercle as it reaches the lateral border of the radius. A second tubercle is present at the junction of this anterior rough margin with the smooth ridge separating the scaphoid and lunate articular facets. The lowermost volar aspect of the radius is concave in the lateral and longitudinal plane for the pronator quadratus muscle (Fig. 4–1).

The detailed description of this region is dictated by the important ligamentovascular relationship investigated by the authors. The medial aspect of the lower end of the radius presents the ulnar notch, a semicylindrical, concave surface directly continuing the hyaline cartilage of the carpal articular surface and separated from it by a sharply demarcated margin. Its width varies in the young adult from 6 mm to 9 mm and it changes its configuration and width considerably in older people.

The lateral aspect is represented by the radial styloid ending distally in a smooth protuberance that can be felt through the skin by palpation; it is an important point of reference.

The lateral surface usually contains two shallow grooves, normally covered by the wide insertion of the brachioradialis tendon, which forms a floor for the passage of the abductor pollicis longus and the extensor pollicis brevis (rarely two tendons, mostly three and more). A small ridge divides the dorsal edge of the styloid process from the dorsal aspect of the distal end of the radius.

Immediately ulnar to the posterior margin of the radial styloid is a smooth and wide area. It serves as the floor for the two radial extensors of the wrist: the extensor carpi radialis longus and the extensor carpi radialis brevis. It is sometimes divided by a slightly elevated, longitudinal crest into two grooves for these two tendons.

Almost in the middle of the dorsal aspect of the distal end of the radius, continuing distally the posterior border of the radius, is a tubercle of significance, the highest point of the posterior aspect of the wrist, called the tubercle of Lister, which is an important surgical landmark (Fig. 3–14). From this high point, the posterior aspect of the radius slopes down laterally into the valley of the radial carpal extensors. The medial side of this tubercle is somewhat excavated, providing a shallow shelf and a deep groove for the passage of the tendon of the extensor pollicis longus. Medial to this groove is the wide longitudinal groove for the tendons of the extensor digitorum and the extensor proprius of the index finger. The tendon of the extensor indicis proprius usually passes obliquely from the ulnar side of the extensor communis to the index finger deep to all the tendons of the extensor communis. The dorsal border of the carpal articular surface of the radius is also separated from the dorsal surface of the radius by a ridge much narrower than the volar. The ridge also exhibits several vascular foramina that are especially evident over the lateral aspect of the styloid process and in the distal part of the groove for the extensor communis tendons.

ULNA

Distally, the ulna ends in a semicylindrical head, with a shallow, semicircular surface facing the carpal and covered with hyaline cartilage. On its radial aspect, the head contains the articular surface for the ulnar notch of the distal radius. The ulnar styloid is found in continuity with the posterior border of the ulna and is separated from the head by a groove for the attachment of the triangular fibrocartilage.

The authors found in the majority of the dry and dissection specimens, two vascular foramina: one is located on the lateral and the other on the medial end of this groove (Fig. 4–1). Injury to the vessels that penetrate into these foramina in fractures of the styloid process and cause interruption of the local blood supply may be responsible for the frequently observed nonunion of the styloid process of the ulna. Part of the groove extends proximally into the shaft on the radial side of the dorsum and serves to lodge the tendon of the extensor carpi ulnaris. The tip of the styloid process is almost constantly free of ligamentous structures; the medial side of the process is easily palpable through the skin in

line with the posterior, subcutaneous border of the ulna. The articular surface of the ulnar head facing the ulnar notch of the radius is slightly narrower than the articular surface of the ulnar notch; it normally varies in width from 5 mm to 8 mm. In older people and especially in the presence of osteoarthritis; the ulnar notch of the radius becomes much wider, irregular and concave in the longitudinal and transverse axis; the ulnar head shows similar changes.

CARPAL BONES

There are eight carpal bones; a thorough knowledge of their configuration, blood supply, and relation to each other, to the bones of the forearm, the metacarpals, and the surrounding soft tissues is essential for adequate diagnosis of injuries and diseases and for efficient surgical treatment. Two rows of carpal bones are described: the proximal and the distal (Figs. 3–8A, 3–9, 4–2, 4–3, 4–4). The proximal row consists of the scaphoid, the lunate, the triquetrum, and the pisiform; the distal row includes the trapezium, the trapezoid, the capitate, and the hamate. A brief description of these bones is necessary; however, it is obvious that in order to better understand the carpus, the practicing surgeon must have an articulated and disarticulated hand of the same side before his eyes constantly. It is surprising how different these little bones look when they are separated from each other (Fig. 4–4) and how much can be learned about the wrist, especially before certain surgical procedures, when each of the carpal bones is examined closely.

The scaphoid

The scaphoid (navicular) bone (Figs. 3–8A, 3–9, 4–2, 4–3, 4–5) is very irregular in shape and very difficult to describe. Its comparison with a boat, which gave this bone its name (*scaphe*—Greek for "dugout, trough or boat"), is strained. It articulates proximally with the radius through a biconvex surface that slopes posteriorly. Immediately distal to this articular surface, running from the ulnar to the radial side on the posterior aspect of the bone, is a narrow rough,

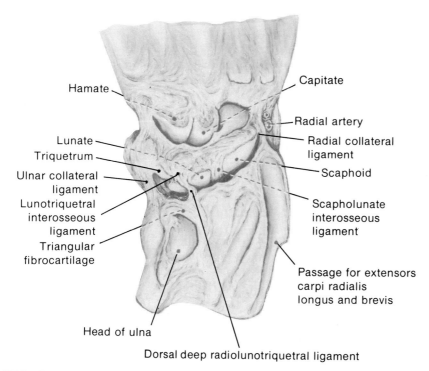

FIG. 4–2   Dorsal aspect of the left wrist in strong volar flexion. In this position, the lunate is the most prominent bone. The scaphoid is also very prominent. The head of the capitate can hardly be palpated; the body of the capitate is felt in a depression.

nonarticulating area with several vascular perforations (Fig. 4–4) that serves as an area of insertion for the posterior radiocarpal ligament. Beyond this, also on the dorsal aspect, the beginning of the distal articulating surface for the trapezium and the trapezoid can be seen (Fig. 4–4).

The volar surface of the scaphoid is a nonarticulating, irregular area with a depression in the middle and an elevation at its distal end. The depression has a large vascular foramen. The elevation is the tubercle of the scaphoid; it is normally almost completely concealed by the tendon of the flexor carpi radialis. This nonarticulating area serves for the insertion of the anterior radiocarpal ligament. The ulnar side of the scaphoid is divided into two equal surfaces. One is located proximally and is small and convex for articulation with the lunate; the other is much larger and is excavated for articulation with the head of the capitate.

The author found that the angle formed by the ulnar and distal borders of the anterior aspect of the scaphoid is approximately 90 degrees. This is probably characteristic of the human scaphoid because this angle is much sharper in the anthropoid hand. It appears to be directly related to the size of the anterior aspect of the trapezoid, which is smaller in the anthropoid hand; therefore, the sharper the angle, the smaller the trapezoid (Fig. 4–3). The size of the trapezoid may in turn be determined by the complexity of function of the thumb-index unit. The lateral aspect of the scaphoid is partially covered by the radial styloid process and by the radial collateral ligament of the carpus, which inserts in the lateral aspect of the tubercle.

The lunate

The lunate bone (semilunar) (Fig. 3–8A, 3–9, and 4–3A and A') owes its name to its distal articular

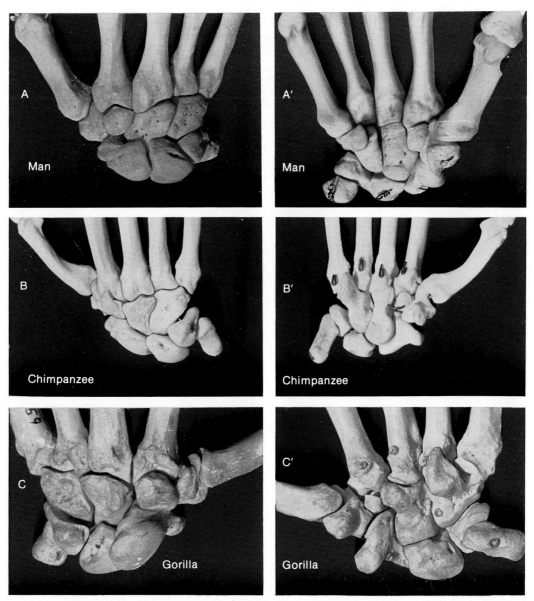

FIG. 4–3 Comparative views of human and anthropoid carpal bones. (**A** to **C**) Dorsal aspect of the carpal bones; (**A′** to **C′**) volar aspect of the carpal bones. The angle formed by the medial and distal borders of the anterior aspect of the scaphoid is considerably sharper in the anthropoid hand (see text); the pisiform is considerably larger in the anthropoid.

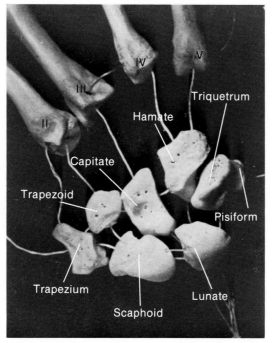

FIG. 4–4 View of separated carpal bones from the dorsal side.

FIG. 4–5 The left wrist joint opened from its proximal aspect, showing the proximal surface of the proximal row of carpal bones. The wrist was separated just proximal to the base of the radius and ulna. The radius and the ulna were divided in the frontal plane; the division was continued into the radial and the ulnar collateral ligaments. The anterior part of the divided bones was reflected forward, and the posterior reflected backward to show the proximal row of the carpal bones from above. The division involved the triangular fibrocartilage, which was also divided in the middle, separating the cartilage into anterior and posterior parts that were reflected with the anterior and the posterior parts of the ulnar collateral ligament, respectively. ▼

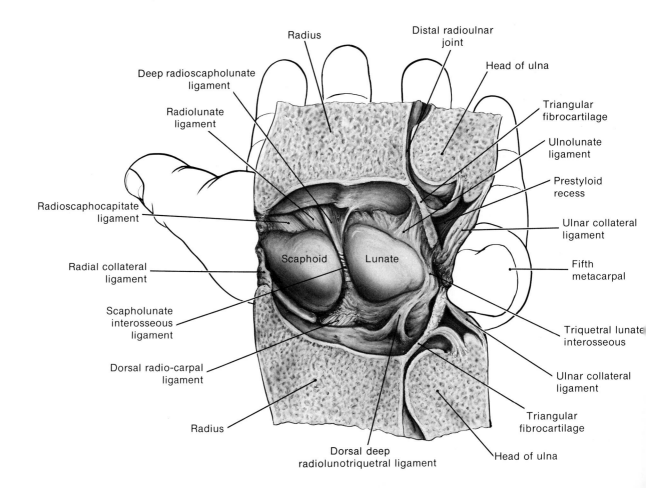

facet, semilunar in shape for articulation with the head of the capitate and the hamate bones. The proximal surface also is articular and extends dorsally in a manner similar to the proximal surface of the scaphoid. The posterior bears multiple vascular foramina of different sizes and doubtless plays a most important role in receiving blood supply through the dorsal radiocarpal ligament. The face in contact with the scaphoid shows two facets. Volar and proximally is a small, round area perforated with vascular foramina for the insertion of a strong ligament, connecting the scaphoid, the lunate, and the radius together in one unit (Fig. 4–5). The remainder of this surface articulates with the corresponding facet in the scaphoid.

The medial side of the lunate connects with the triquetral bone through a small articulating surface. The anterior aspect of the lunate can also be divided into two areas: proximal, perforated by numerous vascular foramina for vessels carried within the anterior radiocarpal ligament, and distal, smooth and almost like an articulating surface. Actually, any ligament connecting the proximal and the distal rows of carpal bones does not adhere to this area of the lunate.

The triquetrum

The triquetral bone (triangular, pyramidal, cuneiform) (Figs. 3–8*A*, 3–9, and 4–4) is wedged between the lunate laterally and the hamate medially and distally. The surface articulating with the lunate is flat and triangular in shape. The surface articulating with the hamate first runs obliquely, distally, and medially, and then turns medially, forming an articular protrusion fitting into a corresponding excavation of the hamate bone. The anterior surface can be divided into two areas: one is proximal, rough, nonarticular, with several vascular foramina; the other is distal, articular, and oval for articulation with the pisiform.

The pisiform

The pisiform is a small, ovoid bone that articulates with the triquetrum through an ovoid, smooth, articulating surface. Its anterior aspect provides insertion to volar carpal and carpometacarpal ligaments. Normally, the pisiform is completely covered by the fibers of the abductor digiti minimi and the tendon of insertion of the flexor carpi ulnaris.

The difference between the human pisiform and the pisiform of the anthropoid hand is striking. The anthropoid pisiform forms a long, round, osseous projection standing out prominently from the volar surface of the triquetrum. This is probably related to the comparative overdevelopment of the flexor carpi ulnaris in the anthropoid (Fig. 4–3).

It is curious to note that incorrect notions sometimes are perpetuated in textbooks. Some still repeat that the radial side of the pisiform has a groove for the passage of the ulnar artery. This is incorrect—the radial side of the pisiform is in contact with the ulnar nerve (Fig. 2–7).

The trapezium

The trapezium (multangular major, greater multangular) plays a significant role in the function of the wrist and the thumb. It is irregular in shape but lends itself to a simple description (Figs. 3–1, 3–8, 3–9, and 4–3*A* and *A'*). It has the configuration of a pentagon, with five sides in addition to its anterior and dorsal surfaces. The two proximal sides are articular surfaces that meet at an angle: lateral for the scaphoid and medial for the trapezoid. Next is a medial facet for the base of the second metacarpal. Distally is the important carpal half of the saddle joint articulating with the base of the first metacarpal (Figs. 3–8, 3–9, and 4–6). The lateral side is nonarticular.

The volar surface has a crest running obliquely in a medial and distal direction—the tubercle of the trapezium. This crest varies in length from 10 mm to 12 mm and in width from 3 mm to 5 mm in the adult hand, as measured in a number of dry specimens by the authors. A line drawn along the crest crosses the head of the third metacarpal distally. The lateral slope of the crest blends with the lateral surface of the trapezium. The medial slope is part of the tunnel for the passage of the tendon of the flexor carpi radialis (Fig. 2–7). The floor of the groove and the

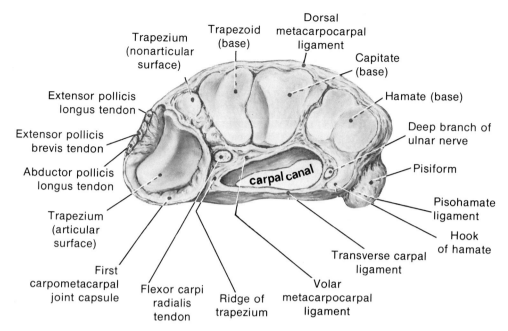

FIG. 4–6 Specimen of the left wrist, showing the distal aspect of the distal row of the carpal bones. The trapezium saddle is shown surrounded by a lax capsule for the trapeziometacarpal joint. The trapezoid is shown to the ulnar side followed by the base of the capitate and the hamate. The location of the flexor carpi radialis is well indicated. The configuration of the carpal canal is shown, wider over the ulnar side and narrower over the radial side. The nerve shown passing to the radial side of the hook of the hamate is an abnormally located deep branch of the ulnar nerve.

rest of the anterior surface show a number of perforations for small vessels.

The dorsal aspect contains two prominent tubercles with an excavation between them. One tubercle is located near the lateral border; the second is near the medial border facing the radial part of the base of the second metacarpal. The excavation between the tubercles shows several small vascular foramina and serves as a shallow groove for the transit of the tendon of the extensor pollicis longus (Figs. 3–1 and 3–8).

The trapezoid

The trapezoid (multangulum minor) (Figs. 3–1, 3–9, and 4–4) articulates with the larger trapezium on the lateral side, with the scaphoid on the proximal side, with the capitate on the ulnar side, and by means of a double surface, with the fork at the base of the second metacarpal on the

distal side (Fig. 4–6). The articular facets are mostly flat and form gliding joints with all the surrounding bones, permitting only very slight motion. The volar aspect is nonarticulating, uneven, and rough, with very few vascular foramina. The borders of this face form a fairly regular pentagonal figure. The apex of the pentagon is directed distally into the fork at the base of the second metacarpal. The dorsal surface is shaped like a falling drop with the rounded bottom directed into the receptacle of the fork of the base of the second metacarpal and the thin proximal end dropping out of the scaphoid (Figs. 3–8A, 4–3, and 4–4). Practically no vascular foramina are found over this surface.

As mentioned previously, the size of the trapezoid is apparently related to the stability of the second metacarpal. The trapezoid is comparatively much larger in the human than in the anthropoid hand. A smaller trapezoid permits the scaphoid to wedge itself deeper distally between the trapezium and the capitate with a corresponding decrease of the mediodistal angle of the scaphoid, as observed in the anthropoid hand (Figs. 1–6 and 4–3).

The capitate

The capitate bone (os capitatum, os magnum; Figs. 4–3 and 4–4) is the largest, most massive carpal bone. It has a well-developed, round head that is responsible for the name *capitate*. Between the head and the distal large body is a narrow portion, the neck. The head of the capitate is similar to the articular head of the long bones. It expands posteriorly more than anteriorly and it is smooth, covered by hyaline cartilage in the fresh state, and presents an oblique anteroposterior ridge separating two facets—one for the scaphoid and one for the lunate. On the ulnar side, the articular surface of the head blends with an articular surface for the hamate.

The neck is not well defined on the ulnar side. It is most evident on the radial side, where it forms a deep depression with several large vascular foramina. The dorsal subcapital region is also depressed and has a number of small vascular foramina. The volar subcapital region shows a deep, narrow furrow that runs directly across the anterior aspect from the medial border to the lateral, then turns distally until it fades into the volar aspect of the base of the body. This furrow is studded with several large vascular foramina. The lateral aspect of the bone is therefore divided into three areas: the articular surface for the scaphoid, the depression corresponding to the neck, and a second articular facet for the trapezoid.

The ulnar aspect is smooth for articulation with the hamate except for an area with several large vascular foramina for the insertion of a strong capitate-hamate interosseous ligament. The dorsal aspect (Fig. 4–4) is nonarticulating and rough. It shows a moderate depression that serves to fit the dorsal lip of the distal radius and the dorsal borders of the lunate and the scaphoid; this surface also has several small openings. The volar surface of the body of the capitate (Fig. 4–4) shows a central elevation located distal to the furrow described with the neck that serves as the area of insertion of volar intercarpal and radiocarpal ligaments.

The entire portion of the bone below the neck is the body of the capitate. It expands and widens distally and ends in a basilar portion. The distal articular surface for the three central metacarpals presents a large central facet for the third metacarpal, a radial facet for the tip of the ulnar part of the fork of the second metacarpal, and an ulnar facet for the radial slope of the base of the ring metacarpal (Fig. 4–6). The dorsal border of the base of the capitate runs in a lateroproximal direction to accommodate the radial hook of the base of the third metacarpal and also the ulnar part of the fork of the second metacarpal.

The hamate

The hamate bone (os hamatum, os unciforme; Figs. 3–8A and 4–4) is distinctly different from the other carpal bones because of the presence of a hook (hamulus or uncus) on its volar-distal surface. The hamate is triangular in configuration with a wide distal base and a proximal apex, as seen from the volar surface. Dorsally in the articulated hand, the apex is completely concealed by the triquetrum. The radial surface articulates with the capitate and presents a small nonarticular area with several vascular openings for the insertion of the capitate-hamate interosseous ligament. The volar surface is uneven; the radial border is vertical; the ulnar border is somewhat spiral. The apex is wedged between the lunate, the capitate, and the triquetrum. The basilar line is angulated slightly.

The anteromedial aspect of the base exhibits a well-defined hook, concave on the radial side and convex on the ulnar side. It measures 8 mm to 10 mm from the volar surface of the hamate bone to the tip; it is from 4 mm to 5 mm thick. The rounded tip together with the pisiform provides ulnar insertion to the transverse carpal ligament. The radial side of the hook forms the medial border of the carpal canal. The ulnar aspect is in contact with the deep branch of the ulnar nerve. The pisohamate ligament, the flexor, and the opponens digiti minimi take the origin from the hook (Fig. 4–6). The medial surface contains an elongated, spiral articular facet occupying approximately three fourths of the surface. The distal fourth represents a nonarticulating area that continues into the dorsal aspect of the bone.

The distal surface articulates with the fourth and fifth metacarpals. It is a saddle joint, concave in the anteroposterior plane, especially in the medial, larger portion, permitting a limited range of flexion-extension of the fifth metacarpal (Fig. 4–6). A minimal amount of rotation around the longitudinal axis of the fifth metacarpal can be actively produced. It may be noted that the perpendicular axis of the concavity of the saddle surface of the hamate for the fifth metacarpal, if continued toward the palm of the hand, will meet at an angle of approximately 90 degrees, a similar perpendicular axis of the concavity of the trapezium (Fig. 4–6). This accounts for the relation of the thumb to the little finger in the position of rest.

Accessory carpal bones

In addition to the normal bones, the carpus may also have accessory bones (Fig. 4–7). It is necessary to be aware of their presence to eliminate diagnostic errors in traumatic or pathologic con-

ditions. Examined from the volar surface, a small ossicle may be present radial to the tubercle of the scaphoid or between the scaphoid tubercle and the trapezium and the first metacarpal on the radial side of the trapeziometacarpal joint; it is known as the *paratrapezium*. The subcapitate bone is very rare and may be found between the capitate and the bases of the second and third metacarpals. A very small accessory bone at the junction of the hamate, the capitate, and the third and fourth metacarpals is known as *Gruber's accessory ossicle*. A small ossicle may also be found in front of the hook of the hamate bone; when present, it may be mistaken for a fracture of the hook. The vesalian bone (os vesalianum) is found between the hamate and the fifth metacarpal; it can be seen from both the volar and the dorsal aspects of the hand.

From the dorsal side, the important (though rare) accessory is the *os centrale*. This is usually located between the scaphoid, the trapezium, and the capitate. It is stated that this bone has a separate ossification center and unites to the scaphoid toward the end of the second intrauterine month. The *epipyramis* is an accessory bone between the triquetrum, the lunate, and the hamate; the *epilunate* may appear between the scaphoid, the lunate, and the capitate. The *os styloideum*, located between the

FIG. 4–7 Accessory bones of the carpus. **A**, Dorsal aspect, from left to right. Proximal row—epipyramis epilunatum, os centrale, radial external. Distal row—os vesalianum, os styloideum, trapezium secundarium, paratrapezium. **B**, Volar aspect, from left to right. Proximal row—radial external. Distal row—paratrapezium, subcapitatum, accessory of Gruber, accessory of the hamate hook, os vesalianum.

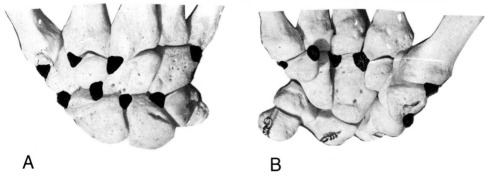

A   B

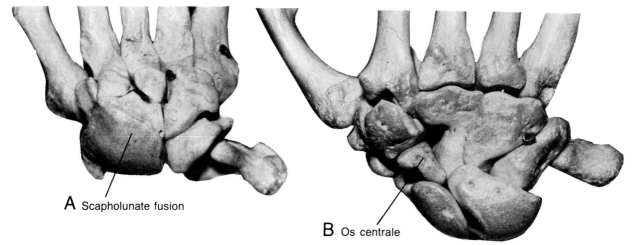

A Scapholunate fusion

B Os centrale

FIG. 4–8 Forepaw of bear (**A**) and hand of orangutan (**B**), dorsal aspect, right wrist, to demonstrate the os centrale of the orangutan and normal fusion of the scaphoid and the lunate in the bear.

FIG. 4–9 Roentgenogram of bilateral lunatotriquetral fusion.

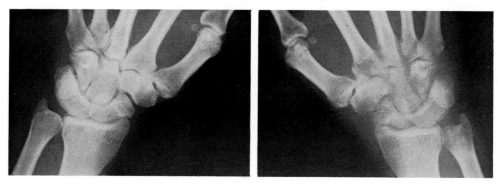

capitate and the trapezoideum, corresponds to the styloid process of the third metacarpal and apparently developed from an independent ossification center that failed to unite. The *trapezium secundarium* may rarely be present between the trapezium and the trapezoid. Very seldom a *bipartite pisiform* is found. In a study based on a review of 6,000 roentgenograms, Mangini reported the os styloideum as the most frequent accessory carpal bone, the paratrapezium was next in frequency.

Fusion of bones of the carpus is not rare. It is known that in the carnivora and other mammals the scaphoid and the lunate normally form one bone (Fig. 4–8). A fusion of the scaphoid and the lunate is very rare in the human wrist. I have personally observed only one case, an accidental finding in an otherwise normal wrist.

Fusions between carpal bones have been described in many conbinations (Figs. 4–9 and 4–10). According to most authors, the most common is between the lunate and the triquetrum (Fig. 4–9). Cockshott states that the overall incidence of carpal fusion is approximately 0.1% among most white groups and over ten times higher among the black races, with certain specific groups reaching as high as 9.5%. Concerning the nature of the fusion, Cockshott states

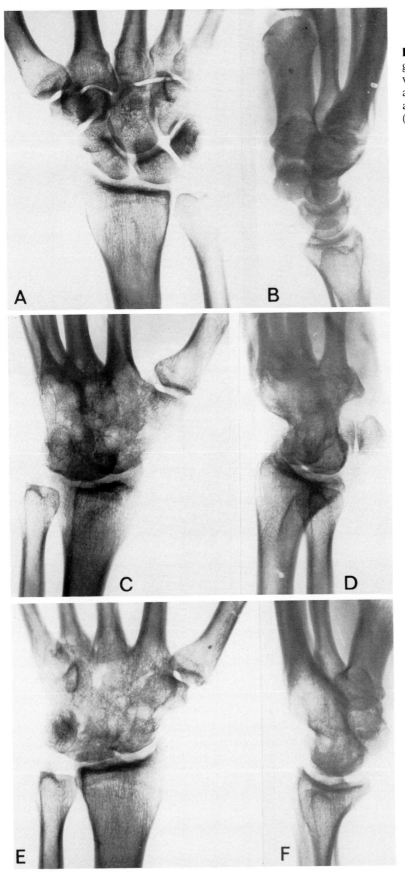

FIG. 4–10 Intercarpal fusion (congenital) of a 35-year-old female, left wrist. **A** and **B**, Normal right wrist. **C** and **D**, Fused left wrist in pronation. **E** and **F**, Fused left wrist in supination. (From Dr. A Rodriguez)

The term fusion is, strictly speaking, incorrect as the basic fault is considered to be a failure of separation. During development the cartilaginous anlages of bones forms around the 5th intra-uterine week. At the site of future joint cavities, a jelly like substance appears proximally and the cartilage becomes cleft into separate structures that will later form the individual bones comprising the articulation. O'Rahilly suggested that it is failure of the formation of these articular interzones that results in persisting continuity of cartilage which later becomes bone. The theory that a bony fusion is due to assimilation of an accessory bone between two bones is no longer seriously held.

LIGAMENTOUS APPARATUS AND JOINTS OF THE WRIST

The joints of the wrist include the radiocarpal, mediocarpal, and intercarpal joints of the proximal and the distal carpal rows. Although it truly belongs to the forearm, the radioulnar joint is also included because of its role in the mechanics of the wrist and the indirect relationship of the head of the ulna to the carpus. The ligaments of these joints retain and hold the bones at rest and during activity. They are also the vehicle for the distribution of the blood vessels and nerves that enter the bones in the areas of ligament insertion. It is essential to be aware of the relationship of the blood vessels to the ligaments for many reasons and especially, to avoid during a surgical approach random incisions that may sever important nutrient arteries and may lead to osteoporosis, nonunion of fractures, or other disturbances.

The articulated hand has two arches: one arch is parallel with the long axis, convex on the dorsum, and concave from the fingers to the wrist on the volar side; the other arch is transverse from the ulnar to the radial side of the palm. Phylogenetically, the longitudinal arch may have developed in connection with function, and the transverse arch may have developed simultaneously for the protection of the moving, regulating, and supplying structures of the hand and the fingers. It is probably similar to the sequence of events in the phylogenetic develop-

ment of the foot. (With due apologies to more expert opinion, the author believes that the subcalcaneotalar passage evolved for protection of the structures of the leg in their course to the forefoot.)

The arches of the hand are maintained by virtue of the configuration of the bones and the tension of the ligaments that hold them together. The transverse arch is evident mostly in the carpal region and at the junction of the carpus with the metacarpus. The volar concavity of the carpus results from the anterior projection of the trapezium on the radial side and the projection of the hamate and the triquetropisiform unit on the ulnar side (Fig. 4–6). The concavity at the base of the metacarpals is determined by the arrangement of the carpal bones. This concavity of the carpus and the bases of the metacarpals is fairly constant and changes only slightly during activity. The metacarpal heads, on the contrary, do not show much transverse arching at rest, but develop a volar concavity during opposition of the thumb and the little finger.

The central axis of the carpal arch coincides with a longitudinal line traced along the axes of the lunate, the capitate, and the third metacarpal. The body of the capitate appears to be the most prominent part along this axis in the carpal canal (Fig. 4–6).

The dorsum of the carpus is correspondingly convex. The most prominent point on the central axis is the posterior aspect of the lunate (Fig. 4–2).

The longitudinal arch with its volar concavity is confined mostly to the metacarpus; it results from the structural curvature of the metacarpals and is fixed. The longitudinal curvature of the phalanges is also caused by the fixed form of the phalanges. The increase of the longitudinal arching of the fingers is functional and obviously caused by the flexion of the fingers in all their joints.

DISTAL RADIOULNAR JOINT

This joint is formed by the radial notch and the ulnar head, as described. Surrounded by a very loose capsule, the bones are held together by the interosseous membrane that descends to the level of the joint, by two ligaments reinforcing the capsule anteriorly and posteriorly, and by the triangular fibrocartilage or articular disk. The triangular fibrocartilage is firmly attached to the distal border of the ulnar notch of the radius. The hyaline cartilage, which covers the articular surface of the radius facing the carpal bones, continues ulnad to also cover the triangular fibrocartilage. The thickness of the articular disk or triangular fibrocartilage is about 2 mm and equals the thickness of the articular radial hyaline cartilage at the notch. The thickness of the fibrocartilage increases to between 4 mm and 5 mm as it approaches the intra-articular side of the ulnar styloid process. The sides of the triangular disk are thickened into anterior and posterior radioulnar ligaments. The apex is inserted into the base of the styloid process on the lateral side (Fig. 4–5). A connection of the triangular disk with the ulnar collateral ligament is so intimate that injuries to the collateral ligament may easily involve the fibrocartilage and cause disturbances of supination and pronation (Figs. 4–2 and 4–5).

The mechanical advantages arising from the interposition of the disk are known. In the distal radioulnar joint, the special arrangment of the fibers of the anterior and posterior radioulnar ligaments creates special conditions for efficient function. The anterior and the posterior radioulnar ligaments reinforce the capsule and connect the radius with the triangular fibrocartilage by transverse fibers. The fibers then change their direction gradually, becoming oblique in a proximal direction toward the ulna. This pattern permits a fixed position of the fibrocartilage and free rotatory motion of the head of the ulna.

The joint has its own synovial membrane, usually completely separated from the radiocarpal joint. A small sacculation of the synovial membrane takes place at the proximal end of the joint between the radius and the ulna in front and posterior to the interosseous membrane. The center of the articular fibrocartilage is occasionally perforated. In these cases, the distal radioulnar joint communicates with the radiocarpal joint.

RADIOCARPAL JOINT

The proximal row of the carpal bones articulates with the radius and the triangular fibrocartilage. From the viewpoint of function, however, to limit this description to the structures of the radiocarpal and distal radioulnar joints is somewhat restricting; therefore, it is important to include the ligaments of the forearm in their relation to the position of the distal ends of the ulna and radius in pronation and supination.

Poirier investigated the role of the interosseous membrane and demonstrated that it prevents displacement of the radius and ulna in a longitudinal direction, even if tremendous force is applied to the ulna with the radius in a fixed position. The oblique direction of the fibers of the interosseous membrane downward and ulnarward from the radius corresponds to the transmission of force when the forearm is in supination and extension and the hand is pressed against a support. The downward force is transmitted from the shoulder through the humerus and the ulna, while the upward force is provided by the pressure of the hand against an obstacle and is transmitted through the radius. The interosseous membrane is relaxed in midposition and is tense in extremes of supination and pronation.

Although it was maintained by some that in pronation and supination the radius is involved in the rotatory movement while the ulna remains motionless, it has been proved that this is incorrect: the ulna also moves but does not rotate. The ulnar styloid process moves laterally in pronation, medially in supination. Poirier* showed that if supination and pronation are examined in reference to the proximal and the distal radioulnar joints, different results are obtained. The axis of rotation of the head of the radius remains fixed throughout pronation and supination; the ulna remains fixed.

At the distal radioulnar joint, any finger held stationary against a surface may serve as the axis of rotation. If the axis passes through the long finger and if the forearm is moved from supination to midposition, the distal end of the

*Vallois HV: Traité d'anatomie humaine. In Poirier P, Charpy A (eds); Traité d'Anatomie, 4th ed, vol 1, p 182, 1926

ulna moves laterally and dorsally, and the lower end of the radius moves in front of the ulna. If pronation is continued from midposition to full pronation, the distal end of the radius passes medial to the distal end of the ulna, although no actual rotation of the head of the ulna has occurred. The only movement of the ulna consists in abduction-extension and abduction-flexion from supination to full pronation and the reverse in return from full pronation to full supination. This movement is almost nil when pronosupination takes place along the long axis of the little finger, but it increases progressively when the axis passes through the ring, middle, and index fingers, or the thumb. This movement of the distal end of the ulna has only a minimal repercussion at the proximal radioulnar joint owing to the length of leverage of the forearm. According to Hultkranz (Poirier), the total extent of movement between the proximal end of the ulna and the humerus does not exceed 2 degrees when the axis of pronosupination passes through the middle finger. During supination there is a limited medial displacement between ulna and humerus; in pronation this movement is lateral.*

At the wrist, the radial articular surface is covered with a thin layer of hyaline cartilage and articulates with the scaphoid and approximately half of the lunate. The other half of the lunate and part of the triquetrum are in contact with the carpal surface of the triangular fibrocartilage; the rest of the triquetrum articulates with the ulnar collateral ligament of the wrist. At the radiocarpal joint, a strong, fibrous capsule reinforced on the radial and the ulnar sides of the carpus unites the radius and the triangular fibrocartilage on one side and with the carpal bones on the other. Two ligaments are described in this region: the volar radiocarpal and the dorsal radiocarpal.

The volar ligament is inserted into the anterior margin of the distal radius, just proximal to the articular surface and to the triangular area over the anterior aspect of the radial styloid process (Fig. 4–1) and also into the anterior border of the triangular fibrocartilage. The fibers of this ligament extend distally and obliquely and insert into the roughened nonarticular areas of the scaphoid, lunate, and triquetral bones. More oblique fibers descend further distally and insert into the body of the capitate. The arrangement of the fibers on the ulnar side is somewhat different. The fibers arise from the triangular fibrocartilage and the inner base of the styloid process and run toward the lunate, triquetrum, and capitate from the ulnar side; thus, the lateral and the medial parts of the volar ligament form a symmetrical pattern.

Testut and Kuenz described a ligament running deep and toward the volar radiocarpal ligament and uniting the distal margin of the radius, just below the insertion of the volar radiocarpal ligament with the interosseous ligament between the lunate and the scaphoid bones. They named it *ligament radio-scapho-lunair profund* (deep radioscapholunate ligament). The author found that in addition to the connection of the three bones, this ligament with its synovial fold permits transmission of blood vessels to the lunate and the contiguous part of the scaphoid. These vessels enter vascular apertures on the ulnar facet of the scaphoid and the anteroradial facet of the lunate. Interruption of the ligament or injury to the anterior margin of the radius in this region may substantially reduce blood supply to scaphoid and lunate, and may be responsible for some of the pathologic lesions that accompany injury to the wrist (Fig. 3–8).

The dorsal radiocarpal ligament is not as dense as the volar ligament. Inserted into the radial margin and the lateral collateral ligament on the radial side and the posterior border of the triangular cartilage and the posterior radioulnar ligament, it descends obliquely and distally toward the triquetrum (Fig. 4–11) and sometimes toward the lunate and the body of the capitate. The ligament is connected intimately with the fibrous compartments for the overlying extensor tendons. A ligamentous extension very similar to the deep radioscapholunate ligament of Testut and Kuenz can be found frequently between the posterior margin of the radius, deep to the dorsal radiocarpal ligament and the interosseous ligament, between the lunate and triquetrum (Figs. 3–8 and 4–2); it could be called dorsal deep radiolunotriquetral ligament.

With its synovial fold, it also serves as a transmitter of blood vessels to these two carpal bones.

The radial collateral ligament originates from the radial styloid and radiates distally to the scaphoid and even the capitate and the crest of the trapezium. It blends with the fibers of the transverse carpal ligament; posteriorly, it joins the fibers of the posterior radiocarpal ligament. The radial artery passes between the ligament and the tunnel for the abductor pollicis longus and the extensor pollicis brevis tendons (Fig.

4–12). The ulnar collateral ligament is attached to the base and the body of the styloid process. Not infrequently, the tip of the process is completely free of ligamentous attachments. The ligament also extends its proximal attachment to the anterior and the posterior borders of the triangular fibrocartilage. From this wide base, the collateral ligament narrows distally and inserts anteriorly into the pisiform and the transverse carpal ligament and medially and posteriorly into the triquetrum where it covers a number of small vascular foramina. It blends

FIG. 4–11 Dorsal aspect of the left wrist joint, showing the collateral ligaments and the capsule enveloping the bones of the carpus. Although separate ligaments can be discerned on very careful dissection and especially distention of the joint by air from within, it is very difficult to discern separate ligaments as shown in the standard treatises of anatomy.

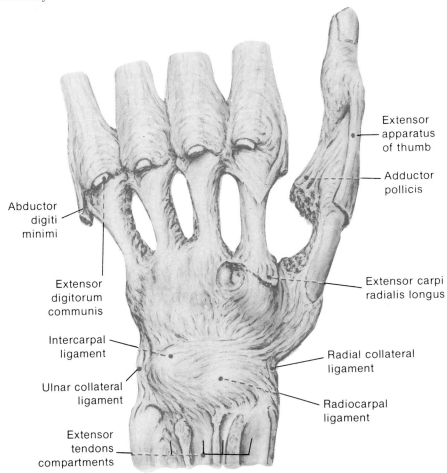

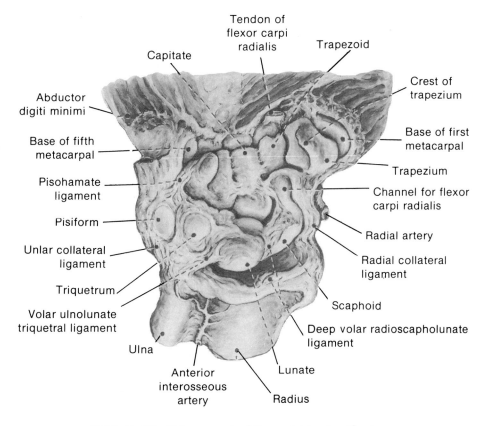

Capitate

Tendon of
flexor carpi
radialis

Trapezoid

Crest of
trapezium

Abductor
digiti minimi

Base of first
metacarpal

Base of fifth
metacarpal

Trapezium

Pisohamate
ligament

Channel for flexor
carpi radialis

Pisiform

Radial artery

Unlar collateral
ligament

Radial collateral
ligament

Triquetrum

Scaphoid

Volar ulnolunate
triquetral ligament

Deep volar radioscapholunate
ligament

Ulna

Anterior
interosseous
artery

Lunate

Radius

FIG. 4–12 Volar aspect of the wrist in dorsiflexion.

anteriorly into the volar radiocarpal ligament and posteriorly into the dorsal radiocarpal ligament.

The distal end of the radius and the adjoining triangular fibrocartilage form a biconcave surface for the biconvex proximal row of the carpus. A synovial membrane covers the intra-articular surface of the radiocarpal joint capsule to form a separate cavity. Except for a communication with the distal radioulnar joint through an opening in the triangular fibrocartilage (which occurs in about 40% of cases), the radiocarpal cavity does not communicate with other joints. Arthrographic studies permit more precise information as to the communication through the triangular cartilage in normal and pathologic cases (Kessler and Silberman).

INTERCARPAL JOINTS OF THE PROXIMAL ROW

The union of scaphoid, lunate, and triquetrum by means of interosseous ligaments constitutes the proximal carpal row. The interosseous ligament between the scaphoid and the lunate is narrow and located near the surface. It spreads from the volar to the dorsal aspects of the proximal articular surfaces of the two bones no deeper than 1 mm to 2 mm. This ligament is covered by a thin layer of cartilage and conceals the line between the two bones to such an extent that to locate the scapholunate joint may be very difficult. It may help to know that the line of separation between the two bones can normally be found by locating Lister's tubercle and the groove of the extensor pollicis longus. A line along the medial (ulnar) ridge of the groove continued distally, with the wrist in neutral position, leads directly into the interosseous space between the lunate and the scaphoid. The interosseous ligament uniting the lunate and the triquetrum is similar in every respect to the interosseous ligament between the scaphoid and the lunate. The line between the two bones may also be concealed but can be found if it is remembered that it is located almost near the apex of the triangular fibrocartilage (Fig. 4–5). Additional short bands connect the bones between themselves on the volar and the dorsal surfaces. These ligamentous bands are known as the volar and dorsal intercarpal ligaments.

The synovial membrane between the carpal bones distal to the interosseous ligaments extends into the synovial membrane of the midcarpal joint; therefore, the articular cavity of the midcarpal joint communicates with the intercarpal spaces between the scaphoid, lunate, and triquetrum but not with the radiocarpal cavity.

The pisiform is articulated with the triquetrum; corresponding more or less flat articular surfaces face each other. The surfaces are covered with hyaline cartilage (Fig. 4–12). The two bones are held together by means of a few strong ligaments: the pisohamate uniting the pisiform with the hook of the hamate, the slip from the ulnar collateral ligament of the wrist, a ligament to the volar surface of the triquetrum, and a ligament to the base of the fifth metacarpal. This joint has a synovial cavity that communicates sometimes with the radiocarpal joint.

MIDCARPAL JOINT

The midcarpal joint is formed by the scaphoid, lunate, and triquetrum in the proximal row and the trapezium, trapezoid, capitate, and hamate in the distal row. The joint between the distal end of the scaphoid and the two trapezial bones is a typical gliding joint. The joints between the concave part of the proximal end of the scaphoid, with the lunate and the triquetrum on one side and the capitate and the hamate on the other side, represent a diarthrodial type. Thus, the midcarpal joint may be considered a complex articulation that may be called an *elipsoidal*

diarthrosis, presenting two components with different degrees of motion: the lateral or radial part is a gliding joint, and the medial or ulnar is a ball-and-socket joint. Motion in a joint of this type will tend to become oblique. The analysis of motion will be presented together with the motion of the other parts of the hand.

The ligaments of the midcarpal joint are deep intercarpal bands uniting these bones in a more or less uniform manner. The capsule is attached to the rough nonarticulating surfaces of the two carpal rows. The volar ligament described mostly is the radiate ligament consisting of thick, fibrous bands connecting the anterior aspect of the body of the capitate in a divergent manner to the scaphoid, lunate, and triquetrum. Short, deep ligamentous bands connect the trapezium and the trapezoid to the scaphoid and the hamate to the triquetrum.

The dorsal ligaments are represented by (1) the transverse dorsal ligament, which starts over the dorsum of the triquetrum and runs in a radial direction over the hamate and the capitate without insertion into these bones, finally inserting into the tubercle of the scaphoid and the dorsal aspect of the trapezium, with an occasional insertion into the dorsum of the trapezoid (this ligament acts as a girth holding the carpal bones together); (2) the dorsal intercarpal ligament, which binds the two rows of bones together by oblique fibers running in a distal direction from the ulnar to the radial side.

The synovial membrane of the midcarpal joint is confined to this joint, extending between the three carpal bones of the proximal row, the four carpal bones of the distal row, and the intermetacarpal joints but not normally communicating with the carpometacarpal joint of the thumb.

DISTAL INTERCARPAL, CARPOMETACARPAL, AND INTERMETACARPAL JOINTS

Distal intercarpal

Three interosseus ligaments unite the trapezium with the trapezoid, the trapezoid with the capitate and the capitate with the hamate. The first is located near the anteroinferior aspect of the joint and is very thin; the second interosseus is located near the posteroinferior aspect of the space between the base of the capitate and the trapezoid; the third is the strongest ligament and is located between the capitate bone and the hamate in the anteroinferior regions of these two bones. The illustration shows the interosseus ligament divided by the section of the hand just in front of the facets of the capitate bone.

Superficial transverse volar and dorsal ligamentous bands unite each of the bones together.

The carpometacarpal joints

These joints are joined by six volar and six dorsal ligaments. They reinforce the small capsules for each joint. The *volar ligaments* are represented by two from the volar surface of the trapezium to the second and third metacarpal bases. Two ligaments unite the capitate with the second, and the third metacarpal bases, and two ligaments descend from the volar surface of the hamate bone for the fourth and fifth metacarpal bases; they are superficial.

The *dorsal ligaments* unite the trapezium with the dorsal base of the second metacarpal; two ligaments unite the trapezoid with the base of the second metacarpal; two ligaments unite the capitate with the bases of the third and fourth metacarpals; and two ligaments unite the hamate bone with the bases of the fourth and fifth metacarpals; they are all superficial.

The *third interosseous carpometacarpal ligament* is found constantly. It is located between the capitate and the hamate bones, immediately distal to the interosseous ligament between these two bones and extends as a strong band to the ulnar side of the base of the third metacarpal and to the radial side of the base of the fourth metacarpal.

Intermetacarpal joints

Between the bases of the metacarpals are four interosseous ligaments uniting transversely the metacarpal bases. The first interosseous ligament between the bases of the first and second metacarpals is on the dorsal side of the metacarpals. It is a strong ligament, placed near the trapezium and the trapezoid just distal to the carpometacarpal joint. It does not restrict abduction but serves to prevent hyperabduction. The ligament also forms a protective tunnel for the branch of the radial artery, which passes from the dorsum to the volar area to contribute to the formation of the deep palmar arterial arch. The ligament between the second and third metacarpal is the strongest; the ligaments between the third and fourth are less resistant. The ligament between the second and third, the third and fourth, and the fourth and fifth are located slightly proximal to the articular junctions. There are also volar and dorsal intermetacarpal ligaments uniting the metacarpal bases from the second to fifth metacarpals. They are usually thin and not very important functionally.

The articular line between the second and third metacarpal bases is concave dorsovolarly toward the radial side of the hand. The articular lines between the third and fourth and between the fourth and fifth are concave toward the ulnar side of the hand.

The synovial membrane of the carpometacarpal joints communicates, as was mentioned before, with the midcarpal joint, with the exception of the carpometacarpal joint of the thumb, which has a separate and independent synovial cavity.

BLOOD SUPPLY TO THE JOINTS OF THE WRIST

The blood supply to the distal radioulnar and radiocarpal joints, to all the carpal bones, the carpometacarpal joints, and the bases of the metacarpals all derive from different arterial branches passing through this area. The radial and the ulnar arteries send direct branches to the radial and the ulnar sides of the wrist; the volar and dorsal interosseous arteries of the forearm contribute directly or indirectly to the formation of the dorsal carpal arterial arch and to the volar carpal and deep palmar arches (Fig. 4–13, 4–14).

A knowledge of the presence and location of the vascular foramina over the end of the radius and ulna, in carpal bones and over the bases of the metacarpals, as shown when these bones were described, is helpful when surgical inter-

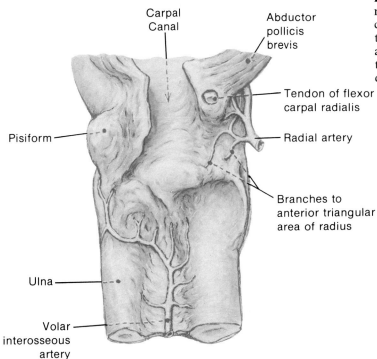

Carpal Canal

Abductor pollicis brevis

Tendon of flexor carpal radialis

Radial artery

Pisiform

Branches to anterior triangular area of radius

Ulna

Volar interosseous artery

A

FIG. 4–13 A, Blood supply to the anterior triangular area of the radius and to the carpometacarpal joint of the thumb, also to the periosteum of the ulna and the anterior aspect of the ulnar head from the volar interosseous artery. **B,** Blood supply to the dorsal aspect of the distal forearm and wrist.

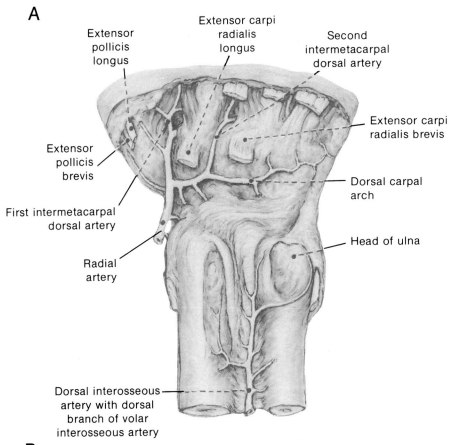

Extensor pollicis longus

Extensor carpi radialis longus

Second intermetacarpal dorsal artery

Extensor carpi radialis brevis

Extensor pollicis brevis

First intermetacarpal dorsal artery

Dorsal carpal arch

Head of ulna

Radial artery

Dorsal interosseous artery with dorsal branch of volar interosseous artery

B

ventions are necessary. The probability of elimination of blood supply when injudicious denudation of the ligaments from both the volar and the dorsal aspects of the joints of the carpus is performed is very great.

Personal investigation by the author demonstrated that the anterior periosteum of the head of the ulna is supplied by branches from the volar interosseous artery; the lower end of the radius is supplied by the dorsal branch of the volar interosseous artery, which penetrates the interosseous membrane and runs on its dorsal surface. The distalmost radius with its triangular volar area shows vascular foramina apparently for the nutrient vessels for this end of the radius and originating from the radial artery itself (Fig. 4–1). The same arterial branches that supply this area apparently carry blood vessels to the volar portion of the interosseous intercarpal ligament to supply the scaphoid and the lunate bones. In fractures occurring in this region, disruption of the blood supply affects multiple areas and may be responsible for the osteoporosis that follows injuries to the wrist.

The distal row of the carpal bones is apparently supplied mostly by branches from the dorsal carpal arch, which is formed by the dorsoradial and the dorsoulnar carpal arteries. These arteries may be of equal caliber, or the radiodorsal artery or the dorsoulnar artery may predominate. The dorsal arch supplies short branches into the distal row and the longer intermetacarpal arteries that apparently supply branches for the bases of the metacarpals.

The scaphoid and the radial collateral ligament receive a fairly large supply of blood from branches of the radial artery. The posterior aspect of the base of the radius also receives its blood supply through this source (Fig. 4–13, 4–14).

A study of the interior of the radiocarpal joint shows that the blood supply is provided through the synovial folds that cover the ligaments that unite the anterior edge of the radius with the proximal row of the carpus. To all appearances, the blood supply to the scaphoid and the lunate is provided by vessels that run

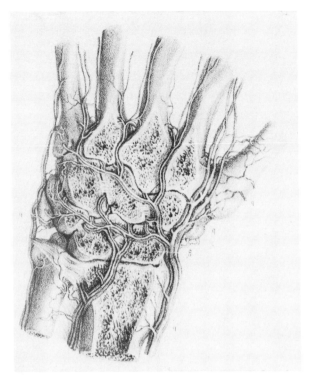

FIG. 4–14 Dorsal aspect of the wrist. Blood supply from the dorsal interosseous artery and the dorsal branch of the volar interosseous to the radius and the ulna and the dorsal carpal arch. Blood supply to the periosteum of the radius from the dorsal arteries, also small branches from the radial artery into the radial collateral ligament.

parallel with the interosseous ligaments of the bones and enter these bones through the previously described vascular foramina. The distribution of these foramina is such that either one or the other bone receives most of the blood. The blood supply to the scaphoid from this source may be very scanty, in which case, most of the blood to this bone will derive from branches of the radial artery running either along or through the radial collateral ligament to the distal end of the scaphoid. The proximal end will therefore not be well supplied. Most of the blood goes to the lunate; however, the reverse may occur, and the entire blood supply from the vessels of the interosseous intercarpal ligament may go to the scaphoid, leaving the lunate practically without blood vessels from this source.*

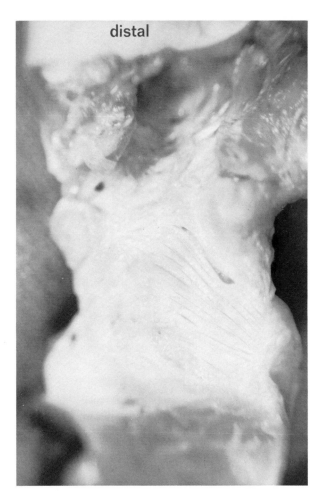
distal

FIG. 4–15 Superficial volar radiocarpal ligaments, right wrist.

Ordinarily, the blood supply between the dorsal edge of the radius and the lunate and the scaphoid through posterior connections is much less important. The interosseous intercarpal ligament between the triquetrum and the lunate is connected to the radius volad and dorsally. Along those ligaments, blood vessels reach both carpal bones; however, the triquetrum is supplied more abundantly than is the lunate, not only through the intercarpal ligament but mostly through the ulnar collateral ligament. This ligament forms a unit connecting the triangular fibrocartilage with the ulnar styloid and the body of the triquetrum. In the majority of wrists examined, a separate blood supply is observed that derives from branches of the volar interosseous artery, penetrating through the capsule and around the ulnar collateral ligament into the base of the styloid process (Fig. 4–13, 4–14). These vessels penetrate into the symmetrically placed foramina found constantly at the base of the styloid process of the ulna between the insertion of the triangular fibrocartilage and the articular end of the head (Fig. 4–1). Apparently, the triangular fibrocartilage of the wrist derives some blood through the same source. It is possible that the frequent occurrence of nonunion of fractures of the styloid process results from the interruption of this blood supply.

The deep palmar arch and the volar carpal arch supply numerous small vessels that penetrate through and between the various fibrous bands and ligaments of the volar aspect of the carpus and richly supply the carpal bones and the anterior aspect of the metacarpal bases (Fig. 4–14 and 4–15).

Further studies of details of carpal circulation are necessary. Travaglini found that there are differences in pattern according to age, presumably connected with the time of appearance of ossification centers and that the intraosseous circulation of carpal bones is widely anastomotic; characteristics of individual arterial bone supply may explain various clinical manifestations connected with injuries and other conditions.

NERVES OF THE ARTICULATIONS OF THE WRIST

It is appropriate to restate the general rule established by Hilton concerning the nerve supply, known as Hilton's law.

The same trunks of nerves, whose branches supply the groups of muscles moving a joint, furnishes also a distribution of nerves to the skin over the insertions of the same muscles; and—what at this moment more especially merits our attention—the interior of the joint receives its nerves from the same source.*

The ultimate distribution of nerves in the

*Hilton J: Rest and Pain, p 166 Philadelphia, JB Lippincott, 1950

joints and their relation to transmission of sensations of orientation and pain requires further study. The large articular branches enter the ligaments and the capsule of the joints according to Hilton's law.

The distal radioulnar joint is under the action of muscles supplied by the volar interosseous (branch of the median), the dorsal interosseous (posterior branch of the radial), and the ulnar nerve. The articular branches derive accordingly from all these sources with variations in distribution.

The radiocarpal joint derives its nerve supply from the deep and dorsal branches of the ulnar nerve, from the volar interosseous nerve, from the dorsal interosseous, and sometimes from the motor thenar branch of the median nerve.

The midcarpal and the carpometacarpal joints receive their nerve supplies from branches of the same nerves that supply the radiocarpal joint.

MUSCLES MOVING THE WRIST

There are three direct motors for flexion and three direct motors for extension of the wrist; these muscles also abduct, adduct, and circumduct the wrist. The other extrinsic muscles of the fingers that have indirect action on the wrist have been described anatomically. Functionally, all these muscles will be considered in a separate chapter. The three flexors are the flexor carpi radialis, the palmaris longus, and the flexor carpi ulnaris.

FLEXOR CARPI RADIALIS

The flexor carpi radialis originates from the medial epicondyle of the humerus, together with the pronator teres lateral to it and the palmaris longus medial to it. It arises from the common tendon and the fascia between the muscles and the fascia that covers the muscles of the epicondylar group. The muscle body that follows the origin descends approximately to the middle of the forearm and ends on a tendon that emerges

on the anterior surface of the muscle. The muscle fibers are arranged in a bipennate pattern. The muscle is the most superficial of the forearm, running anterior to the flexor digitorum superficialis. The tendon gradually becomes cylindrical and runs superficial and radial to the tendon of the flexor pollicis longus (Figs. 2–31 and 3–16). It engages in a special tunnel under the protection of the crest of the trapezium (Figs. 2–7 and 3-16). The tendon of the flexor pollicis longus, which was on the ulnar side, crosses the front of this tunnel to enter the thumb (Fig. 2–7). Completely separated from all the other tendons in the carpal canal, the tendon of the flexor carpi radialis emerges from its tunnel and inserts into the base of the second metacarpal sending a strong, oblique, tendinous slip to the third metacarpal (Fig. 2–7).

Variations. The tendon of the muscle frequently extends its insertion to the base of the third and even the fourth metacarpal base. An additional insertion into the trapezium, which takes place within the groove of passage under the crest, is so frequent that some anatomists consider it to be constant. The tendon frequently has an insertion into the scaphoid or the volar transverse carpal ligament.

The Arterial Supply. The arterial supply of the muscle is provided by two groups of arteries: superficial, deriving from several accessory branches from the ulnar artery, and deep, formed by the principal artery to the muscle deriving from the common trunk of the ulnar recurrent arteries. The muscle may also be supplied by branches from the radial, ulnar, and anterior interosseous. No intramuscular anastomoses were found in the depth of the muscular body. The artery of the median nerve, which assumes a large diameter as a rare variation, is sometimes responsible for the blood supply to the muscle. The arteries usually enter the muscle body on the deep surface of the muscle near the elbow.

The Nerve Supply. Innervation of the flexor carpi radialis comes from the median nerve. Several small branches penetrate the muscle on the deep surface slightly proximal to the middle of the muscular body.

PALMARIS LONGUS

The palmaris longus originates, together with the pronator teres, the flexor carpi radialis, and the flexor carpi ulnaris, from the medial epicondyle of the humerus. It arises from the common tendon, the intermuscular septum, and the overlying fascia and runs distally toward the wrist, parallel with the medial side of the flexor carpi, and in or near the midpalmar fascia.

Approximately in the middle of the forearm, the slender, flat muscle belly begins to show a tendon on the volar surface. The tendon is flat throughout its course and spreads out on reaching the midpalmar fascia, into which it continues directly. It is a decidedly variable muscle, frequently absent, either unilaterally or bilaterally. According to most anatomists it is absent in about 11 to 12 cases per 100.

When present and normal, its relationship to the median nerve is helpful to the surgeon because the median nerve is found immediately under the tendon in the midline of the proximal part of the wrist (Fig. 2–31). The tendon serves as a key guide to the structures of the wrist, as described by the author in a previous study. The tendon is good material for tendon graft because it is easily accessible, and its loss does not adversely affect function.

Variations.   Although the palmaris longus tendon is a guide to the structures of the wrist when it is normal, its multiple variations may confuse even the experienced. The following eventualities should be kept in mind: division of the terminal tendon into two or three separate tendons; transformation of the terminal tendon into a muscular sheet; division of the tendon into a thin muscle body descending to the transverse volar carpal ligament and a tendon running parallel with the muscle (*see Fig. 9–21*); deviation of the tendon with insertion into the pisiform or the abductor pollicis brevis (Fig. 2–30); insertion of the tendon into the antebracial fascia without any continuity with the midpalmar fascia.

The variations of the origin are concerned mostly with the ascent or the descent of the area of origin on the epicondyle or on muscle bellies of other muscles in this region. The variations are probably of more importance to the surgeon than to the comparative anatomist who attempts to solve the problem of the phyogenetic derivation of the palmaris longus in connection with the midpalmar fascia.

Blood and Nerve Supply.   The blood supply is derived from the same arterial branches that supply the flexor carpi radialis. The nerve supply comes from the median nerve, frequently from a common trunk which supplies the flexor carpi radialis and the palmaris longus.

FLEXOR CARPI ULNARIS

The origin of the flexor carpi ulnaris is double. One head arises from the common mass of the muscles of the medial epicondyle medial to the palmaris longus and anterolateral to the origin of the flexor digitorum sublimis; it is very superficial. The second head originates from the medial border of the olecranon, the upper part of the posterior border of the ulna, and from the area just distal to the ulnar insertion of the medial collateral ligament of the elbow. A tendinous arch unites the two heads. Dorsal to this arch the ulnar artery and the posterior recurrent ulnar artery pass into the forearm.

The muscle descends vertically in the forearm. The tendon appears approximately in the middle third of the forearm over the anterior aspect of the muscle. The muscle fibers descend obliquely on the posteromedial aspect of the tendon almost to its insertion into the pisiform.

The insertion into the pisiform is very extensive and as mentioned before, it appears to continue superficially directly onto the fibers of the abductor digiti minimi (Figs. 2–30 and 2–65). On removal of the abductor digiti minimi, the tendon shows an extension into the anterior aspect of the base of the fifth and sometimes the fourth metacarpal. The tendon sends a lateral expansion that runs to the hook of the hamate bone (Fig. 2–63) and to the medial side of the anterior transverse carpal ligament, forming a roof for the ulnar nerve and artery that pass between the expansion of the tendon and the transverse volar carpal ligament (Fig. 2–30). A few fibers of the tendon slip around the ulnar border and connect with the dorsal transverse carpal ligament.

Variations of the Flexor Carpi Ulnaris. The variations of origin usually involve the size of the humeral or ulnar heads. The variations of insertion affect the various expansions of the tendon near the pisiform bone with accentuation and overdevelopment of these expansions.

Blood and Nerve Supply. The arterial supply derives from three arteries, all branches of the ulnar artery: the superior, middle, and inferior. The inferior is the most important and runs parallel with the muscle belly until the muscle belly joins the tendon. The nerve supply is from the ulnar nerve either by a single trunk or several twigs entering the muscle belly near the elbow joint.

EXTENSORS OF THE WRIST

The three extensors are the extensor carpi radialis longus, the extensor carpi radialis brevis, and the extensor carpi ulnaris.

Extensor Carpi Radialis Longus. The muscle originates from the lateral epicondylar ridge of the humerus and from the epicondyle, together with the common tendon of the extensors, and in front of these tendons. Proximal to the origin of this muscle lies the origin of the brachioradialis; distal to the origin of the extensor carpi radialis longus is found the origin of the extensor carpi radialis brevis.

The tendon appears on the deep surface of the extensor longus muscle and runs together with the tendon of the extensor carpi radialis brevis to the wrist. The junction of the muscular fibers to the tendon occurs at about the proximal half of the middle third of the forearm.

Extensor Carpi Radialis Brevis. This muscle originates from the lateral epicondyle and distal to the extensor longus in front of the common tendon of the extensors, and from the intermuscular septum and the fascia which covers all of these muscles. The muscle belly that follows runs toward the middle of the forearm where it

joins a tendon on the deep lateral surface of the muscle. The tendon is strong and flat and runs together with the tendon of the extensor carpi radialis longus toward the wrist.

The tendon of the extensor longus is lateral, and the tendon of the extensor brevis is medial. The two tendons are deep to the abductor longus and the extensor pollicis brevis, which cross them in the lower third of the forearm. At the wrist, the tendons run in a special compartment formed by a groove on the radius located lateral to the groove for the extensor pollicis longus and medial to the tunnel for the tendons of the abductor pollicis longus and the extensor pollicis brevis (Fig. 3–14). These compartments are covered by the dorsal transverse carpal ligament. In the passage under the transverse carpal ligament, the tendons are crossed by the tendon of the extensor pollicis longus (Fig. 3–14). Upon emergence from under the distal edge of the dorsal retinaculum the two tendons insert into the bases of the second and the third metacarpals.

Extensor Carpi Ulnaris. The extensor carpi ulnaris originates from the dorsal aspect of the lateral humeral epicondyle, distal and posterior to the tendon of the common extensor, and from the intermuscular septum that separates this muscle from the anconeus and the supinator; from the fascia covering all these muscles and from the posterior border of the ulna distal to the insertion of the anconeus to about 6 cm to 8 cm proximal to the styloid process.

The entire muscle belly is enclosed in an osteofibrous tunnel formed by the ulna and the different fascial coverings. The tendon begins at about the middle of the forearm, but the muscle fibers descend in a penniform manner to a level slightly proximal to the wrist.

The tendon free of muscle fibers runs toward the radial groove of the distal end of the ulna that is transformed into a special tunnel by the dorsal transverse carpal ligament. The tendon pursues its course to the ulnar tubercle at the base of the fifth metacarpal into which it is finally inserted.

Variations of the Extensors of the Wrist. Complete or incomplete union of the extensors radialis longus and brevis at the point of their origin is encountered frequently. At the distal end, a supernumerary tendon may be inserted into the third metacarpal when it comes from the extensor radialis longus or to the second metacarpal when it comes from the radialis brevis. The extensor radialis brevis may be absent or extended to the fourth metacarpal.

An additional muscle with origin between the extensor longus and brevis from the humerus and insertion into the first metacarpal, known under the name of *extensor carpi radialis accessorius*, was described by Wood. In this case, it may present several variants and terminate on the radial part of the abductor pollicis brevis, between the first and second metacarpals with extension to the interosseous muscle, or into the flexor brevis of the thumb.

Testut observed a muscle that originated between the brachioradialis and the extensor carpi radialis longus from the medial epicondyle of the humerus. After a short run as a flesh mass, it formed a cylindrical, long tendon, running along the radial side of the brachioradialis and ending in a muscular mass alongside the radial side of the abductor pollicis and inserted into the base of the proximal phalanx. It could be called the humeral abductor of the thumb.

The extensor carpi ulnaris has a very constant insertion, and the only frequent variation is a persistent expansion that runs alongside the radial border of the tendon toward the base of the fourth metacarpal. This insertion sometimes extends to the dorsal carpal ligament of the wrist; sometimes there is a double tendon inserting into the fifth metacarpal. Extension of the tendon to the proximal phalanx or to the extensors of the little finger digit may occur.

Blood and Nerve Supply to the Extensors of the Wrist. The blood supply to the extensors longus and brevis derives mostly from the anterior recurrent radial artery which penetrates the muscles from their deep surfaces and supplies them at several levels with proximal and distal branching. There is an abundant intramuscular communication between the arterial branches.

The nerves to the extensor longus originate from the radial nerve before its division into anterior and posterior branches. The nerve to the extensor brevis derives from the same source, or occasionally from the posterior branch before it penetrates the supinator muscle.

The blood supply to the extensor carpi ulnaris appears to be less abundant than to the other muscles. A few small arterial branches come to the proximal part of the muscle from the recurrent radial, and a few branches come from the posterior interosseous.

The nerve supply is provided by branches of the posterior interosseous (posterior branch of the radial nerve) on its emergence from the supinator muscle. Several small branches enter the deep surface of the muscle approximately 10 cm distal to the tip of the olecranon near the posterior border of the ulna.

Current Concepts of the Anatomy of the Wrist

Julio Taleisnik

LIGAMENTS

The volar radiocarpal and intercarpal ligaments are thick and strong and are covered by a homogeneous soft tissue layer that must be removed for the fascicular structure of the volar capsule to be seen (Fig. 4–15). The dorsal ligaments are comparatively thin, reinforced by the floor and septae of the fibrous tunnels for the six dorsal wrist compartments, which normally provide much of the support to the dorsum of the wrist. A proposed classification of these ligaments divides them into two major groups: *extrinsic* and *intrinsic*.

EXTRINSIC LIGAMENTS

Extrinsic ligaments course between the carpus and the radius (proximal or radiocarpal ligaments) and the carpus and the metacarpals (distal or carpometacarpal ligaments. Proximal extrinsic ligaments cover all four quadrants of the joint: radial, volar, ulnar, and dorsal.

Radial collateral ligament

The radial collateral ligament (Fig. 4–16) is more volar than lateral. It originates from the volar margin of the styloid process of the radius and attaches on the tuberosity of the scaphoid and into the walls of the tunnel for the flexor carpi radialis tendon. It courses volar to the transverse axis of motion of the wrist joint, and is the most lateral of the volar radiocarpal ligaments.

Radiocarpal ligaments

The radiocarpal ligaments are disposed in superficial and deep layers. The superficial volar radiocarpal ligaments (Fig. 4–15) are arranged in a complex and seemingly disorganized pattern. Most fibers assume, however, a V shape; the apex is attached to the capitate and lunate and the two arms diverge toward the radius and ulna. Although not well defined, these fascicles provide some restraint and support, and they function as true ligaments. Their radial attachment is on a bony crest on the volar aspect of the distal radius (Fig. 4–17). The three strong volar radiocarpal ligaments can be seen best from within the joint (Fig. 4–18). They are named according to their points of origin and insertion. The most lateral bundle is the radiocapitate ligament (or radioscaphocapitate ligament; so named because of a weak additional, central attachment to the volar aspect of the scaphoid). Immediately medial to this is the radiolunate ligament. Both of these fascicles, the radiocapitate and the radiolunate ligaments, originate from a rough triangular facet located in the distal radius between the crest for the origin of the superficial radiocarpal layer and the volar margin of the articular surface of the radius (Fig. 4–17). Still more medial and slightly deeper is a third fascicle, the deep radioscapholunate ligament (Figs. 4–18 and 4–19*B*). It originates from a small tubercle on the anterior margin of the radius where the proximal bony crest and the border of the radius meet at the apex of the previously described triangular surface. This ligament inserts primarily into the lunate and secondarily into the scaphoid and then continues along the scapholunate interspace. Together with the radiocapitate ligament, it tethers the proximal pole of the scaphoid to the volar margin of the radius.

Ulnocarpal complex

The ulnocarpal complex is an intricate complex of ligaments and supportive structures of considerable functional significance that occupies the ulnar quadrant of the wrist joint. Lewis and co-workers (1970) observed in the lower primate that the styloid process of the ulna articulates

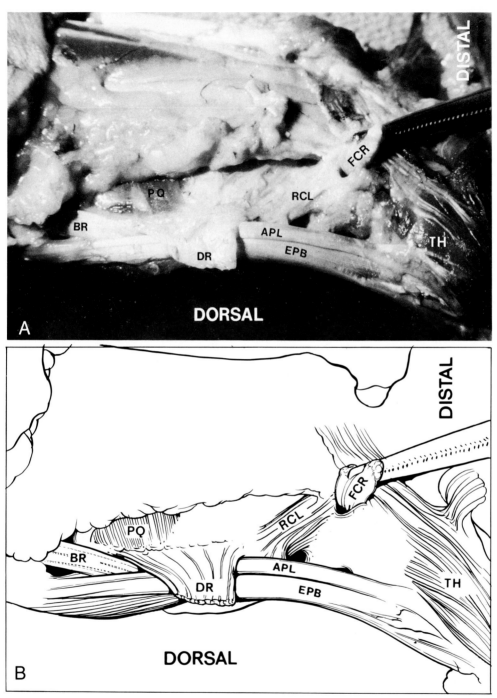

FIG. 4–16 Volar radial aspect of a right wrist. FCR is flexor carpi radialis; TH is thenar muscles; RCL is radial collateral ligament; PQ is pronator quadratus; BR is brachioradialis; EPB is extensor pollicis brevis; APL is abductor pollicis longus; DR is radial origin of dorsal extensor retinaculum.

with the triquetrum. Phylogenetic development is accompanied by a progressive recession of the ulnar styloid from the carpus, and in humans, the space is replaced by a cartilaginous filler, the *ulnocarpal meniscus homologue* (Fig. 4–20). This structure is frequently separate from the *triangular fibrocartilage* (Fig. 4–21), and the two should not be confused. In these cases, both the meniscus and the triangular fibrocartilage share a strong origin from the dorsal and ulnar corner of the radius. From here the meniscus swings volar and around the ulnar border of the wrist to insert into the triquetrum (Fig. 4–22).

Proximal to the meniscus, the triangular fibrocartilage extends horizontally from the distal border of the sigmoid fossa of the radius into the radial base of the ulnar styloid. Between the two is the prestyloid recess (Fig. 4–19*A*), a

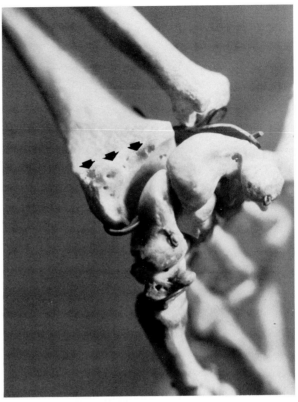

FIG. 4–17 Volar surface of distal right radius. Arrows delineate ridge for origin of superficial radiocarpal ligaments. Triangular surface between ridge and articular margin is for the origin of the deep volar radiocarpal ligaments.

FIG. 4–18 Deep volar radiocarpal ligaments (right wrist) seen from within the joint. U is ulna; R is radius; UL is ulnolunate ligament; RL is radiolunate ligament; UCL is ulnar collateral ligament; RSC is radioscaphocapitate ligament; RSL is deep radioscapholunate ligament; L is lunate; S is scaphoid.

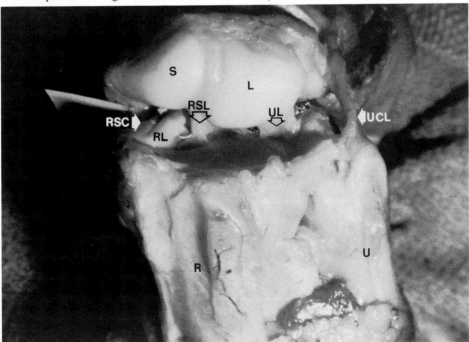

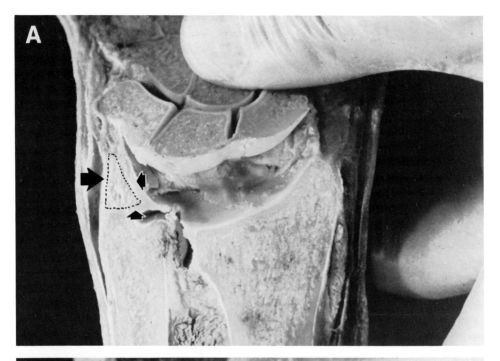

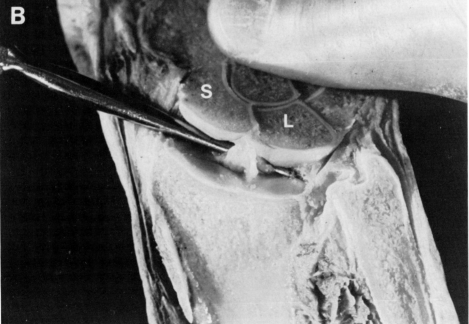

FIG. 4–19 Sagittal section, right wrist. **A**, Dorsal half shows prestyloid recess (*large arrow*). Conjoined origin of triangular fibrocartilage and ulnocarpal meniscus homologue (*small arrows*) is seen. **B**, Volar half. Hemostat is under the radioscapholunate ligament. S is scaphoid; L is lunate.

triangular area filled with synovium that surrounds the tip of the ulnar styloid. In other specimens, triangular fibrocartilage and meniscus homologue cannot be as clearly differentiated and remain fused into a larger mass. This mass separates medially to insert in part into the caput ulna and to continue in part along the ulnar border of the wrist to attach on the volar aspect of the triquetrum. These two portions of the complex represent the triangular fibrocartilage and the ulnocarpal meniscus homologue. The triangular fibrocartilage itself is usually thinner at its midportion (Fig. 4–19*A*), at times presenting a perforation linking the radiocarpal joint with the distal radioulnar synovial pouch (recessus sacciformis).

In a recent study by Palmer (1981), all specimens showing this type of perforation presented a kissing area of lunate chondromalacia, at times deep enough to show the subchondral bone. Two other associated anomalies found frequently in specimens with a perforated triangular fibrocartilage have been an ulna-plus variant of distal radioulnar relationship and a tear of the lunotriquetral ligament. The anterior and posterior margins of the triangular fibrocartilage itself are

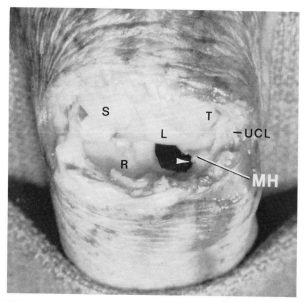

FIG. 4–20 Right wrist specimen opened from the dorsum. The dark marker was placed under the free undulating border of the ulnocarpal meniscus homologue (MH) (*arrow*). S: scaphoid; L: lunate; T: triquetrum; R: radius; UCL: unlar collateral ligament.

FIG. 4–21 Triangular fibrocartilage, right wrist.

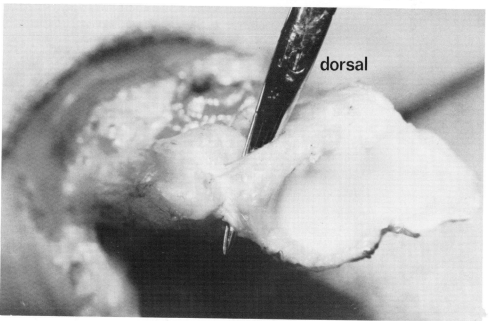

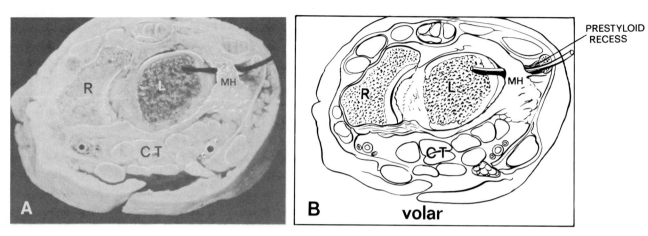

FIG. 4–22   **A** and **B**, Transverse section. Specimen shows cut ulnocarpal meniscus homologue, with dark marker placed underneath, from radiocarpal joint to prestyloid recess. R is radial styloid; L is lunate; MH is meniscus homologue; CT is carpal tunnel.

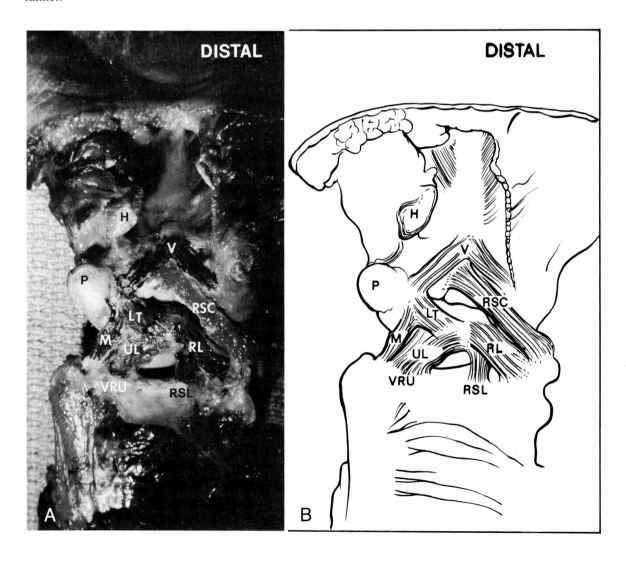

reinforced by fasicular thickenings constituting the *volar* (Fig. 4–23) and *dorsal distal radioulnar joint ligaments* (Fig. 4–24). The triangular fibrocartilage is also connected to the carpus by the *ulnolunate* ligament (Figs. 4–18), another component of the ulnocarpal complex originating from the volar border of the triangular fibrocartilage and inserting into the lunate.

The last component of the ulnocarpal complex is the *ulnar collateral ligament* (Fig. 4–18) which is usually poorly developed, although it has been described as originating from the tip of the ulnar styloid and attaching in the medial carpus. More than an actual ligamentous fascicle, it can best be considered as a thickening of the joint capsule produced by the close relationship of the capsule itself and the sheath of the overlying extensor carpi ulnaris (Fig. 4–25). The tip of the ulnar styloid is covered by hyaline cartilage and frequently lies free within the prestyloid recess (Fig. 4–19A). The functional ulnar collateral is actually the very strong ulnocarpal meniscus homologue, with additional dynamic support derived from the exten-

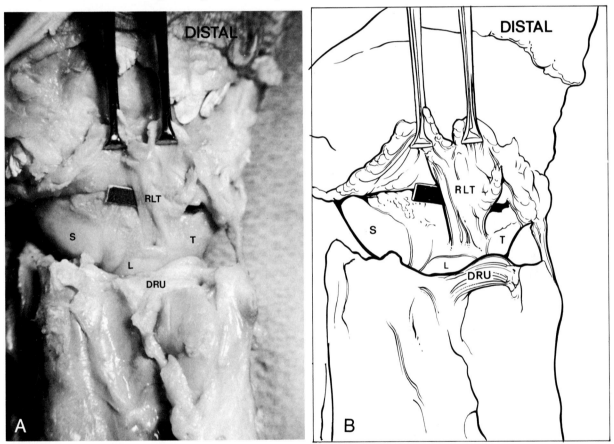

FIG. 4–24 **A** and **B**, The dorsal deep radiolunotriquetral ligament (RLT) and detached from its proximal origin, folded distally, and held by two clamps. Insertion in lunate (L) and triquetrum (T) is seen. S is scaphoid; DRU is dorsal radioulnar ligament.

◀ **FIG. 4–23** **A** and **B**, Volar ligaments. VRI is volar (distal) radioulnar ligament; RSC is radioscaphocapite ligament; RL is deep radiolunate ligament; RSL is radioscapholunate ligament; UL is ulnolunate ligament; LT is lunotriquetral ligament; M is ulnocarpal meniscus homologue; V is V or deltoid ligament.

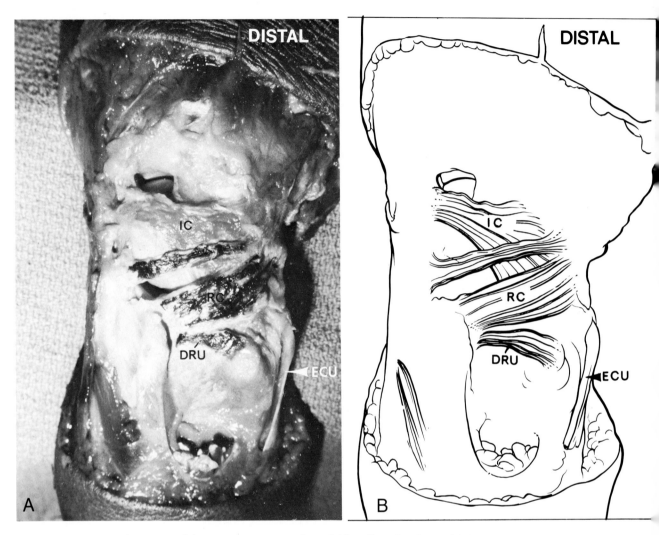

FIG. 4–25 A and **B**, Dorsal ligaments. DRU is dorsal (distal) radioulnar; RC is dorsal radiocarpal; IC is dorsal intercarpal; ECU is extensor carpi ulnaris tendon.

sor carpi ulnaris sheath, which in fact is a part of the fibrous system of the ulnocarpal complex. Except for the medial attachment of the triangular fibrocartilage into the head of the ulna, the actual medial support to the carpus arises from the dorsal and ulnar corner of the radius and attaches into the volar surface of the carpus through the triquetral insertion of the ulnocarpal meniscus and the lunate insertion of the ulnolunate-triangular fibrocartilage complex. The volar and radial corner of the radius is diagonally connected to the carpus by all the

deep radiocarpal volar ligaments; thus the carpus is mostly "suspended" from the radius, by a fibrocartilaginous ligament "sling" (Fig. 4–26) positioned diagonally within the radiocarpal joint because of its oblique origin from the distal radius and its insertion on the volar aspect of the carpus.

Dorsal radiocarpal ligament
The dorsal radiocarpal ligament (Fig. 4–25) originates from the dorsal margin of the distal radius, coursing distally and medially to insert

into the lunate and triquetrum. In contrast to the strong volar support, this is a rather thin ligament, heavily reinforced by the fibrous sheaths of the extensor tendon compartments. This anatomic disposition of the dorsal radiocarpal ligament leaves an area of capsular weakness at the level of the proximal pole of the scaphoid. There is frequently a fascicular fold arising from the dorsal border of the radius together with the dorsal radiocarpal ligament, which inserts into both the lunate and the triquetrum in a manner similar to that of the volar deep radioscapholunate ligament. Because of this similarity this structure has been called the *dorsal deep radiolunotriquetral ligament* (Fig. 4–24).

INTRINSIC LIGAMENTS

Intrinsic ligaments of the wrist originate and insert on the carpal bones. The intrinsic and volar ligaments are also thicker and stronger than the dorsal ligaments. According to their length and the relative intercarpal mobility they allow, these ligaments may be classified as short, intermediate and long. The *short intrinsic ligaments* are stout and unyielding dorsal, volar, and interosseous fibers binding the four bones of the distal carpal row into a single functional unit.

Intermediate intrinsic ligaments
The *lunotriquetral ligament* (Fig. 4–23) lies between the lunate and the base of the pisiform facet of the triquetrum and continues the overall direction of the radiolunate ligament. Both these ligaments have been considered a single radiotriquetral fascicle. The *scapholunate ligaments* are found on both the volar and dorsal surfaces, with the dorsal ligament shorter and more dense than the volar ligament. These ligaments course obliquely and distally from the lunate to the scaphoid and permit considerable motion of the scaphoid on the lunate. From neutral to full dorsiflexion, the lunate rotates approximately 28 degrees and the scaphoid approximately 30 degrees. From neutral to complete volar flexion, the lunate rotates 30 degrees and the scaphoid 60 degrees. The scapholunate ligaments are twisted as rotation proceeds to

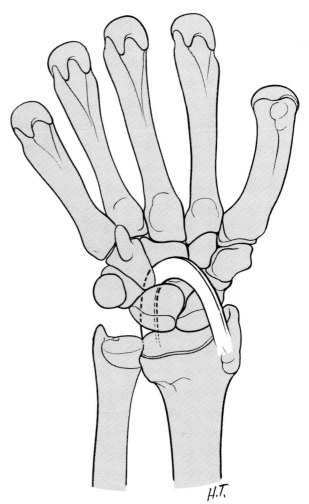

FIG. 4–26 Radiocarpal sling.

unwind as scaphoid and lunate return to a neutral position. Associated with this differential rotation is a proximal-distal shift between the scaphoid and the lunate by which the scaphoid moves proximally during volar flexion and distally in dorsiflexion. This shift is more apparent between the volar surfaces of these two bones as they are brought into closer contact in full volar flexion and is necessitated by the difference in the degrees of curvature of the proximal poles of the scaphoid and the lunate. The greater curvature of the scaphoid requires that it shift proximally in relation to the lunate to maintain contact with the articular surface of the radius.

Three *scaphotrapezium ligaments* (Fig. 4–27) allow considerable volar-to-dorsal rocking of the distal pole of the scaphoid on the biconcave surface formed by the trapezium and trapezoid.

Long intrinsic ligaments

The long intrinsic ligaments are volar and dorsal. The *volar intrinsic intercarpal ligament* is the most important of the two and has been called *deltoid, radiate,* and *V* ligament (Fig. 4–23). It stabilizes the capitate, because it is attached to the neck of the capitate and fans out proximally to insert into the scaphoid, the triquetrum, and at times the lunate. When its central fibers to the lunate are absent, it is no longer a deltoid or radiate structure; rather, it forms a V with the lunate cradled in its opening. The lateral fascicle of the V or deltoid ligament contributes to the support of the distal pole of the scaphoid, while the medial fascicle between the capitate and the triquetrum is the only structure other than the scaphoid that crosses and therefore stabilizes the midcarpal joint. The *dorsal intercarpal ligament* (Fig. 4–25) is a thin structure originating from the triquetrum and coursing laterally and obliquely to insert on the scaphoid. It presents a stronger distal fascicle that attaches to the trapezium and trapezoid as well. There is an area of weakness between the fibers of the dorsal radiocarpal and intercarpal ligaments, corresponding to the capitolunate joint.

THE FUNCTIONAL IMPORTANCE OF THE LIGAMENTS OF THE WRIST

The four carpal bones with strong volar ligamentous attachments are the capitate, lunate, scaphoid, and triquetrum (Fig. 4–23). Originating proximally from the radius, scaphoid, and triquetrum, V-shaped fibers converge to the *capitate.* Contained within this V is a second V consisting of the radiolunate and ulnolunate ligaments converging toward the volar surface of the *lunate.* The space of Poirier is an area of weakness on the volar aspect of the radiocarpal capsule, caused by the absence of a volar lunocapitate ligament. Poirier (quoted by

Destot) actually described a "small hernia of synovial membrane" between the two V ligaments. When a volar lunocapitate ligament is present, the long intrinsic V changes into a radiate or deltoid structure; conversely, the absence of the capitolunate support may be responsible for some forms of wrist instability. Already in 1935 Navarro suggested that this absence was to a great extent, the "explanation of carpal subluxations." Fisk believed that the stability of the carpus depended on the integrity of the volar capsule between the capitate and the lunate and that the midcarpal joint did not become unstable until this capsule was divided. It also has been suggested that a systemic articular laxity or hypermobility in otherwise normal individuals may predispose them to wrist instability. The combination of ligamentous deficiency and systemic joint hypermobility may explain why some normal wrists are somewhat unstable to a dorsal stress applied to the hand in a direction similar to that of the floor reaction force exerted on the hand during a fall with the wrist in dorsiflexion (Fig. 4–28). In these cases the capitate can almost be subluxed dorsally on the lunate by manipulation alone, as observed by Destot. Volar stress applied to such a "lax" but otherwise normal wrist reproduces the volar intercalated segment instability (VISI) deformity described by Linscheid and co-workers. On dorsal stress, a dorsiflexed intercalated segment instability (DISI) deformity is produced, except that the scaphoid, instead of shifting into an abnormal position perpendicular to the longitudinal axis of the radius, remains aligned with it. The response of a wrist to injury probably depends on its intrinsic stability, and this, in turn, depends not only on the bony elements but also on the muscular, tendinous, and ligamentous supports, and their relative strength or laxity. Excessive dorsal midcarpal laxity is frequently found in the uninjured wrists of patients with carpal subluxations or dislocations and may be essential to whether an injury produces carpal dislocation or subluxation rather than a fracture without ligament disruption.

The volar aspect of the scaphoid has three clearly defined ligamentous zones: *proximal,* for

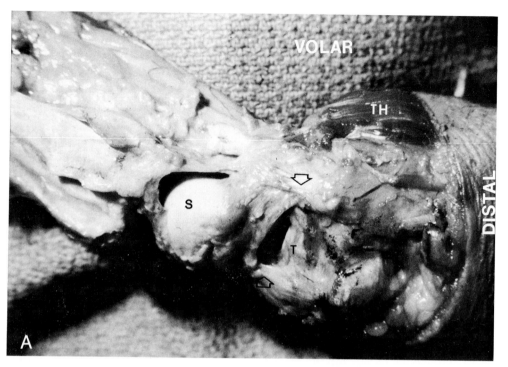

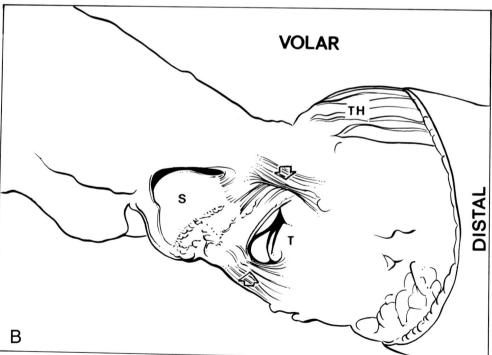

FIG. 4–27 A and **B**, Scaphotrapezium ligaments, volar and dorsal *(arrows)*. The thin lateral scaphotrapezium ligament has been excised to expose the joint. S is scaphoid; TH is thenar muscles; T is trapezium.

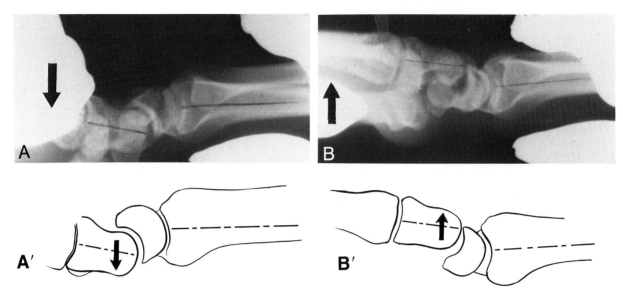

FIG. 4–28 Manual stress applied to lax wrist demonstrates normal midcarpal instability. **A** and **A**′, Force applied on the hand in a volar direction with the radius stabilized. **B** and **B**′, Force applied in a dorsal direction.

the insertion of the ligaments controlling the motions of the scaphoid on the radius (deep radioscapholunate ligament) and the lunate (intrinsic lunoscaphoid ligaments); *distal,* connected to the radius by the radial collateral ligament and to the capitate by the volar intercarpal or V ligament; and *central,* for attachment of the radiocapitate ligament. The scaphoid rotates on the central ligament as a gymnast balancing on a horizontal bar when executing a hip circle. The contact point of the scaphoid with the ligament coincides with the transverse axis of scaphoid rotation. Both the radiocapitate and the deep radioscapholunate ligaments tether the proximal pole of the scaphoid to the volar margin of the radius. If these two fascicles are intact, dorsal rotatory subluxation of the scaphoid cannot occur (Fig. 4–29). There is nothing dorsally to prevent or cushion this displacement because the proximal pole of the scaphoid is essentially unprotected.

The ulnocarpal meniscus homologue, the lunotriquetral ligament, and the capitotriquetral fascicle of the V ligament (Fig. 4–23) insert on the *triquetrum* in a single pivot area around the base of the pisiform facet. From here, these multiple fascicles radiate toward the ulnocarpal complex, the lunate, and the capitate, respectively. A similar but less developed pattern is found on the dorsal aspect (Fig. 4–25). This ligament distribution is ideally suited to the successive control of the smooth progression of the triquetrum on the helicoidal surface of the hamate from a low position in dorsiflexion to a high position (Fig. 4–30). The triangular disc (Fig. 4–21) is involved with distal radioulnar support during pronation and supination. As rotation occurs, there is deformation of this ulnocarpal disc (Kauer, 1977), with an associated shift of the dorsal extensor tendons. Kauer described a roof-tile arrangement of the dorsal tendons in which a definite stratification is present, with the more ulnar tendons running deeper to the radial tendons on the dorsum of the wrist. In supination, they all come closer together, their stratification allowing the respective sheaths to shift partially, one on the other.

Both volar, V-shaped ligamentous structures bring into play an exquisite system of alternating tension forces (Fig. 4–31) that controls both

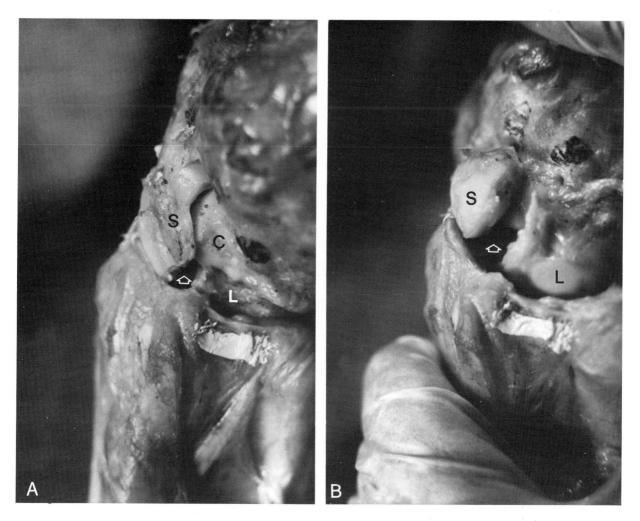

FIG. 4–29 A, Division of scapholunate interosseous ligaments allows gap (*arrow*) between the scaphoid (S) and lunate (L), but full rotatory subluxation is not possible until all volar tethering ligaments are divided. (**B,** *arrow*). C is capitate.

the extent of intercarpal displacements and the smooth progression of individual carpal bones from one clinical extreme of wrist movement to the opposite. For instance, during ulnar deviation, the lunate deviates ulnad, but it also migrates radially and dorsiflexes. The amount of radial displacement is checked by the ulnolunate ligament, while lunate dorsiflexion is controlled by the radiolunate ligament, which now courses longitudinally rather than obliquely; therefore, these two fascicles, normally oriented obliquely when the wrist is in neutral position, change the

direction of their fibers, the more *medial* ulnolunate becoming largely *transverse* and the *lateral* radiolunate assuming a *longitudinal* alignment. The shape of the proximal ligamentous V is changed into an L. The distal V undergoes similar but opposite changes: the *lateral* capitoscaphoid fascicle becomes *transverse* to control capitate migration ulnarward, while the *medial* capitotriquetral fascicle appears more *longitudinal*. The volar flexing capitate pulls down on the triquetrum, bringing it along the volar surface of the hamate. In this

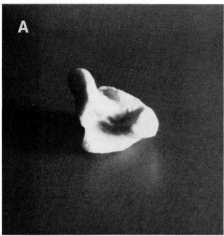

FIG. 4–30 **A**, Helicoidal surface of hamate for articulation with triquetrum. **C** and **D**, show high position of triquetrum; **E**, **F**, and **G** show low position of triquetrum.

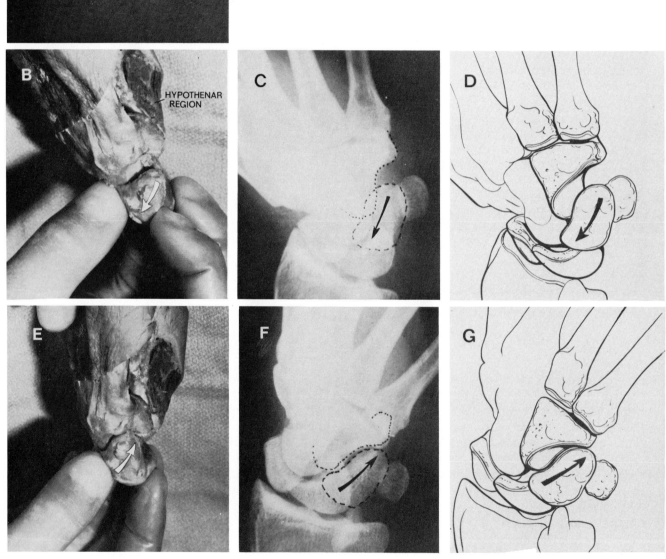

HYPOTHENAR
REGION

position, the triquetrum occupies what Weber (1980) calls a "low position" on the helicoidal facet of the hamate (Fig. 4–30). Thus the distal V ligament has also changed its shape into an L, facing opposite to the proximal L complex.

The medial or capitotriquetral fascicle of the deltoid ligament is the only structure, other than the scaphoid, to cross the mid-carpal joint in a position to stabilize the medial half of the carpus. Loss of this support is believed to be the cause of medial carpal instability. Patients with this instability can voluntarily and consistently reproduce a painful, sudden "snap" or "jerk" which is palpable between the triquetrum and the hamate dorsally (Fig. 4–32). At this point, the wrist assumes a position of longitudinal collapse that can be recognized clinically.

Lewis (1970) and Kauer (1980) have de-emphasized the functional value of a collateral ligament system in the human wrist. The radial collateral is actually the most lateral of the volar radiocarpal ligaments (Fig. 4–16), while the ulnar collateral is poorly defined. Furthermore, Kauer pointed out that during ulnar deviation, a true radial collateral ligament would need to bridge an increasingly wider distance, as would a true ulnar collateral ligament during radial deviation. If these ligaments were this long in the midposition of the wrist during volar and dorsiflexion, they would be lax and therefore nonfunctional. Kauer stressed that, instead, there is an "adaptable collateral system," a dynamic muscular support provided by the extensor carpi ulnaris on the ulnar side (Fig. 4–25) and by the extensor pollicis brevis and abductor pollicis longus tendons on the radial side of the wrist (Fig. 4–16). Poirier (quoted by Navarro) has already pointed out that the radial collateral ligament and tendon of the abductor pollicis longus are so adherent to each other that their separation is extremely difficult.

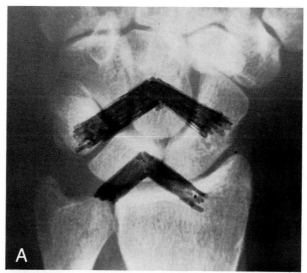

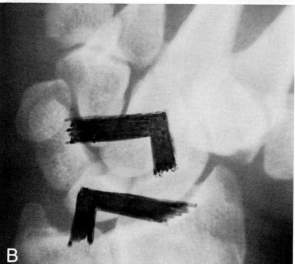

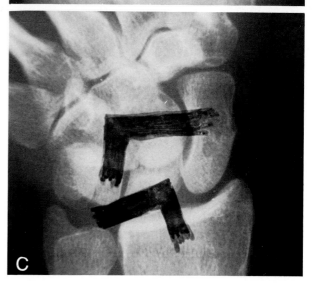

FIG. 4–31 Changes of volar radiocarpal and intercarpal ligaments during radial and ulnar deviation (see text). **A**, Neutral deviation; **B**, radial deviation; **C**, ulnar deviation.

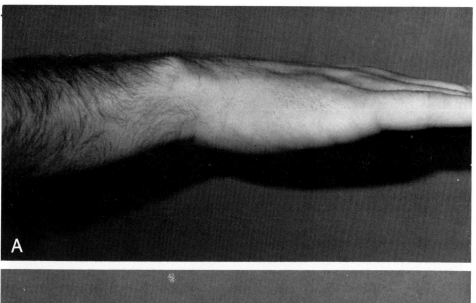

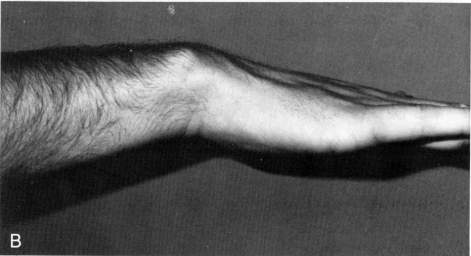

FIG. 4–32   Midcarpal instability. **A** shows normal clinical alignment; **B** demonstrates position of carpal collapse.

CARPAL KINEMATICS

Navarro introduced in 1919 the concept of a vertical or columnar carpus different from the traditional concept of a carpus represented by two horizontal or transverse rows of four bones each. Navarro postulated that the carpus is composed of three vertical columns: a *central* or flexion-extension column formed by the lunate, capitate, and hamate; a *lateral* or mobile column composed of the scaphoid, trapezium, and tra-

pezoid; and a *medial* or rotation column consisting of the triquetrum and pisiform, which he called the pisotriquetral system. Navarro believed that the influence of the radius on the carpus ended on the scaphoid, "while the disposition of bones and ligaments in the medial column explained the continuation along the medial column of the movements of the forearm." This concept was recently modified (Taleisnik, 1976) by expanding the central column to include the lunate and the entire distal carpal row (Fig. 4–33). This limited the mobile column to the scaphoid and the rotation column to the triquetrum. In 1939, Ghia observed that because scaphoid displacements in a dorsovolar direction were greater than the lunate and nonexistent for the triquetrum, the proximal row showed a "rotation movement around a proximal-distal axis which passes through the pyramidal (triquetrum) bone." This concept of the triquetrum as a pivot point is reinforced by the disposition of the carpal ligaments in relation to this bone and by the helicoidal shape of the triquetral facet of the hamate (Fig. 4–30).

In summary, the wrist may be viewed as a central flexion-extension longitudinal link composed of the radius and the flexion-extension carpal column onto which attach two V-shaped ligament structures. Wrist motions are produced by muscles that attach beyond this column into the metacarpals. The distal carpal row of the carpal bones is firmly attached to the hand and moves with it; therefore, during dorsiflexion the distal carpal row dorsiflexes, during volar flexion it volar flexes, and during radial and ulnar deviation, it deviates radially or ulnarly. Scaphoid and triquetrum displacements are directly determined by their connections with the distal carpal row. The lunate's indirect response is dictated by the pull of its ligaments and by the pressures exerted on it by the scaphoid and triquetrum. The connecting rod within this link is of course the scaphoid, which is a lateral mobile column with three ligamentous zones. The triquetrum is the medial or rotation column. Both the scaphoid and the triquetrum, as well as the medial or capitotriquetral fascicle of the deltoid ligament that crosses the midcarpal joint, contribute to the smooth transition of movement between the radiocarpal and midcarpal joints and to their stability, particularly when the link systems between the radius and the flexion-extension column is subjected to longitudinal compression loads.

With its multiple, small articular surfaces, the wrist allows all the movements of an enarthrodial joint without its intrinsic structural weakness. Both the radiocarpal and mid-

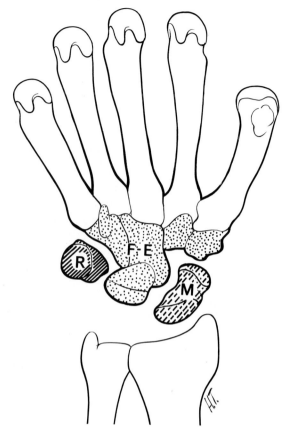

FIG. 4–33 Columnar carpus. M is mobile or lateral column; F–E is flexion–extension or central column; R is rotating or medial column.

carpal joints contribute to the total range of wrist motion, their relative participation largely determined by the location and orientation of the scaphoid (Fig. 4–34). The scaphoid is considered to be in longitudinal position when it reaches maximum dorsiflexion and its long axis is closely parallel to the long axis of the radius (Fig. 4–34B). Both the proximal and distal poles of the scaphoid are snugly applied to the lunate and to the trapezium-trapezoid facets, respectively. Midcarpal motion is largely eliminated, and the entire carpus is effectively changed into a single functional unit that moves on the radius at the radiocarpal joint level. Normally, the scaphoid becomes longitudinal during dorsiflexion and ulnar deviation. Both these motions take place predominantly at the level of the radiocar-

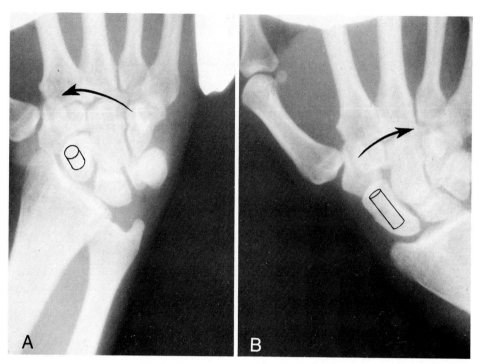

FIG. 4—34 **A**, Perpendicular position of the scaphoid when the wrist is volad flexed and radially deviated. **B**, Longitudinal position of the scaphoid when the wrist is dorsiflexed and ulnad deviated.

pal joint. In the opposite end-position of the scaphoid, its axis is transverse or *perpendicular* to the long axis of the radius (Fig. 4–34A) and is foreshortened when seen from the palm. The midcarpal joint is "unlocked," and the distal carpal row is allowed to migrate radially. The perpendicular scaphoid is found in radial deviation and in volar flexion, both predominantly midcarpal motions. There is a third degree of radiocarpal motion. In 1896, Meyer (quoted by Bryce) and later on Cyriax and Capener, suggested that there is some carpal rotation independent of forearm pronation and supination. During wrist dorsiflexion and ulnar deviation the hand tends to pronate on the forearm. There is apparent additional clinical pronation of the hand owing to the extension of the mobile fourth and fifth metacarpals at the metacarpal joints; conversely, during dorsiflexion and radial deviation there is supination of the hand. These motions can best be appreciated in patients with surgically created one-bone forearms. This additional degree of wrist motion may be an important factor in the mechanism of wrist injuries, as well as in their treatment.

VASCULAR ANATOMY OF THE CARPUS

The blood vessels that supply the carpus arise directly or indirectly from the radial, ulnar, and interosseous arteries. Classic descriptions show that anastomosis of these branches results in the formation of a volar carpal arch, a dorsal carpal arch, and superficial and deep palmar arches (*see Figs. 5–1 and 5–2*). According to these descriptions, the *superficial palmar arch* is formed by the superficial palmar branch of the radial artery and the termination of the ulnar artery and does not actually supply the bony carpus. The *volar carpal arch*, formed by the anastomosis of the volar carpal branches of the radial and ulnar arteries, is traditionally described as a transverse anastomotic loop running along the distal border of the pronator quadratus. The *dorsal carpal arch* courses across the midcarpus and is formed by a large vessel arising from the radial artery (the ramus carpus dorsalis) and a similar dorsal carpal branch from the ulnar artery. Smaller vessels from the convexity (distal) and concavity (proximal) of this arch anastomose with perforating metacarpal vessels and with branches from the interosseous arteries, thereby forming a dorsal vascular plexus called the *dorsal carpal rete*. The *deep palmar arch* is a most important supplier of blood to the carpus. It is formed by the deep palmar branch of the ulnar artery and by the termination of the radial artery in the palm. This arch traverses the hand slightly distal to the bases of the metacarpals and projects 1.5 cm to 2.0 cm proximal to the superficial palmar arch. Ascending (recurrent or articular) branches arise from the concavity of this arch, and traverse proximally on the volar surface of the carpus to join descending vessels from the volar carpal arch and from the volar division of the anterior interosseous artery.

Although the anterior interosseous artery is an important supplier of blood to the carpus, it is generally agreed that the dorsal interosseous artery does not significantly share in the carpal supply. The anterior interosseous artery divides proximal to the pronator quadratus into a volar branch and a larger, dorsal branch, which is considered by most to be the actual continuation of the main trunk of the anterior interosseous. In 1923, Lawrence and Bachuber described an anastomosis between volar terminal vessels from the anterior interosseous artery and recurrent rami from the deep palmar arch. This was also reported by Lawrence (1937) and by Quiring (1940). Since 1940, there have been reports of preservation of hand viability after ligation of both the radial and ulnar arteries, depending to a considerable extent on the completeness of this volar anastomosis.

Variations from the classic description of the deep palmar and the dorsal carpal arches have

been seen. Coleman and Anson classified deep palmar arches into two groups: complete (group I), present in 97% of their specimens, and incomplete (group II), in which the radial artery and branches of the ulnar artery did not join. Two types were then described within group II: type A, in which the radial was the sole contributor to the thumb and the radial aspect of the index finger, and type B, in which the area solely supplied by the radial artery extended to include the third digit.

A review of the literature suggests that the classic description of a dorsal carpal arch formed by anastomosis of the radial, ulnar, and interosseous arteries is far from constant. Coleman and Anson (1961) and Mestdagh and co-workers (1979) studied the dorsal carpal vessels. In their experience, the dorsal plexus resulted most frequently from anastomosis of branches of the radial and interosseous arteries. The classic radial-interosseous-ulnar configuration was in fact second in frequency.

The use of standard dissecting techniques for the study of these small vessels, even with the assistance of magnification, is difficult and may produce conflicting results. Fracassi (1945) reported the successful use of corrosion of perivascular tissues to demonstrate striking examples of the bare vascular trees. Recent technical improvements involving the use of perivascular debridement by chemical means have allowed more accurate study of the fine extraosseous arteries. These techniques make the dissection of the minute vessels within capsule and ligaments unnecessary; furthermore, the three-dimensional orientation of the pericarpal vascular lattice is preserved, and the vascular access to each carpal bone can be determined more precisely. Gelberman and collaborators injected specimens with either diluted Ward's blue latex or Batson's compound.* Batson's compound sets up as a rigid material that retains a three-dimensional orientation. Both latex and Batson's compound resist bleach digestion of the perivascular soft tissues, allowing the tridimen-

*Polyscience Incorporated, Paul Valley Industrial Park, Warrington, PA 18910

sional vascular pattern to emerge virtually intact.

EXTRAOSSEOUS VASCULARITY

The pericarpal arterial network is formed by the anastomosis of three dorsal and three volar arches, connected longitudinally along their medial and lateral borders by the ulnar and radial arteries. Additional longitudinal anastomoses are provided by the volar and dorsal divisions of the anterior interosseous artery.

The three dorsal arches (Fig. 4–35) are located at the radiocarpal, intercarpal, and basal metacarpal levels; the first two are the most constant. The more proximal *radiocarpal*

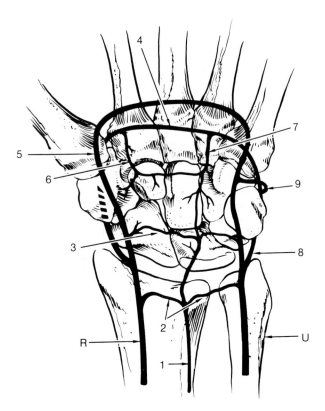

FIG. 4–36 Schematic drawing of the arterial supply of the volar aspect of the wrist. (R) radial artery; (U) ulnar artery; (1) volar branch anterior interosseous artery; (2) volar radiocarpal arch; (3) volar intercarpal arch; (4) deep palmar arch; (5) superficial palmar arch; (6) radial recurrent artery; (7) ulnar recurrent artery; (8) medial branch, ulnar artery; (9) branch of ulnar artery contributing to the dorsal intercarpal arch. (Gelberman RH, Panagis JS, Taleisnik J, Baumgaertner M: The arterial anatomy of the human carpus, Part I: The extraosseous vascularity, J Hand Surg 8:367, 1983)

FIG. 4–35 Schematic drawing of the arterial supply of the dorsum of the wrist. (R) Radial artery; (U) ulnar artery; (1) dorsal branch, anterior interosseous artery; (2) dorsal radiocarpal arch; (3) branch to the dorsal ridge of the scaphoid; (4) dorsal intercarpal arch; (5) basal metacarpal arch; (6) medial branch of the ulnar artery. (Gelberman RH, Panagis JS, Taleisnik J, and Baumgaertner M: The arterial anatomy of the human carpus, Part I: The extraosseous vascularity, J Hand Surg 8:367, 1983)

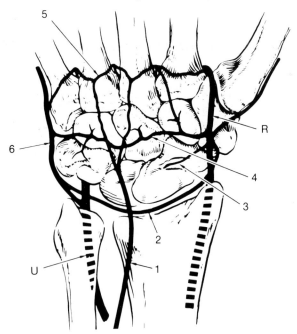

arch courses across the wrist at the level of the radiocarpal joint and is most frequently formed by branches of the radial, ulnar, and anterior interosseous arteries. Radial-ulnar and radial-interosseous combinations were seen in fewer than one third of specimens. The dorsal interosseous artery was judged not to be a significant contributor. The *intercarpal arch* is similar to the dorsal carpal arch of previous studies. It runs transversely at the level of the intercarpal joint. Contrary to previous reports by Coleman and Anson (1961) and Mestdagh and associ-

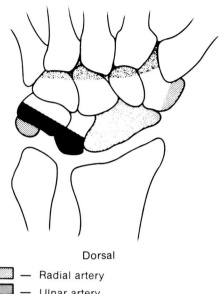

Dorsal

▨ — Radial artery

▩ — Ulnar artery

■ — Radiocarpal arch

☐ — Intercarpal arch

▨ — Basal metacarpal arch

FIG. 4–37 Schematic drawing of the dorsum of the wrist showing contributions to the carpal bones. (Gelberman RH, Panagis JS, Taleisnik J, Baumgaertner M: The arterial anatomy of the human carpus, Part I: The extraosseous vascularity, J Hand Surg 8:367, 1983)

ates (1979), the classic radial-interosseous-ulnar pattern was found to be most frequent (53% of specimens). The distal or *basal metacarpal arch* was complete in only 27% of specimens, partially present in 46%, and absent in the rest. This smaller dorsal arch traverses the bases of the second through fifth metacarpals.

The three volar arches (Fig. 4–36) are the radiocarpal, the intercarpal, and the deep palmar. The volar *radiocarpal* is similar to the classic volar carpal arch. It is formed as a radial-interosseous-ulnar system in 87% of specimens and as a radial-ulnar arch in 13%. The volar *intercarpal arch*, the smallest and least consistent, is present in slightly more than half of specimens. In most cases, it is formed by branches of all three major contributing arteries. The volar *deep palmar arch* is present in all specimens. Of its numerous branches,

those arising from its concavity and traversing in a recurrent proximal direction are most important. The two main recurrent arteries are the radial and ulnar. As previously stated, survival of the hand after major arterial injury proximal to the wrist may depend on the effectiveness of this system of volar recurrent vessels.

All three volar arches are connected longitudinally by the radial, ulnar, and interosseous arteries and by the deep palmar recurrent vessels. In general, with the exception of the scaphoid and the pisiform, the dorsal supply to the carpus is provided mainly by the dorsal intercarpal arch (Fig. 4–37). There are additional contributions to the lunate and triquetrum from the radiocarpal arch proximally

FIG. 4–38 Schematic drawing of the volar aspect of the wrist showing the contributions to the carpal bones. (Gelberman RH, Panagis JS, Taleisnik J, Baumgaertner M: The arterial anatomy of the human carpus, Part I: The extraosseous vascularity, J Hand Surg 8:367, 1983)

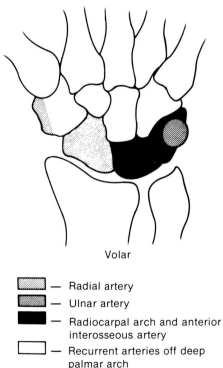

Volar

▨ — Radial artery

▩ — Ulnar artery

■ — Radiocarpal arch and anterior interosseous artery

☐ — Recurrent arteries off deep palmar arch

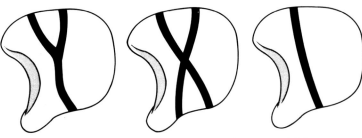

FIG. 4—39 Schematic representation of Y, X, and I intraosseous vascular patterns to the lunate (Gelberman RH, Bauman TD, Menon J, Akeson WH: The vascularity of the lunate bone and Kienböck's disease, J Hand Surg 5:272, 1980)

and to all bones of the distal carpal row from the basal metacarpal arch distally. The scaphoid is supplied by branches of the radial artery; the pisiform receives one to three small vessels directly from the ulnar artery; while circulation to the trapezium is reinforced by direct branches from the radial artery trunk. The volar pattern again shows that the scaphoid and pisiform receive their major branches directly from the radial and ulnar arteries, respectively, rather than from the transverse arches (Fig. 4–38). The volar radiocarpal arch provides the main supply to the lunate and triquetrum, while the recurrent branch from the deep palmar arch supplies all bones in the distal carpal row.

INTRAOSSEOUS VASCULARITY

Most carpal bones are exclusively supplied by branches of the transverse arches rather than by direct branches of the main arteries. Exceptions are the scaphoid and pisiform, and partly the trapezium, which receive some of their arterial supply from the main trunks of the radial and ulnar arteries. All vessels enter bone in nonarticular surfaces in areas of ligamentous and capsular attachments. The carpal vessels can be classified into three major groups, based on the presence or absence of intraosseous

anastomoses, the size and location of nutrient vessels, and the dependence of large areas of bone on a single intraosseous vessel. Group I includes the scaphoid, capitate, and some lunates, each with vessels entering only one surface or with large intraosseous areas dependent on a single intraosseous vessel. The carpal bones in this group are considered to be at greater risk to develop avascular necrosis after fracture. The blood supply to the scaphoid enters the bone at and distal to its waist and extends proximally. The vessels to the capitate also penetrate the distal portion of the bone and spread proximally to supply the head and neck. Seventy percent of capitates do not have intraosseous anastomosis; 50% of these have nutrient vessels supplying the head from the volar surface only.

In a 1963 study of the intraosseous arterial pattern of the lunate, Lee reported that in 66% of 53 normal specimens there were dorsal and volar vessels that anastomosed within bone. In 26% there was only a single volar or dorsal vessel; in 7.5% there were volar and dorsal vessels that failed to connect with each other. In a more recent study by Gelberman and co-workers (1980), three major intraosseous patterns were found and were named Y, X, or I, according to their configuration (Fig. 4–39). The Y design was the most common, with a single stem arising from either the volar or the dorsal facets of the lunate. The I pattern was next in frequency, whereas the X was observed in only 10%.

Rarely, the lunate is supplied by a single volar vessel. About 20% of lunates have this type of single blood supply and belong with this group of bones (Group I), which is more susceptible to avascular changes after injury. Group II includes the trapezoid and hamate, both of which have at least two areas of vessel entry but lack significant intraosseous anastomosis. The probability of avascular necrosis occurring in these carpal bones is fairly remote. The carpal bones in group III, like those in group II, present two surfaces for vessel entry and no large area depends on a single nutrient artery. In group III, intraosseous anastomoses are consistently found; the trapezium, triquetrum, and pisiform and 80% of lunates belong to this group. Groups II and III both show very low incidences of avascular necrosis, suggesting that the presence or absence of intraosseous anastomosis, which is the only anatomic difference in blood supply between the carpal bones in both groups, may be entirely irrelevant from a clinical standpoint.

5
The Blood and the Nerve Supply of the Hand

The Blood Supply of the Hand

E. F. Shaw Wilgis
Emanuel B. Kaplan

In the embryo lymphatics, veins and arteries are all developed as tissue spaces that become confluent and form a connected system of channels. These channels communicate freely among themselves in a plexiform arrangement and function as conduits for any of these fluid types. During development, these vessel systems are isolated and become separate entities. Persistence of various patterns of the embryonic vascular channels results in lymphangiomas, hemangiomas, and arteriovenous fistulae.

The main arterial supply to the forearm and hand is derived from the continuation of the axillary to the brachial artery. At the elbow or just distal to it, the brachial artery divides into the radial and ulnar arteries and the anterior and posterior interosseous arteries. These vessels course through the forearm with the interosseous branches terminating at the wrist.

ARTERIES

The hand is supplied by the radial and ulnar arteries and is supplemented by the anterior interosseous artery and its posterior branch. The artery of the median nerve, which normally arises from the proximal part of the anterior interosseous artery, runs as a long, slender twig over the volar aspect of the median nerve. In the infrequent cases when it is very large, the artery of the median nerve also contributes to the blood supply of the hand (*Fig. 5–7*). The presence of a large artery in front of the median nerve and running into the carpal canal may be confusing if its significance and derivation are not known.

The radial and the ulnar arteries, with contributions from the other arteries, form the arterial arches of the hand. The variations observed in the formation of the arches and the digital branches result from differences in the sizes of the five contributing arteries: the radial, the ulnar, the anterior interosseous, the dorsal branch of the anterior interrosseous, and the artery of the median nerve. The retention of the embryonal type with predominance of one of these arteries is responsible for the variations. The radial and ulnar arteries form the main arterial supply to the hand.

The general pattern of the hand's arterial supply consists of two systems for the volar aspect and a single system for the dorsal aspect. The volar supply is arranged into a superficial and a deep group (Fig. 5–1).

RADIAL ARTERY

The radial artery can be palpated just anteromedial to the tendons of the abductor longus and the extensor brevis muscles, proximal to the styloid process of the radius. It frequently has a volar branch (volar carpal artery), that passes transversely toward the ulna and

FIG. 5–1 Standard type of the superficial and the deep arterial arches formed by the superficial branch of the radial artery and the ulnar artery and by the deep branch of the radial and the ulnar arteries (modified from Henle).

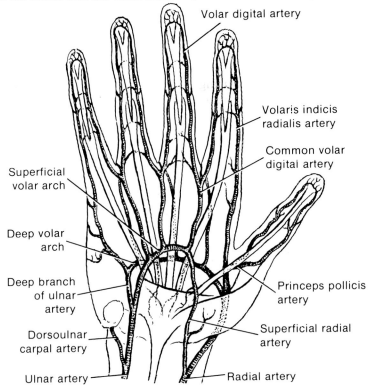

Volar digital artery

Volaris indicis radialis artery

Common volar digital artery

Superficial volar arch

Deep volar arch

Deep branch of ulnar artery

Dorsoulnar carpal artery

Ulnar artery

Princeps pollicis artery

Superficial radial artery

Radial artery

anastomoses with a similar branch from the ulnar artery (volar ulnar carpal). This transverse anastomosis forms an arch that functions as an arterial landmark at the distal border of the pronator quadratus.

Transverse arch

The transverse arch may be of sufficient volume to cause considerable bleeding when divided. Its importance lies in its contribution of blood to the distal end of the radius and carpal bones through a network (volar carpal rete) with contributory small branches from the anterior interosseous artery and from the ascending branches deriving from the deep volar arch.

The radial artery also supplies a dorsal carpal artery (dorsal radial carpal) that forms a dorsal arterial arch with a similar branch of the ulnar artery (dorsal ulnar carpal). The dorsal branch of the radial artery branches off, very deeply, under the tendons of the anatomic snuff-box and the carpal extensors. The dorsal branch of the ulnar artery arises from the medial side of the artery distal to the head of the ulna and runs under the tendons of the flexor carpi ulnaris, the medial collateral ligaments, and the tendon of the extensor carpi ulnaris toward the distal carpal bones.

Dorsal carpal arch

The dorsal carpal arch, which is formed by the union of the radial and the ulnar dorsal carpal arches, forms a network that supplies the carpal bones (Fig. 4–14 and Fig. 5–2). The network

FIG. 5–2   Dorsal arterial arch formed by a branch of the radial artery and a branch of the ulnar artery with extensive anastomosis with branches of the posterior interosseous artery of the forearm. The dorsal metacarpal arteries to the thumb and the radial side of the index finger branch off from the radial artery. The second, third, and fourth metacarpal arteries supply the corresponding digits. The fifth metacarpal artery comes off from the ulnar and supplies the ulnar side of the fifth finger (modified from Henle).

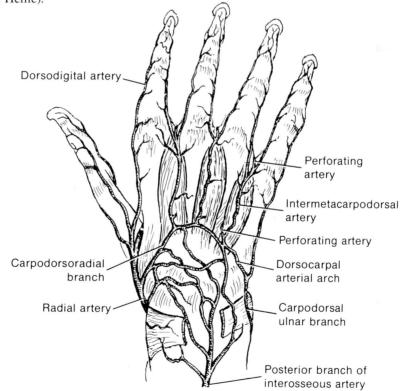

(dorsal carpal rete) receives contributory branches from the dorsal branch of the volar interosseous and occasionally receives small branches from the deep palmar arch as perforating branches passing between the proximal ends of the metacarpals. The structure of the volar carpal rete over the volar aspect of the carpus resembles the dorsal carpal rete, but the dorsal carpal rete differs from the volar rete because of the dorsal metacarpal arteries to the second, third, and fourth intermetacarpal spaces (Fig. 5–2).

The first dorsal metacarpal supplies the dorsum of the thumb and the radial side of the index finger and is a separate branch that usually originates just before the radial artery penetrates between the two heads of the first dorsal interosseous distal to the emergence of the dorsal radial carpal artery. The first dorsal metacarpal runs quite superficially on the dorsal surface of the index head of the first dorsal interosseous muscle (Figs. 3–14 and 5–2). In places it is fairly large and thus can be easily palpated. This artery can be easily injured in intervention over the metacarpomultangular joint of the thumb, when approached from the dorsum of this joint.

During surgery in this region, the radial artery must be carefully identified and protected. The radial artery passes into the palm of the hand (Fig. 2–63) between the oblique and transverse heads of the adductor pollicis and forms the deep palmar arch by anastomosing with the deep branch of the ulnar artery.

Deep palmar arch

The radial artery becomes the deep palmar arch as it enters the palm between the two segments of the first dorsal interosseous muscle (Fig. 2–63). Before the radial artery is covered by the oblique head of the adductor pollicis muscle, the *princeps pollicis artery* branches from it and runs on the volar aspect of the adductor pollicis muscle between the flexor pollicis brevis and the tendon of the flexor pollicis longus. The princeps pollicis divides at various levels near the metacarpophalangeal joint of the thumb into the two volar arteries of the thumb. The *volar indicis radialis* artery arises slightly more medial or from the same trunk as the princeps pollicis. It runs parallel with the second metacarpal between the first dorsal interosseous and the adductor pollicis. Three *metacarpal* arteries run in the second, third, and fourth intermetacarpal spaces, respectively, and digital branches by division into two branches for each finger.

Other arterial branches contribute to a rich anastomosis among all of these arteries. Some branch off the deep arch as ascending twigs to the carpal rete; others form two sets of perforating branches, uniting the deep volar arch with the dorsal arch. The perforating arteries are usually located in the interbasal and intercapitular areas between the metacarpals. The perforating between the heads of the metacarpals is probably less constant than in the others.

ULNAR ARTERY

The ulnar artery passes into the hand from behind the expansion of the tendon of the flexor carpi ulnaris. The expansion of the tendon fused with the antebrachial fascia covers the ulnar artery and the ulnar nerve, which repose in a triangular channel formed by the anterior carpal ligament and the unciform process medially. The artery is accompanied by the two veins; the ulnar nerve is on its medial side.

The ulnar artery sends out a large branch that pierces the muscles of the hypothenar group and enters the retrotendinous midpalmar. This branch is accompanied by the deep branch of the ulnar nerve, which is somewhat more proximal, becoming dorsal to the deep arch. The nerve and the artery both pass to the radial side of the hand through the fascial foramen between the transverse and oblique parts of the adductor pollicis and enter the space dorsal to the adductor pollicis. In their passage, the deep branch of the ulnar nerve and the deep palmar arch are well protected by the midpalmar fat pad described by the author as the *paniculus adiposus volaris profundus*. The nerve and the arch are protected in their radial halves by the adductor pollicis muscle. A few smaller branches derive from the ulnar artery proximal to the deep ulnar branch and supply hypothenar

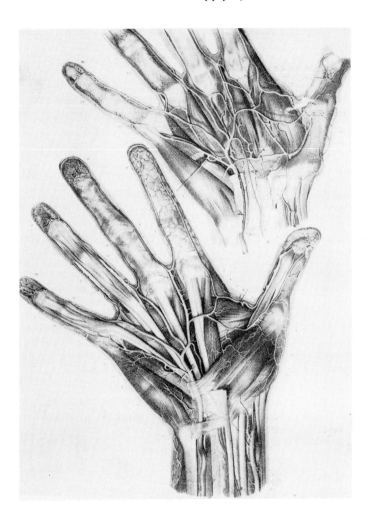

FIG. 5–3 Superficial and deep arterial palmar arches. (Bourgery JM: Traite complet de l'anatomie de l'homme. Vol. 4. Paris, L. Guérin, 1867–1871)

muscles. If one of these branches is unusually large, it can easily be mistaken for the true deep branch of the ulnar artery.

About 2 cm to 3 cm from the proximal apex of the pisiform, the previously described dorsal ulnar carpal artery passes underneath the tendon of the flexor carpi ulnaris, the collateral ligament, and the extensor carpi ulnaris to unite with a similar dorsal radial carpal and thereby form the dorsal carpal arterial arch.

Superficial palmar arch

The ulnar artery itself continues superficially and passes under the midpalmar fascia, where it forms the superficial arterial arch by anastomosis with the *superficial branch of the radial artery*, which passes either above or at the same depth as the abductor pollicis brevis (Fig. 5–3). The superficial arch supplies the second, third, and fourth intermetacarpal arteries, which bifurcate at the roots of the fingers to supply the two contiguous fingers: the ulnar side of the index and the radial side of the middle finger, the ulnar side of the middle and the radial side of the ring finger, the ulnar side of the ring and the radial side of the little finger, and a separate branch for the ulnar side of the little finger.

The dorsal arterial supply derives from the dorsal carpal rete. The rete is formed by the dorsal radial carpal branch of the radial artery at the point where it passes under the abductor

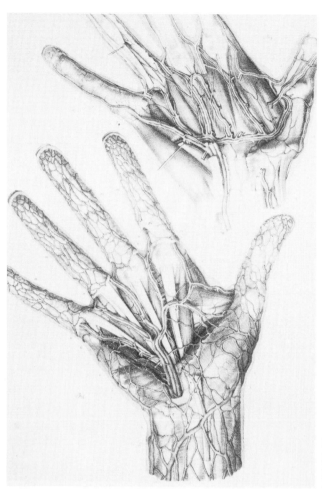

FIG. 5–4 Superficial and deep veins of palm of the hand. (Bourgery JM: Traite complet de l'anatomie de l'homme. Vol. 4. Paris, L. Guérin, 1867–1871)

pollicis longus and passes medially beneath the extensor carpi radialis longus and brevis and the extensor pollicis longus to anastomose with the dorsal carpal branch of the ulnar artery. From this rete, the second, third, and fourth dorsal metacarpal arteries emerge and run on the surface of the dorsal interosseous muscles to the interdigital folds. These arteries then each divide into two dorsal digital branches for the contiguous fingers. Between the bases of the metacarpal bones, the dorsal metacarpal arteries anastomose with the perforating branches of the deep volar arch. Distally, between the metacarpal heads, they are connected by perforating branches to a volar common digital artery of the corresponding spaces.

Although this is the commonly accepted pattern of the hand's arterial supply (Fig. 5–4), the pattern does not always correspond to the true arterial arrangement. Studies by Dubreuil–Chambardel (1926) are the most comprehensive and accurate. Other dynamic anatomic studies have been done in living subjects. Mozersky and associates (1973), stimulated by the development of hand ischemia in a young man after cannulation of the radial artery, studied 70 subjects with the directional Doppler ultrasonic flow detector to determine the adequacy of the normal palmar anastomosis of blood vessels. They found that 17 (12.1%) of 140 palmar arches displayed radial-dominant circulation and had incomplete volar palmar arches. In two of these, no collateral flow was detectable when the radial artery was occluded. The collateral circulation was judged poor in 11 of the 14 radial-dominant palms. Twenty-five of the 122 hands (20.5%) with ulnar-dominant circulation had incomplete palmar arches. In 20 hands, there was no detectable circulation upon ulnar artery occlusion. Twelve patients with incomplete palmar arches were found to have poor collateral supply. The dominant circulation was symmetrical in all but two cases.

These clinical studies correlate well with the anatomic studies mentioned earlier and emphasize the importance of understanding anatomic variations. For microvascular repair and replantation, a thorough knowledge of possible variations is necessary so that the surgeon will not be misled by a confusing clinical picture.

VARIATIONS

Variations of the superficial palmar arch

The superficial palmar arch may have three variants. The first variant, in which the ulnar artery is responsible for the formation of the superficial palmar arch, occurs in about 66% of cases. It has seven types.

Type 1. The ulnar artery is responsible for the formation of all the digital arteries (Fig. 5–5A).

Type 2. The ulnar artery ends as the radial collateral of the index finger; the two collaterals of the thumb are formed by the first volar metacarpal of the radial artery (Fig. 5–5B).

Type 3. The most frequent variation, the ulnar artery ends in the second intermetacarpal space; the two volar collaterals of the thumb and the collateral radial of the index are furnished by the radial artery (Fig. 5–5C).

Type 4. The ulnar artery runs vertically from the pisiform bone to the third intermetacar-

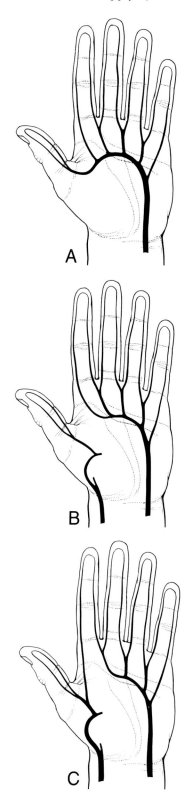

FIG. 5–5 Variations of the superficial palmar arch with the ulnar artery dominant in its formation to varying extent.

(Continued)

Fig. 5–5 (Continued)

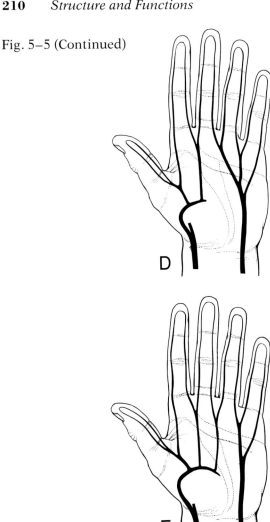

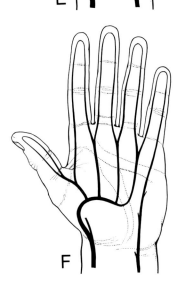

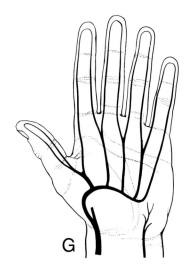

pal space. It supplies only five collateral arteries to the fingers; the other five collateral arteries are furnished by the first and the second volar metacarpal branches of the radial artery (Fig. 5–5D).

Type 5. The ulnar artery runs vertically and reaches the fourth intermetacarpal space, furnishing only three collateral arteries for the fingers; the other seven are supplied by the metacarpal branches of the radial artery (Fig. 5–5E).

Type 6. The ulnar artery, much reduced in volume, supplies only the ulnar collateral to the fifth finger (Fig. 5–5F).

Type 7. The ulnar artery gives only insignificant branches to the digital arteries, and the main supply derives from the radial artery (Fig 5–5G).

The ulnar artery at first forms the entire superficial blood supply to the palm, then regresses in favor of the radial artery to the point that the radial artery is responsible for the entire blood supply. In these cases the superficial branch of the radial artery does not participate in the formation of the superficial arch at all and is completely lost in the blood supply of the thenar muscles.

The second variant of the superficial palmar arch, in which the superficial radial palmar artery participates in the formation of the arch, occurs in about 30% of cases.

Type 1 (very frequent). Before the anastomosis with the ulnar artery, one or two colaterals for the thumb are furnished (Fig. 5–6*A*).

Type 2. In addition to the collateral of the thumb are a radial collateral or two collaterals for the index (Fig. 5–6*B*).

Type 3 (the most frequent). Regular anastomosis occurs between the superficial radial palmar and the ulnar artery (Fig. 5–6*C*).

Type 4. The superficial radial branch supplies the collateral to the thumb, the index finger, and the radial side of the middle finger, terminating directly in the radial branch of the middle finger and supplying five digital branches, while the ulnar supplies also the remaining five digital arteries and ends vertically and independently in the ulnar branch of the middle finger (Fig. 5–6*D*).

Type 5. The ulnar artery supplies only the fifth and fourth fingers or none at all, in which case the superficial branch of the radial artery supplies all the fingers, and the ulnar artery supplies mostly the hypothenar muscles (Fig. 5–6*E*).

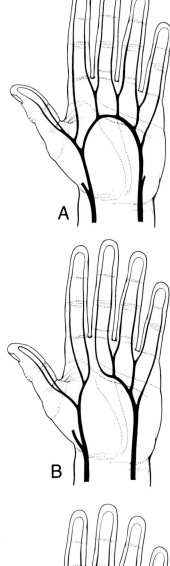

FIG. 5–6 Variations of the superficial palmar arch in which the superficial radial palmar artery participates in its formation.

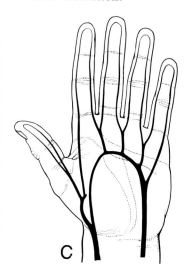
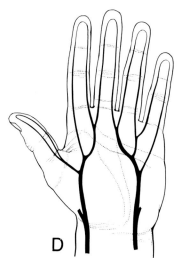
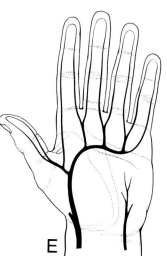

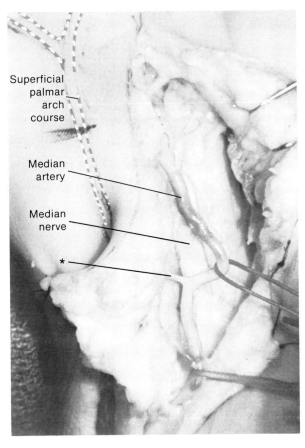

Superficial
palmar
arch
course

Median
artery

Median
nerve

*

FIG. 5–7 Right hand. Well-developed median artery coursing along the median nerve, anastomosing (∗) with the superficial palmar arch.

The third variant of the superficial arch, in which the median artery contributes to the information of the arch (Fig. 5–7), was seen in only 4% of the 1,200 cases reported by Dubreuil–Chambardel. In this variant, types similar to those previously described, in which arteries participate in the formation of the arch, may be encountered. Very infrequently, an additional subcutaneous transverse anastomosis with a subcutaneous branch of the superficial branch of the ulnar artery is found. If this is present it will lie on top of the midpalmar aponeurosis and may be taken for the superficial arterial palmar arch, if its position is not assessed properly.

Variations of the deep palmar arch
The most frequent variation of the deep palmar arch is a regular anastomosis between the radial artery and the deep branch of the ulnar artery. Several variations occur in the distribution and number of metacarpal arteries provided by the radial deep branch of the ulnar artery; the interior interosseous artery may participate in the formation of the deep palmar arch with the radial artery or the deep branch of the ulnar artery. An interesting variant was described in which the dorsal arch contributed to the deep palmar arch through a larger artery penetrating from the dorsum through the second intermetacarpal space to furnish the second, third, and fourth intermetacarpal arteries of the palm.

Variations of the dorsal carpal arch
The dorsal carpal arch as generally described is not constant. According to Dubreuil–Chambardel, several types are observed. One of the most frequent is the so-called radial type in which the radial dorsal carpal branch alone forms the dorsal carpal arch (see Fig. 4–14); this type is seen in about 58% of cases. A second type is formed by the confluence of the radial

carpal and the ulnar carpal arteries and the corresponding arteries, which may contribute equally or unequally to the dorsal arch. A third type is formed by the anterior or posterior branch of the anterior or posterior interosseous arteries of the forearm. This type is seen in about 19% of cases.

Variations caused by age

The configuration of the arteries varies with age. In children, the arteries are more or less straight, and the anastomotic branches are small; in adults, the arteries are more arched, with branches arising from the concave or sometimes from the convex side of the arch. In the elderly, the arteries are much larger and are tortuous and elongated; they are observed most frequently in anatomic laboratories. It has been justly stated that most of the illustrations of the arteries in the classic treatises by the earlier anatomists were drawn from dissections of old subjects and do not conform to the appearance of the arteries of younger individuals.

Variations of the brachial and antebrachial arteries

Several studies of interest consider the blood supply of the hand and are concerned with the brachial and antebrachial patterns (McCormack, Cauldwell, and Anson). The brachial artery presents varied levels of origin, bifurcations, and duplications. There were major variations in the brachial and the antebrachial arteries in 18.53% of 750 upper extremities. In 364 cadavers, arterial variations were observed in 6.23% bilaterally and in 24.45% unilaterally. Generally, variations were observed more often on the right than on the left side of the hand. In 628 upper extremities, the most common variations were high origin of the radial artery, high origin and unusual course of the ulnar artery, and formation of a common trunk for both radial and ulnar arteries by the superficial brachial artery. The surgeon must be aware of these variations by thorough exploration before any surgical procedure.

Variations of the superficial volar arch

The superficial volar arches in the 650 specimens of Coleman and Anson were found to be either of the complete or incomplete group. In the complete arch group (80%), all the contributing branches anastomose; five types were observed:

Type 1. The arch is formed by the superficial volar branch of the radial artery and the larger ulnar artery. This was found in 34.5% of the specimens.

Type 2. The arch is formed entirely by the ulnar artery; this was present in 37% of specimens.

Type 3. The arch is formed by the enlarged median nerve artery; this was present in 3.8% of specimens.

Type 4. The arch is formed by the radial artery, median nerve artery, and the ulnar artery; it is found in only 1.2% of specimens.

Type 5 (an unreported type). The arch is formed by an ulnar artery joined by a large vessel from the deep palmar arch joining the superficial arch at the base of the thenar eminence.

No contribution to the superficial arch by the volar interosseous artery was observed in this series. The incomplete group is divided into four types similar to those of the complete group. The median nerve artery is always deep to the transverse carpal ligament. The deep volar arch is less variable than the superficial and was complete in 97% of specimens. Four types of perforating arteries passed from volar vessels through the metacarpal interspaces to anastomose with the dorsal metacarpal arteries and provide the principal arterial supply to the dorsal surface of the hand.

NERVES OF THE ARTERIES AND VEINS

Pick has described the sympathetic nerves as they innervate the vessels in the forearm and hand. All surgeons should be familiar with the innervation of the arteries and veins.

Each spinal nerve carries a variable number of autonomic fibers that originate from cells of autonomic centers or enter the spinal nerve through the rami communicantes. Among these fibers are vasomotor fibers that leave the branches of the spinal nerve and form the nervi vasorum. At various levels of the peripheral nerve, the spinal nerve forms fine branches that penetrate the perivascular tissues and pass into the vascular walls. Therefore it is clear that the blood vessels are supplied by branches of the spinal nerves; the level of nerve supply varies. Either a long branch comes off and penetrates the wall of a vessel where a division into terminal branches takes place, or many small branches penetrate a vessel segmentally a short distance from each other.

Maximenkow found that the superficial veins of the extremities are supplied by all of the cutaneous nerves, although at times only a limited number of the cutaneous nerves supplied the veins. This applies to the deep veins, which are mostly supplied by all the nerves of the extremity. The vascular nerves usually branch from the main trunks at a sharp angle, pass through the perivascular tissue, and finally penetrate the adventitia of vessels. Not infrequently, the nervi vasorum are found in the muscular, articular, and periosteal branches adhering to the outside of the vascular wall before penetrating the vessel. When the vascular nerve reaches the vessel, it is usually divided into ascending and descending branches in the perivascular tissues before it penetrates the arterial and venous walls. At times, short vascular branches penetrate the wall at various levels as secondary branches.

The length of the nerve corresponds to the diameter of the blood vessel: the larger diameter vessels have the longer nerves. The distribution of the nerve endings is irregular, and the branches frequently form arches and circles. The nerves supply the arteries and the veins, although more nerves enter the arteries. The nerves penetrating the veins sometimes enter at the level of the valves. *Note that alongside the nervi vasorum there are usually found arterial and venous branches that supply the nerves—vasa nervorum; this indicates an intimate morphologic and functional relationship between these structures* (Fig. 5–8).

The problem of intramural vascular distribution of terminal organs was studied by Dolgo Sanburow. In connection with this, another observation of the role of the epineural veins in diagnosis of interruption in injured nerves was made by Margorin. Enlarged and twisted epineural veins in the region of fibrous union between the peripheral and central segments of a nerve indicate a total interruption of the nerve.

The distribution of the nerve branches to the larger arterial trunks can be dissected and followed (Fig. 5–9). The *ulnar artery* is supplied in the forearm by a special nerve called the *nerve of Henle*, or the arterial branch of the ulnar nerve. It arises high in the forearm from the ulnar nerve and follows the ulnar artery in several filaments down to the palm of the hand. Lazorthes mentions that this nerve was found to be one of the longest arterial nerves in the extremities. The *radial artery* receives branches from the superficial branch of the radial nerve and multiple twigs from the lateral cutaneous nerve of the forearm.

The *interosseous arteries* are supplied in the following manner: The *anterior interosseous artery* is frequently reached by the anterior interosseous nerve and also by a branch from the median nerve. The *nutrient arteries* for the radius and the ulna are accompanied by branches of the anterior interosseous nerve. The *posterior interosseous artery* is supplied by the posterior interosseous nerve, a branch of the radial nerve.

The *palmar arterial arches* are supplied by the median and the ulnar nerves. Obviously many variations may exist in the relative distribution of the branches from these two nerves; however, the radial part of the superficial arterial arch is supplied mostly by the median nerve. The ulnar part of the superficial arterial arch is supplied by the ulnar nerve, as is the deep arch. The radial artery at its entrance into the deep structures of the palm and over the dorsal arterial arch is supplied mostly by branches of the median nerve. Apparently, any large trunk in the vicinity of the radial or the ulnar part of the arches is capable of sending one or several twigs

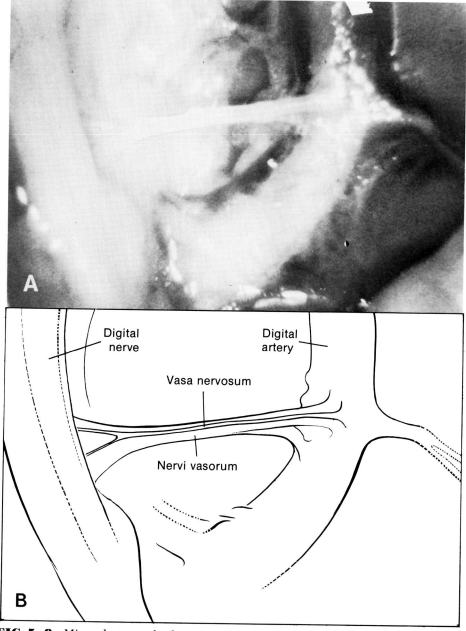

FIG. 5–8 Microphotograph of nervi vasorum and vasa nervorum coursing between digital nerve and digital artery.

to the corresponding part of the deep or superficial arch. The digital arteries apparently receive minute twigs from the accompanying digital nerves (Fig. 5–9).

The connections of the autonomic efferent fibers with the arterial and the venous walls form a part of the vasomotor system. The fibers reach their destinations in the vessels through the peripheral nerves (the branches of the median and ulnar nerves). The autonomic fibers join the peripheral nerves from the stellate and the second and third thoracic sympathetic

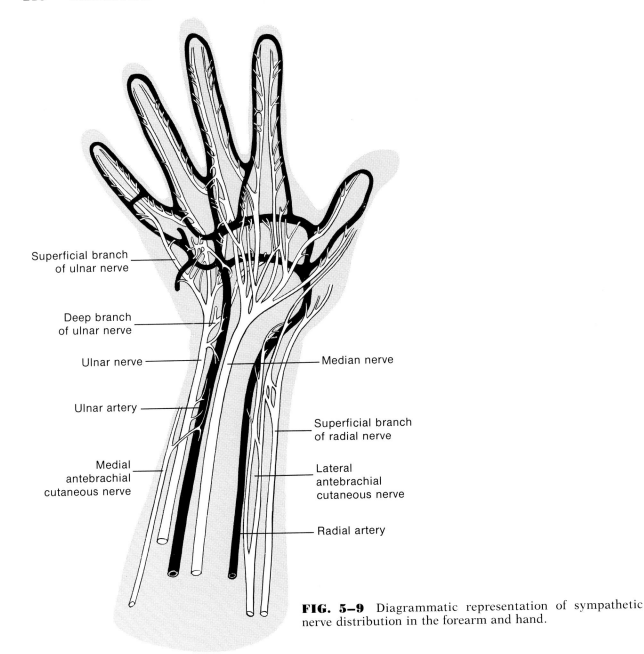

Superficial branch
of ulnar nerve

Deep branch
of ulnar nerve

Ulnar nerve

Ulnar artery

Median nerve

Superficial branch
of radial nerve

Medial
antebrachial
cutaneous nerve

Lateral
antebrachial
cutaneous nerve

Radial artery

FIG. 5–9 Diagrammatic representation of sympathetic nerve distribution in the forearm and hand.

ganglia. The sensory fibers of the vascular walls pass through the same peripheral branches and probably follow the usual sensory pathways through the posterior roots of the peripheral nervous system.

THE VENOUS SYSTEM

The venous system of the hand may be divided into deep and superficial veins; the deep veins usually accompany the palmar arches and the dorsal arterial arch. Veins usually are double and may run either parallel with or across the arteries at various angles; they usually are of much smaller caliber than the arteries. Veins anastomose freely through the perforating branches between the volar and the dorsal aspects of the hand. In young adults and children, veins are quite well defined and can be easily separated from the arteries. In older individuals and in the very old, the venous

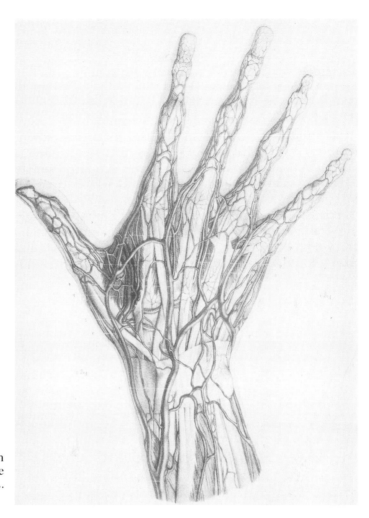

FIG. 5–10 Superficial veins of the dorsum of the hand. (Bourgery JM: Traite complet de l'anatomie de l'homme. Vol. 4. Paris, L. Guérin, 1867–1871)

system is usually more abundant; veins in the elderly are dilated and present an annoying problem in surgery of the hand. Most of the drainage is directed toward the radial and ulnar veins, although some of the blood is directed into the superficial system (Fig. 5–10).

Surprisingly the volar digital arteries in the fingers are usually not accompanied by double veins. The digital nerves and arteries run together with the nerves more superficial than the arteries. The absence of veins accompanying these volar digital arteries must be taken into account in the surgical approach to the digital nerves.

Recent experiences with transplantation of fingers, when the entire finger is carried into a

new position and depends for its survival on transplantation of the neurovascular pedicle, indicate that in addition to the artery and the nerve, an adequate venous system is most important. This means that the digital artery requires two venae comitantes; however, even in the most extensive anatomic atlases the venae comitantes are not demonstrated. The veins are usually shown up to the interdigital folds. The deep and superficial arterial palmar arches are shown to have venae comitantes, but the veins are not extended into the fingers. These omissions in atlases result from the technical difficulties presented by injections of the digital veins. These difficulties were thought to be not caused by the presence of valves in the small veins of fingers but by the extremely small diameters of these veins.

We have several times attempted to inject these small veins in order to see their distribution in relation to the digital arteries, but these attempts were unsuccessful. Some success was achieved in very fresh specimens, in which most of the veins returning from the fingers and thumb represent a crisscross network that surrounds the neurovascular bundle in the fingers, the palmar arteries, and the dorsal anastomotic veins proximal to the arterial arches. In several specimens, a single long vein followed the digital artery, although this was uncommon. In the embryologic sections, the same pattern of distribution of the veins was found (Fig. 5–11).

Most of the veins were centered around the neurovascular bundle at a certain distance from the artery and the nerve. A similar arrangement is represented in *Practice Anatomie* by Lanz and Wachsmuth.

A number of small veins in the superficial layers of the palm and fingers bleed profusely when divided during surgery; however, a vessel divided inadvertently near a digital nerve is probably a digital artery. The superficial veins of the dorsum of the fingers run in a pattern of several trunks parallel with the long axis of the finger. This is especially evident over the middle phalanges when transverse incisions are made. These trunks collect the veins from the irregular plexus of the volar and lateral sides of the fingers.

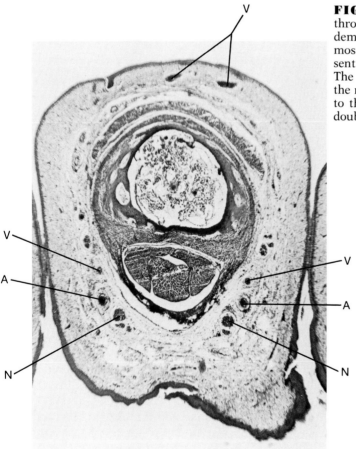

FIG. 5–11 Full-term infant. Section through the ring finger (middle phalanx) to demonstrate the distribution of veins. The most volar part shows numerous dots representing sectioned superficial veins in the skin. The next large sections are digital nerves (N); the next represent digital arteries (A). Dorsal to the artery is a single vein (V). The usual double venae comitantes are not found.

Very rarely, a single vein for an artery is found (Figs. 2–59 and 2–60). Most frequently, small veins unrelated to the arteries are found in the subcutaneous layers; they drain either into the superficial system or into the deep veins of the palmar arches. The superficial venous system is more abundant; the veins collect most of the subungual and terminal volar plexuses. They collect into lateral veins over the dorsum of the fingers and finally are directed toward the interdigital spaces to form a venous network over the dorsum of the hand.

In a recent superb anatomical study of the venous system of the digits Moss, Schwartz, Ascher, Wheeler, Ogden, and Lister demonstrated by microdissection, histological and corrosive techniques that the digital veins have valves which prevent the flow of blood from the dorsum to palmar aspect, proximal to distal and ulnar to radial digits in the proximal venous

FIG. 5–12 A·F The presence and distribution of valves in digital veins has been demonstrated by: (A) Microdissection—here, a vein over the proximal phalanx has been opened longitudinally to demonstrate the two valve cusps; (B) Histology—the cusps of a valve over the proximal phalanx are shown in cross-section (arrow indicates dissection of venous flow); (C) Corrosion specimens—a valve over the proximal phalanx is shown here in relief by the technique of Batson. The venous flow patterns imposed by the valves were shown by radiographs in cadaveric digits after digital microcannulation. (D) illustrates the free movement of dye from palmar injection to dorsal veins and from digit to digit via the natatory veins (see arrow). (E) demonstrates that dye injected in the dorsum of the digit and obstructed by a tourniquet (see double arrow) does not pass to the palmar surface. The valves preventing such flow (see solid arrows) appear as circular opacities, notably at the palmar end of the web-space vein (see open arrow) (F) shows a composite schematic of the left ring finger prepared from all sources demonstrated, in which the distribution of valves is notably preventing flow from dorsal to palmar, from proximal to distal, and from ulnar to radial digits in the proximal venous arches. (From Moss SH, Schwartz KS, Von Drasek-Ascher G, Ogden LL, Wheeler CS, Lister GD: Digital venous anatomy. Submitted to J Anat)

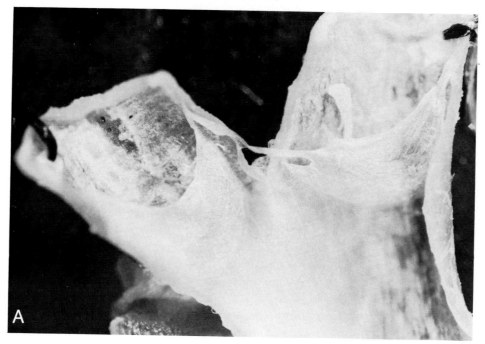

A

(Continued)

Fig. 5–12 (Continued)

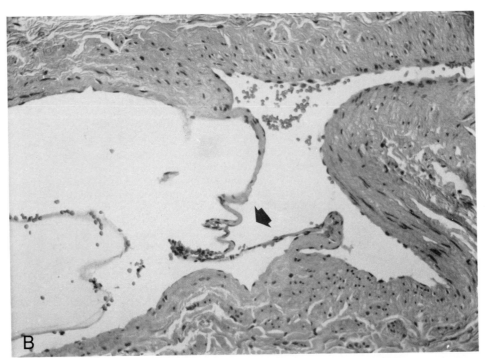

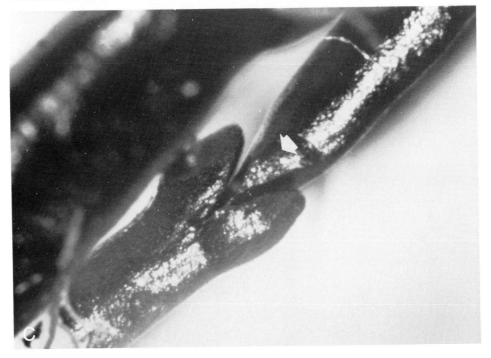

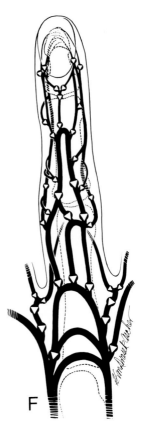

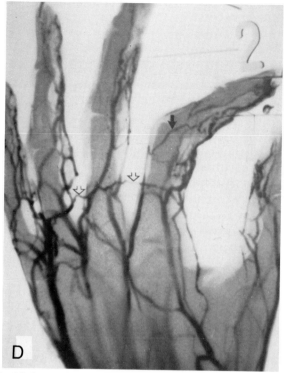

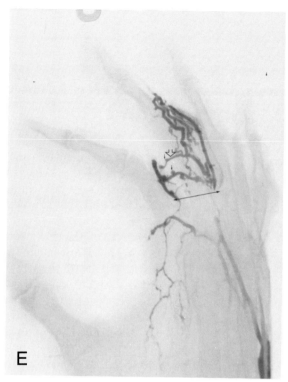

Fig. 5–12 (Continued)

arches (Fig. 5–12*A*–*F*). The clinical implications of this study are not only related importantly in digital replantation surgery but also the study adds to our understanding of the basic pathomechanics of reducing postoperative edema with vigorous exercises. Furthermore, the dangers of circumferential dressings of individual digits are further emphasized.

There exists great variability in the dorsal veins of the hand. Nevertheless, they all connect finally in the cephalic and basilic veins of the forearm and arm. The identification of valves in the digital veins is a recent anatomical observation with significant clinical application.

LYMPHATIC SYSTEM

General description of the lymphatic system follows the principles established by the early anatomists. The studies of Sappey are still of great importance. The superficial lymphatics of the fingers form two or three collateral channels that follow the corresponding collateral digital artery. These channels are directed dorsally in the interdigital spaces and along the medial and lateral borders of the hand. The sub-

cutaneous lymphatic network is very dense over the volar surface of the hand and less dense over the dorsal surface. The superficial lymphatic vessels collect on the forearm on the dorsal and volar aspects and continue into the arm; the deep lymphatic vessels accompany the deep arteries and veins and follow the deep channels that are the satellites of the arteries and veins of the forearm. The interphalangeal and metacarpophalangeal joints are apparently supplied by lymphatic vessels joining the digital arteries, which communicate with the collectors on the dorsum of the hand.

The lymphatics of the anterior surface of the carpus present a unique picture, forming a very dense network of which the proximal lymphatics are connected with the anterior interosseous lymphatic trunks and the distal lymphatics are connected with the collectors of the lymph trunks that accompany the volar arteries. The ulnar collectors pass to the ulnar lymphatic trunks, and the radial collectors terminate in the trunks that accompany the radial vessels. The posterior aspect of the carpus directs its lymphatics into the posterior interosseous trunk of the forearm.

Nerve Supply to the Muscles and Skin of the Hand

Robert J. Schultz
Emanuel B. Kaplan

Observations by the classic anatomists demonstrated that innervation to the skin and the short and the long muscles of the hand originates from the radial, median, musculocutaneous, and ulnar nerves.

Dissections by anatomists of the 19th century revealed the presence of variations in the nerve supply. Thompson, in 1891 to 1893, described in great detail the variations and the anastomoses between the nerves of the forearm and the hand. In 1867 and later, Gruber investigated the subject of nerve variations. The material made available by these two anatomists was very extensive, but their valuable contributions were not appreciated sufficiently until the experiences of World War I. It was at this time that many discrepancies were found in the interpretation of nerve function because of the examination of patients as based on the standardized descriptions of the nerve supply. Many investigations have been conducted since World War I and in conjunction with observations following World War II, have demonstrated the wealth and value of the findings made by the earlier anatomists.

Embryologically, three nerves supply the ventral musculature of the upper extremity: the median, ulnar, and musculocutaneous. One nerve, the radial, supplies the dorsal musculature; therefore, it is appropriate that anastomoses between the radial nerve (which supplies the dorsal musculature) and the three ventral nerves would be less common than anastomoses and substitutions between the three nerves supplying the ventral musculature.

It has been found that besides anastomoses through visible branches, there are numerous internal plexuses with frequent interchange of fibers from different funiculi. Stoffel maintained that there is a definite topographic arrangement of the nerve fibers to the various muscles. According to Stoffel, in a cross-section the topographic relationship of a nerve at different levels remains relatively constant, permitting a very accurate approximation of different specific pathways in case of accidental or experimental interruption of a nerve trunk. He based his opinion on physiologic, pathologic, histologic studies and nerve dissections after formalin fixation. Before Stoffel's investigation, Russels, in 1891, believed and maintained that each nerve fasciculus that produces a simple movement runs separately from other fasciculi from the root of the nerve to the muscle without interconnection with other motor fasciculi. Stoffel's views were confirmed by other investigators such as Pierre Marie, Meige, and Gosset, who by means of electric stimulation of nerve trunks made studies of the wounded in World War I. Other investigators, including Tinel, also found evidences of intratruncular localization of nerve fasiculi. The views that isolated noninterconnecting pathways for fasciculi exist have been challenged with the belief that instead of specific disposition of fasciculi, there are multiple interchanges between the various fasciculi.

By using different methods of investigation (maceration, special dissociation of fibers, interstitial injections of Mercury), Heineman, Compton, Velt, Goldberg, Borchardt, and Wjasmenski found the existence of the internal plexuses.

Dustin (1918) examined the nerve trunks of the upper extremity and concluded that the fascicles of a nerve vary not only in different people but in the same person between both sides, that the fasciculi of a nerve divide and reunite to form an elongated, wide plexus with the result that transverse sections even a few millimeters apart do not show the same topography, and that the fasciculi tend to fuse along their courses and separate at points of branching or termination. These interchanges forming intertruncular internal plexuses are not exceptional arrangements in that they reflect the general tendency of the nervous system to constitute plexuses throughout its entire course from the central nervous system through the juncture of the roots to the peripheral system. The brachial plexus, for instance, demonstrates the anastomoses between the larger and the smaller trunks of the nerves and their terminal anastomoses.

Sunderland, in detailed anatomic studies, has demonstrated specific predictable topographic distribution of nerves at different cross-sectional levels. He also demonstrated that multiple interchanges occur between the various fasciculi, eliminating the concept of isolated pathway transmission (Fig. 5–13). Jabaley and associates confirmed and amplified Sunderland's findings, noting that despite the funicular plexus formation and interchange within the nerves of the forearms, these communications are not of a degree that preclude such procedures using microsurgical techniques, as internal neurolysis, funicular nerve repair and nerve grafting.

The existence of internal plexus, together with the variations of the nerve supply and the anastomoses of different nerve trunks must be kept in mind for proper interpretation of normal and abnormal muscle function caused by injuries of the nerve trunks.

The wrist and the hand are supplied by four nerves: the musculocutaneous, radial, median, and ulnar nerves. The musculocutaneous nerve is responsible mostly for supplying the skin and the joints over the radial part of the forearm, wrist, and the proximal part of the thumb. The radial nerve supplies part of the dorsal skin over the wrist and the hand, the joints of the carpus, and the radial metacarpophalangeal joints, as well as the long extensors of the wrist, fingers, and thumb. The median nerve supplies most of the flexors of the wrist, the long flexors of the fingers, and a part of the intrinsic muscles of the hand, including the muscles of the thenar eminence and the greatest number of the joints of

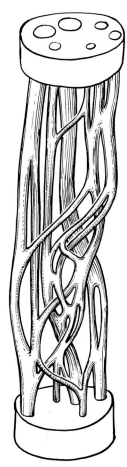

FIG. 5–13 Funicular pattern of a 3-cm segment of the musculocutaneous nerve. (Adapted from Sunderland)

the fingers. It further provides sensation to more than half of the palmar skin and a part of the dorsal skin of the fingers and thumb. The ulnar nerve supplies two of the deep long finger flexors, one flexor of the wrist, most of the intrinsic muscles of the hand, all the hypothenar muscles, some of the thenar muscles, and some of the joints of the fingers and the wrist. It supplies sensation to part of the palmar and the dorsal skin of the wrist and fingers.

INDIVIDUAL NERVE DESCRIPTIONS

Although a study of an entire nerve is interesting

in its discussion of distribution, anastomoses, and terminal innervation, the description of each nerve is here limited to only the wrist and hand as delineated by the title of the book.

MUSCULOCUTANEOUS NERVE

The terminal branch of the musculocutaneous nerve, upon piercing the fascia in the proximal region of the elbow, continues into the forearm and divides into anterior and posterior branches. The anterior branch is located slightly more medial and the posterior slightly more lateral over the radial aspect of the forearm. The branches are sensory throughout their courses.

The anterior branch ends in the skin of the proximal part of the thenar eminence. Sometimes a slender branch runs along the radial side of the eminence to the proximal phalanx. Cruveilhier described a deeper branch emanating from the anterior branch to the radiocarpal joint and the radial artery. Frequently, it unites with a branch of the radial nerve. The posterior branch descends to the distal part of the forearm and supplies the skin, mostly the region of the anatomic snuff-box, and rarely, the proximal part of the dorsum of the hand.

The musculocutaneous nerve has several important anastomoses. In the arm anastomoses with the median nerve are not directly concerned with the innervation of the hand. Over the thenar eminence, however, the palmar cutaneous branch of the median nerve forms a frequent anastomosis with the thenar branch of the musculocutaneous. The ulnar nerve, through its dorsal cutaneous branch may form an anastomosis with the musculocutaneous nerve when the musculocutaneous nerve extends its branches over the proximal dorsal part of the hand. The anterior branch of the radial nerve can also form a connection with the anterior and posterior branches of the musculocutaneous nerve in the region of the carpus.

MEDIAN NERVE

The median nerve is a large trunk emanating from the union of the lateral and the medial cords of the brachial plexus. It assumes important relations in the axilla and over the anteromedial aspect of the arm in its course toward the forearm. In the forearm, it passes between the two heads of the pronator teres and then descends in the midline between the flexor digitorum superficialis and the flexor digitorum profundus. It enters the carpal canal superficial to the flexor superficialis of the index and long fingers or the flexor profundus of the index finger and divides into its terminal branches (Figs. 5–14 and 2–31C).

As the nerve leaves the arm and passes into the forearm, it supplies branches to the elbow joint and the pronator teres. Slightly more distal, it gives off the branches that affect the function of the wrist and the fingers. Of two major branches of the median nerve, one supplies the superficial muscles and the other the deep muscles of the forearm. Each of these trunks may divide into several smaller branches:

1. The superficial or muscular trunk commonly provides a branch for the pronator teres; a branch to the flexor carpi radialis, which arises approximately 1 cm to 2 cm below the articular line of the elbow; and a branch for the palmaris longus, which appears on the anteromedial side of the nerve. A few branches arise more distally and penetrate the flexor digitorum superficialis; these branches frequently supply the other muscles. Variations in nerve branching are frequent. From the distal part of the superficial trunk, a separate branch is given off to the superficialis indicis. An injury to the median nerve just proximal to this branch will not involve any of the flexors but may produce an isolated paralysis of the index finger superficialis.

2. The deep group of branches supplies the flexor pollicis longus, the flexor digitorum profundus to the index and long fingers, and the pronator quadratus. The branch supplying the profundus indicis is constant, but the long finger may have only a partial supply from the median nerve. At times, the entire flexor digitorum profundus is supplied by the median nerve. The anterior interosseous

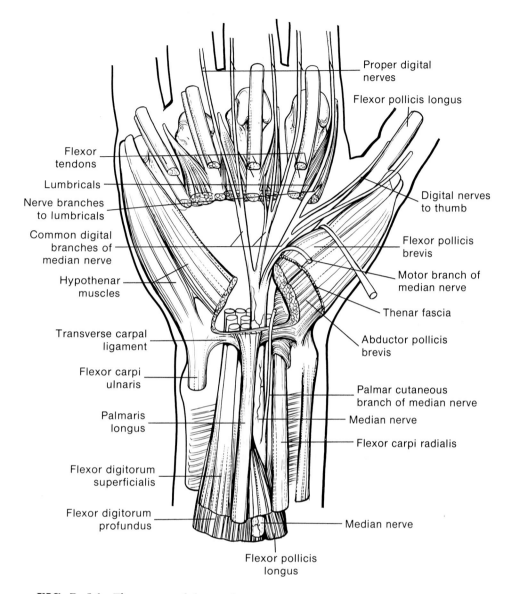

FIG. 5–14 The course of the median nerve and its branches in the palm. Note the branch to the lumbrical and thenar muscles. There is often a fascial band where the recurrent motor branch enters the thenar musculature.

nerve is the main trunk of the deep layer, supplying the flexor pollicis longus and the flexor digitorum profundus to the index finger, in addition to innervation by the branches of the deep trunk. The nerve may supply the posterior aspect of the radiocarpal joint through the branches traversing the interosseous membrane. The terminal part of

the anterior interosseous nerve supplies the pronator quadratus and the anterior surface of the radiocarpal joint.

3. The palmar cutaneous branch arises from the anterior surface of the median nerve at various levels, proximal to or at times through the transverse carpal ligament between the tendon of the flexor carpi radialis

and the palmaris longus. Its distribution is to the volar skin of the wrist and palm. Anastomosis can occur with the anterior branch of the musculocutaneous nerve or the anterior branch of the radial nerve.

Terminal branches

The terminal branches of the median nerve divide in the majority of hands at the distal border of the transverse carpal ligament (Fig. 5–14). The nerve is most frequently split into one radial and one ulnar division, but this arrangement may vary. The radial division is the larger of the two and provides the motor branch for the thenar muscles, the proper digital nerve to the radial side of the thumb, and the first common digital nerve, which forms the volar proper digital nerve to the ulnar side of the thumb and the proper digital nerve to the radial aspect of the index finger.

The proper digital nerve on the radial side of the thumb lies on the palmar surface of the abductor pollicis brevis and as it goes distally, takes a lateral course in which it crosses the flexor pollicis longus tendon and runs parallel with the flexor brevis, volar to its corresponding digital artery until it reaches the tip of the distal phalanx (Fig. 5–15). It provides branches to the pulp of the thumb, the dorsal subungual area, as well as articular branches to the metacarpophalangeal and the interphalangeal joint.

The first common digital nerve lies on the palmar surface of the abductor pollicis brevis and is crossed volad by the superficial branch of the radial artery. The nerve divides immediately into two branches: the proper digital nerve to the ulnar aspect of the thumb and the proper digital nerve to the radial aspect of the index finger (Fig. 5–16). The ulnar proper digital nerve of the thumb or the radial proper digital nerve of the index finger may give a branch to the adductor pollicis, thus providing median nerve supply to a muscle that usually is supplied by the ulnar nerve.

The proper digital nerve to the ulnar aspect of the thumb runs on the ulnar side of the metacarpophalangeal joint, crosses the insertion of the adductor pollicis, and terminates, provid-

ing articular branches to the metacarpophalangeal joint and the proximal interphalangeal joint, and further distally, a branch to the pulp and the subungual region of the tip of the thumb.

The proper digital nerve to the radial aspect of the index finger runs parallel to the first lumbrical and may be considered its faithful satellite (Fig. 5–14). It provides one or two twigs to the lumbrical (Fig. 2–66; *see also Fig. 9–13*). Branches of this nerve are distributed to the palm, the radial half of the palmar aspect of the finger, the metacarpophalangeal and the interphalangeal joints, as well as the dorsal skin on the radial side of the index finger over the middle and the distal phalanges.

The motor branch of the median nerve, commonly referred to as the recurrent branch, arises from the anterior aspect of the nerve, crossing part of the main nerve trunk and the transverse carpal ligament before it enters the substance of the thenar muscles (Figs. 5–15 and 5–16). As it enters the thenar muscles, it pierces a thickened fascial band (Fig. 5–14). The author of this chapter has found this band at times to constrict the nerve, producing isolated entrapment of the motor branch. The branches of the motor nerve supply the abductor pollicis brevis, the opponens pollicis, and the superficial head of the flexor pollicis brevis. The nerve to the abductor brevis enters the muscle on its deep surface, whereas the nerves to the other muscles enter on their palmar surfaces near the middle of the muscle belly.

Medial branches

The medial division of the median nerve forms two branches: a common digital nerve to the second intermetacarpal and one to the third intermetacarpal space.

The common digital nerve of the second space provides one or two twigs to the second lumbrical. It then runs toward the deep transverse intermetacarpal ligament and on the surface of the ligament, bifurcates into two proper digital nerves—one to the ulnar side of the index finger, and the other to the radial side of the long finger (Fig. 2–66). In the palm, the common digital nerve lies dorsal to the superfi-

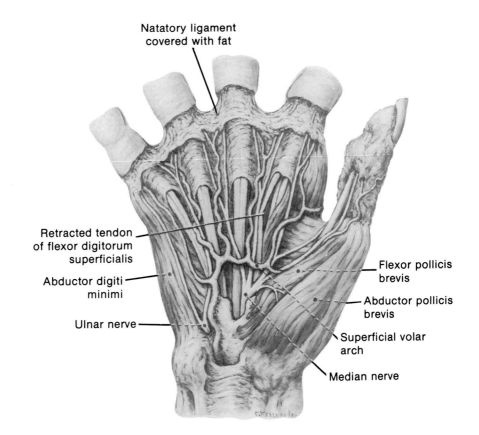

FIG. 5–15 Volar surface of the hand with midpalmar fascia and subfascial fat removed. The interdigital or natatory ligament is left intact. The branches of the superficial palmar arch cover the common digital nerves; both are directed toward the fingers to provide proper digital branches for the fingers. The prolongation of the interdigital or natatory ligament into the fingers provides special cylindrical covering for the digital vessels and nerves. The digital nerve to the radial aspect of the index finger is parallel with the first lumbrical. This is a constant relationship. This hand shows the branching of the digital nerve to the ulnar aspect of the thumb from the digital branch directed toward the radial side of the index finger. There is usually a separate branch of the median nerve that is divided into an ulnar and a radial branch to the thumb. The lumbrical muscle belly at its origin is very frequently covered by the tendon of the flexor superficialis. To demonstrate the lumbrical, the superficialis tendon was retracted.

The ulnar digital branch of the ulnar nerve to the little finger is most frequently parallel with the abductor digiti minimi and is covered by the aponeurosis of the hypothenar muscles. In the undissected hand it is protected by the thick fat pad. The arterial branches of the arch are usually more superficial than are the common digital nerves.

cial palmar arch (Fig. 5–15) covered by the palmar fascia. Over the deep transverse metacarpal ligament, its divisions are well protected by the fat pads that fill the spaces between the pretendinous bands of the palmar fascia (Fig. 5–16). In the fingers, each proper digital nerve

lies volar to the corresponding artery and is protected by a tunnel of fat reinforced by the Cleland's skin ligaments (Fig. 2–24). The nerve supplies the skin of the corresponding area of the palm of the hand, the palmar surfaces of the corresponding halves of the index and the long

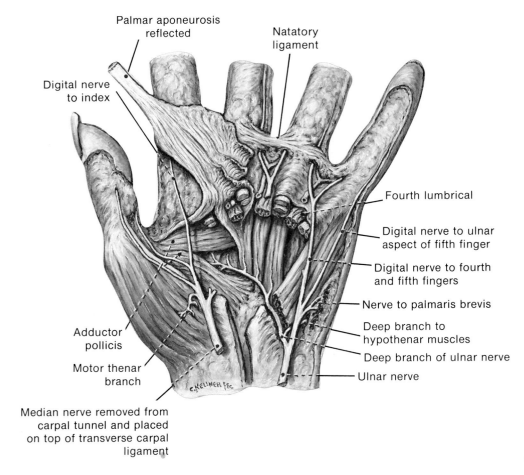

Palmar aponeurosis reflected

Natatory ligament

Digital nerve to index

Fourth lumbrical

Digital nerve to ulnar aspect of fifth finger

Digital nerve to fourth and fifth fingers

Nerve to palmaris brevis

Deep branch to hypothenar muscles

Deep branch of ulnar nerve

Ulnar nerve

Adductor pollicis

Motor thenar branch

Median nerve removed from carpal tunnel and placed on top of transverse carpal ligament

FIG. 5–16 The ulnar nerve is left in its normal relationship; the median nerve is removed from its normal position in the carpal canal and placed anterior to the volar carpal ligament. The midpalmar fascia is resected and reflected. The deep branch of the ulnar artery is demonstrated. In this specimen, the ulnar digital nerve of the thumb originates from the radial branch of the index finger. The midpalmar fascia shows the connection to the vaginal ligament and to the lumbrical canals in the distal part of the hand.

fingers, articular branches to the corresponding sides of the metacarpophalangeal, proximal, and distal interphalangeal joints, and dorsally the subungual regions and the dorsal skin on the corresponding sides over the middle and distal phalanges (Figs. 5–17 and 5–18).

The common digital nerve of the third intermetacarpal space has the same general characteristics as the nerve of the second space, except that it crosses the flexor tendons of the long finger over their synovial bursa (Fig. 5–15). The

nerve supplies the ulnar side of the long and the radial side of the ring finger and the palmar skin overlying the nerve. The division into the two proper digital nerves may occur more proximally than the digital nerve of the second intermetacarpal space. An anastomotic branch uniting the common digital nerve of the third intermetacarpal space with the common digital nerve of the fourth intermetacarpal space (a branch of the ulnar nerve) is almost constantly present (Figs. 5–19 and 5–20).

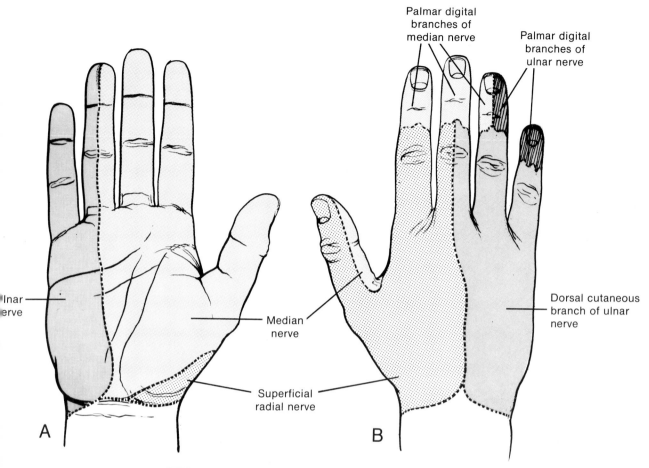

FIG. 5–17 Normal pattern of sensory distribution on the palmar and dorsal surfaces of the hand. Note that the palmar nerves provide sensation distal to the midportion of the middle phalanges on the dorsum of the fingers.

The cutaneous innervation to the dorsal aspect of the proximal and the distal phalanges is not emphasized sufficiently. This feature of volar nerves providing dorsal sensation is extremely important because it can be a trap to the unwary. There are usually three collateral branches arising at different levels from the palmar proper digital nerve. One arises near the metacarpophalangeal joint and then turns laterally around the joint, reaching the dorsum of the proximal phalanx where it forms an overlapping innervation with the sensory branch forearm and hand. The second arises slightly more distal and passes dorsally, and the third

branches off near the distal interphalangeal joint to supply the dorsal skin and the subungual space of the distal phalanx.

The sensory pattern of the median nerve (Figs. 5–17 and 5–18) includes the hand, radial to the midline of the ring finger from the base of the palm to the tip of the finger, the entire palmar surface and the dorsal subungual region of the thumb, the entire palmar surface of the index, long, and the radial half of the ring finger, as well as the dorsum of these fingers from the mid-middle phalanx distally.

In view of the complex architecture, topography, and fascicular patterns of the

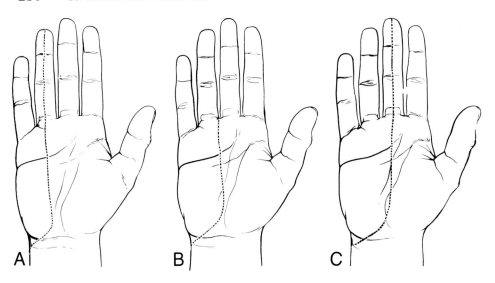

FIG. 5–18 Variations of the sensory pattern of the ulnar nerve on the palmar aspect of the hand.

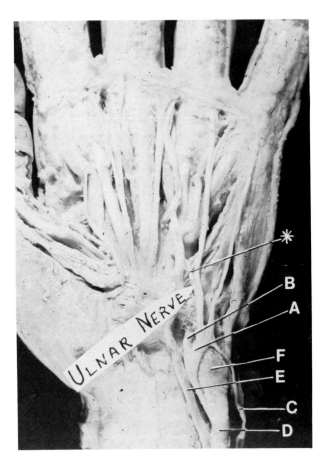

FIG. 5–19 Variation of the ulnar nerve over the base of the hypothenar eminence of the left hand. A, Ulnar nerve distal to the pisiform; B; deep motor branch; C; additional branch of ulnar nerve; D, flexor carpi ulnaris tendon; E, ulnar artery; F, pisiform bone; (*) communicating sensory branch.

median nerve in the forearm (especially in the distal third), whenever surgical repair of the nerve is required, the surgeon should use microsurgical fascicular technique and avoid twisting or distorting the divided ends. The possibility of accurate opposition of specific tracts is influenced by so many uncertain factors (especially in old injuries) that it requires the expertise and patience of the skilled surgeon.

ULNAR NERVE

The ulnar nerve is the largest nerve of the medial cord of the brachial plexus and starts its long journey in the axilla. It passes through the posterior compartment of the arm, then behind the medial epicondyle of the elbow to the anteromedial aspect of the forearm, and reaches the lateral aspect of the pisiform. In the forearm, the nerve rests on the surface of the flexor digitorum profundus and is covered by the flexor carpi ulnaris. Just distal to the elbow joint, the nerve is separated from the ulnar artery which lies 4 cm to 5 cm lateral to the nerve. The ulnar artery runs toward the ulnar nerve at the junction of the proximal fourth with the distal three fourths of a line uniting the pisiform with the medial epicondyle (about 6 cm to 8 cm from the medial condyle of the humerus). Beyond this point, the ulnar artery becomes a steadfast companion on the lateral side of the nerve, descending together toward the pisiform, where the deep branch of the nerve is accompanied constantly by the deep branch of the artery into the hand.

At the wrist, the ulnar nerve passes, with the artery on its lateral side, through a tunnel called the *loge de Guyon*. The loge is bounded by the pisiform and the hook of the hamate and covered volarly by the volar carpal ligament, an expansion from the tendon of the flexor carpi ulnaris, and the fascia of the forearm (Fig. 2–31C). The tendon itself deflects medially (Figs. 2–30, 2–66, and 5–15).

In its course through the forearm, the ulnar nerve gives articular branches to the elbow joint, a proximal nerve to the flexor carpi ulnaris, the nerve for the flexor digitorum profundus, a small distal branch to the flexor carpi ulnaris, the long nerve to the ulnar artery (nerve of Henle), and the dorsal cutaneous branch of the hand. The branch or branches to the flexor profundus enter the muscle near the elbow joint and innervate the medial half of the muscle. The nerve of Henle, or the long nerve to the ulnar artery, runs along the volar surface of the artery and at times perforates the antebrachial fascia to supply the skin of the hypothenar eminence and the area slightly lateral to it.

The dorsal cutaneous branch of the ulnar nerve leaves the ulnar nerve about 5 cm to 6 cm proximal to the styloid process of the ulna or infrequently, at the level of the ulna head. It perforates the fascia in its course toward the dorsum of the wrist, but before perforating the fascia, it sends a few twigs to the radiocarpal joint and perhaps to the dorsal carpal arterial arch. After perforating the fascia, it supplies the

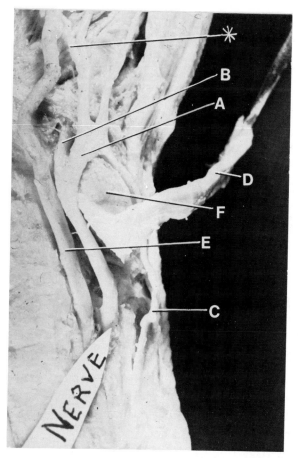

FIG. 5–20 Same specimen as in Figure 5–19, magnified with tendon of flexor carpi ulnaris (D) divided and retracted distally.

ulnar side of the hand with small branches. Running in the subcutaneous fascia in company with the dorsal superficial veins, it gives an ulnar digital nerve, which provides sensation up to the mid-middle phalanx, and at times it may supply the entire dorsal length of the little finger. Another branch runs toward the fourth intermetacarpal space and divides into two digital branches. One supplies the radial side of the little finger up to the mid-middle phalanx, or at times the entire radial dorsal side of the little finger, and the other branch supplies the dorsal ulnar side of the ring finger up to the mid-middle phalanges. From the mid-middle phalanx to the

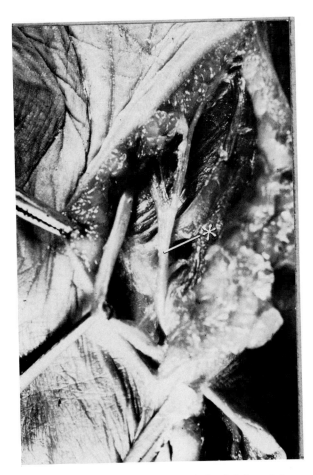

FIG. 5–21 Hypothenar area of the left hand demonstrating the ulnar artery retracted by a hook on the left. The ulnar nerve (*) in the center on top of the abductor of the little finger with the superficial digital branch on the right and a deep branch penetrating the short flexor of the little finger.

tip of the little finger and the ulnar side of the ring finger, the innervation arises from the dorsally directed branches of the palmar proper digital nerves.

Multiple anastomoses occur between branches of the sensory branch of the radial and posterior branch of the musculocutaneous nerve over the dorsum of the hand. It is useful to remember that an interval exists between the branches of the dorsal cutaneous branch of the ulnar nerve, which descends along the ulnar aspect of the dorsum of the hand, and the sensory branch of the radial nerve, on the radial side of the dorsum of the wrist and hand, providing an area comparatively free of important nerves. This area lies approximately between the tendon of the extensor pollicis longus and the tendon of the extensor carpi ulnaris; here, the possibility of injury to the nerves supplying the dorsum of the metacarpophalangeal joints and the proximal phalanx is reduced.

Terminal branches

In the palm, the ulnar nerve divides into two terminal branches: superficial and deep. The division occurs in the loge de Guyon approximately midway between the distal and the proximal borders of the volar carpal ligament medial and posterior to the artery and almost against the radial side of the pisiform (Fig. 5–16). In this region the two branches are covered by a very thick fat pad and the palmaris brevis muscle. The dissection of these branches in the living hand under proper hemostasis is not difficult but is quite confusing to the inexperienced. (Fig. 5–21).

Superficial Branch.   Distal to the palmar carpal ligament, the superficial branch, which is almost entirely sensory, is covered by the thin fascia of the hypothenar eminence, the fat pad, and the palmaris brevis muscle. Small single or multiple twigs supply the palmaris brevis muscle, after which the nerve divides into three branches: one sensory, for the ulnar aspect of the little finger, one for the central ulnar aspect of the palm, and one to form the common digital nerve for the fourth intermetacarpal space. This nerve is located deep (dorsal) to the superficial palmar arterial arch; it crosses the tendons of the flexors to the little finger very obliquely and divides into two proper digital nerves that rest on the surface of the deep transverse intermetacarpal ligament and pass to and innervate the radial side of the little finger and the ulnar side of the ring finger. The common digital nerve is covered by the palmar fascia, whereas the site of bifurcation is covered and protected by the interdigital fat pad.

The proper digital nerve to the ulnar side of

the ring finger has one or two small collateral branches that arise approximately at the metacarpophalangeal joint and supply, in a pattern similar to the digital nerves of the median nerve, the corresponding half of the dorsal surface of the middle and the distal phalanges (Fig. 5–22). Articular branches arise from the proper digital nerve as previously described.

Deep Branch.   The deep branch of the ulnar nerve is the motor branch. Immediately after its emergence, the deep branch penetrates between the abductor digiti minimi and the flexor digiti minimi brevis (Figs. 2–66, 5–16 and 5–22). It is usually accompanied by the deep branch of the ulnar artery, which penetrates into the interval of the abductor and the flexor digiti minimi brevis. The French anatomists Delorme and Farabeuf called attention to a small artery that

replaces the deep branch of the ulnar artery. This small artery penetrates together with the deep nerve but instead of following the path of the deep nerve, completely exhausts its supply in the muscles of the hypothenar eminence. In this case, the deep branch of the ulnar artery is given off more distally and usually enters the retrotendinous midpalmar space between the flexor tendon sheath of the little finger and the flexor digiti minimi brevis and thus joins the course of the deep ulnar nerve.

Before the deep motor branch penetrates into the depth of the hypothenar eminence, it supplies the abductor digiti minimi and the flexor digiti minimi brevis. While passing through the opponens muscle, it supplies it with several small twigs. After passing through the hypothenar muscles, it enters the midpalmar

FIG. 5–22   The deep branch of the ulnar nerve demonstrating its course and branches to the interossei and medial two lumbrical muscles.

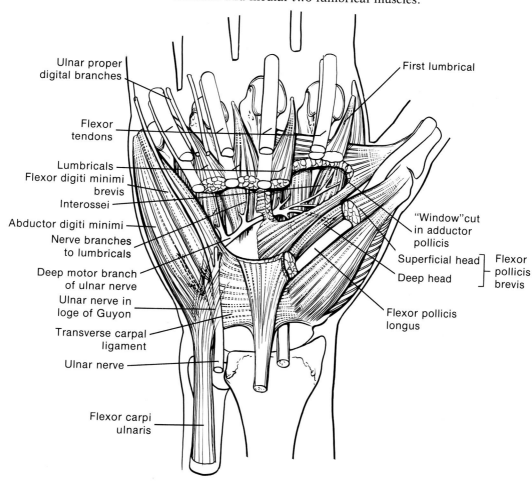

space dorsal to the flexor tendons. The deep branch runs deep to the palmar interosseous fascia in a slightly curved arch and is covered by the deep fat pad (described by Dr. Kaplan). The nerve continues its course with the artery until it passes through the arch of the adductor pollicis and terminates in the deep head of the flexor pollicis brevis (Fig. 5–16).

According to Rauber, the concave side of the nerve arch supplies articular branches to the carpal joints. These branches are probably inconstant or are perhaps so tenuous that they are easily lost.

The deep branch of the ulnar nerve gives off branches that supply the interosseous muscles and the two ulnar lumbricals. The nerve fibers to the third and the fourth lumbricals arise by a common trunk with the branches to the corresponding interosseous muscle and then separate to pass to the lumbrical (Fig. 5–22). In this position, they are palmar in relation to the deep branch of the ulnar nerve and enter on the dorsal surface of the lumbrical (Fig. 5–22). This can be contrasted with the first and the second lumbrical muscles, which are usually innervated on their palmar surfaces from the digital branches of the median nerve, because the first and second lumbricals are dorsal to these branches of the median nerve (compare Figs. 2–66 and 5–16).

The nerves to the interossei enter the palmar surfaces of the muscles under cover of the deep fat pad and the fascia, which covers the interosseous muscles in the ulnar half of the palm and under cover of the adductor muscle in the radial half of the palm. The deep branch of the ulnar nerve penetrates through the opening of the adductor pollicis to supply the first dorsal interosseus and the adductor muscle itself on its dorsal aspect (Fig. 5–16). A very similar arrangement is found in the hand of the gorilla (Fig. 1–3).

Variations

At the entrance of the ulnar nerve into the hand, several variations may be found, some of which may present problems during surgical procedures. The path of the dorsal cutaneous branch of the ulnar nerve, which most commonly passes proximal to the ulnar head, may at times be found crossing the ulnar head; in this position, it may be jeopardized during surgical procedures involving the ulnar head. A rare variation found by Kaplan occurs when the dorsal and main trunk of the ulnar nerve encircle the pisiform; in this variation, the dorsal cutaneous branch gives off an additional branch, 2-cm proximal to the ulnar styloid, that passes about the ulnar side of the pisiform to join the palmar sensory branch of the ulnar nerve. The pisiform is therefore bounded on three sides by the branches of the ulnar nerve (Figs. 5–19 and 5–20). The additional branch of the dorsal cutaneous nerve continues directly into the palmar ulnar digital artery of the little finger distal to the pisiform. A branch from the main trunk of the ulnar nerve is also observed coming off proximal to the origin of the abductor digiti minimi, passing under the muscle to join the dorsal cutaneous branch.

In surgical procedures involving the pisiform, this variation may pose definite hazards. In fractures of the pisiform, there may be immediate injury to these branches of the ulnar nerve, or during healing of a fracture, entrapment in scar or callus with resultant constant pain.

Muscle anomalies such as variant hypothenar muscles can alter the usual relationships of the ulnar nerve in this region. An aberrant abductor digiti minimi with a high origin may cross volar to the ulnar nerve. Dr. Kaplan's anatomic notes of 1927 depict a dissection specimen with a variant abductor digiti minimi and lumbrical ringing the ulnar nerve at Guyon's tunnel (Fig. 5–23).

The topography of the fasciculi of the ulnar nerve has been described by several authors. Stookey stated that "the funiculus for the flexor carpi ulnaris and flexor profundus may be identified in the ulnar nerve 4 to 5 cm above the medial condyle lying in the medial and dorsal parts of the nerve." Others, such as Hovelacque, Pierre Marie, Meige and Gosset, and of Déjerine and Mouzan, Tinel, Anderle, and Sunderland and Jabaley, also established the relationship of pathways in the trunk of the ulnar nerve in the arm.

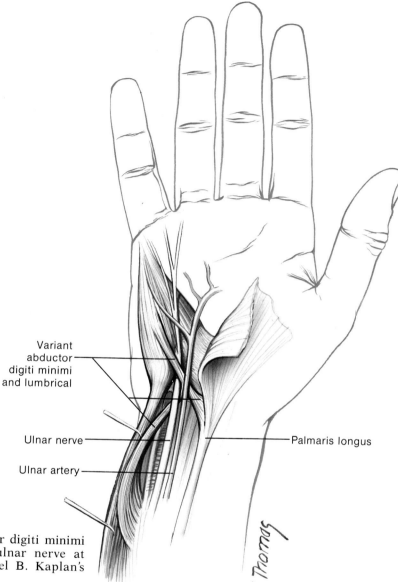

Variant
abductor
digiti minimi
and lumbrical

Ulnar nerve

Ulnar artery

Palmaris longus

FIG. 5–23   An anomalous adbuctor digiti minimi lumbrical almost encircling the ulnar nerve at Guyon's tunnel. (From Dr. Emanuel B. Kaplan's anatomical sketches, 1927)

RADIAL NERVE

The radial nerve is one of the largest nerves of the brachial plexus. It is a branch of the posterior cord and descends from the axilla to the posterior aspect of the arm, crosses the humerus in the spiral groove, and exits into the anterior aspect of the distal arm, passing into the proximal forearm, where at the level of the radial head it terminates in two branches—one predominantly motor and the other sensory. Only those branches and characteristics that

have bearing on the function of the hand and the wrist will be considered.

The radial nerve in its distal course passes over the lateral epicondylar ridge of the humerus to enter the anterior compartment of the arm. This crossing occurs almost exactly 10 cm proximal to the tip of the lateral epicondyle and can be located easily by measurement and palpation. To outline the course of the radial nerve as it passes from the arm towards the elbow, a horizontal line is traced uniting the lateral and the medial epicondyles of the humerus. This transverse line is divided into three parts, and the point of junction of the lateral and the middle third is marked. The point of intersection of the radial nerve on the lateral epicondylar ridge (10 cm proximal to the epicondyle) and the point of junction of the lateral and the middle third of the transverse line are united. This line marks almost the exact course of the radial nerve towards the forearm.

About 4 cm to 5 cm proximal to the point of intersection of the radial nerve with the interepicondylar line of the humerus, the radial nerves gives off its branch to the brachioradialis and the extensor carpi radialis longus. This branch emerges just distal to the nerve of the brachioradialis and runs distally, entering the extensor carpi radialis longus in the vicinity of the lateral epicondyle.

The nerve to the extensor carpi radialis brevis arises from the main trunk of the radial nerve, or at times, from the deep muscular division (posterior interosseus nerve), and enters the muscle on its medial aspect in the upper third of the forearm. After supplying the brachioradialis and the extensor carpi radialis longus, and at times, the extensor carpi radialis brevis, the radial nerve divides into its two terminal branches; the level of this division varies.

The superficial branch is thinner than the deep motor branch. As it passes into the forearm, it is bounded by the brachioradialis muscle laterally, the tendon of the biceps brachias (which is medial), and the brachialis muscle, which forms a bed for it. This area is filled with fatty areolar tissue that protects the division of the radial nerve and also makes it easier for the surgeon to recognize the location of the division. The superficial branch passes under cover of the brachioradialis muscle, being attached to its deep surface by a thin fascial layer until it reaches the lower third of the forearm. About 8 cm from the tip of the radial styloid, the nerve emerges from under the tendon of the brachioradialis between this tendon and the tendon of the extensor carpi radialis longus. It perforates the fascia more distally and divides into a lateral and a medial branch.

The lateral branch runs toward the anatomic snuff-box, superficial to the abductor pollicis longus and extensor pollicis brevis, passing to and innervating the radial half of the dorsum of the thumb (excluding the subungual area, which as previously described, is supplied by branches of the median nerve). Lejars described small twigs from the branch to the abductor pollicis brevis muscle. This was also considered by Frohse, Frankel, and Hovelacque, because of the frequent tendinous connections of the abductor pollicis longus (supplied by the radial nerve) with the abductor pollicis brevis.

The medial branch supplies the dorsum of the radial part of the hand, the dorsum of the ulnar side of the thumb (not including the subungual region), and the dorsum of the proximal and mid-middle phalanges of the index, long, and the radial half of the ring finger. It communicates freely with the dorsal branch of the ulnar nerve.

The motor division of the radial nerve, referred to as the *posterior interosseous nerve*, separates from the superficial branch in the volar part of the upper forearm and penetrates the supinator muscle, passing under the arcade of Froshe; before its penetration or immediately afterwards, it emits one or two branches to the supinator muscle.

The relationship of the deep branch to the radial head and neck in pronation and supination changes with the position and is of importance in surgery of the region. Upon emerging from the supinator, the posterior interosseous nerve divides into short muscular branches and a long slender branch, which continues on the interosseous membrane in company with the posterior interosseous artery. The short branches of the posterior interosseous nerve supply the extensor digitorum communis, the extensor digiti minimi, and the extensor carpi ulnaris. The long branch supplies the abductor pollicis longus, the extensor pollicis brevis, the extensor pollicis longus, and the extensor indicis proprius.

The terminal part of the deep nerve, which runs on the posterior surface of the interosseous membrane, becomes somewhat nodular (referred to as a *ganglion*) and divides into numerous twigs to supply the ligaments of the radiocarpal, carpal, and carpometacarpal joints. Hovelacque cites Froment (1846) and Rauber (1865) as describing perforating twigs passing through the proximal intermetacarpal spaces for anastomosis with the deep branch of the ulnar nerve.

CUTANEOUS INNERVATION OF THE HAND AND FINGERS AND THEIR VARIATIONS

The standard description of the cutaneous innervation of the hand and fingers divides the territories of each nerve into clearly defined areas (Fig. 5–17). The sensory distribution on the palmar surface of the hand and the fingers is divided primarily between the median and the ulnar nerves, with minor contributions by the medial antebrachial cutaneous, the musculocutaneous, and even the radial nerves.

To determine the sensory pattern, the hand can be divided longitudinally through the midline of the ring finger, extending proximally to the flexion crease of the wrist (Fig. 5–17). The entire palmar skin on the radial side of this line is supplied by the median nerve, including the tip of the thumb and the dorsal subungual area of the thumb. The cutaneous innervation to the ulnar side is by the ulnar nerve. A small area at the base of the thenar eminence may be supplied by the radial nerve. The musculocutaneous nerve supplies the skin on the radial side of the distal forearm, just proximal to the carpal crease. On the ulnar side, the area proximal to the volar carpal crease is supplied by the medial antebrachial cutaneous nerve.

The sensory pattern of the dorsum of the hand is divided between the radial, ulnar, and median nerves. The longitudinal line of division is similar to the palmar surface, but there is a transverse line at the level of the mid-middle phalanx, distal to which is innervated by branches of the proper digital nerves (Fig. 5–17). The radial aspect of the dorsum of the hand, including the dorsum of the thumb and the

entire dorsum of the proximal phalanx of the index, long, and the radial half of the dorsum of the ring finger, is supplied by the radial nerve. The dorsum of the distal and middle phalanges of the index, the dorsum of the distal and the middle phalanges of the long finger, and radial half of the distal and middle phalanges of the ring finger are supplied by branches of the proper digital nerves of the median nerve.

The ulnar cutaneous distribution of the dorsum of the hand includes the dorsal aspect of the small finger and the ulnar half of the dorsum of the ring finger. This sensory distribution is by the dorsal cutaneous branch of the ulnar nerve and by dorsal branches of the proper digital nerves of the ulnar nerve. The branches of the palmar nerves supply the skin distal to the mid-middle phalangeal level, whereas the dorsal cutaneous branch provides sensation up to this point.

VARIATIONS OF SENSORY AND MOTOR NERVE SUPPLIES

Variations in sensory and motor distribution of nerves have important clinical significance; these variations must be known in order for the physician to understand the complex deficit patterns that occur in injury and plan surgical treatment. On examination of the hand following injury to the nerves, consideration variations may be encountered. The studies of Tinel, Stopford, and Pitre on known injuries of the nerves showed considerably less anesthesia than would be expected from the distribution of the nerves. According to Stopford, the palmar distribution of the median nerve is remarkably constant; however, slight variation of sensibility may occasionally occur in the palm or in the fingers with a shift either radially or ulnad.

Although the clinical problems of nerve variations were in the past not extensively elaborated upon, the actual documentation of anatomic variations by earlier anatomists was extensive. The clinicians of the 19th century were at a disadvantage in contrast with contemporary clinicians in that they did not have the abundant clinical material provided by the advances in civilization and expressed in the "improved" methods of mutilation such as high-speed vehicles. In many of the shorter contemporary clinical reports, the findings of the earlier anatomists are not sufficiently mentioned, while other authors left the impression that very little was known in the past concerning the now rediscovered variations. This lack of recognition of early researchers may have resulted from the relative inaccessibility of the earlier texts and papers.

The most common communications are found between the median, musculocutaneous, and the ulnar nerves. The radial nerve, which embryologically belongs to a separate region, does not enter into many anastomoses with the three volar nerves. The median nerve establishes anastomoses with the musculocutaneous nerve at many points along its course. In the arm, the median nerve may carry sensory and motor fibers that are most commonly carried by the musculocutaneous nerve. In the hand, the musculocutaneous nerve may provide the sensory innervation over the thenar eminence.

Connections of the median nerve with the ulnar nerve, found by many clinicians and anatomists, are of special interest and are more complicated. Several times, Kaplan observed various anastomoses between the median and the ulnar nerves, especially in the forearm on the surface of the flexor digitorum profundus. Similar anastomoses were observed by Kaplan in the forearm of a young gorilla. In one case of an accidental division of the ulnar nerve proximal to the medial epicondyle, the patient was examined on the day following the accident. He had no paralysis of any of the intrinsic muscles but had complete anesthesia of the ulnar side of the hand and the entire little finger.

SENSORY VARIATIONS

The most common sensory variations occur on the dorsum of the hand and have been described by Learmonth and Hutton (Fig. 5–24). According to Stopford, commonly radial nerve anesthesia does not extend beyond the second metacarpal. When the radial distribution is restricted, the musculocutaneous nerve provides sensation to the dorsum. The interchange and anastomoses between the various nerves supplying the dorsum of the hands restrict to very small areas the extent of sensory loss caused by injury to a single nerve. Injuries to the ulnar nerve produce constant and complete anesthesia to the ulnar border of the hand and the entire little finger.

MOTOR VARIATIONS

Standard descriptions of the innervation of the abductor pollicis brevis, the opponens, part of the flexor pollicis brevis, and the first and the second lumbricals by the median nerve and all the other intrinsic muscles by the ulnar nerves express the most common pattern of innervation.

Gruber and Thompson reported communications between the median and the ulnar nerves in large series of cadaver dissections. The Martin–Gruber anastomosis is a motor anastomosis going from the median to the ulnar nerve in the forearm (Fig. 5–25). It occurs basically in two patterns: from the median nerve in the proximal forearm to the ulnar nerve in the middle to distal third of the forearm and from the anterior interosseous nerve to the ulnar nerve.

Thompson described four types of motor anastomoses: from the anterior interosseous to the middle third of the ulnar nerve; from the main trunk of the medial to the ulnar nerve; the same type with formation of a sling between the two nerves and branches from this sling supplying the ring and small fingers of the flexor digitorum profundus; and superficial anastomosis volar to the flexor muscles joining the ulnar nerve at its midportion. Of the four types described, the first three all lie on the surface of the flexor digitorum profundus muscle. The studies of Borchardt and Wjasmenski demonstrated that occasionally the anastomotic connection from the median nerve went mainly into the deep branch of the ulnar nerve and only a small part into the superficial branch. Kaplan found similar connections in his dissections.

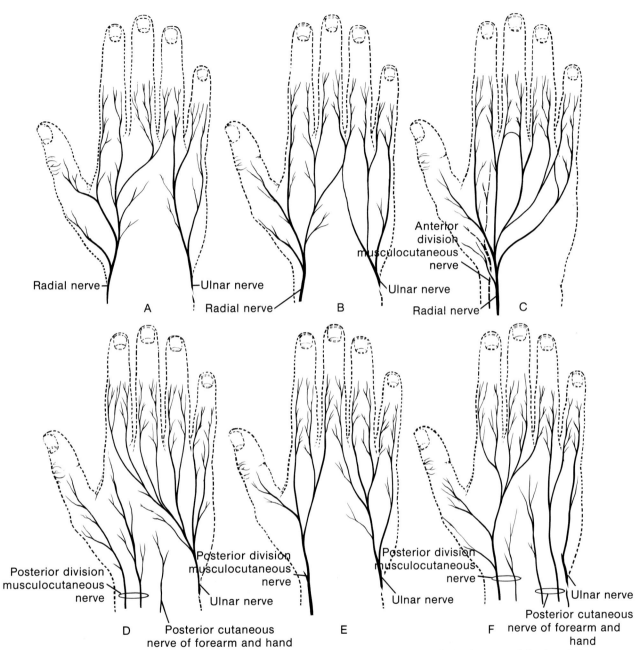

FIG. 5—24 Variations of the sensory distribution of the dorsum of the hand. [From Boileau Grant JC: Grant's Atlas of Anatomy. Baltimore, Williams & Wilkins, 1962. Adapted from Learmonth (1919), Hutton (1906), and Appleton (1911)]

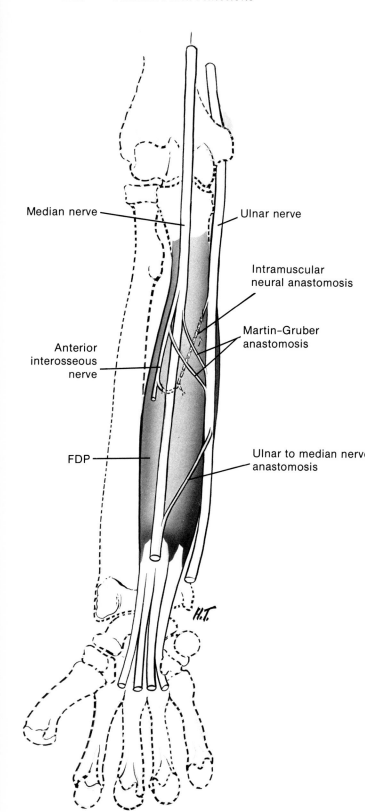

Median nerve

Ulnar nerve

Intramuscular
neural anastomosis

Martin–Gruber
anastomosis

Anterior
interosseous
nerve

FDP

Ulnar to median nerve
anastomosis

Riche and Cannieu described motor anastomoses between the median and ulnar nerves in the palm (Fig. 5–26). They described three variations: an inconstant anastomosis occurring deep in the palm between the motor branch of the median nerve to the superficial head of the flexor pollicis brevis and the ulnar nerve to the deep head of the flexor pollicis brevis; an anastomosis of the median and ulnar motor branches through the first lumbrical or through the innervation of the adductor pollicis; and a similar anastomosis that may take place through a slender branch of the median nerve to the third lumbrical joining the neural twig to this muscle from the deep branch of the ulnar nerve.

As previously stated, the median nerve may form anastomoses with the branches of the radial nerve in the vicinity of the abductor pollicis brevis through a special branch of the radial nerve, which according to Lejars may innervate the abductor pollicis brevis.

The ulnar nerve may anastomose with the terminal branches of the posterior interosseous nerve. This may take place between the terminal branches of the posterior interosseous through penetrating branches passing between the metacarpals and joining branches of the deep motor division of the ulnar nerve.

These innervations of the muscles of the thenar eminence, the lumbricals, and the interossei demonstrate that in spite of minor discrepancies, the anatomic studies of the past and present show general agreement. (Stookey, Pollock, and Loyal Davis; Murphey and Kirklin; and Finlayson, Clifton, Rowntree, and others).

Other motor variations that occur involve an extension of the ulnar nerve to innervate all the

FIG. 5–25 Martin–Gruber anastomosis between median nerve or its anterior interosseous branch and the u nerve. The commonly occurring intramuscular neural cor tion within the flexor digitorum profundus (FDP) betwee anterior interosseous branch of the median nerve and motor branch of the ulnar nerve to this muscle is also re sented. A less frequent ulnar-to-median nerve anastomos the distal forearm is also seen. (Reproduced from Kaplan Spinner M: In Omer G, Spinner M (eds): Normal Anomalous Innervation Patterns in the Upper Extremit Management of Peripheral Nerve Problems, Philadelphia, Saunders, 1980)

intrinsic muscles or participating equally with the median nerve in the innervation of the intrinsic muscles. The median nerve, on the other hand, may take over the entire nerve supply of all the intrinsic muscles. Either the median or the ulnar nerve may shift their innervation. For example, the first dorsal interosseous, the third lumbrical, the adductor pollicis, or even the abductor digiti minimi may get their innervation from the median nerve.

ARTICULAR INNERVATION

The articular innervation of the small joints of the hand has been studied by many investigators. Head maintained that no loss in the perception of movement in any joint occurs when the median or the ulnar nerves are divided at the level of the wrist, provided the injury is not complicated by division of the tendons. He felt that "deep sensibility" runs mainly with the

FIG. 5–26 Riche–Cannieu (R–C) anastomosis between the ulnar and median nerves in the palm. (Kaplan EB, Spinner M: In Omer G, Spinner M (eds): Normal and Anomalous Innervation Patterns of the Upper Extremity, Philadelphia, WB Saunders, 1980)

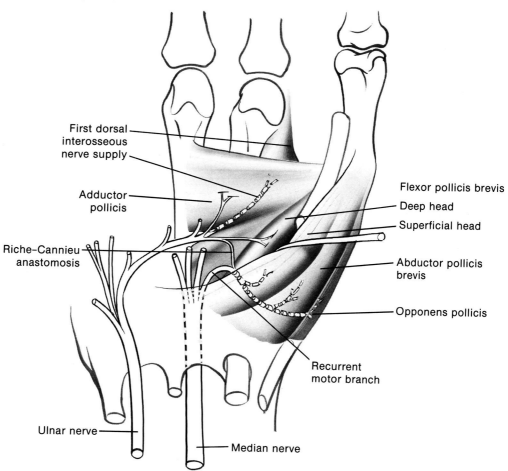

motor nerves and passes into the joints along the tendons and possibly the blood vessels.

Stopford made a significant contribution on the subject of stereognosis. He found that normally the ulnar nerve conducts afferent impulses that excite consciousness from all of the three joints of the little and the ring fingers, but noted in the case of the ring finger, variations were found. The median nerve was noted to provide the only pathway of transmission of afferent impulses from interphalangeal joints of the index and long fingers and the interphalangeal joint and frequently the metacarpophalangeal joint of the thumb. It may supplement the distribution of the ulnar nerve to the articulation of the ring finger. He felt that the radial nerve supplements the supply of the median nerve to the joints of the thumb and the metacarpophalangeal joints of the index and long fingers. The radial nerve may at times provide the only supply to the metacarpophalangeal joint of the thumb. Stopford emphasized the close relationship between variations in the cutaneous and the articular distributions of the various nerves, and felt that the nerves are either afferent or vasomotor in function.

Dr. Kaplan felt that the innervation to the metacarpophalangeal and interphalangeal joints were from the collateral branches of the proper digital nerves. The exact nature of this innervation was not clear. Recently, studies by Schultz and Krishnamurthy by gross dissections and microscopic cross-sections demonstrated that the articular branches to the proximal interphalangeal joint arise from the palmar proper digital nerves (Fig. 2–28). They noted that the proximal interphalangeal joints are innervated by a single articular nerve that arises from the proper digital nerves on the radial and ulnar sides of the finger. These articular branches arise proximal to the proximal interphalangeal joint and pass in a dorsolateral direction superficial to the articular artery. Just before entering the joint, the nerve bifurcates. The superior branch is most often thicker and longer and enters the joint in the midlateral plane. The inferior branch has a shorter course and enters the joint at the

lateral border of the palmar plate at its junction with the capsule. In the capsule, the nerve fibers are found grouped predominantly in a lateral and palmar location. Those which enter in the midlateral plane then descend palmarward, whereas those from the inferior branch pass into the palmar plate. No articular branches were noted to enter the capsule from the nerves passing dorsal to the joints. Nerves lay dorsal to the extensor mechanism in the finger and did not provide branches to the joint. The innervation of the proximal interphalangeal joint was found to be congruous with the palmar sensory innervation and had no relationship to the dorsal sensory innervation.

Stilwell found that there is a probably large source of proprioceptive afferents from various deep structures of the hand with proprioceptive triad, consisting of Ruffini organs, small Pacinian corpuscles, and free endings. According to Stilwell, the deep hand tissues are innervated by both deep and cutaneous nerves, and the afferents may follow both paths. He noted that abundant sources of proprioceptive signs are related to all motor mechanisms of the fingers and the wrist and that they probably constitute in part a neuroanatomic basic for normal mammal motor control and hand sensation. Free endings, some of which probably transmit pain sensations, are not more numerous in the deep structures of the hand than in other corresponding tissues of the limbs or the trunk; however, the skin of the hand has a more abundant supply of free endings than does any other skin region of the body. This means that the skin of the hand is considerably more sensitive than the skin of other regions, while sensation from the deeper parts would be similar to deep sensation in other parts of the body.

Gambier, Asvazadurian, and Venturini studied the nerve supply to the tendons and indicated a complex mechanism, whereby the nerve supply enters along with the vascular supply. Willgis and associates studied the sympathetic innervation in the hand using histofluorescence techniques; they demonstrated small twigs passing from the digital nerve to the digital artery. Schultz and Krishnamurthy found branches of the proper digital nerves in the vinculi and are proceeding with further studies. Studies by Potenza showed that the nerve and the vascular supply to tendons come from the surrounding tissues.

An important study was made by Rabischong on the proprioceptive innervation of lumbrical muscles in the human hand. He found that this innervation was extensive, more extensive than in other muscle system. This very rich nerve supply in the lumbricals apparently assures the complicated tensiometric activities that control the flexion-extension action of the fingers as the important regulatory activity of the lumbrical muscles.

6
The Retinacular System of the Hand

Emanuel B. Kaplan
Lee W. Milford

The muscles and the tendons of the hand, the vessels, the nerves, and the joints are invested in a system of connective, fatty and serous tissues. The functions of the various parts of this system are expressed in several ways: the retention of the moving parts in definite locations, the extension of action beyond the insertion of the tendons, and the protection of the moving parts or the delicate structures from injury. It is represented by fascial layers, expansions, reinforcing bands, fat pads, and synovial sheaths.

The role of some of these structures is static, dividing the hand into a functional or structural compartment, so thoroughly studied by Kanavel; the role of others is dynamic, extending or limiting action or creating mechanical advantages for better application of force. For practical purposes, all will be described as a retinacular system or retinacular apparatus of the hand, although some of the structures may not be directly related to each other.

There are a few fascial layers in the palm and over the dorsal aspect of the hand. They are comparatively simple, if followed systematically through the longitudinal and the cross-sections of the hand and also in simple dissections.

Upon dissection and removal of the skin of the palm of the hand, a very thin layer of fat is observed in the midpalmar region of the hand with fibrous strands uniting the skin to the underlying fascial sheet. The creases of the palmar skin appear to be joined even more firmly than the rest of the palmar skin.

The thin layer of subcutaneous fat becomes much thicker toward the thenar and the hypothenar eminences, forming thick fat pads over each eminence. These pads may be of considerable thickness but become thinner toward the marginal borders of each eminence to continue with the subcutaneous fat of the dorsum of the hand.

The pad of the thenar eminence expands distally into the first intermetacarpal space and thins out almost completely proximally toward the metacarpocarpal joint of the thumb (Fig. 2–64). The pad over the hypothenar eminence may be especially thick and contains the fibers of the palmaris brevis muscle. It extends to the distal crease of the palm distally, and proximally, it covers the pisiform abundantly (Figs. 2–64, 6–1, and 6–2). The two pads extend toward the center of the palm, where they blend with the thin subcutaneous fat layer of the midpalmar area. The pads of the eminences play their role as protectors of the nerves, blood vessels, and muscles of the thenar and the hypothenar areas (Fig. 2–64).

FIG. 6–1 Palmar aponeurosis of the hand. The pretendinous band to the little finger and the pretendinous band to the index finger appear to surround the metacarpal heads instead of going directly into the anterior surface of the fingers. This direction of the pretendinous band to the index finger with absence of a superficial transverse ligament extending toward the thumb is similar to the arrangement of the pretendinous bands of the midplantar aponeurosis of the gorilla foot and denotes complete functional independence of the first digit. The interdigital or natatory ligament is shown. It is partly responsible for limitation of flexion of a finger when the other fingers are extended. Three windows are shown between the metacarpal heads, exhibiting the digital vessels and nerves, which are usually completely covered by small fat pads that protect the digital vessels and nerves and stand out prominently in the palm of the normal hand, when the fingers are hyperextended, as slight elevations between the fingers just below the digital skin folds.

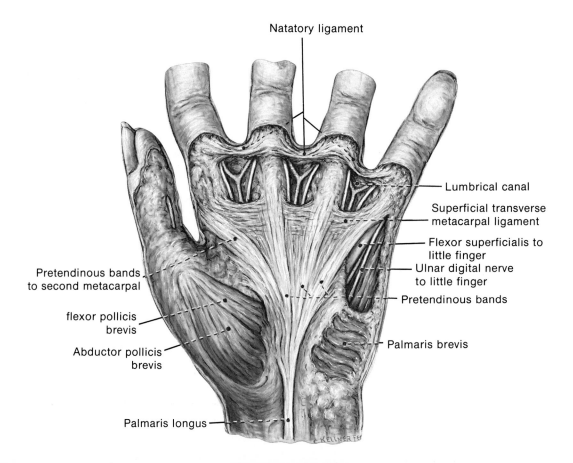

Natatory ligament

Lumbrical canal

Superficial transverse metacarpal ligament

Flexor superficialis to little finger

Ulnar digital nerve to little finger

Pretendinous bands

Palmaris brevis

Pretendinous bands to second metacarpal

flexor pollicis brevis

Abductor pollicis brevis

Palmaris longus

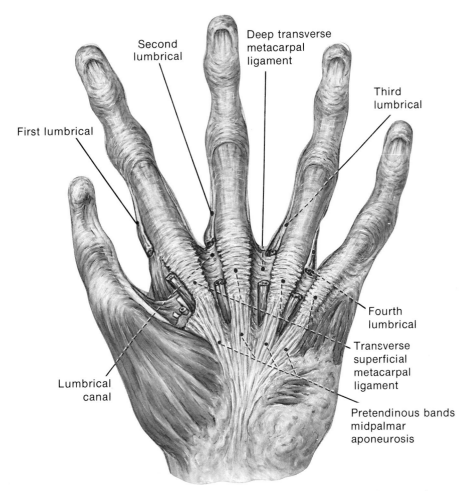

First lumbrical

Second lumbrical

Deep transverse metacarpal ligament

Third lumbrical

Fourth lumbrical

Transverse superficial metacarpal ligament

Pretendinous bands midpalmar aponeurosis

Lumbrical canal

FIG. 6–2 Midpalmar aponeurosis. The transverse fibers over the intermetacarpal spaces are excised. The deep transverse metacarpal ligament is seen forming the floor of the lumbrical canal. The superficial transverse metacarpal ligament extends more distally than usual. It is removed from the intermetacarpal spaces where it forms the volar cover of the lumbrical tunnel. The distal part of the lumbrical canal usually is covered with fat only. The proximal part of the lumbrical canal is covered also by the superficial transverse metacarpal ligament of the palmar aponeurosis. The natatory or interdigital ligament is located further distal in the web and is not shown here.

THENAR AND HYPOTHENAR FASCIAE

When the fat pads are removed completely, the muscles of the thenar and the hypothenar eminences show a thin fascial cover that turns around the radial side of the hand for the thenar area and around the ulnar side of the hand for the hypothenar area and continues directly with the fascia that covers the interosseous muscles over the dorsum of the

hand (Fig. 2–64). The fascia covering the interosseous muscles in the back of the hand represents the posterior interosseous fascia; it adheres to the exposed posterior aspect of each metacarpal and is free over the interosseous muscles (Fig. 2–6).

The adductor pollicis muscle is covered by its fascia on the volar surface of the muscle in continuity with the thenar fascia. The fascia turns around the free border of the muscle to the deep surface of the adductor muscle, covers this muscle, and separates it from a fascial layer covering the first and the second intermetacarpal spaces with their interosseous muscles. The fascia covering the interosseous muscles of the second intermetacarpal space represents the volar interosseous fascia of the radial half of the hand. This fascia runs around the radial side of the second metacarpal and the metacarpophalangeal joint and the first dorsal interosseous muscle and blends with the posterior interosseous fascia. A potential space is formed between the volar interosseous fascia of the radial half of the hand and the deep dorsal fascia of the adductor pollicis muscle.

Thus, in the first intermetacarpal space the dorsal interosseous fascia covers, as described, the first dorsal interosseous and continues into the volar interosseous fascia. The adductor pollicis is covered by its own fascia on the dorsum. This fascia continues from the dorsal to the volar aspect of the adductor pollicis. Thus, the potential space is formed between the volar interosseous in front of the first dorsal interosseous muscle and the fascia covering the dorsal part of the fascia of the adductor pollicis muscle. The fasciae of the dorsum of the hand and the wrist will be described with the dorsal carpal ligament; however, it may be mentioned now that another fascial structure is found in the first intermetacarpal space. The fascia that is found between all the extensor tendons of the hand and is named *intertendineal fascia* (Anson) extends to the first intermetacarpal space and forms a layer connecting the tendons of the extensors of the fingers with the extensors of the thumb. It covers the fasciae of the first dorsal interosseous muscle and of the adductor pollicis; it extends toward the first interdigital fold and forms a distinct edge in the form of an arch between the tendon of the extensor digitorum of the index and the tendon of the extensor pollicis brevis. This edge blends into the subcutaneous fat of the skin of the fold. A similar fascial layer was observed in the foot of a chimpanzee and was noted several years previously in a gorilla foot by Raven of the American Museum of Natural History, although he believed it to repre-

sent a modified, deep transverse metatarsal ligament.

The thenar fascia extends distally and blends with the ligaments of the metacarpophalangeal joint of the thumb. The hypothenar fascia extends distally into the ligaments of the metacarpophalangeal joint of the little finger. Proximally, both fasciae blend with the transverse volar carpal ligament.

The thenar and the hypothenar fasciae are joined in the center of the palm by the dense fibrillar, shiny central fascia named the *midpalmar fascia*, or midpalmar aponeurosis. Thus, the fascia of the volar aspect of the hand is described as the thenar, the hypothenar, and the midpalmar fasciae or aponeuroses.

MIDPALMAR FASCIA

The midpalmar fascia is a dense fascial sheet extending from the transverse carpal ligament (the anterior annular ligament of the wrist) to the metacarpophalangeal joints of the index, middle, ring, and little fingers (Fig. 6–1). It is triangular in shape, with the base oriented toward the fingers and the apex attached approximately in the midline of the transverse carpal ligament. The apex is frequently adherent to the volar surface of the transverse carpal ligament and continues directly into the tendon of the palmaris longus, when the palmaris longus is present.

When the palmaris longus is absent, the apex of the midpalmar fascia either blends directly into the transverse carpal ligament or ends in a pointed, short fascial appendix or continues into the antebrachial fascia. The connection of the apex with the transverse carpal ligament is covered normally by a thick fat pad that connects the thenar and the hypothenar fat pads.

When the apex of the midpalmar fascia is dissected and lifted off the transverse carpal ligament, it sometimes shows that the distal border of the transverse carpal ligament continues deeply toward the midpalmar fascia for a short distance and blends with a layer of loose, cellular connective tissue mixed with fat. This layer of loose, fat tissue continues distally and covers the superficial palmar arterial arch, the common digital nerves of the median to the index, middle and ring finger, the ulnar nerve to the ring finger and the radial side of the little finger, and the synovial bursa of the flexor tendons of the fingers.

The distal part of the midpalmar fascia gradually becomes wider as it runs toward the fingers. It is very dense and shows a system of longitudinal fibers diverging as they approach the metacarpophalangeal joints. The longitudinal fibers run exactly parallel with and anterior to the flexor tendons of the middle and ring fingers, forming distinct bands. These bands were named *pretendinous bands* because of their location.

The pretendinous bands to the index and little fingers have a slightly different course. Instead of running directly over the volar surface of the metacarpophalangeal regions, the band over the index finger deflects radially and appears to run around the radial side of the index; the pretendinous band of the little finger appears to run in a similar manner around the ulnar side of the little finger (Fig. 6–1).

The longitudinal bands continue distally and adhere firmly to the fibrous tunnels or the sheaths of the flexor tendons of the four fingers (Fig. 6–2). Sometimes, they continue into the fingers; however, the continuation of the pretendinous bands into the anterolateral sides of the fingers is observed mostly in pathologic fasciae of Dupuytren's contracture. The pretendinous bands are connected by short fibers with the overlying skin of the palm of the hand and with the skin of the volar root of the fingers. When the fingers are hyperextended, the pretendinous bands become tense and depress the skin along the flexor tendons over the metacarpal heads in the distal part of the hand. Simultaneously with the depression produced by the pretendinous bands, slight elevations appear between the depressed areas. These elevations are caused by the protruding fat pads in the distal parts of the intermetacarpal spaces.

The functional relation of the midpalmar aponeurosis (midpalmar fascia) to the palmaris longus is of great interest. The author has found that traction in a proximal direction applied to the apex of the palmar fascia or to the palmaris longus produced slight flexion of the fingers at the metacarpophalangeal joints in the cadaver. Occasionally, even in the cadaver, traction produced no flexion of the fingers, although tension of the midpalmar fascia was observed almost constantly. In the living, on exposure of the midpalmar fascia during surgical procedures, only tensing of the fascia could be produced by traction applied to the palmaris longus. Electric stimulation of the palmaris longus never produced flexion of the fingers in the cases observed by the author.

In the proximal part of the midpalmar fascia between the four pretendinous divergent bands, a few longitudinal, thinner fasciculi fill the interpretendinous spaces. These longitudinal fasciculi stop approximately at the level of the distal crease of the palm. They are interrupted by superficial transverse fibers running from the ulnar to the radial border of the palm of the hand.

The transverse fibers are thin, strong, shiny, stringlike structures running between the pretendinous bands, over the pretendinous bands, and even through them, interlacing with them and appearing to hold the pretendinous bands together (Fig. 6–1). In certain cases of Dupuytren's contracture, they form a dense transverse band (*see Fig. 9–18*). Normally, the approximate longitudinal width of the area occupied by the transverse fibers is about 1 cm. It does not form a continuous band. Pellets of fat can be seen penetrating from under the fascia through the transverse fibers toward the palmar skin. The transverse fibers stop more or less abruptly at the level of the distal crease of the palm of the hand. The width of the combined fibers, their course from the second to the fifth metacarpal, the superficial location, and the approximate similarity to the location of the deep transverse ligament justify the name of the superficial transverse ligament of the palm for this structure.

The fibers of the superficial transverse ligament of the palmar aponeurosis, together with the pretendinous bands, firmly adhere to the fibrous tunnels or sheaths of the flexor tendons over the metacarpophalangeal joints of the four fingers (Fig. 6–2).

Distal to the course of the transverse fibers of the superficial transverse ligament and distinctly separated from them, there is another group of fibers immediately under the skin of the interdigital folds. These fibers can span the spaces between the fingers in the interdigital folds by short and long strands forming a band named the *ligamentum natatorium* by Braune. A brief mention of this ligament can be found in Grapow's work done under the direction of Braune and mentioned by Eycleshymer.

The *ligamentum natatorium* or the interdigital ligament (Figs. 2–24 and 6–1) continues directly into the fingers and invests the digital artery and nerve on each side in a fatty tunnel reinforced by fibrous strands, described by Cleland and Grayson as skin ligaments. The pretendinous bands on each side, the superficial transverse ligament proximally, and the natatory or the interdigital ligament distally contribute to the formation of three windows between the index and the middle intermetacarpal area, between the middle and ring fingers, and between the ring and little fingers. These windows are closed by three large fat pads that were mentioned previously. They stand out as intermetacarpal elevations when the pretendinous bands are tense and depress the palmar skin over the metacarpal heads on hyperextension of the fingers. When removed, they expose the digital arteries and nerves in their course from the palm of the hand to the fingers in company with the lumbricals. The fat pads covering the windows are in direct connection with the loose cellular, fatty tissue found under the midpalmar fascia as mentioned before, covering the superficial arterial arch, the common digital nerves and the flexor digital bursa (Fig. 2–64).

Braune and Grapow believed that the physiologic significance of the natatory ligament or interdigital ligament and the superficial transverse metacarpal ligament resides in the possible aid of movement of blood through the passing veins. It is probable that the natatory (interdigital) ligament restricts excessive independent flexion of a finger when the others are extended, or vice versa. The superficial transverse ligament is probably a purely retinacular ligament similar to the deep transverse ligament, reinforcing the fixation of the metacarpals.

To remove the midpalmar fascia, it is necessary to separate it from the transverse carpal ligament in the proximal part of the hand. As was described previously, the fascia adheres to the transverse carpal ligament. Immediately under (dorsal to) the midpalmar fascia, the transverse carpal ligament extends the fibers of its distal border toward the cellular layer of the fat, which varies in thickness and protects the superficial arch and other structures. This layer of cellulo-fatty tissue extends distally under the pretendinous bands to the line where the bands adhere firmly to the fibrous tunnels of the flexor tendons of the fingers. In the spaces between the pretendinous bands the fatty layer extends distally under the palmar fascia, covering the lumbrical muscles and the common digital nerves and vessels, until it reaches the superficial transverse ligament and the windows described previously. It then protrudes through these windows and contributes to the formation of the fat pads that protrude through the windows and cover the structures dorsal to them.

The only area where the midpalmer fascia adheres firmly to the underlying structures is in the region of the fibrous tunnel of the flexor tendons. It was found in serial sections of fetal hands that the flexor tendon tunnels develop much earlier than do the midpalmar fascia and that the pretendinous bands of the midpalmer fascia adhere to the flexor tunnels at a later date (Fig. 6–3). In the 40-mm to 60-mm fetus (Fig. 2–18), the midpalmar fascia is not visible, while the flexor tendon tunnel is in full formation even before the actual splitting of the tendons into the superficialis and the profundus. The deep transverse metacarpal ligament is just in the process of formation but does not as yet form a continuous band. No septa are visible between the lumbricals with the neurovascular bundle and the flexor tendons, except the wall of the tunnel itself.

In older fetal hands (Figs. 2–19 and 2–22), further development of the deep transverse metacarpal ligament is evident. This development continues with more delimitation of the tunnels of the flexors but without obvious adherence of the midpalmar fascia to them (Fig. 2–20). The midpalmar fascia appears to be an independent and older development, establishing later connections with the fibrous tunnels of the flexor tendons (Figs. 6–4 and 6–5).

The hand of a premature 7-month baby shows very little evidence of pretendinous bands (Fig. 6–3). Dissection of hands of full-term babies begins to show well-defined pretendinous and transverse fibers and also interdigital ligaments and adherence of longitudinal bands to the fibrous tunnels.

Transverse sections through adult hands show the relation of the midpalmar fascia to the tunnels of the flexors. There is adherence of the midpalmar fascia to the tunnels but no septa extending to the deep transverse ligament, unless the walls of the tunnels are considered as septa (Figs. 2–21, 2–23, and 6–2). The pretendinous bands of the midpalmar fascia may be dissected off the tunnels with comparative ease, or the tunnels may be opened and the anterior wall lifted with the dissected midpalmar fascia, giving an impression of septa extending from the midpalmar fascia into the depth of the hand (Fig. 5–16).

The midpalmar fascia can be separated by cutting from the thin thenar fascia on the radial side and the thin hypothenar fascia on the ulnar side. When this is done, it can be observed that the hypothenar fascia continues directly with the fascia covering the interosseous muscles of the ulnar half of the volar aspect of the hand; the thenar fascia continues over the adductor pollicis muscle toward the fascia covering the interosseous muscles of the ulnar half of the hand. Both are actually one continuous, thin, fascial sheet from the thenar eminence over the adductor muscle, over the ulnar half of the interosseous muscles toward and over the hypothenar muscles.

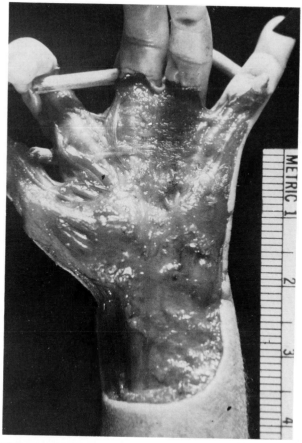

FIG. 6–3 Hand of a 7-month premature infant. The pretendinous bands of the midpalmar aponeurosis are indistinguishable. The superficial transverse fibers of the palmar aponeurosis are clearly seen, as are the fibers of the natatory interdigital ligament.

The crest of the third metacarpal is the meeting line of the origin of the transverse part of the adductor pollicis muscle with its volar and dorsal fasciae, the interosseous fascia of the ulnar half of the hand, and the interosseous fascia of the radial half of the hand. This line also is joined by the adhesion of the posterior wall of the ulnar bursa of the flexor tendons. The frequently thickened fascia covering the volar surface of the adductor muscle running toward the crest creates an impression of a septum between the midpalmar fascia and this line. *Actually, the septum is nothing but the continuation of the fascia of the thenar muscles* (Fig. 2–64), which

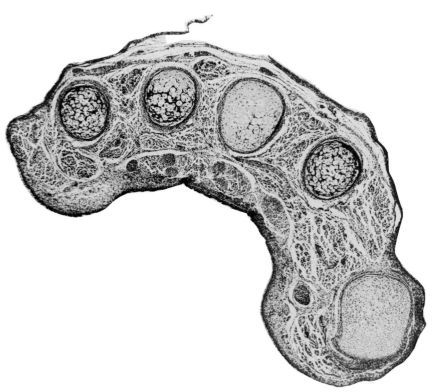

FIG 6—4 Transverse section through the palm of a fetal hand through the shaft of the metacarpals. The midpalmar aponeurosis is still indistinguishable.

sometimes passes over the synovial sheath of the index flexors when these have a separate synovial sheath. There are no septa from the midpalmar fascia to the fascia of the deep volar aspect of the hand.

The flexor tendons that occupy the palm in their passage to the fingers are enclosed in synovial bursae. One is located in the ulnar part of the hand and usually includes the index, middle, ring, and little fingers. It is frequently separated from the synovial bursa enclosing the flexor pollicis longus.

The ulnar synovial bursa is separated from the midpalmar fascia by the arterial superficial arch, the common digital nerves, and the cellular, fatty, fascial layer mentioned before; however, the deep dorsal surface of the ulnar bursa is not free. It adheres firmly to the volar interosseous and the adductor fascia in the

region of the crest of the third metacarpal where the transverse fibers of the adductor pollicis muscle take origin. This connection of the bursa persists through the entire length of the crest of the third metacarpal and extends proximally with the ulnar bursa into the carpal canal, stopping at varying levels. It does not adhere to the interosseous fascia ulnar to the crest, neither does it adhere to the adductor fascia radial to the crest.

In a transverse section through the midhand, the connection of this bursa with the crest divides the hollow of the palm into two halves: the ulnar palmar half and the radial palmar half. The radial half is located over the adductor muscle; the ulnar half, over the interossei of the third and the fourth intermetacarpal spaces (Fig. 2–64), covered with their volar interosseous fascia.

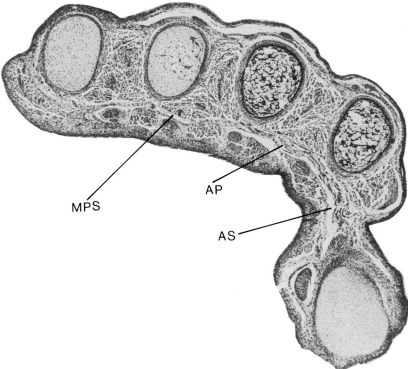

FIG 6–5 Section through a 5-month fetal hand, through the middle of the hand and the proximal phalanx of the thumb. The adductor space (AS) between the flexor tendons and the adductor muscle (AP) is apparent. The midpalmar space (MPS) between the interosseous fascia and the flexor tendons also is obvious. The tendons of the extensor digitorum communis, with their intertendinous connection, are indicated over the dorsum of the hand. The separation between the adductor space and the midpalmar space is formed by an intimate connection of the ulnar bursa with the third metacarpal. In this section as well as in other sections of the fetal and the adult hands, no septum could be found in direct continuation with the midpalmar aponeurosis or as a derivative of the midpalmer aponeurosis.

The first impression obtained when the transverse hand section is studied is of a septum between the midpalmar fascia and the crest of the third metacarpal. Further dissection of the structures of the transverse section shows the actual situation (Fig. 6–6). The ulnar bursa, when dissected and reflected from the hand, adheres to the crest of the third metacarpal approximately in the region of the flexor tendons to the middle finger. The midpalmar fascia is separated from the volar side of the bursa by a layer of fat. The adductor pollicis fascia is continuous with the fascia of the interosseous muscles of the ulnar half. No septum between the

midpalmar fascia and the crest of the third metacarpal exists.

The present description of the midpalmar fascia differs fundamentally from the accepted forms and from a study made and reported by the author several years ago. At that time, it appeared to the author that small, longitudinal septa united the pretendinous bands of the midpalmar fascia with the fascia of the adductor pollicis over the radial half of the hand and with the volar interosseous fascia of the third and the fourth intermetacarpal spaces. This was not confirmed. The author believes now that only fatty, fibrous tissue fills in these areas and that there

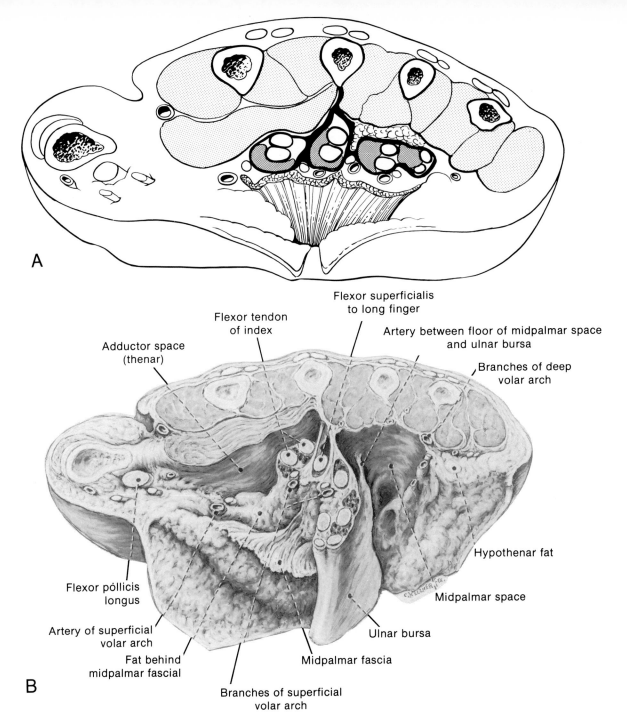

A

B

Adductor space
(thenar)

Flexor tendon
of index

Flexor superficialis
to long finger

Artery between floor of midpalmar space
and ulnar bursa

Branches of deep
volar arch

Hypothenar fat

Midpalmar space

Ulnar bursa

Midpalmar fascia

Branches of superficial
volar arch

Fat behind
midpalmar fascial

Artery of superficial
volar arch

Flexor póllicis
longus

FIG. 6–6 **A**, Line drawing of the cross-sectional anatomy of a left hand transverse through the level of the middle of the second, third, fourth, and fifth metacarpals and obliquely through the proximal phalanx of the thumb (see Fig. 2–64). **B**, Further dissection of the cross-section of this specimen. The palmar fascia is separated from the retroaponeurotic fat. The skin is completely removed. The illustration shows no direct continuation of the midpalmar fascia around the flexor tendons of the index finger or between the index and the middle finger flexors. There is a visible separation between the midpalmar space and the adductor space, but the separation is caused mostly by adherence of the ulnar bursa to the crest of the third metacarpal. All the flexor tendons are displaced from the midpalmar space. The septa surrounding the flexor superficialis of the middle finger are synovial folds of the ulnar bursa (see Fig. 2–64).

are no actual septa between the midpalmar fascia and the volar interosseous and the adductor fascia.

This view does not agree with most of the descriptions of the relation of the midpalmar fascia to the deep structures. The experiences of the surgeons who have occasion to remove the midpalmar fascia for the treatment of Dupuytren's contracture show that some septa are found and must be excised from the deeper parts of the hands. In order to find the reason for this discrepancy, the author dissected a number of hands in cadavers afflicted with Dupuytren's contracture. The result of the investigation showed several important facts. The fascia in the hand afflicted with Dupuytren's contracture is not a normal fascia and does not reflect or exaggerate a normal condition; therefore, the bands of contracture may assume the most bizarre ways: they may stop at the metacarpophalangeal joints, extend to the skin of the fingers or penetrate between the tendons for attachment into the interosseous fascia, may extend toward the thumb or form double bands, or may branch from one band into two fingers (*see Fig. 9–18*).

In view of the material usually available in the anatomic laboratories for dissection (older people), the incidence of Dupuytren's contracture of the hands is high; therefore, a question may arise as to whether the reported increase in the number of pretendinous bands, as described by some writers, results from observations on hands afflicted with Dupuytren's contractures in a mild form.

The penetration of the midpalmar contracted bands into the deeper parts of the hands and the increase in the number of bands is probably not a normal condition but a result of pathologic changes that do not follow normal patterns. Consequently, in surgery of Dupuytren's contracture, when excision is necessary, it is more logical to remove visible extensions of the contracted bands and not look for hypothetical septa.

Further studies of the midpalmar fascia reveal other interesting facts that may throw some light on the significance and the functional role of the fascia.

The midpalmar fascia in the primate hand has been described. In the dissection of a hand of a gorilla, Duckworth* found that the antebrachial fascia continued over the transverse carpal ligament, consisting mostly of transverse fibers and thin longitudinal fibers. About 5 mm proximal to the metacarpal heads, the fascia splits into four portions that run along the line of the digits and are wrapped around the tendon sheaths and attached to the metacarpals.

Strauss found a definite midpalmar aponeurosis in the hands of two lowland gorillas.† Strauss and Howell found a "a structure that was 'clear cut' enough to be termed a natural palmar aponeurosis."

The author dissected three gorilla hands with special attention paid to the midpalmar fascia and studied the model of the specimen in the anatomic museum of the College of Physicians and Surgeons of Columbia University (Fig. 6–7). It was found that a dense fibrolipomatous layer covered the whole subcutaneous surface of the palm. Over the hypothenar area, distinct transverse fibers corresponding to the palmaris brevis were found in two hands. The midpalmar fascia consisted of a thick, amorphous sheet without differentiation into longitudinal bands, adherent to the flexor tunnels in the region of the metacarpophalangeal joints.

These dissections, literary references, and additional dissection of hands of the rhesus monkey by the author produced a general impression that the midpalmar fascia of the dissected primates is somewhat similar to that in humans but perhaps not as well differentiated (Fig. 6–8). In contrast, the plantar fascia of the foot of the gorilla appears to be defined much better (Fig. 6–9).

The pretendinous bands of the gorilla foot stand out well. the pretendinous band to the second toe appears to have a course similar to

---

*Duckworth WLH: Studies from the Anthropological Laboratory. London, Cambridge University Press, 1904

---

†Strauss WL, Jr.: Personal communication

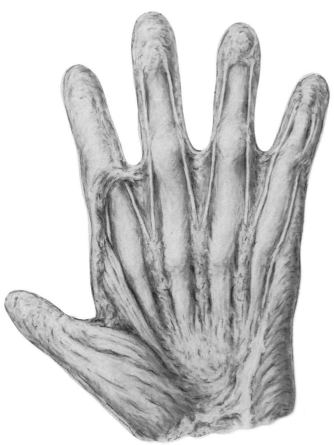

FIG. 6—7 The hand of a gorilla with the skin removed, showing the subcutaneous fat and an absent midpalmar aponeurosis, which was probably removed in the process of dissection. (Specimen from the Museum of the Department of Anatomy, College of Physicians and Surgeons, Columbia University, New York, NY)

the pretendinous band of the index finger of the human hand (compare with Fig. 6–1), separating the second toe from the active big toe (Fig. 6–10) in the same way as the index is separated from the active thumb in the human hand.

The plantar fascia of the human foot also exhibits longitudinal pretendinous bands similar to the pretendinous bands of the hand, but the pretendinous band to the big toe appears to run around the big toe similar to the band that runs around the index finger of the hand or the second toe of the gorilla foot (Fig. 6–11). Thus, a

strong impression is created that the midpalmar fascia with its pretendinous fibers serves mostly to fix and immobilize the metacarpals.

In the presence of a strong and independent flexor pollicis or hallucis longus, the differentiation becomes more distinct; therefore, the midpalmar fascia of the human hand is more differentiated than the midpalmar fascia of the anthropoid hand. In the foot of the bear, the midplantar fascia apparently shows no differentiation whatsoever and is simply fused with the flexor digitorum brevis.

In the dissection of human hands, the author never found an instance where the midpalmar fascia was absent. There was no reference in the available literature to absence of the midpalmar fascia. In contrast, the palmaris longus has been found absent in a comparatively large number of cases (11% to 23%).

If the midpalmar fascia together with the palmaris longus represented a remnant of a flexor superficialis (third flexor in addition to the flexor sublimis and profundus), there would have

FIG. 6—8 Small chimpanzee hand, showing the arrangement of the midpalmar fascia.

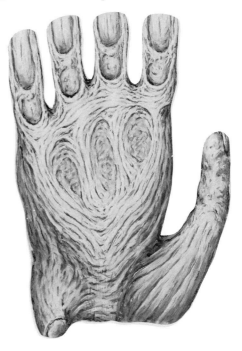

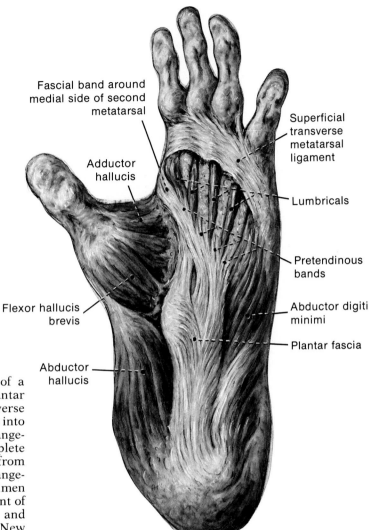

Fascial band around medial side of second metatarsal

Adductor hallucis

Superficial transverse metatarsal ligament

Lumbricals

Pretendinous bands

Abductor digiti minimi

Plantar fascia

Flexor hallucis brevis

Abductor hallucis

FIG. 6–9 The plantar surface of a gorilla foot, showing the midplantar fascia and the superficial transverse metacarpal ligament, which blends into the interdigital ligament. The arrangement of the fibers indicates a complete separation of the movable big toe from the other toes, similar to the arrangement of the human hand. (Specimen from the Museum of the Department of Anatomy, College of Physicians and Surgeons, Columbia University, New York, NY)

been, perhaps occasionally, instances where the midpalmar fascia was absent in a way similar to the absence of the palmaris longus.

The author believes that this discrepancy, the comparatively late appearance of the mid-palmar fascia in the fetal hands and the relation of the pretendinous longitudinal bands to the fixed metacarpals or metatarsals and their probable relation to the independent flexor pollicis or hallucis longus indicates that the midpalmar fascia is only a superficial retinaculum having no other function and not intended for any other

function than fixation of the metacarpals (Fig.6–12). In support of this view, it may be added that in a dissection of two hands of a young chimpanzee, a well-formed palmaris longus was found in each hand, but the palmar aponeurosis was absent.

The connection of the midpalmar fascia with the palmaris longus tendon is incidental, inconstant and without particular significance. Although the midpalmar fascia is present constantly, its complete surgical removal does not produce any significant alterations in the func-

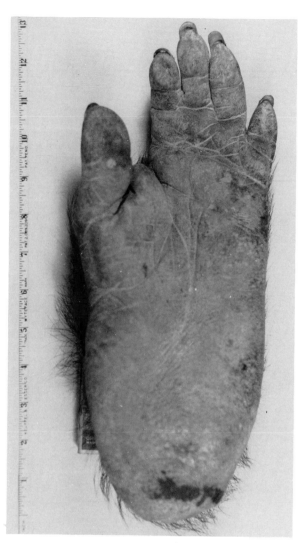

FIG. 6—10 Plantar surface of the foot of a full-grown female gorilla. The pattern of the plantar creases is somewhat similar to the pattern of the creases of the human hand. The strong big toe, with its position of opposition is also similar to the position of opposition of the human hand.

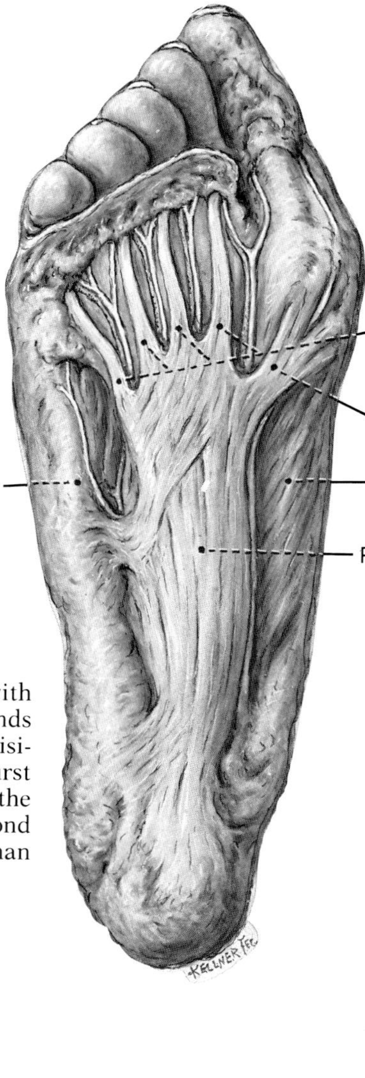

Pretendinous bands

Pretendinous band medial side of first metatarsal

Abductor digiti minimi

Abductor hallucis

Plantar fascia

FIG. 6—11 Plantar fascia of human foot in comparison with Figure 6-9. The fascia is more dense, the pretendinous bands are shorter, and their transverse superficial fibers are not visible. The plantar fascia extends medial to the head of the first metatarsal, in contrast with the foot of the gorilla, in which the most medial extension of the fascia goes around the second metatarsal, similar to the extension of the fascia in the human hand.

tion of the hand or in the power of the flexor muscles.

DEEP PALMAR FAT PAD

The floor of the palm between the thenar and the hypothenar eminences, as mentioned before, is divided by the insertion and the adhesion of the posterior (dorsal) surface of the ulnar flexor bursa into two compartments: the radial and the ulnar. The fascia that covers this floor is a continuation of the hypothenar fascia over the interosseous muscles and over the adductor pollicis toward and over the muscles of the thenar eminence. The fascia of the floor continues distally and merges with the deep transverse metacarpal ligament (Fig. 2–13). Proximally, the fascia spreads over the ligaments of the carpus and continues directly with the fascia of the anterior surface of the pronator quadratus muscle.

When the ulnar bursa of the flexor tendons of the hand is completely removed from the palm, the interosseous fascia is always found to be covered by a layer of encapsulated fat. This encapsulated fat conceals the anterior interosseous fascia of the third and the fourth intermetacarpal spaces and overlaps slightly the origin of the adductor pollicis muscle (Fig. 2–30 and 6–13).

This fat pad was always present in human hands dissected by the author and in hands dissected by the first-year medical students of the College of Physicians and Surgeons for the past 10 years. Despite its constant presence, the pad has not been described, to the knowledge of the author, as a definite structure in any of the old or the new anatomic treatises.

The size and the width of the fat pad vary little. The length is about 4 cm to 5 cm; the width, about 2 cm. It extends distally almost to the palmar end of the fibrous tunnels of the flexor tendons of the long, ring, and little fingers. Proximally, it extends into the carpal canal, midway between the palmar and the antebrachial borders of the transverse carpal ligament. On the ulnar side, it extends to the

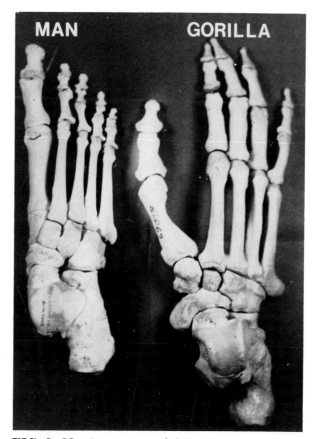

FIG. 6–12 Comparison of skeletal structures of the foot of a gorilla and of a human. The gorilla foot shows a combination of a fairly good supportive mechanism with an excellent grasping device in the forefoot. The big toe of the gorilla articulates with the medial cuneiform, permitting motion of the big toe similar to the motion of the opposable human thumb. The opposition of the big toe in the gorilla foot is produced essentially by the peroneus longus, which apparently has no counterpart in the hand. The flexor hallucis longus is strongly developed in the gorilla; the flexor hallucis brevis is also well developed for opposition of the big toe.

muscles of the hypothenar eminence; on the radial side, it overlaps slightly the crest of the third metacarpal with the origin of the adductor pollicis. The distal end of the fat pad is well defined and rounded; the proximal part is less defined and thins out gradually.

The pad is firmly adherent to the ulnar volar interosseous fascia but can be lifted

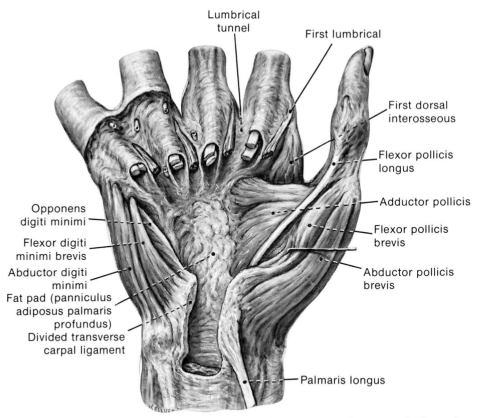

Lumbrical tunnel

First lumbrical

First dorsal interosseous

Flexor pollicis longus

Adductor pollicis

Flexor pollicis brevis

Abductor pollicis brevis

Opponens digiti minimi

Flexor digiti minimi brevis

Abductor digiti minimi

Fat pad (panniculus adiposus palmaris profundus)

Divided transverse carpal ligament

Palmaris longus

FIG. 6–13 The deep midpalmar fat pad covers, conceals, and protects the branches of the deep ulnar nerve and the deep palmar arch in the midpalmar space. Note the distance of the interdigital fold from the distal border of the deep transverse intermetacarpal ligament.

slightly from the fascia covering the origin of the adductor pollicis because in this area the posterior wall of the ulnar bursa of the flexor tendon adheres to the crest of the third metacarpal. The fat pad actually serves as the floor of the ulnar half of the space of the palm, named midpalmar space of Kanavel.

The author dissected three gorilla hands and found the fat pad present in all of them in the same location of the palm as in the human hand; however, the size of the pad was smaller in relation to the size of the midpalmar space. In two chimpanzee hands dissected by the author, the fat pads were absent. In human fetuses over 10 cm and in premature infants, the deep pad was always present.

The fat pad, which provides a soft elastic cushion for the bursa of the flexors, apparently plays an important role in the protection of the deep branch of the ulnar nerve, which the pad covers completely from its point of entry into the midpalmar space to its exit through the opening in the adductor pollicis muscle. The deep branch of the nerve is protected from the constant motion of the flexor tendons in their bursa and also from external pressure exerted by the fingers or by tools held in the hand. Its development may also be related to the development of the thumb, because a thumb that is longer, more active, and stronger than normal may produce more pressure in the palm of the hand and require more adequate protection of the deep branch of the ulnar nerve. This is perhaps the reason for the absence of the deep palmar fat pad in the chimpanzee with its underdeveloped thumb.

The fat pad can be seen well in all sections of the hand (Fig. 2–64) through the area of its location. The fat pad is important and constant enough to deserve a name. The author suggests *the deep palmar fat pad* or *panniculus adiposus palmaris profundus.*

In infections of the midpalmar space, the panniculus may be the most vulnerable element of the space and the first to undergo necrosis. It is also the origin of deep lipomas of the hand.

DEEP TRANSVERSE METACARPAL LIGAMENT

In the Nomina Anatomica Tokyo nomenclature (1975), the ligament is known as the *Lig. metacarpeum transversum profundum.* It has been known as the deep transverse intermetacarpal ligament and as the capitular ligament, but in order to eliminate confusion it is better to refer to it as the deep transverse metacarpal ligament, which conforms with the newest nomenclature of the International Federation of Hand Surgery.

The deep transverse metacarpal ligament forms a continuous band from the ulnar side of the little finger to the radial side of the index finger, transversely across the proximal parts of the heads of the second, the third, the fourth, and the fifth metacarpals. On the ulnar side of the little finger, it blends with the ulnar collateral ligament of its metacarpophalangeal joint; on the radial side, it blends with the radial collateral ligament of the metacarpophalangeal joint of the index finger. Over the metacarpophalangeal joints, it represents the posterior wall of the fibrous tunnel of the flexor tendons blending with the capsule of the metacarpophalangeal joint; between the joints it forms a narrow band holding the metacarpals together (Figs. 2–21 and 6–2). Proximally, the ligament continues uninterruptedly into the volar interosseous fascia.

The thickness of the ligament is about 1 mm to 2 mm; its width between the metacarpals is about 5 mm to 6 mm; its height does not exceed 1 cm. Although proximally it gradually becomes thinner toward the volar interosseus fascia, it behaves differently at the distal border. The distal border is sharp (Fig. 3–2) and ends approximately 2 cm to 4 cm proximal to the interdigital skin fold, making it possible to feel the distal edge of the deep transverse ligament by palpation. The space between the distal edge of the deep transverse ligament and the skin fold is filled by the interdigital or natatory ligament (Fig. 2–24).

The volar surface of the transverse intermetacarpal ligament has transverse markings; it is smooth and shiny. The lumbrical muscle lies on this surface in company with the digital nerves and arteries, which are more volar. The whole group is covered volad by the intermetacarpal fat pad. The interosseous muscles (Fig. 2–23) pass on the dorsal side of the deep ligament.

From the viewpoint of the surgical approach, the deep transverse ligament is nearer to the volar surface of the hand and is much more accessible than from the dorsal side. The function of the deep transverse ligament consists of retaining the metacarpals together and establishing mechanical advantages for the action of the lumbrical muscles.

TRANSVERSE CARPAL LIGAMENT

The carpal bones of the volar aspect of the wrist are joined together, forming a deep excavation for the passage of the tendons, vessels, and nerves from the forearm into the hand. The transverse carpal ligament transforms the excavation into a closed passage named the *carpal canal.*

The transverse carpal ligament is a dense, wide transverse band. It is inserted into the hook of the hamate bone and the pisiform on the ulnar side; on the radial side it is inserted firmly into the crest of the trapezium, the tubercle of the scaphoid, and sometimes to the styloid process of the radius (Fig. 6–14). The ligament varies in height from about 22 mm to 32 mm; its thickness varies from 1 mm to

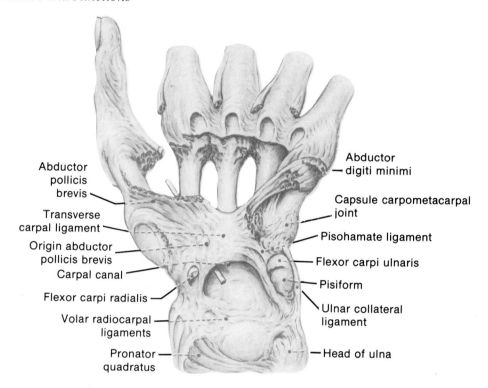

Abductor pollicis brevis

Transverse carpal ligament

Origin abductor pollicis brevis

Carpal canal

Flexor carpi radialis

Volar radiocarpal ligaments

Pronator quadratus

Abductor digiti minimi

Capsule carpometacarpal joint

Pisohamate ligament

Flexor carpi ulnaris

Pisiform

Ulnar collateral ligament

Head of ulna

FIG. 6–14 Demonstration of the transverse carpal ligament, showing its width in connection with the abductor brevis and the opponens pollicis and its relation to the flexor carpi radialis, also the flexor and the abductor of the little finger. A small rod is introduced into the carpal canal to show that on the radial side the wall of the canal runs obliquely, parallel with the first metacarpal.

2 mm. Distally, it blends with the fibers under the midpalmar fascia; proximally, it continues with the antebrachial fascia. Volad, it is covered by the midpalmar fascia and the palmaris longus tendon.

On the radial side, the transverse carpal ligament bridges the crest of the trapezium, creating a tunnel for the tendon of the flexor carpi radialis, and serves as an area of origin for the thenar muscles (Figs. 3–18 and 6–14). On the ulnar side, it is reinforced by the pisiform-hamate ligament and serves as an area of origin for the hypothenar muscles (Figs. 3–18 and 6–14).

An extension from the tendon of the flexor carpi ulnaris to the hook of the hamate bone creates an additional channel between the transverse carpal ligament and the extension, outside of the carpal canal, for the passage of the ulnar vessels between the hook of the hamate

and the pisiform (Fig. 2–7). This channel is known in the French literature as the channel of Guyon. Actually, the fascial extension from the tendon of the flexor carpi ulnaris represents a continuation of the superficial fibers of the dorsal carpal ligament, which pass from the dorsum of the wrist around the ulnar side of the wrist to the transverse carpal ligament. The transverse carpal ligament corresponds to an area covering the distal row of the carpal bones and the bases of the metacarpals.

In transverse section, the carpal canal is somewhat triangular with rounded angles. The apex of the triangle is directed toward the radial side and the base toward the ulnar side (Fig. 4–6). The ulnar side of the carpal canal is represented by the concavity of the hook of the hamate. The ulnar part of the canal is occupied by the tendons of the flexor superficialis of the ring and the little fingers and the flexor profundus of the little finger. The apex of the triangle on the radial side is invariably occupied by the tendon of the flexor pollicis longus (Fig. 2–31).

The direction of the canal on the ulnar side is almost parallel with the ulnar border of the hand. The direction on the radial side is oblique distally and radially (Fig. 6–14), parallel with the direction of the first metacarpal. The inside of the carpal canal is lined by an extension of the volar interosseous fascia (Fig. 4–6), which covers the entire inner surface of the canal.

The structures that pass through the carpal canal are the median nerve and all the flexor tendons of the fingers in their synovial bursae. The median nerve is invested in a cellulo-adipous layer, making it difficult to separate the nerve from the synovial bursa of the flexor tendons. The tendon of the flexor carpi radialis is outside the carpal canal. The ulnar artery and nerve are also outside the carpal canal (Fig. 2–31).

The functional role of the transverse carpal ligament is in the maintenance of the carpal arch. It also serves as a most important retinacular pulley for the flexors of the fingers, and for this reason it is also called the flexor retinaculum. The transverse carpal ligament serves as a guard for the median nerve, which it protects in the passage from the forearm to the hand; however, it may also cause compression of the median nerve. Many observations were made on the nature and the morphology of the contracture (Newman, Marie and Foix, Moersch, Zachary, Phalen, Bunnell, Mangini, and others). An anatomic study of the carpal canal was reported lately by Robbins who also showed how in some conditions extreme positions of volar flexion or dorsiflexion compress the median nerve against the transverse carpal ligament.

RETINACULAR APPARATUS OF THE DORSUM OF THE HAND AND THE FINGERS

The retinacular apparatus of the dorsum of the hand and the fingers presents a complicated system of bands and fibers that unite into a functional group—the dorsal structures of the hand with the deep transverse metacarpal ligament and with the fibrous tunnels of the fingers.

There was a tendency after the work of Legueu and Juvara, in 1892, to describe an intimate interconnection between the mid-palmar fascia and the tendons of the extensor communis of the hand. The original diagram of Legueu and Juvara (Fig. 6–15) was reproduced constantly with many modifications, especially in the French anatomic textbooks, including the very latest treatises. A modified diagram of Legueu and Juvara was described by Dr. Kaplan, in 1938, in a study of the palmar fascia in connection with Dupuytren's contracture.

The diagram of Legueu and Juvara and all subsequent modifications show that special fibers from the midpalmar fascia run along the sides of the fibrous tunnels of the flexor tendons in a dorsal direction, perforate the deep transverse metacarpal ligament, and continue after perforation into the extensor apparatus of the dorsum of each finger. In the illustration of Paturet, a sagittal septum is shown from the tendon of the extensor communis of the middle finger on its radial side running between the metacarpophalangeal joint and the tendons of the interosseous and the lumbrical to the subcutaneous layer of the skin of the palm; it is called *cloison sagittal (fibres perforantes).**

This illustration apparently emphasizes the description given by Legueu and Juvara, who state, "There are fibers which we call perforating, because instead of stopping at the deep aponeurosis, they traverse, perforate this aponeurosis—to encircle the metacarpophalangeal joints."†

This description, which was accepted by Dr. Kaplan in the past, was reinvestigated subsequently by dissection of normal adult and fetal hands by embryologic and pathologic studies; unfortunately, it could not be confirmed. There was not a single instance where perforating

*Paturet G: Traité d'anatomie humaine, vol. 2, p 324. Paris, Masson, 1951

†Legueu F, and Juvara E: Bulletins de la Société Anatomiques de Paris, p 392. 1892

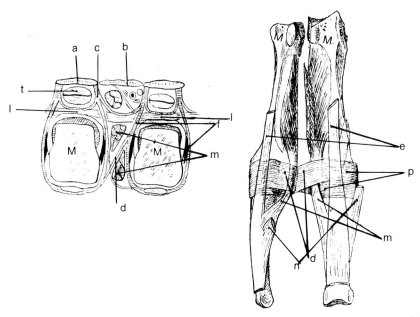

FIG. 6–15 Copy of illustration given in the article of Legueu and Juvara, in which the fibers of expansion of the extensors digitorum communis (p) are shown penetrating (f) directly through the deep transverse metacarpal ligament. This illustration is reproduced frequently in anatomic textbooks in the French language. In the author's investigation, the fibers of extension from the tendon of the extensor digitorum communis were never found to perforate the deep transverse metacarpal ligament.

fibers were found running from the dorsum to the palm of the hand in the spaces between the metacarpophalangeal joints through the deep transverse metacarpal ligament. Humphrey's views on the development of the pronator flexor and the supinator extensor parts of the forearm probably would not support such perforating fibers. There is a definite separation in the development of the two groups, and although in the lower animals of the zoologic scale a fusion between the two occurs in the mammals and especially in man, it is not common. Each group is comparatively independent, the interossei remain with the extensors over the dorsal part, and the lumbricals over the flexor part of the hand.

The probability of perforating fibers is not great, according to the developmental factors.

The development of the deep transverse metacarpal ligament (Figs. 2–18, 2–19, 2–20, and 2–22) shows that embryologically it probably consists of a dorsal and a volar part. The dorsal part develops with the extensor tendons and their expansions, and the volar develops with the tunnel of the flexor tendons. No perforating fibers can be visualized. Distal to the deep transverse metacarpal ligament in the interdigital folds and over the fingers, the expansions of the extensor communis definitely spread toward the fibrous tunnels of the flexor tendons (Figs. 2–14 and 2–26).

In a larger magnification over the head of the metacarpal, which is 1 cm to 2 cm distal to the distal edge of the deep metacarpal transverse ligament, the expansion of the extensor communis digitorum passes around the metacarpophalangeal joint; the tendon of the interosseous muscle remains between the capsule and the extensor expansion (Fig. 2–27). The extensor expansion continues its encircling volar course toward the fibrous tunnel of the flexor tendons (Fig. 2–59) and ends in this vicinity.

In the transverse section through the metacarpophalangeal joints of the adult hand, the deep transverse metacarpal ligament does not show any perforating fibers coming from the expansion of the extensor digitorum through the deep transverse metacarpal ligament (Fig. 2–23).

The thumb has no deep transverse ligament uniting its metacarpal with the other metacarpals. The space between the first and the second metacarpals is filled with fat that expands from the previously described fat pad of the thenar eminence. In view of the special function of the thumb, a retaining deep transverse metacarpal ligament would constitute an impediment to its function; however, the dorsal apparatus of the thumb follows a pattern observed over the dorsum of the other fingers.

The expansions of the extensor pollicis longus and brevis encircle the metacarpophalangeal joint and fuse with the tunnel of the flexor pollicis longus and the sesamoids connected with the tunnel (Fig. 3–3).

In the description of the insertion of the extensor communis tendon and the tendons of the interossei and the lumbricals, their connection with the metacarpophalangeal and the interphalangeal joints was given.

EXTENSOR RETINACULUM

The antebrachial fascia of the forearm extends and blends into the extensor retinaculum of the wrist (Figs. 3–14 and 6–16). The extensor retinaculum represents a structure of thickened oblique and transverse fibers running over the dorsum of the wrist from the radial side to the ulnar side, covering all the extensor tendons and separating the subcutaneous fascia. On the radial side, the extensor retinaculum blends into the transverse carpal ligament after passing over the grooves of the abductor pollicis and the extensor pollicis tendons. On the ulnar side, it passes over the head and the styloid process and the ulnar collateral ligament to join the transverse carpal ligament over the pisiform and the tendon of the flexor carpi ulnaris.

It is important to mention that the extensor retinaculum consists of a superficial and a deep layer. The fibers of the superficial and the deep layers do not insert into the ulnar head and the styloid process but pass over these structures to insert into the medial side of the pisiform and the triquetrum. The details of this insertion were studied and described by Deleeuw, who also explained the relationship of the extensor retinaculum to the mechanism of rotation and supination of the distal radioulnar joint. Personal studies were made by Dr. Kaplan.

The extensor retinaculum is about 2 cm to 3 cm wide. It is formed by a superficial and a deep layer that can be separated by dissection. The superficial and the deep layers can be differentiated with greater ease over the ulnar side of the wrist. The deep layer contributes to the formation of the tunnels for the abductor longus and the extensor brevis pollicis, the two radial extensors, and the extensor minimi. All these tunnels adhere to the radius. The tendon of the extensor indicis proprius passes deep to the tendon of the other extensors in the same tunnel. The deep layer then continues its course toward the extensor carpi ulnaris but does not adhere to the ulna. It passes over the tendon of the extensor carpi ulnaris and inserts into the ulnar side of the pisiform and over the dorsum of the triquetral and the ulnar base of the fifth metacarpal.

In its passage, the deep layer forms a tunnel for the tendon of the extensor carpi ulnaris from the groove for the tendon of the extensor carpi ulnaris on the ulnar head to the base of the fifth metacarpal. This tunnel also extends proximally over the groove for the extensor tendon of the ulnar head. The extension is thinner than the fibers of the deep layer running to the pisiform and the triquetrum. This extension over the groove is inserted into the medial edge of the groove. On the lateral side of the groove, the extension is inserted into the side of the tunnel for the tendon of the extensor digiti minimi. The tunnel for the extensor carpi ulnaris permits limited radial and lateral motion of this tendon but does not permit its dislocation from the groove (Fig. 6–17).

(Text continues on page 268.)

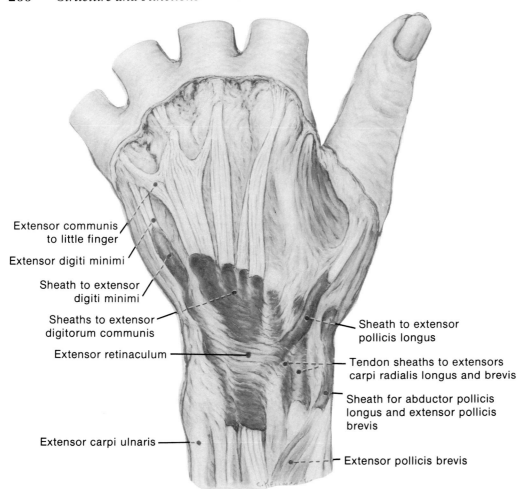

Extensor communis
to little finger

Extensor digiti minimi

Sheath to extensor
digiti minimi

Sheaths to extensor
digitorum communis

Extensor retinaculum

Extensor carpi ulnaris

Sheath to extensor
pollicis longus

Tendon sheaths to extensors
carpi radialis longus and brevis

Sheath for abductor pollicis
longus and extensor pollicis
brevis

Extensor pollicis brevis

FIG. 6–16   Demonstration of the extent of the synovial sheaths of the extensors of the hand and the fingers, showing separate tunnels for the various tendons within the extensor retinaculum. The tendons of the extensor digitorum communis show a common variant with multiple interconnections. Compare illustration with the dorsum of the hand of the gorilla (see Fig. 2–57).

FIG. 6–17   **A**, Left wrist. Extensor retinaculum in pronation. The oblique fibers of the ligament are directed toward the pisiform and the triquetral bone. There is a space between the tendon of the extensor digiti minimi and the tendon of the extensor carpi ulnaris at the level of the distal radioulnar joint.

Extensor retinaculum in supination. In supination, the tendon of the extensor carpi ulnaris moves radially toward the tendon of the extensor digiti only a few millimeters within the ulnar tunnel. The radius rotates toward the ulna, which does not rotate but shifts toward the radius. The rotation of the radius moves the tendon of the extensor digiti minimi toward the tendon of the extensor carpi ulnaris because the extensor digiti minimi remains in its dorsal tunnel attached to the radius by the extensor retinaculum. Thus, the distance between the tendon of the extensor digiti minimi and the extensor carpi ulnaris disappears. In supination, the tendon of the extensor digiti minimi becomes placed dorsal to the extensor carpi ulnaris because of the absence of attachment of the superficial fibers of the extensor retinaculum to the ulna and tunnel of the extensor carpi ulnaris. **B**, Left wrist with the superficial fibers of the extensor

(Continued)

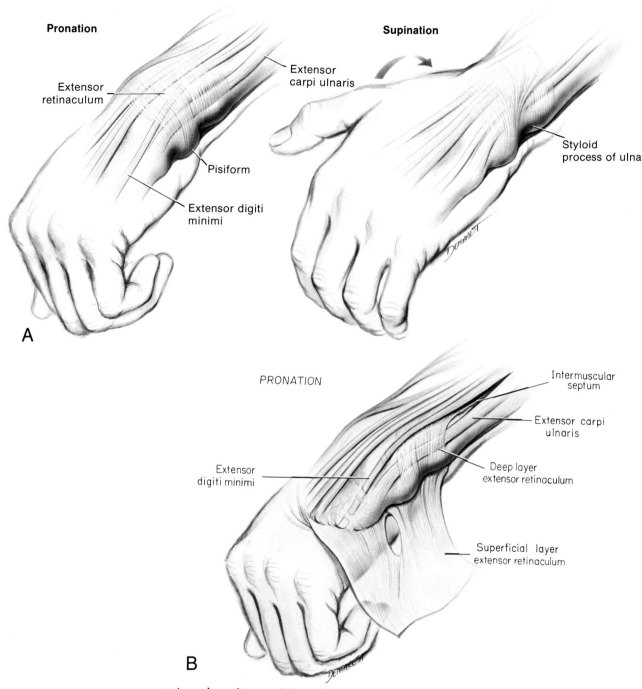

retinaculum dissected from the deep fibers of this ligament. The deep fibers of the dorsal carpal ligament are attached to the ulna but also are directed toward the pisiform and the triquetral without attachment to the ulna. Fibers of the deep ligament form a roof over the ulnar tunnel of the extensor carpi ulnaris. The antebrachial intermuscular septum between the digital extensors and the extensor carpi ulnaris is attached to the ulnar shaft but is not attached to the distal end of the ulnar shaft and the head of the ulna under the extensor retinaculum. Thus, the extensor retinaculum does not interfere with free movement between the radius and the ulna in pronation and supination; at the same time, it forms a dorsal roof over the ulnar tunnel preventing dorsal displacement of the extensor carpi ulnaris tendon.

It was explained in the preceding pages that in pronation and supination of the forearm, the ulna does not rotate. It moves from side to side. In pronation, it moves medially and dorsally, and in supination, it moves laterally and volarly. In its medial shift, the tunnel of the extensor digiti minimi prevents the displacement of the tendon of the extensor carpi ulnaris; in its lateral shift, the tensing of the superficial and the deep layers of the dorsal carpal ligament also prevents displacement.

The superficial layer of the dorsal carpal ligament has the same direction of the fibers and inserts similarly to the deep layer except that it blends its fibers on the ulnar and the radial sides with the fibers of the transverse carpal ligament. The dorsal carpal ligament continues over the dorsal aspect of the extensor tendons in the form of a thinned-out sheet that gradually fades away in its dorsal course before it reaches the metacarpophalangeal joints. The diverging tendons of the extensor communis digitorum are connected together by a thin, fascial, intertendinous sheet (Fig. 2–6).

The continuation in a very thinned-out form of the extensor retinaculum over the tendons of the extensor communis acts as a weak anchor, preventing overstretching of the extensors of the fingers when strong flexion of the fingers is exerted. The dorsal carpal ligament, through its tunnel formation, acts as a very strong retinacular apparatus for the extensor tendons.

The combination of all the retaining and connecting bands of the dorsal apparatus permits a unified system of the entire retinacular dorsal apparatus in the following manner. The tendons of the extensors of the fingers have a retinaculum over the carpus formed by the osteofibrous tunnels. In addition to the ligament represented by the extensor retinaculum, the extension of the fascia over the divergent extensor tendons forms an anchorage restraining overstretching of these tendons in flexion. The tendons are held together by the intertendinous fascia, which may be continuous or interrupted and is reinforced by tendinous interconnections near the distal part of the metacarpals. The intertendinous band, which becomes thinner in

its course toward the heads of the metacarpals, runs into the sharp proximal edge of the expansion of each tendon of the extensor communis over the dorsum of the metacarpophalangeal joint (Fig. 2–6).

The expansion of the extensor tendon turns around the sides of the corresponding joint obliquely and distally and becomes connected with the collateral ligaments of each joint, and further distally, with the fibrous tunnel of the flexor tendons. An oblique anchorage is formed, permitting extension and flexion but fixing the extensor tendon so that it cannot slide off from its position in relation to the axis of the finger. Further distally, the extensor tendon is fixed firmly to the base of the middle phalanx. The expansion of the extensor tendon, together with the interossei and the lumbricals, establishes connections with the ligaments and the capsule of the proximal interphalangeal joint and the tunnel of the flexor tendons, anchoring the entire apparatus by oblique fibers and again permitting extension and flexion.

A similar arrangement occurs over the distal interphalangeal joint (Fig. 2–6), anchoring the dorsal apparatus to the distal interphalangeal joint and the distal part of the fibrous tunnel of the flexors. The extensor apparatus of the thumb has a very similar pattern in relation to the metacarpophalangeal and the interphalangeal joints (Fig. 2–66 and 3–21). Thus, the extensor tendons of the extensor communis have four areas of anchorage, and the extensors of the thumb have three areas of anchorage.

Any injury to the retinacular anchorage, be it at the carpus or the metacarpophalangeal and the interphalangeal joints, will produce a more or less serious disruption of the functioning of the fingers and the thumb.

RETINACULAR SYSTEM OF THE DIGITS
(Milford)

RETAINING LIGAMENTS OF THE SKIN

The retaining or retinacular ligaments of the digits are those that maintain the position of the skin over the digits and those attached to or associated with the extensor mechanism over the dorsum of the fingers. These ligaments are Cleland's cutaneous ligament; Grayson's ligament; the oblique retinacular ligament, described first by Weitbrecht and later by Landsmeer and by Haines; the transverse retinacular ligament, called the fascial band by Bunnell; and the sagittal band, also known as the shroud or sling ligament (Fig. 6–18). Another retaining ligament can be called the peritendinous cutaneous fibers and was described by Cleland and later by Stanislavjevic.

Cleland's cutaneous ligament

Cleland's cutaneous ligament consists of four slightly flattened, conelike structures arising on each side of the digit or thumb from the interphalangeal joint (see Figs. 6–19 and 6–20). These ligaments consist of dense fibrous bundles that diverge from their origin to insert into the skin. In dissection, these bundles seem at first to constitute a sheet of tissue or a septum, but this is true only of the stronger fibers. In fact, the fibers are not arranged in one plane, but radiate to two planes to form a structure shaped somewhat like a flattened cone.

The largest of the four bundles of fibers originates from the lateral margin of the middle phalanx over its proximal fourth, from the capsule of the proximal interphalangeal joint, and from the flexor tendon sheath. These fibers project in a generally straight line and are quite strong, requiring sharp dissection to rupture. Most of them project outward obliquely from the phalanx, diverging into two planes to insert into the skin, and are somewhat larger than they are in their area of origin. There are also weaker fibers that project to the skin on the palmar surface. Most of these fibers originate deep to the transverse retinacular ligament and eventually pass dorsal to the digital nerves and vessels. The fibers of this bundle with most dorsal origin become taut when the proximal interphalangeal joints is flexed because they are stretched over the condyle of the proximal phalanx. This tautness seems to lend some stability to the otherwise relaxed skin. Similarly, the more volad originating fibers become taut when the proximal interphalangeal joint is extended. The volar skin is obviously less mobile in such extension, principally because of the tightening of the volar fibers. This strongest bundle is also represented in the thumb, where it arises from the junction

FIG. 6–18 Schematic representation of the retinacular ligaments of the digit as viewed from the lateral aspect. Grayson's ligament is not represented. (From Milford, LW: Retaining Ligaments of the Digits of the Hand. Philadelphia, WB Saunders Co., 1968)

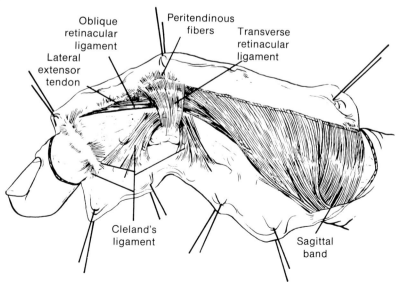

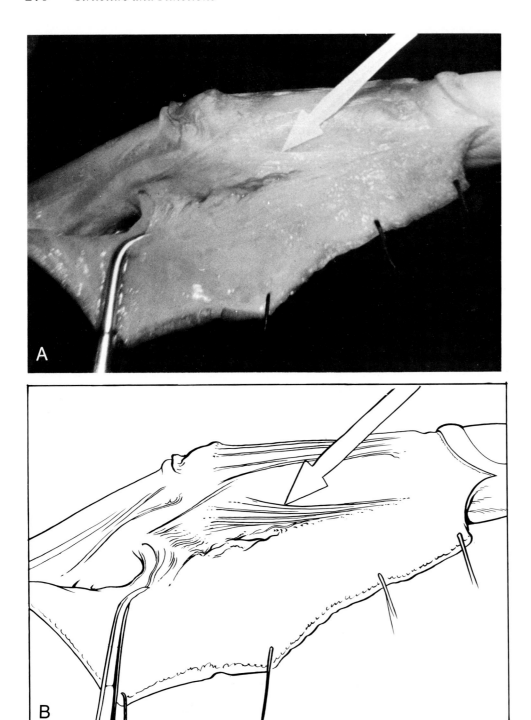

FIG. 6–19   **A** and **B**, Cleland's ligament at the proximal interphalangeal joint. The bundles are seen between the arrow and probe. (From Milford, LW: Retaining Ligaments of the Digits of the Hand. Philadelphia, WB Saunders Co., 1968)

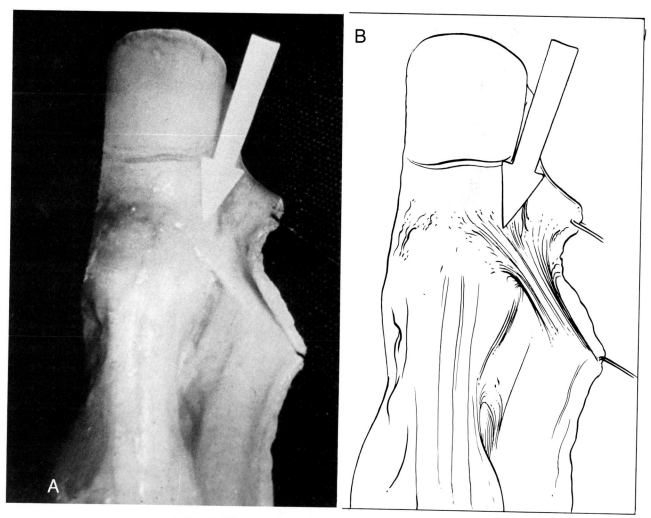

FIG. 6–20 **A** and **B**, Cleland's ligament dissected at the interphalangeal joint of the thumb. The arrow notes the origin of this cutaneous ligament from the joint level. (From Milford, LW: Retaining Ligaments of the Digits of the Hand. Philadelphia, WB Saunders Co., 1968)

of the flexor tendon sheath and this sheath's insertion into bone. The fibers project distally and laterally to insert into the skin.

The next largest of these four bundles consists of a set of fibers, one on each side of the proximal phalanx, originating from the distal fourth of this phalanx, from its lateral border, and from the capsule of the proximal interphalangeal joint. These fibers radiate into two planes and therefore are more than just a septum; however, they diverge in a direction proximal and opposite from the fibers of the largest set of bundles. Because these fibers are more perpendicular to the axis of the phalanx they insert more promptly into the surrounding skin and are therefore shorter than the fibers of the largest bundles that are just distal.

In addition to the two bundles just described, two distal bundles originate from the lateral aspect of the distal interphalangeal joint.

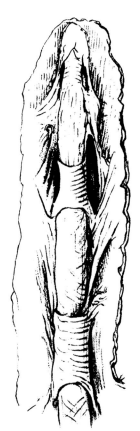

FIG. 6–21 Cleland's ligament, original drawing. (J Anat Physiol **12**:526, 1878)

These fibers originate from the bone and capsule over a very small area of 1 mm to 2 mm just proximal and distal to the distal interphalangeal joint. They pass almost immediately into the skin laterally and dorsally over the distal interphalangeal joint, which is possible because the skin lies almost against the bone at this level with minimal intervening fat. These fibers interlace with those of the largest bundle from the proximal interphalangeal joint area as they project distally and with the distal fibers as they project proximally. The fibers pass dorsal to the digital nerves and vessels, as do all fibers of Cleland's ligament.

The above description is based on dissection performed by Dr. Milford, the results of which were published in a 1968 monograph entitled

Retaining Ligaments of the Digits of the Hand, it differs somewhat from Cleland's original description (Fig. 6–21).

Grayson's ligament

Grayson's ligament (Fig. 6–22) originates from the volar aspect of the flexor tendon sheath. Its fibers project at right angles to this sheath, pass volar to the digital nerves and vessels, and insert into the skin at the same level as their origin. The fibers do not spread or fan out like those of Cleland, but tend to be parallel. The strongest of the fibers are those of the middle three fourths of

FIG. 6–22 Schematic presentation of Grayson's and Cleland's ligaments. Grayson's ligament is volar to the neurovascular bundle, while Cleland's ligament is dorsal. (From Milford, LW: Retaining Ligaments of the Digits of the Hand. Philadelphia, WB Saunders Co., 1968)

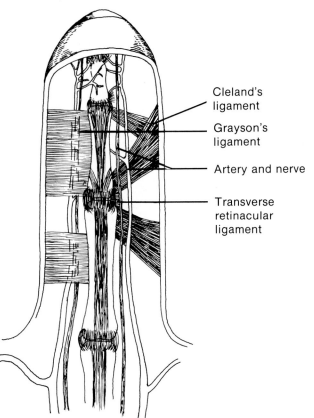

Cleland's ligament

Grayson's ligament

Artery and nerve

Transverse retinacular ligament

the middle phalanx in the finger and those just proximal to the interphalangeal joint in the thumb. The fibers are continuous across the midline with those of the opposite side. A similar set of tranverse fibers proximal to the proximal interphalangeal joint arises in the midportion of the proximal phalanx. These fibers are not as dense or as frequent and are probably not strong enough to hold the digital nerves and vessels in place and keep them from bowstringing in the finger during flexion. Along with the dorsally located fibers of Cleland, they form a tube in which the digital vessels and nerves are encased.

The above description differs considerably from Grayson's original description, and is based on microdissection and cross-section studies performed by Dr. Milford and published in *Retaining Ligaments of the Digits of the Hand.*

Peritendinous cutaneous fibers

Cleland accurately described the function of the peritendinous cutaneous fibers, but not their anatomy. (He did not, in fact, call them *peritendinous cutaneous fibers.*) These fibers arise from the extensor mechanism, especially over the distal interphalangeal and proximal interphalangeal joints, and insert almost entirely to the dorsal skin folds over these two joints (see Fig. 6–23). The fibers are much less distinct over the metacarpophalangeal joint. Many of these fibers are easily disrupted by blunt dissection, and they are almost nonexistent over the central tendon of the extensor mechanism. Their insertion corresponds to the creases of the skin over the proximal interphalangeal and distal interphalangeal joints. At these levels the fibers are very strong and short and require sharp dissection to disrupt. When the fibers are cut, the skin over the dorsum of the finger can be shifted easily, as can a glove. These fibers are also found in the thumb, especially at the interphalangeal joint.

Transverse and oblique retinacular ligaments

The retaining ligaments at the level of the proximal interphalangeal joint associated with the extensor mechanism have been called the *retinacular ligaments*, with transverse and oblique components as described by Landsmeer (Fig. 6–24); the oblique component was called the *link ligament* by Haines (Fig. 6–25) and was originally named the *retinaculum tendoni longi* by Weitbrecht (Fig. 6–26); the transverse component was called the *fascial sheath* by Bunnell.

Transverse retinacular ligament

The transverse retinacular ligament is composed of thin, strong fascia easily perforated by a dissection probe but difficult to tear. Its fibers originate from the volar aspect of the capsule in the flexor tendon sheath at the level of the proximal interphalangeal joint. The fibers then pass superficial to the fibers of Cleland's ligament, which arise in the same area and act as a sling. Some fibers also arise in the skin at the anterior lateral aspect of the finger at the level of the flexor crease. Normally they are destroyed during sharp dissection; however, those fibers originating from the skin do broaden the origin of the ligament by passing dorsally with the other fibers to form a sheet of fascia that inserts mainly at the lateral margin of the lateral tendon of the extensor mechanism. The fibers are already perpendicular to the longitudinal axis of the finger, thus passing over the condyle of the proximal phalanx. Some fibers pass distally and obliquely as they curve around the joint capsule and attach further distally on the lateral tendon, making the ligament trapezoidal when its origin has been detached. Most of the fibers insert in the lateral margin of the lateral tendon, but a few pass dorsally over the extensor tendon and become continuous with those of the opposite side.

The ligament seems to act as a stabilizer for the lateral tendon. It also seems to pull the lateral tendon volad when the proximal interphalangeal joint is flexed. As this joint is flexed, those fibers that pass just distal to the greatest width of the condyle of the proximal phalanx are tightened because they are pulled over this area of the condyle. The lateral tendon lies dorsal to the fulcrum of the proximal interphalangeal joint, and as flexion occurs, the tendon tenses until it may slide from the apex of

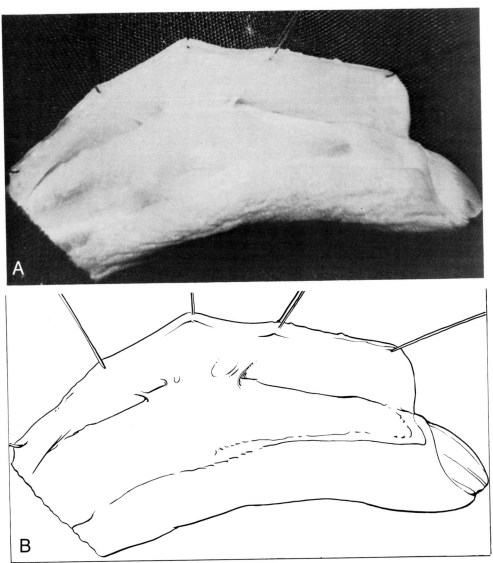

FIG. 6—23 **A** and **B**, Peritendinous cutaneous fibers at the dorsal aspect of the proximal interphalangeal joint. (From Milford, LW: Retaining Ligaments of the Digits of the Hand. Philadelphia, WB Saunders Co., 1968)

the joint and subluxate laterally. Because of this action, the tendon can be considered to be pulled laterally by the transverse retinacular ligament, which does not yield to the demand of the lateral tendon to lengthen so that the lateral tendon may remain in its original position. Of course, the lateral tendon itself becomes increasingly tight because of the flexing of the joint. Because

of their eccentric insertion, the distalmost fibers of the transverse retinacular ligament act under the same influence as does the collateral ligament of the metacarpophalangeal joint. This is not to imply that the transverse retinacular ligament alone is responsible for lateral subluxation of the lateral tendon because if this ligament is divided, the lateral tendon still subluxates

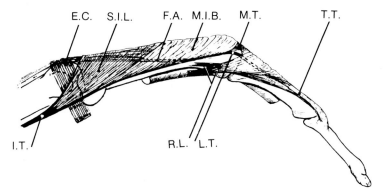

FIG. 6—24 Landsmeer's original illustration. R. L. (*arrowhead*) represents both the transverse and oblique retinacular ligaments. (Landsmeer JF: The anatomy of the dorsal aponeurosis of the human finger and its functional significance. Anat Rec 104:31, 1949)

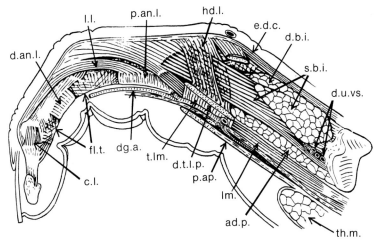

FIG. 6—25 Haines' "link ligament," the oblique retinacular ligament, 1.1 (*arrowhead*). (Haines RW: The extensor apparatus of the finger. J Anat **85**:251, 1951)

FIG. 6—26 Weitbrecht's representation of the retinacular ligament (f) termed by him, *retinaculum tendini longi*. He also described the skin ligament (g), which is today called *Cleland's ligament*. (Weitbrecht O: Syndesmologia sive Historia Ligamentum Corporis Humani, 1742)

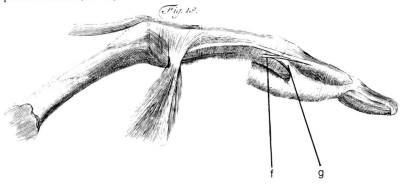

volad when the proximal interphalangeal joint is flexed.

All fibers of this ligament lie slightly against the capsule of the proximal interphalangeal joint, and their course is over the volar origin to dorsal insertion. They stand out in relief only after the plane of dissection is found and the sheet is elevated from its bed. Those strong, discrete, well-ordered fibers can be seen in this thin ligament.

Oblique retinacular ligament

In 1949, Landsmeer called attention to an oblique component of the retinacular ligament (Fig. 6–24); a year later, Haines described the same ligament (Fig. 6–25) and called it the "link ligament" for functional reasons. Neither knew that this ligament had been described 200 years earlier by Weitbrecht in a work entitled *Syndesmology* in which he named it the "retinaculum tendoni longi" (Fig. 6–26). Subsequent work by Landsmeer, Haines, Stack, Tubiana, Valentine, and others has added to the understanding of the function of this ligament.

In contrast to the fibers of the transverse retinacular ligament, those of the oblique retinacular ligament are tendinous in character. This probably was recognized by Weitbrecht when he named the ligament retinaculum tendoni longi. The fibers arise from the bone of the distal fourth of the proximal phalanx, the junction of the phalanx, and the flexor tendon sheath. They form a narrow, strong tendinous band that passes parallel to the lateral margin of the lateral extensor tendon and along the longitudinal axis of the phalanx. The origin is at times covered by the border of the extensor tendon.

Fibers of the oblique retinacular ligament cross the proximal interphalangeal joint deep to those of the retinacular ligament and are generally quite separate. A few of the oblique fibers insert into the middle of the transverse retinacular ligament; most of them pass deep to it and finally join the lateral margin of the lateral tendon. The fibers project distally parallel to those of the lateral tendon, of which the band becomes an integral part at about the level of the proximal interphalangeal joint.

These fibers can sometimes be seen to continue at the lateralmost part of the lateral tendon as it inserts into the distal phalanx. The oblique retinacular ligament consistently passes just volar to the axis of rotation of the proximal interphalangeal joint when the joint is flexed; it thus becomes quite tight when the joint is extended. Because of this, easy active or passive flexion of the distal interphalangeal joint is not possible when the proximal interphalangeal joint is extended. In some cases of arthritis, this ligament may be selectively contracted, causing constant hyperextension of the distal interphalangeal joint when the proximal interphalangeal joint is only partially extended.

The oblique retinacular ligament may be represented in the thumb by a small tendinous band originating from a discrete muscle bundle deep within the mass of the abductor pollicis brevis and also in the adductor pollicis. It then passes parallel to the extensor pollicis longus and inserts along with this tendon into the distal phalanx.

The sagittal band

The sagittal band, also known as the sling or shroud ligament, may be considered a homologue of the transverse retinacular ligament (Fig. 6–18). Its fibers originate from the deep transverse metacarpal ligament and flexor tendon sheath and constitute the most proximal part of the dorsal expansion of the extensor mechanism. The fibers form a strong, thin, tendinous sheet, and the major fibers project perpendicular to the longitudinal axis of the finger as it inserts on the lateral margin of the extensor tendon. Some fibers can be seen to continue to the dorsum of this tendon to become continuous with those of the opposite side. The proximal border of the band is free or melds gently into the dorsal fascia of the hand. The distal portion of the band fuses with aponeurotic expansion of the interosseous and lumbrical muscles.

Down the radial side of the index finger, the sagittal band originates from the base of the proximal phalanx, the metacarpal head and the side of the flexor tendon sheath, the volar plate, and passes along the metacarpal head outside the capsule. Its major fibers pass over the bone insertion of the first dorsal interosseous muscle and tendon. A similar arrangement is found on the ulnar side of the little finger for the abductor digiti minimi tendon. The sagittal band passes deep to the tendon of those other intrinsic muscles and inserts into the aponeurotic expansion of the extensor mechanism. Fibers do not perforate the transverse metacarpal ligament or the flexor tendon sheath.

SYNOVIAL SHEATHS OF THE HAND

The synovial sheaths invest the extensor tendons mostly over the carpus. The flexor tendon sheaths can be divided into two groups: the digital and the palmocarpal sheaths.

SYNOVIAL SHEATHS OF THE EXTENSOR TENDONS

The largest sheath encloses the tendons of the extensor digitorum communis and the extensor indicis (Fig. 6–16). It is separate from the others and extends proximally from about 10 mm to 15 mm above the extensor retinaculum. Distally, it surrounds separately and descends along each tendon. Its total height is from about 4 cm to 4.5 cm.

The sheath of the abductor pollicis longus and the extensor pollicis brevis starts at the intersection of these muscles with the tendons of the radial extensors. It is approximately 5 cm long and extends to the metacarpophalangeal joint of the thumb. It is most frequently a common sheath for both tendons but may be separated distally and proximally.

The sheath of the extensor carpi radialis longus and brevis starts at the intersection of the extensor brevis and extends to a point just proximal to the insertion of the extensors into the metacarpal bases. The sheath communicates freely with the sheath of the extensor pollicis longus. The total length of the sheath is about 5 cm.

The extensor pollicis longus sheath is very long; it measures about 6 cm and includes some of the fleshy fibers of the muscle proximal to the dorsal carpal ligament. Distally, the sheath extends over the trapezium and even the first metacarpal.

The extensor digiti minimi also has a separate, long sheath measuring from about 6 cm to 7 cm from the proximal border of the extensor retinaculum to the middle of the fourth metacarpal where it divides. It sometimes communicates with the distal radioulnar joint in its passage over this joint.

The sheath to the extensor carpi ulnaris is confined between the proximal end of the dorsal carpal ligament and the insertion of the tendon.

SYNOVIAL SHEATHS OF THE FLEXOR TENDONS

The flexor tendons of the fingers possess digital sheaths that envelop the tendons from the line of insertion of the flexor profundus to a line about 10 mm proximal to the proximal border of the transverse carpal ligament (Fig. 6–27). This arrangement usually is observed in the index, middle, and ring fingers. The little finger has a similar arrangement but less frequently. The thumb has a separate digital sheath that extends through the carpal canal into the forearm.

The palm of the hand shows two large synovial sacs. One is connected with the thumb and is known as the radial bursa. It starts at the insertion of the flexor pollicis longus at the base of the distal phalanx. It invests the tendon of the flexor pollicis longus and passes through the carpal canal, through the extreme radial apex of the carpal canal, and reaches the distal line of the pronator quadratus muscle or lies on the volar aspect of the pronator quadratus, deep in the forearm.

The other ulnar palmocarpal synovial sac or bursa is the largest and invests the tendons of the flexors about 1 cm to 3 cm proximal to the ends of the digital sheaths. The distance between the proximal end of the digital sac and the distal end of the palmar varies considerably for each finger. The longest sac is usually for the index

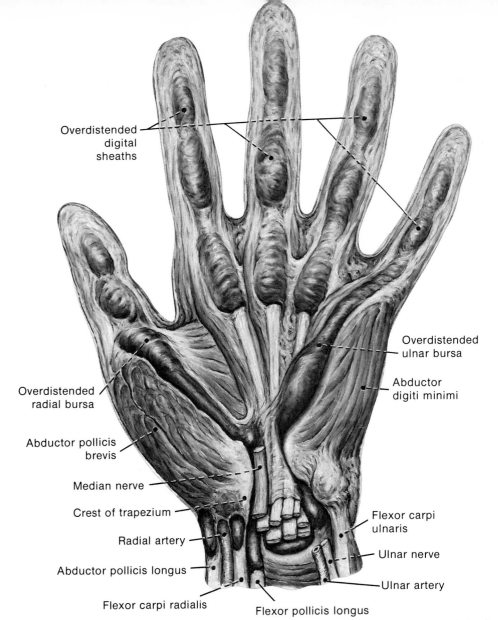

Overdistended
digital
sheaths

Overdistended
ulnar bursa

Abductor
digiti minimi

Overdistended
radial bursa

Abductor pollicis
brevis

Median nerve

Crest of trapezium

Radial artery

Abductor pollicis longus

Flexor carpi radialis

Flexor pollicis longus

Flexor carpi
ulnaris

Ulnar nerve

Ulnar artery

FIG. 6–27 Demonstration of the synovial sheaths of the flexor tendons of the fingers. The three separate sheaths for the index, middle, and ring fingers extend through the length of the digits and end approximately at the distal crease of the palm. A so-called ulnar bursa extends through the length of the little finger and communicates with the common synovial bursa, which usually encloses more proximally the index, middle, and ring finger flexor tendons. In this specimen an intercommunication is found between this bursa and the so-called radial bursa, which is a synovial sheath enclosing the flexor pollicis longus throughout the length of the thumb to the retro-tendinous Parona's space in the distal forearm. Not infrequently, there is partitioning of the ulnar bursa into three separate compartments: one behind the deep flexors, which is the longest one and extends into Parona's space proximal to the transverse carpal ligament; the other compartment is slightly shorter and is located between the deep and the superficialis flexors; the third compartment is located in front of the flexor superficialis. This is the shortest compartment and may not extend beyond the distal edge of the transverse carpal ligament. Not infrequently, they are separated from each other. A mixture of lamp black and gelatin was used for distension of the synovial sheaths.

finger and the shortest for the little finger, unless the digital sheath of the little finger communicates directly with the unlar palmar sac.

The ulnar sac or bursa is arranged in three communicating, superimposed invaginations or compartments. The most superficial lies in front of the tendon of the flexor superficialis, the middle extension between the tendons of the superficialis and the profundus and the posterior behind the tendons of the flexor profundus. The common part of the three partitions is on the ulnar side of the tendons. This arrangement leaves the origin of the lumbrical muscles completely outside of the ulnar sac. The most superficial compartment may be the shortest and is confined between the proximal and the distal borders of the transverse carpal ligament. It is also the shallowest and usually does not extend in the radial direction beyond the ring finger. The middle invagination is slightly longer and may extend slightly more radially. The posterior compartment is the longest and extends beyond the index tendon or, in cases of a separate bursal sac for the index tendons, beyond the middle finger.

It was stated previously that the ulnar bursa fuses firmly with the fascia covering the ulnar interosseous muscles and the adductor pollicis in the region of the crest of the third metacarpal and divides the palm of the hand into two halves. The posterior compartment of the ulnar bursa forms the connection with the crest of the third metacarpal. The ulnar sheath extends into the forearm and rests on the surface of the pronator quadratus or just distal to it. The most common pattern of digital and palmocarpal synovial sheaths shows separate digital sheaths for the index, middle, and ring fingers, a separate digitopalmocarpal sheath for the thumb, and a separate digitopalmocarpal sheath for the little finger; however, not infrequently variations occur showing communications between all the digital sheaths and the ulnar palmocarpal, or extension of one of the sheaths of the ring, middle, or index fingers into the ulnar palmocarpal sheath. A separate carpal sheath is sometimes found for the index tendons between the radial and the ulnar sheaths. There is frequent communication between the ulnar and the

radial sheaths, so that air or liquid injected into the ulnar sheath will spread into the radial sheath or the reverse.

The digital synovial sheaths are contained in the tunnel of the flexor tendons. Under the slightest pressure, the synovial sheaths distend in places where they are not compressed and become bulbous—very seldom do they present the cylindrical, regular appearance seen in illustrations (Fig. 6–27).

Inside the digital sheaths, the tendons are not attached by a continuous mesotendon to the synovial wall.* Instead, there are separate synovial bands called *vincula tendinum brevia* and *longa*. There are usually two types of vincula brevia. One vinculum is found at the insertion of the tendon of the flexor profundus into the distal phalanx; it is triangular and unites the dorsal surface of the tendon with the synovial wall. The other short vinculum is quadrilateral and runs between the synovial wall of the proximal phalanx and the two tendons. The long vinculum is represented also by two types: one group unites the two tendons near the midline; the other group unites the sublimis tendon with the periphery of the synovial wall (Figs. 2–8 and 2–33).

Each tendon has its own separate synovial investment. The vincula serve to carry blood vessels and nerves that probably run in the walls of the small arteries. The radial synovial bursa has a wide, interrupted synovial fold that connects the tendon in the thumb with the synovial wall. The blood and the nerve supply of the ulnar synovial sac is provided through the interspaces on the radial, extrasynovial side of the sac.

The synovial membrane between the tendons and the walls of the osteofibrous tunnels and the wall of the sac have several folds that permit free motion of the tendons.

In addition to all the synovial sacs on the palmar surface, there is another small sac covering the tendon of the flexor carpi radialis in its passage under the crest of the trapezium. This synovial covering extends for a distance of about

---

*Mayer L: Tendons, Ganglia, Muscles, Fascia. Lewis Practice of Surgery, Vol. 3. Hagerstown, Prior, 1942

1.5 cm to 2 cm between the scaphotrapezial and trapeziometacarpal joints.

HAND SPACES

Although the structures of the hand are compactly arranged together, there are potential spaces of constant limitations that can be brought into evidence by injections of fluids or air. These spaces are of importance in the spread of infections. The investigations of Kanavel were responsible for the thorough understanding of the significance of these spaces, for the anatomic description, and for the logical treatment of infections of the hand.

The spaces of the dorsum of the hand are potential areas between the fascial layers. As indicated previously, the antebrachial fascia continues into the extensor retinaculum, which has a superficial and a deep layer. The carpal ligament thins out distally, covering the extensor tendons. An intertendineal fascia includes all the extensor tendons. Sometimes a fascial layer is found under and above the intertendineal fascia; these layers are called supratendinous and infratendinous fascia, respectively. A fascial layer covers the interosseous muscles and is known as the interosseous fascia. Immediately under the skin, a superficial and a deep fascia are described. The extent and the separation of all these fasciae vary. The spaces often intercommunicate (Figs. 2–6).

SPACES OF THE PALM OF THE HAND

The most important spaces were named by Kanavel as the thenar and the midpalmar spaces. They are deep, potential spaces located between the flexor tendons in front (volad) and the adductor-anterior interosseous fascia behind (dorsally). These names were accepted and used profitably by the clinicians and the anatomists; however, objections were raised, especially concerning the thenar space. The anatomic location of the thenar space is not over the thenar eminence, but over the adductor muscle; therefore, it was considered propitious to call it the adductor space. In the same line of reasoning, the midpalmar space is not located over the mid-palm and therefore should not be called midpalmar space.

Perhaps, the corresponding spaces should be called the deep retrotendinous radial and the deep retrotendinous ulnar palmar spaces, but these descriptive, more precise names make them much longer.

THENAR SPACE—ADDUCTOR SPACE, DEEP PALMAR RADIAL

The thenar space is limited on the ulnar side by the fusion of the ulnar bursa to the crest of the third metacarpal; on the radial side, the fusion of the thenar fascia with the midpalmar fascia forms its limit. On the volar side, it is limited by the flexor tendons of the middle and index fingers in their covers, by the branches of the median and superficial arterial arch in their lipocellular layer, and the midpalmar fascia.

On the dorsal side, the space is limited by the adductor fascia, which joins the anterior interosseous fascia in the region of the deep transverse metacarpal ligament between the index and the middle fingers. Proximally, it is stopped by the junction of the ulnar and the radial synovial bursa and the extension of the interosseous fascia in the carpal canal. Distally, it is open toward the first and the second interdigital folds, following the course of the first and the second lumbrical muscles.

MIDPALMAR SPACE—DEEP PALMAR ULNAR

The midpalmar space is located between the flexor tendons and the anterior interosseous fascia.

Its limits are as follows:

Anterior—the flexor tendons in their ulnar bursa, the branches of the superficial arterial arch and the median and the ulnar nerves in their lipofibrous layer, and the midpalmar fascia

Posterior—the anterior interosseous fascia covering the interosseous muscles of the third and the fourth intermetacarpal spaces and the deep palmar fat pad, which protects the deep ulnar artery and nerve

Ulnar—the continuation of the anterior

interosseous fascia with the fascia of the hypothenar muscles and fusion of this fascia with the midpalmar fascia

Radial—the fusion of the third metacarpal with the ulnar bursa

Proximal—the contact of the ulnar bursa with the continuation of the anterior interosseous fascia in the carpal canal

Distal—the space is open along the course of the third and the fourth lumbrical muscles into the third and the fourth interdigital folds.

The midpalmar space may communicate freely with the thenar space, and infections of either space may spread early and easily into each other. The midpalmar space may be the site of large lipomas that develop in the deep palmar fat pad and present problems of approach and removal.

PARONA'S SPACE

Parona's space was described comprehensively in 1876 by Parona.* Following the recent traditional trend, a Russian clinical investigator claims that the space was first described by Pirogoff.† Be that as it may, it was known as Parona's space even in Russia.

The space is important because infections from the deep parts of the hand mostly from the radial and the ulnar bursae, when uncontrolled or fulminating, may spread into this space. It is located in the lower end of the forearm and is limited anteriorly by the deep flexors to their origin on the forearm; posteriorly, by the pronator quadratus covered by its fascia; radially, by the flexor carpi radialis, and ulnad, by the flexor carpi ulnaris and the antebrachial fascia. Distally, it communicates with the hand through the carpal canal, which is normally closed by the contact of the ulnar and the radial synovial sacs with the extension of the anterior interosseous and the adductor fascia covering the posterior wall of the carpal canal.

Other potential but less significant spaces may be found in the palmar subcutaneous area or in front of the flexor tendon. The fingers have a closed space over the tip and the volar aspect of the distal phalanx.

*Parona F: Dell'oncotomia negli accessi profundi diffusi dell'avambrachio. Annali Universali di Medicina e Chirurgia, Milano, 1876

†Lubotsky DN: Priority of N. I. Pirogoff in problems of surgical anatomy of the extremities. Khirurgiia **12**:11, 1950 (Russian)

7

Kinesiology of the Hand and Wrist and Muscular Variations of the Hand and Forearm

Mechanism of Action of the Fingers, the Thumb, and the Wrist

Emanual B. Kaplan
Richard J. Smith

Most actions of the fingers, thumb, or wrist require the participation of groups of muscles. The action of these muscles is determined by their insertions, the courses of their tendons, and their relation to the joints and ligaments. In order to fully appreciate the mechanism of muscle function, we must first understand the details of their anatomic structures.

In flexing one joint there may be a complex interplay of several muscles; on the other hand, a muscle will generally not fully participate in the act of flexion. Only parts of a muscle are activated, and with increased demand, all the other parts of a muscle join together with parts or all of other muscles. This establishes an important principle: A muscle produces graded participation in response to need and combines its partial activity with either total or partial activities of other muscles coacting in the same movement. This principle is of special significance in electromyographic investigation of muscular activity.

Accomplishment of any motion may require multiple adaptations that may depend upon the insertions of the muscles, muscular combinations, or the nerve supply with anastomoses between nerve trunks.

Experiments with muscle action in cadavers, the stimulation of individual muscles in living patients, and observations of various nerve injuries demonstrate the difficulties of interpreting the function of the muscles involved.

It must be mentioned that although the muscles play the paramount role in the movement of the fingers and the thumb, the role of the sensory nerves to the skin for tactile and thermic perception and to the joints and the bone for proprioception are most essential. The disturbances caused by the dysfunction in these organs may overshadow the muscle disabilities and must never be neglected.

THE MOTORS AND MECHANISMS OF ACTION OF THE FINGERS

Normal flexion of the finger includes contraction of the following muscles:

Flexor digitorum profundus
Flexor digitorum superficialis
Palmar and dorsal interosseous muscles
Lumbricals
Two radial carpal extensors
Ulnar carpal extensor
Indirect participation of the extensors of the fingers

Normal extension of the finger includes contraction of the following:

Extensor digitorum communis
Extensor proprius of the index and little fingers
Palmar and dorsal interosseous muscles
Lumbricals
Extrinsic flexors of the fingers
Palmaris longus
Flexor carpi radialis
Flexor carpi ulnaris

Normal abduction of the fingers includes contraction of:

Dorsal interosseous muscles
Abductor digiti minimi
Extensor digitorum communis
Extensor proprius of the little finger (abducts the little finger)
Lumbricals (in some instances)

Abduction of the fingers is most efficient when the long axes of the fingers are in continuation with the long axes of their corresponding metacarpals. The dorsal interossei are responsible for this abduction. Abduction in hyperextension of the fingers is produced by the dorsal interossei with the assistance of the extensors of the fingers, the abductor digiti minimi, and the extensor proprius of the little finger. Abduction of the fingers is also possible in flexion of the fingers at the metacarpophalangeal joints. This is accomplished by the dorsal interossei and the abductor digiti minimi and can be verified easily by palpating the first dorsal interosseous in active abduction of the index finger flexed at the metacarpophalangeal joint, or the abductor digiti minimi in abduction of the flexed little finger.

Normal adduction of the fingers is produced by the palmar interossei, assisted by the extensor proprius of the index finger and the long flexors of the fingers. Adduction in the neutral position is performed by the palmar interossei and the extensor proprius of the index finger. Adduction in extension of the metacarpophalangeal joints is produced by the palmar interossei and the extensor proprius of the index finger. Adduction in extension of the metacarpophalangeal joints is produced by the palmar interossei and the extensor proprius of the index finger. Adduction in flexion is produced by the natural pull of the long flexors, which adduct the fingers simultaneously with flexion, with some assistance from the palmar interossei. Patients with complete division of all the flexor tendons can flex their metacarpophalangeal joints with adduction of the fingers. The adduction of the fingers in this instance is produced by the palmar interossei and not by the configuration of the metacarpophalangeal joints or pull of the interdigital natatory ligaments.

FLEXOR DIGITORUM PROFUNDUS

The flexor digitorum profundus is a flexor of the distal phalanx; however, flexion of the distal phalanx cannot be accomplished by the average person without simultaneous flexion of the middle phalanx. Exceptionally, certain people are able to extend or hyperextend the middle phalanx by active contraction of the middle band of the extensor digitorum communis, thus preventing flexion of the middle phalanx by the flexor superficialis. Then the flexor profundus can act on the distal phalanx and can flex it independently. In testing the normal action of the flexor profundus, the middle phalanx must be held firmly by the examiner to eliminate the action of the flexor superficialis on the middle phalanx. The distal phalanx can then be flexed actively without simultaneous flexion of the middle phalanx.

Although the action of the flexor profundus is closely associated with the action of the flexor superficialis in flexion of the middle phalanx; it does not ordinarily flex the metacarpophalangeal joint. Under certain special conditions, the flexor profundus may produce flexion at the metacarpophalangeal joint:

1. In complete hyperextension of the wrist and fingers, the flexor profundus in association with the flexor superficialis will actively flex the two distal phalanges and at the completion of this flexion, will produce weak flexion of the proximal phalanx.
2. In old cases of injury or paralysis of the deep branch of the ulnar nerve, the long flexors may actively produce weak flexion at the metacarpophalangeal joint of the ring and little fingers, but only after flexing the distal and middle phalanges. If the distal and the middle phalanges are held passively extended, isolated active flexion of the proximal phalanx at the metacarpophalangeal joint is very weak. It becomes practically impossible if the injury to the nerve is located proximal to the nerve supply of the ulnar half of the flexor profundus muscle.
3. In the cadaver, traction applied to the divided tendons of the flexor profundus may produce many abnormal reactions, including complete flexion of the distal phalanges, the proximal phalanges, and even flexion of the wrist. These reactions could not be reproduced in the living because complete flexion of all the joints of the finger requires extension of the wrist, although in extreme contractures of the muscle, especially in the presence of weak or paralyzed wrist extensors, permanent flexion of the fingers and wrist may occur.

The effect of loss of action of the flexor profundus on the distal phalanx differs in cases caused by tendon divisions and in cases caused by paralysis of the median and ulnar nerves. In cases of high median nerve paralysis, the distal phalanx of the index finger cannot be flexed actively, and frequently the distal phalanx of the middle finger cannot be flexed. Occasionally, the distal phalanx of the middle finger can be flexed owing to an additional nerve supply to the flexor profundus of the middle finger from the ulnar nerve. Although no active flexion of the distal phalanx of the index finger can be produced, mild flexion of the distal phalanx will occur if the middle phalanx is hyperextended by the contraction of the intrinsics; the passively overstretched tendon of the flexor profundus, induced by hyperextension, returns to its normal length and creates an impression of flexion. The same reaction sometimes applies to the middle finger.

In cases of high ulnar nerve paralysis, this false flexion cannot be produced because the paralysis involves the interossei and the lumbricals to the ring and little fingers, eliminating the possibility of hyperextension of the middle phalanx of these fingers. In cases of division of the tendons of the flexor profundus, no overstretching of the tendon is possible; the distal phalanx remains in extension or hyperextension, and no false flexion of the distal phalanx of the index or the middle finger can be observed.

The flexor profundus is intimately related to the flexor superficialis, not only in a common passage from the origin through the carpal canal and the hand, but especially in their common formation of a special unit in the tunnels of the fingers described as a perforating and perforated combination of tendons. The relation of these tendons (Figs. 2–8, 2–32, and 2–33) with a difference of functional length (full flexion to full extension) varying between 3 mm and 5 mm at the proximal phalanx at the level of perforation is of functional importance. Their independent motion is restricted by the vincula, the close contact between the two tendons, and the enclosure in the tunnel; they act simultaneously on the two distal phalanges of a finger, producing synchronous flexion of the distal and middle phalanges. In cases of complete elimination of either muscle, the remaining muscle acts independently and fairly satisfactorily. The action of the profundus may be considered more advantageous because it acts on the distalphalanx.

Separation of the deep flexor tendon of the fingers or the thumb distal to the forearm is determined using a simple method suggested by T.C. Thompson* for diagnosis of the tendon of the triceps surae in the leg. With the dorsum of the forearm placed on a flat resistant surface, press on the anterior distal third of the forearm toward the radial side for the flexor pollicis longus and toward the middle for all the flexors of the fingers. If there is no interruption of the continuity of the tendons, the distal phalanx of the thumb and the two phalanges of the other fingers flex with considerable force.

FLEXOR DIGITORUM SUPERFICIALIS

The flexor digitorum superficialis is a flexor of the middle phalanx; it flexes the middle phalanx independently, without producing simultaneous flexion of the distal phalanx. It never has any action on the distal phalanx.

To test the flexor superficialis, it is necessary to relax the distal phalanx completely and make

*Thompson TC, Doherty JH: Spontaneous rupture of tendon of Achilles: New clinical diagnostic test. J Trauma 2:126, 1962

sure that the distal phalanx can be passively, freely moved from flexion to extension and from extension to flexion. If the distal phalanx is free and the middle phalanx is strongly flexed, it indicates action of the flexor superficialis. Sometimes it is difficult to decide whether the flexor profundus is responsible for the flexion of the proximal interphalangeal joint; close observation of the following points will help:

1. When the flexor superficialis is inactive, either through paralysis or division of the tendon, the activation of the flexor profundus produces a strong initial flexion of the distal phalanx, followed by secondary flexion of the middle phalanx.
2. In older cases of flexor superficialis inactivity, the middle phalanx often becomes hyperextended at the proximal interphalangeal joint, and the distal phalanx assumes a constant flexed position.

The flexor superficialis produces only very weak flexion of the proximal phalanx, very similar to that of the flexor profundus.

The long flexors of the fingers are comparatively short, so that extension of the wrist and the metacarpophalangeal joints is required for efficient flexion of the distal and proximal interphalangeal joints. For this reason, the extensors carpi radialis longus and brevis and the extensor carpi ulnaris contract strongly with contraction of the long flexors of the fingers. This important relation between the action of the long flexors of the fingers and the extensors of the wrist can be observed in patients with paralysis of the long finger flexors and in cases of complete division of the long finger flexors. When these patients are asked to flex the fingers, they extend the wrists instead.

For effective, strong, isolated flexion of the distal and middle phalanges only, the proximal phalanx must be extended. Extension of the proximal phalanx at the metacarpophalangeal joint is effected by the extensor communis digitorum, which thus assists in flexion of the distal and middle joints of the finger and provides strong stability in actions requiring clawing of the fingers.

INTEROSSEOUS, LUMBRICAL AND EXTENSOR MUSCLES

Flexion of the metacarpophalangeal joints of the fingers is produced by the interosseous muscles and the lumbricals and is very closely connected with other activities of these muscles (Fig. 7–1). The interosseous muscles work together with the *lumbricals* and the *extensor digitorum communis* in extending the interphalangeal joints. They act together with the lumbricals in flexing the metacarpophalangeal joints and frequently in abduction; in adduction of the fingers, the palmar interossei act together with the long flexors without the extensor communis.

Dr. Kaplan reviewed the literature and made personal investigations on the action of these muscles and concluded that it is impossible to assign a rigidly standardized function to a lumbrical or an interosseous muscle or even to the extensor digitorum communis. Each muscle may have a slightly different function in different people, just as each intrinsic muscle may have a varying nerve supply or a different type of insertion. In one person, the lumbrical may even act as an abductor of a finger; in another, it has no action of abduction. The interosseous may have excellent extensor action of the two distal phalanges in one person and very weak or no extension in others. The extensor digitorum may produce almost complete extension of all the phalanges in some, but very limited extension of the two distal phalanges in others. No investigations concerning racial differences are known to the author, but it is not inconceivable that structural peculiarities described by a French anatomist based on findings in the anatomic laboratories in France may differ from the material obtainable in Philadelphia, Canada, or England. It has sometimes been suggested that the lumbrical extends the distal phalanx, only, that the extensor digitorum extends only the proximal phalanx, that the middle phalanx is extended by the palmar interossei, and that the extensor proprius of the index and the little fingers extends all the phalanges of the corresponding fingers.

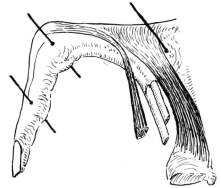

FIG. 7–1 Flexion of the proximal phalanx and of the middle phalanx. In this position, flexion of the proximal phalanx is maintained mostly by the fibers of the interossei, inserted into the lateral bases of the proximal phalanx. The fibers of the interossei that insert into the lateral bands are not activated. This permits further flexion of the two distal phalanges by the long flexors or extension of these phalanges by the fibers of the interossei inserted into the lateral bands, and by the action of the lumbricals. If the middle phalanx is flexed before flexion is attempted in the metacarpophalangeal joint, the flexor superficialis may act as a flexor of the metacarpophalangeal joint.

STUDIES CONCERNING DIGITAL MOTION

In 1948, Braithwaite, Channell, Moore and Willis, in a combined investigation, concluded that the "current conception of the role of the lumbrical and digital movement is incorrect." They believed that "it is unnecessary to postulate a direct pull of the lumbricals on the dorsal extensor expansion to produce extension of the interphalangeal joints." They also stated that if a constant tone is maintained between the flexors and the extensors, "flexion of the first phalanx by contraction of lumbricals and interossei will automatically produce the necessary relaxation of the flexors and tightening of the extensor to enable extension of the interphalangeal joints to occur." Apparently, they believed also in strong abductor action of the lumbrical and in stabilization of the extensor apparatus over the metacarpophalangeal joint by the balancing action of the interossei on each side of the tendon of the extensor digitorum.

In 1912, Willan found that the lumbricals

extend only the distal phalanx. He also mentioned that the extensor indicis and the extensor proprius of the little finger extend all the phalanges of the corresponding fingers. McKenzie claimed that the lumbricals are flexors of the proximal phalanges but do not extend the distal phalanges.

The most important modern contribution to the understanding of the mechanism of digital motion was made by Duchenne of Boulogne. He found that the true anatomic description of the lumbricals was first given by Columbus, successor of Vesalius in Padua before Fallopius; the action of the lumbrical was first suspected by Fallopius in his *Observations Anatomicae* published in 1561. Fallopius was apparently also the first to discover the action of extension of the distal and middle phalanges of the finger by the interosseous muscles, although Fallopius disputed the action of flexion of the promixal phalanx by the interossei as noted by Vesalius. According to Duchenne, Bouvier, in 1851, was the first to accurately report the insertion of the interosseous into the base of the proximal phalanx and into the dorsal expansion.

It is of great interest to consider Duchenne's findings in reference to Galen. It is very difficult to decipher some of Galen's statements in the Greek text because of differences in anatomic terms, but Daremberg, who translated Galen's work into French, made the part concerning the lumbrical muscles and the extensors very clear. Galen stated that, in addition to the extensor digitorum, there was an extensor proprius for each finger. According to Galen, abduction of the fingers was produced by the extensor proprius of the little finger and the extensor proprius of the ring finger in conjunction with the first and the second lumbricals and adduction by the extensor proprius of the index and middle fingers in conjunction with the third and fourth lumbricals. He did not suspect the action of the interossei on abduction and adduction of the fingers, but he knew that the proper extensor was acting in lateral deviation of the fingers.

Duchenne was apparently the first to establish the action of the proper extensors of the index and little fingers as adductor of the index finger and abductor of the little finger,

respectively. He was probably the first to clearly explain the action to the extensor communis on the proximal phalanx and the relation of the extensor communis to the extension of the middle and distal phalanges.

In 1734, Albinus, in his *Historia Musculorum Hominis*, stated that *"extensor communis digitorum manus extendit digitos et quidem ossa eorum prima, secunda, terita: prima etiam in exteriora flecsit."* He knew of the abductor action of the extensor communis but apparently thought that the interossei were secondary in their extension action on the middle and distal phalanges.

Recently a number of new observations have clarified further the mechanisms of digital motion (Baumann, Bunnell, Haines, Hauck,[*] Kaplan, Landsmeer, Mason,[†] Montant and Baumann, Salsbury, Sunderland, Walsh).

In the following description a unified explanation of the mechanism of finger and hand motion will be attempted, based on personal experience, personal experimentation, and mostly on the fundamental, valuable investigations of others. Electromyographic studies, further anatomic and clinical investigations supplemented by cinematographic demonstrations, and mechanical analyses have increased our understanding of movements of the fingers and of the hand as a whole. The electromyographic investigations of Long and Brown, Backhouse and Catton, anatomomechanical analyses of Landsmeer and Stack, anatomic and clinical studies by Tubiana and Valentin, and clinical application of new principles by Boyes, Littler, Riordan, Verdan and Michon, Fowler and Zanolli and others have solved a number of problems and opened up new vistas for further studies. Therefore, it is essential to present their most pertinent findings.

Long and Brown
In 37 individuals Long and Brown studied the muscles of the middle finger using coordinated

[*] Hauch G: Arch Klin Chir p 123, 1923
[†] Mason ML: Rupture of the tendons of the hand with a study of the extensor tendon insertions in the fingers. Surg Gynecol Obstet 50:611, 1930

electromyograms and electrogoniograms. *The extensor digitorum* is always active in the extension of the metacarpophalangeal joint and also functions as a brake on the metacarpophalangeal joint or control at moderate or maximal levels during flexion. *The lumbrical muscle* is always active in extension of the interphalangeal joints and is apparently the major extensor of these two joints. It is inconstant as a flexor of the metacarpophalangeal joint. It does not contract when both interphalangeal joints are flexed. The muscle acts as a true synergist to the extensor digitorum, supplying a graded flexor force for proper action of the extensor digitorum. The lumbrical action predominates if the metacarpophalangeal joint is flexing or flexed; the extensor digitorum equals or predominates when the metacarpophalangeal joint is extending or held extended.

They believed that *the interossei* have no flexion component on the metacarpophalangeal joints and are primarily extensors of the two interphalangeal joints through the dorsal expansion. They are reserve extensors of the interphalangeal joints and act in synergy with the lumbrical in extension of the interphalangeal joints, especially during simultaneous flexion of the metacarpophalangeal joints, when the extensor digitorum acts as a stabilizer of this joint. In opening the full hand, the interossei play a secondary role because the combination of the extensor digitorum-lumbrical is sufficient to produce full extension of the finger at all of its joints.

The flexor digitorum profundus is active when flexion of all joints is required. It is very active when flexion of the metacarpophalangeal joint is required with the interphalangeal joints flexed. The muscle does not contract in synchrony with the lumbrical except under special circumstances. In whole-hand closing and opening, the flexor profundus and the lumbricals are out of phase with each other. In some cases, they become synergists in simultaneous metacarpophalangeal flexion and interphalangeal extension. *The flexor digitorum superficialis* is subservient to the flexor profundus and varies in electromyographic response with the position of the

wrist, with least response in extension and greatest response in flexion.

The authors conclude that the interosseous lumbrical mechanism cannot be considered as a unit but represents two kinesiologic entities. The interossei are involved in interphalangeal extension only when the metacarpophalangeal joint is flexing or held flexed; the lumbrical is always active in interphalangeal extension. Neither the interossei nor the lumbricals are active during closure of the hand. The extensor digitorum is active in extension of the metacarpophalangeal joint or when this joint is held extended, but it also acts as a brake in many flexor movements of the metacarpophalangeal joint. The flexor profundus is the most active flexor and is joined by the flexor superficialis when the wrist is flexed. Its maximum action is when the hand is closed without flexion of the distal phalanx.

Backhouse and Catton

Backhouse and Catton studied the action of the lumbricals electromyographically and by direct stimulation and found that the lumbrical muscles act primarily as extensors of the interphalangeal joints, accompanied by active contraction of the extensor digitorum. The lumbricals are efficient extensors of the interphalangeal joints in association with a normal extensor digitorum. The lumbricals prevent hyperextension of the proximal phalanx by the extensor digitorum by flexor action on the metacarpophalangeal joint, thus allowing an efficient pull to the dorsal expansion, which then acts directly on the interphalangeal joints. The lumbrical muscle is an active extensor of the interphalangeal joints, and its action is assisted considerably by the extensor digitorum, but only when the extensor digitorum hyperextensor effect on the metacarpophalangeal joint is neutralized by the lumbrical. The metacarpophalangeal flexion is carried out by the lumbrical muscle only when the interphalangeal joints are extended. On electrical stimulation of the lumbricals, flexion of the metacarpophalangeal joint occurs only after extension of the interphalangeal joints. The lumbrical does not show any activity when the finger is opposed to the thumb and apparently does not act as a radial deviator.

Tubiana and Valentin

Tubiana and Valentin studied the action of the finger muscles by observation, experimentation, and slow-motion cinematography.

Action of the extensor digitorum is analyzed in reference to the proximal and distal interphalangeal and to the metacarpophalangeal joints. In experiments on cadavers with the wrist in neutral position and the three finger joints flexed, traction applied to the extensor tendon at the metacarpophalangeal joint produced extension of the metacarpophalangeal joint followed by limited extension of the interphalangeal joints; as soon as the metacarpophalangeal joint becomes extended, the interphalangeal joints stop their extension and remain flexed. Flexion of the interphalangeal joints increases when the metacarpophalangeal becomes hyperextended.

To produce full extension of the interphalangeal joints experimentally by traction on the extensor digitorum tendon at the metacarpophalangeal joint, it is necessary either to detach the insertion of the extensor digitorum into the capsule of the metacarpophalangeal joint and the lateral extensions sagittal band running on each side to the deep transverse intermetacarpal ligament or to divide the flexor tendons. It is also possible to extend the distal and middle phalanges by traction of the extensor digitorum tendon, simultaneously maintaining the proximal phalanx in very slight flexion, which permits relaxation of the flexor tendon and also of the dorsal aponeurosis extension to each side of the metacarpophalangeal joint.

The action of the extensor digitorum on the proximal phalanx was ingeniously explained by the presence of the two insertions of the midband of the extensor digitorum, namely, the insertion to the base of the middle phalanx and the insertion to the base of the proximal phalanx. When the interphalangeal joints are flexed, the insertion to the base of the proximal phalanx is relaxed. When the interphalangeal joints begin to extend by pull on the extensor

digitorum tendon, the flexed base of the middle phalanx and the tensing insertion of the midband of the extensor digitorum push up the head of the proximal phalanx into extension; the insertion of the extensor digitorum to the base of the proximal phalanx starts to become tense, producing hyperextension of the proximal phalanx, but the tension of the flexor tendons does not permit the interphalangeal joint to extend.

Analysis of the intrinsic muscles, the interossei, and lumbricals based on experiments on cadavers confirmed the findings of Long and Brown and Backhouse and Catton.

Extension of the fingers in a normal hand begins with extension of the proximal phalanx. As soon as the proximal phalanx reaches an individually variable angle of extension, the interphalangeal joints begin to extend; their full extension is prevented by the tension of the flexors. The actions of the extensor digitorum and the intrinsic muscles complete each other and can even replace each other in extending the interphalangeal joints under certain circumstances of stabilization of the metacarpophalangeal joint in neutral position or flexion. The retinacular ligament assures the interdependence of the two distal phalanges by producing extension of the distal interphalangeal joint, when the proximal interphalangeal joint is extended.

Landsmeer

The analysis of finger movement by Landsmeer introduced new factors based on mechanical principles. He stated that the function of a muscle on a definite joint must be considered in the light of action of tendons bridging more than one joint. For the finger, one unit is represented by the interarticular unit of the two interphalangeal joints; the other unit represents the bi-articular system of the metacarpophalangeal and proximal interphalangeal joints. Landsmeer introduced the term *intercalated bone*. In the interphalangeal joints' bi-articular unit, the middle phalanx represents the intercalated bone. In the metacarpophalangeal and proximal interphalangeal system, the proximal phalanx represents the intercalated bone. The complicated action of the various parts of the dorsal expansion, the extensor tendon, the flexors, and the intrinsic muscles is explained.

The action of the retinacular system, which was mentioned by others, was also described by Landsmeer, who offered a mechanical explanation of certain functional peculiarities and phenomena of finger movement. The ingenious explanations of some of the finger movements only emphasized the necessity of further investigations with addition of other factors not immediately considered.

The character of the retinacular ligaments varies in different hands, and in some fresh anatomic specimens and on surgical exposure in living individuals, they do not produce the limitations and characteristic movements ascribed to their retinacular systems. It is interesting that in some of the pathologic conditions found in certain finger deformities, the retinacular ligaments may be found thickened, retraced, and obvious. It may not be coincidental that in Dupuytren's contractures, instead of the normal four pretendinous bands, more contracted bands are formed running to the thumb, extending from one finger to the other, or even forming transverse bands between the index finger and thumb.

The extension of the pretendinous bands over each side of the finger to the extensor expansion of the middle phalanx, as frequently observed in Dupuytren's contracture, cannot be considered as a retinacular ligament because it runs from the pretendinous band and not from the sheath of the flexor tendon, as the retinacular ligament usually does. Thus, it is possible that some of the thickened structures of the fingers connected with the extensor apparatus, like the additional pretendinous bands in Dupuytren's contracture, may simply represent pathologic expressions of a connective tissue disease. It may involve also the so-called cutaneous ligaments of Cleland (first reported by him in 1867 at the meeting of the British Association in Dundee and then described in the *Journal of Anatomy and Physiology* in 1878).

Stack

Stack's description of the muscle function of the fingers was based on anatomic studies and elaborated by models that demonstrated the complicated mechanism involved in the participation of the components of the extensor apparatus combined with the action of the flexors and the lumbricals. According to Stack, the extensor assembly consists of three pairs of components: the rectinacular ligaments that coordinate the movements of the interphalangeal joints; the "wing" tendons (lumbrical on the radial side and an interosseus on the ulnar side); and the phalangeal tendons or dorsal interossei. The retinacular ligaments are relaxed in full extension of the proximal interphalangeal joints and in this position cannot extend the distal joint fully because the surfaces of the joint are eccentric. The pull of the wing tendons (lateral bands) transfers the pull of the extensor tendon from the base of the middle phalanx to the base of the distal phalanx, permitting full extension of the distal joint. The lumbricals are extensors of the interphalangeal joints. The interossei act as flexors and abductors of the metacarpophalangeal and extensors of the interphalangeal joints.

In analyzing the complex of interossei-lumbricals-extensors of the fingers it must be emphasized that just as the long flexors are too short to permit full extension of the fingers and wrist against them, the extensors digitorum and proprius of the fingers are too short to permit full flexion of the fingers and wrist against them. Thus, complete flexion of the wrist often will not permit full flexion of the fingers because of shortness of the extensors, and complete extension of the wrist will not permit full extension of the fingers because of shortness of the flexors.

A clear picture of the tendinoligamento-aponeurotic ensemble is necessary to comprehend the mechanism of motion. Therefore, in addition to the earlier description of the anatomy of the muscles (Figs. 2–9, 2–11, 2–61, 2–62, and 2–63) certain details will now be emphasized (Figs. 7–2 and 7–3). It is important to remember the arrangement of the tendons and the ligaments around the metacarpophalangeal joint.

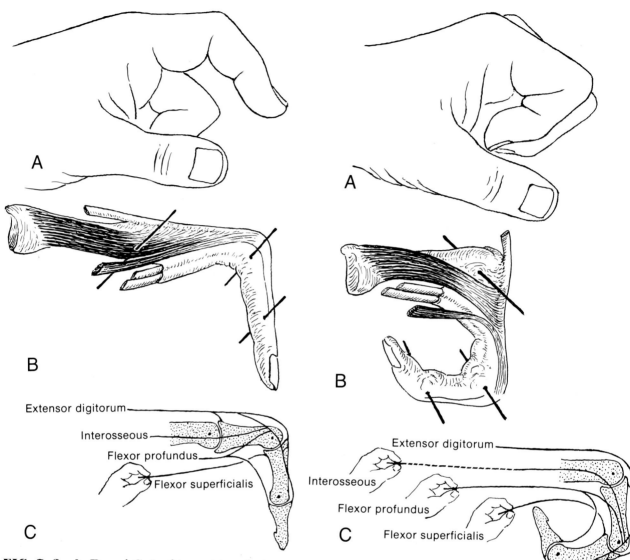

Extensor digitorum
Interosseous
Flexor profundus
Flexor superficialis

Extensor digitorum
Interosseous
Flexor profundus
Flexor superficialis

FIG. 7–2 **A**, **B**, and **C**, In this position, flexion is produced by the long flexors only exerting their action on the two distal phalanges, while the proximal phalanx is fixed simultaneously by the extensor digitorum; the interossei are not acting. When extension of the two distal phalanges is required with extension of the proximal phalanx, the extensor digitorum in the area of the metacarpophalangeal joint predominates over the interossei attached to the lateral bands and into the lateral bases of the proximal phalanx. The long flexors are almost inactive. The subordinated interossei are able to extend the two distal phalanges without producing flexion at the metacarpophalangeal joint; however, their subordinated action contributes to the stabilization of the metacarpophalangeal joint.

FIG. 7–3 **A** and **B**, Complete flexion at the metacarpophalangeal, proximal, and distal interphalangeal joints. This action results from the activity of the lateral bands of the interosseous muscle on the metacarpophalangeal joint and independent action of the flexor superficialis and profundus on the distal and the proximal phalanges.

C, The lateral bands of the interossei are probably exerting some hyperextensive action on the distal phalanx, but this action is subordinated to the stronger action of the flexors profundus and superficialis. The subordinated action of the interossei on the dorsal aspect of the distal and the middle phalanx probably contributes to stabilization of the distal and the proximal interphalangeal joints.

1. The insertions of the interossei into the dorsal apparatus and the base of the proximal phalanx are similar for the palmar and dorsal interossei, although some difference is seen in the insertion of the third palmar interosseous and the first dorsal interosseous. Most of the first dorsal interosseous is inserted into the lateral aspect of the base of the proximal phalanx, and most of the tendon of the third palmar is inserted into the dorsal apparatus; however, each interosseous contributes to the formation of the dorsal apparatus (Figs. 2–61 and 2–62).

2. The interosseous tendon of insertion is usually double. The part inserted into the base is responsible for lateral motion; the part inserted into the dorsal apparatus induces flexion of the proximal phalanx with simultaneous extension of the distal and middle phalanges.

3. Normally, the interosseous tendon is placed volar to the transverse axis of the metacarpophalangeal joint (Figs. 6–16 and 7–4).

4. The sagittal bands of the dorsal apparatus, which centralize the extensor digitorum tendon in the region of the metacarpophalangeal joint and link it to the deep transverse metacarpal ligament and volar plate, hold the interosseous tendons adjacent to the sides of the metacarpophalangeal joint. The fibers permit interosseous tendon motion only in the distal and proximal directions, but not dorsally or volad. The interosseous tendon is always volar to the axis of metacarpophalangeal motion.

5. The extensor digitorum tendon is always maintained over the midline of the metacarpophalangeal joint by the sagittal bands and by the connection of the volar aspect of the tendon with the capsule of the metacarpophalangeal joint. Transection of either the radial or ulnar tendon of the interosseous will not cause displacement of the extensor to one side.

6. The lumbrical muscle is inserted into the radial side of the dorsal aponeurosis slightly more distally than the part of the interosseous that contributes to the dorsal apparatus.

7. The extensor digitorum tendon is connected to the dorsal capsule of the metacarpophalangeal joint by slender or more dense fibers, permitting slightly limited, independent motion of the tendon over the joint.

8. Proximal to the area of connection of the extensor tendon with the capsule of the joint, the dorsal apparatus has a free, curved edge (Fig. 2–6).

9. The lumbrical and the interosseous muscles are located volar to the axis of flexion and extension of the metacarpophalangeal joint.

At the proximal interphalangeal joint, the following points are important:

1. The central slip of the extensor tendon is fused with the dorsal capsule of this joint. With the lateral slips of the extensor tendon, it covers the entire width of the dorsal aspect of the joint to the dorsal edge of the collateral ligament. The central slip is inserted into a wide ridge of the dorsal base of the middle phalanx.

2. From this group of tendons, oblique anchoring fibers (the transverse retinacular ligaments) descend on each side of the finger to the fibro-osseous tunnel of the flexors (Figs. 2–11 and 2–13).

3. The lateral bands of the interossei and the lumbricals are intimately connected with the lateral slips of the extensor tendon. The entire apparatus is normally dorsal to the axis of flexion-extension of the proximal interphalangeal joint (Fig. 7–4).

4. The anchoring fibers of the transverse retinacular ligaments maintain the relation of the dorsal apparatus over the dorsum of the proximal interphalangeal joint and prevent dorsal subluxation of the lateral bands.

5. The connection of the central slip and the lateral slips of the extensor digitorum with the dorsal capsule of the joint prevents the descent of the lateral bands to the side of the joint volar to the axis of flexion-extension. Only disruption of the dorsal capsular arrangement of the extensor tendon longitudinally or transversely causes a descent of the lateral bands volar to the axis of flexion-extension.

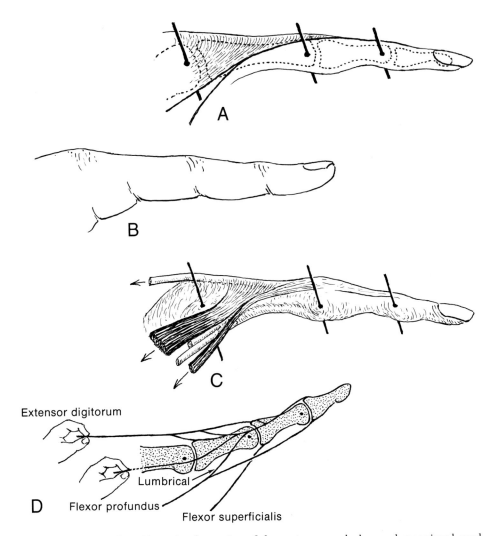

Extensor digitorum

Lumbrical

Flexor profundus

Flexor superficialis

FIG. 7–4 **A** and **B**, The axis of rotation of the metacarpophalangeal, proximal, and distal interphalangeal joints in relation to the dorsal apparatus of the finger. **C**, The dorsal apparatus of extension is placed entirely dorsal to the axis of rotation of the proximal and the distal interphalangeal joints. The axis of rotation of the metacarpophalangeal joint is so placed that the interossei and the lumbricals are volar to the axis of rotation. The entire dorsal apparatus constitutes a unit. Traction applied to this unit just distal to the metacarpophalangeal joint will be transmitted through the entire unit simultaneously, volar to the axis of rotation of the metacarpophalangeal joint and dorsal to the axis of rotation of the interphalangeal joints.

D, In complete extension of the three phalanges, the lateral bands of the interossei and the lateral bands of the extensor digitorum communis act very strongly. The interossei inserted into the lateral bases of the proximal phalanx are somewhat less tense, but the lumbricals act especially strongly in this position. If there is complete flexion of the two distal phalanges, while the metacarpophalangeal joint just begins to flex, the flexion of the metacarpophalangeal joint is produced by the long flexors with participation of the interossei inserted into the lateral bases of the proximal phalanx.

At the distal interphalangeal joint, the relation of the extensor apparatus to the joints is as follows:

1. The two contained lateral bands fuse to form a wide, resistant band that crosses the joint and actually represents the dorsal capsular ligament of this joint. It inserts widely into the dorsal base of the distal phalanx.
2. Oblique fibers connect the terminal part of the extensor apparatus with the collateral ligament of this joint and with the terminal part of the flexor tunnel (Figs. 2–11 and 2–13).
3. The entire apparatus is completely dorsal to the axis of flexion-extension of the joint (Fig. 7–4). Injuries in this area, irrespective of how they are produced (avulsion, fracture, hyperextension, or hyperflexion), usually involve the entire articular apparatus.

The dorsal apparatus then, shows a definite relation to the axes of flexion-extension of the three joints of the finger. At the *metacarpophalangeal joint*, the extensor communis produces longitudinal dorsal axial traction, but the interossei and lumbrical produce traction volar to the axis of flexion-extension. At the *proximal and the distal interphalangeal joints*, traction applied either to the extensor communis or to the lumbrical-interosseous unit will produce traction dorsal to the axes of flexion-extension (Fig. 7–4).

The transverse fibers of the dorsal apparatus unite the lateral bands of the interossei and lumbricals with the central slip of the extensor digitorum in the middle third of the proximal phalanx. These fibers run across the tendon of the extensor communis from one side to the other of the dorsal apparatus and permit the lateral bands a degree of independent movement. After complete extension is exerted by the extensor digitorum communis on the proximal and middle phalanges, there remains the possibility of more extension of the middle and distal phalanges by tension of the lateral bands. This tension changes the direction of the transverse and oblique fibers of the dorsal apparatus into curved or arciform fibers (Fig. 7–5).

The changes of the fibers of the dorsal apparatus can be produced easily in the cadaver, but the author observed it also in fingers exposed for surgical procedures under local anesthesia, when the patient produced it by active extension of the proximal phalanges first, followed by hyperextension of the middle and distal phalanges. Also, the author observed it in patients under general anesthesia by faradic stimulation of the extensor digitorum and added stimulation of the interossei.

In order to establish the role of each component of the dorsal aponeurosis, the author studied the behavior of the extensor digitorum, the interossei, and the lumbricals in many experiments on the cadaver, in the live rhesus monkey under faradic stimulation and during surgical operations, and in cases of known nerve injuries.

EXPERIMENTS IN THE CADAVER

Experiments in the cadaver have only relative value, but when performed judiciously with proper recognition of their limitations, are very informative. Such experiments are of little value when performed on preserved and long dead subjects because stiffness of joints and restrictions of motion interfere with proper estimation of normal activity.

The experiments on the cadaver revealed the following information:

1. The hand was held in moderate flexion at the wrist with the fingers completely flexed into a fist; the extensor digitorum tendon of any finger divided over the metacarpal. Traction applied to the distal segment produced extension of the distal, middle, and proximal phalanges. After a varying angle of extension of the distal and middle phalanges, if the flexion of the wrist was maintained by the examiner, the distal and middle phalanges stopped their extension and flexed, but the proximal continued its hyperextension. With increase of the hyperextension of the proximal phalanx, the flexion of the distal and middle phalanges increased proportionately (Fig. 7–6).

If the wrist was acutely dorsiflexed, the

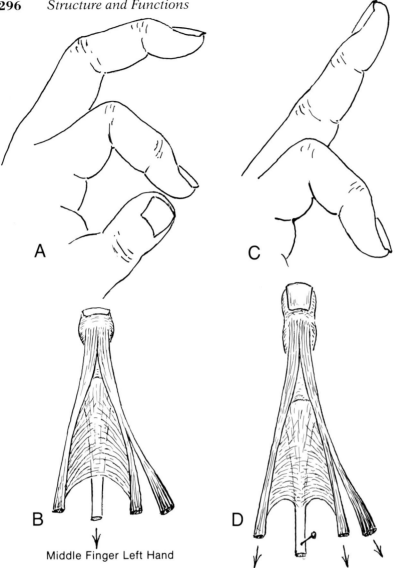

B
Middle Finger Left Hand

FIG. 7–5 Demonstration of why the lateral bands produce more extension through the dorsal aponeurosis after the tendon of the extensor digitorum communis exhausts its full functional length on hyperextension of the proximal phalanx and incomplete extension of the middle phalanx. The obliquity and the curvature of the fibers uniting the lateral bands of the dorsal aponeurosis with its central portion, represented by the tendon of the extensor digitorum, permit enough independent motion of the lateral bands to effect further extension of the distal and the middle phalanges when the tendon of the extensor digitorum is at maximum active stretch.

A, The proximal phalanx extended and the middle and the distal phalanges slightly flexed, this corresponds to **B**, which represents schematically the dorsal apparatus of the middle finger of the left hand. An arrow shows that traction is applied to the tendon of the extensor digitorum communis. The fibers of the dorsal apparatus between the central slip and the lateral bands show a wide curve.

C shows hyperextension at the metacarpophalangeal joint and the proximal and the distal interphalangeal joints. **D** shows the extensor tendon fixed in hyperextension with a pin, while traction is applied to the interossei and the lumbricals, producing hyperextension of all the joints. The fibers of the dorsal apparatus form a double curve instead of a single curve, as in **B**.

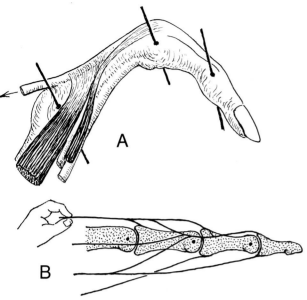

FIG. 7–6 **A** and **B**, When the action of the extensor digitorum alone predominates, the proximal phalanx of the metacarpophalangeal joint extends mostly through the anchorage of the tendon to the capsule of the joint, but also through transmission of force to the middle band, which is inserted into the dorsal base of the middle phalanx and extends the middle phalanx and partly the distal phalanx. The two distal phalanges cannot be completely hyperextended by the action of the extensor digitorum, although in certain individuals this is possible. These individuals are able to hyperextend the middle phalanx through the middle band of the extensor communis, simultaneously flexing the distal phalanx. This attitude of the finger resembles the finger deformity known as mallet finger.

distal and middle phalanges flexed considerably, the proximal phalanx remaining hyperextended. If the wrist was kept in palmar flexion with the proximal phalanges hyperextended, the distal and middle phalanges extended considerably but still could not be hyperextended. If traction on the extensor digitorum continued with the wrist strongly hyperextended (dorsiflexed), the distal and middle phalanges extended almost completely, but the dorsiflexion of the wrist diminished. This remained true when additional traction was applied to the lumbrical in certain hands or to the interossei on each side of the finger in most hands.

Examination of the transverse and the arciform fibers of the dorsal apparatus showed that the fibers forming a wide curve from one interosseous lateral band to the other interosseous band over the extensor tendon (Fig. 7–5B) formed shorter curves between one interosseous band and the extensor tendon, and the extensor tendon and the other interosseous band (Fig. 7–5D). This experiment proved that the extensor communis tendon was able to extend the distal, middle, and proximal phalanges from the position of a fist but not into complete extension of the distal and middle phalanges. It also proved that the interossei (or the lumbrical in certain hands) were able to hyperextend almost completely the flexed distal and the middle phalanges. The comparative independence of action of the extensor digitorum tendon and the lateral bands of the dorsal apparatus results from the special disposition of the fibers of the dorsal apparatus.

2. If in addition to the division of the extensor digitorum tendon, as in the previous preparation, the two long flexors also were divided and the previous experiment repeated, traction applied to the tendon of the extensor produced almost complete hyperextension of the distal and middle phalanges and very strong hyperextension of the proximal phalanx in most hands (Fig. 7–4). If the connection of the anterior aspect of the extensor communis tendon with the capsule of the metacarpophalangeal joint was severed, complete, unrestricted hyperextension of the middle and proximal phalanges and extension of the distal phalanx occur.

This experiment showed that hyperextension of the distal and middle phalanges by the extensor communis does not occur for two reasons: because of the relative shortness of the long flexors of the fingers and because the connection of the extensor communis tendon with the posterior capsule of the metacarpophalangeal joint does not permit full utilization of the functional length of the extensor on the middle phalanx.

The extensor digitorum communis in its incomplete extension of the distal phalanx does not act directly on the distal phalanx but indirectly through the tension of the middle slip of the extensor communis inserted into the middle phalanx and the oblique anchoring fibers (transverse retinacular ligament) that pull on the dorsal apparatus over the middle and distal phalanges. Normally, hyperextension of the distal phalanx cannot be produced under the strongest action of the extensor communis tendon, even by persons who can actively produce hyperextension of the middle phalanx by the extensor digitorum.

3. Experiments with fingers dissected out of the hand and disarticulated at the base of the metacarpals were performed to establish the action of the lumbricals and interossei. The extensor communis tendon was divided over the metacarpal; the long flexors were divided just proximal to the origin of the lumbrical muscle. Traction applied to the extensor tendon produced almost unrestricted extension of the distal and middle phalanges with hypertension of the proximal phalanx, but there was considerable instability of the metacarpophalangeal joint. Traction simultaneously applied to the lumbrical produced hyperextension of the distal phalanx with slight radial inclination of the finger. If additional traction was applied to the corresponding radial interosseous (first dorsal to the index, second dorsal to the middle, second volar to the ring, and third volar to the little), the radial inclination of the finger became extreme with maximum hyperextension of the middle and distal phalanges. If additional traction was applied to the radial and ulnar interosseous of each finger, the stability of the finger at the metacarpophalangeal joint became very effective with hyperextension of the proximal, middle, and distal phalanges (Fig. 7–4).

This experiment showed that the lumbrical is an excellent extensor of the distal phalanx and a good radial abductor of the finger; that the lumbrical with its corresponding interosseous produces even more effective abduction and more effective extension of the middle and distal phalanges; and that the interossei acting on both sides of a finger simultaneously with the lumbrical and extensor communis produce the extension of all the phalanges of the finger with most effective stability. In a few hands, the first lumbrical did not produce any extension of the distal phalanx; in others, the interossei occasionally did not contribute either on one or the other side to the extension of the middle and the distal phalanges; however, in all the hands the interossei contributed to radial deviation of the extended finger and when pulled on both sides, to the stability of the metacarpophalangeal joint.

4. In the experiments on the isolated fingers, with the traction of the extensor tendon omitted, traction on the lumbrical produced flexion of the metacarpophalangeal joint with simultaneous extension of the distal and the proximal interphalangeal joints with slight radial deviation. Additional traction applied to the radial interosseous produced stronger flexion of the metacarpophalangeal joint and sometimes, stronger extension of the distal and the proximal interphalangeal joints (Fig. 7–7). In some fingers, the traction of the dorsal or volar interosseous would produce less extension of the distal and the proximal phalanges than the lumbrical; in others, the reverse occurred. In all fingers, the simultaneous traction on the interossei of each side of the finger produced much more effective extension of the distal and middle phalanges than did the lumbrical alone and very much more effective flexion of the metacarpophalangeal joint. In all experiments, traction on each interosseous produced correspondingly, either radial or ulnar deviation, irrespective of whether the finger was in flexion, extension, or neutral position.

This experiment showed that the lumbrical and the interossei are simultaneous flexors of the metacarpophalangeal joint and extensors of the distal and proximal interphalangeal joints. The lumbricals are abductors of variable strength; the interossei are valuable abductors and adductors of the fingers. When combined on each side of the finger, they are much more effective flexors of the metacarpophalangeal joints than the lumbricals.

5. The lumbrical muscle apparently has considerable power of traction. When the muscle is divided near its tendinous part, in a fresh cadaver, it reacts proximally 3 cm to 5 cm from

its tendon. If the flexor profundus is divided just proximal to the origin of the lumbrical, the gap between the divided ends of the tendon is wide because the lumbrical pulls the distal end of the divided tendon distally, and the proximal end of the flexor tendon retracts under the normal pull of the divided profundus muscle.

It was difficult to observe the distal advance of the tendon of the flexor profundus in the cadaver, whereas this was observed effectively in the surgical experiment and in experiments in living rhesus monkeys.

6. Experimental traction applied to all the extensor tendons simultaneously produced the same effect as did traction of isolated tendons. There was considerable abduction of the fingers at maximum extension of the proximal phalanges.

The extensor indicis produced adduction of the index finger in some instances. The extensor proprius of the little finger exhibited marked abduction of the little finger. These two tendons did not otherwise behave differently from the extensor digitorum.

It was clear to the author that effectiveness of the digital mechanism, among other factors, results from the specific balance between the muscles at the distal and proximal interphalangeal and the metacarpophalangeal joints and the specific arrangement of the dorsal apparatus in relation to the transverse axes of these joints.

The following factors are prerequisites for normal action of the finger:

1. *Balance* is required at the distal interphalangeal joint between the muscles of the dorsal apparatus inserted into the dorsal base of the distal phalanx and the flexor profundus tendon inserted into the volar base of the same phalanx. At the proximal interphalangeal joint, the balance is between the midportion of the extensor digitorum inserted into the dorsal base of the middle phalanx and the flexor superficialis inserted into the lateral volar ridges of the middle phalanx. At the metacarpophalangeal joint, the balance is between the tendon of the extensor communis

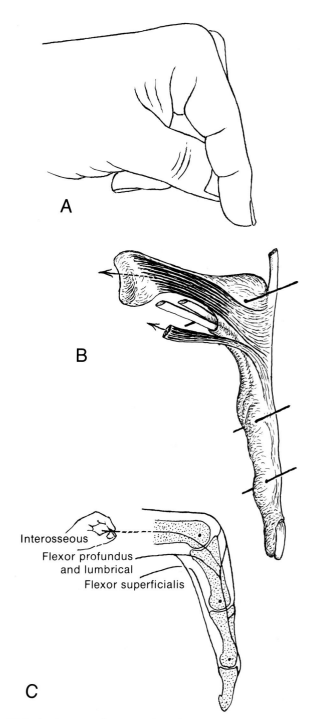

FIG. 7–7 **A** and **B**, Results of simultaneous strong action of the lateral *base* insertion of the interossei and the lateral *band* insertion of the interossei with strong action of the lumbrical and inaction of the long flexors **C**.

loosely inserted into the capsule of the metacarpophalangeal joint or the dorsal base of the proximal phalanx and the interossei and the lumbricals aided by the long flexors in special instances.

2. *Arrangement* of the dorsal apparatus dorsal to the transverse axes of flexion-extension at the distal and the proximal interphalangeal joints and volar to the transverse axis of the metacarpophalangeal joint with free motion of the apparatus over the dorsum of the finger.

3. *Normal joints.*

4. *Normal nerve supply* to the functioning muscles, irrespective of variations in the derivation of the nerve supply.

Tendon injuries

To establish the significance of injuries to different tendons in relation to muscular action, injuries were reproduced in a number of cadavers. In experiments on cadavers with normal joints and normal arrangement of the dorsal apparatus, dorsal or volar tendinous injuries were made on five series of tests:

Injury Of Dorsal Apparatus Between the Distal and Proximal Interphalangeal Joints.   Division or avulsion of the dorsal apparatus, complete or incomplete, in the area included between the distal interphalangeal joint and the proximal interphalangeal joint (Fig. 7–8C) breaks the balance of this joint. The flexor profundus is unopposed, the distal phalanx flexes, and extension of the distal phalanx is abolished either completely or partially. This results in the baseball or mallet finger deformity (Fig. 7–8A). If the division of the tendon persists, the tendon retracts proximally and transfers its action to the dorsum of the proximal interphalangeal joint, where it unbalances the forces acting over this joint in favor of the dorsal motors, inducing a secondary hyperextension of the proximal interphalangeal joint (Fig. 7–8B and D).

The function of the various components of the dorsal apparatus of the fingers becomes clearer in the presence of various injuries and diseases afflicting the fingers. Several factors produce hyperflexion of the distal phalanx with accompanying hyperextension of the middle phalanx. When the insertion of the extensor apparatus is detached from the base of the distal phalanx, the distal phalanx cannot be extended and remains flexed. With persistence of this deformity, hyperextension develops in the region of the proximal interphalangeal joint; however, the same deformity also may develop differently when there is a tear of the flexor superficialis tendon, proximal to the proximal interphalangeal joint. In this instance, hyperextension of the proximal interphalangeal joint appears first, and flexion deformity of the distal phalanx develops subsequently. In spastic paralysis of the hand, simultaneous development of flexion of the distal phalanx with hyperextension of the proximal interphalangeal joint is observed.

In hands afflicted with rheumatoid arthritis, hyperextension of the proximal interphalangeal joints with simultaneous flexion of the distal phalanx is observed frequently. In each of these instances, the sequence of development of deformities results from involvement of the same structural factors but at different times. Thus, a combination of several factors may produce this deformity: interruption of continuity of the extensor apparatus at the distal joint, rupture of the flexor superficialis at the middle phalanx, disruption of the volar plate at the proximal interphalangeal joint, muscular imbalance, as in spastic paralysis, arthritic disintegration of the capsule of the proximal joint, and individual physiologic control of muscles.

Injury Of Dorsal Apparatus at the Proximal Interphalangeal Joint or Over the Proximal Phalanx.   Division of the dorsal apparatus at the proximal interphalangeal joint from one lateral band through the midportion of the extensor to the other lateral band without division of the lateral bands, or over the proximal phalanx between the proximal interphalangeal and metacarpophalangeal joints produces a deformity frequently observed after injury. The deformity is reproduced in the cadaver when after the division of the tendon, traction is applied to the extensor communis and the interosseous-lumbrical unit.

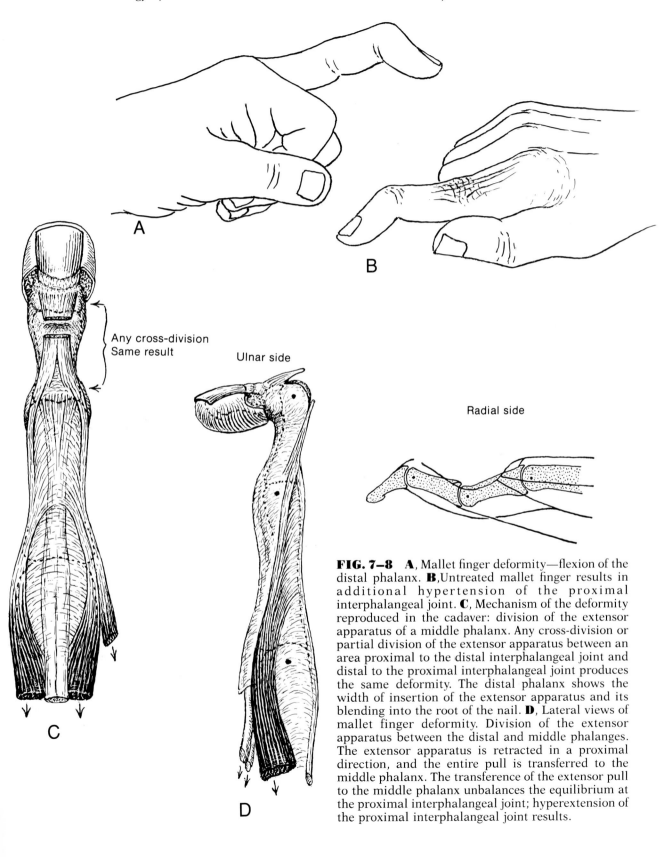

FIG. 7–8 A, Mallet finger deformity—flexion of the distal phalanx. **B**, Untreated mallet finger results in additional hypertension of the proximal interphalangeal joint. **C**, Mechanism of the deformity reproduced in the cadaver: division of the extensor apparatus of a middle phalanx. Any cross-division or partial division of the extensor apparatus between an area proximal to the distal interphalangeal joint and distal to the proximal interphalangeal joint produces the same deformity. The distal phalanx shows the width of insertion of the extensor apparatus and its blending into the root of the nail. **D**, Lateral views of mallet finger deformity. Division of the extensor apparatus between the distal and middle phalanges. The extensor apparatus is retracted in a proximal direction, and the entire pull is transferred to the middle phalanx. The transference of the extensor pull to the middle phalanx unbalances the equilibrium at the proximal interphalangeal joint; hyperextension of the proximal interphalangeal joint results.

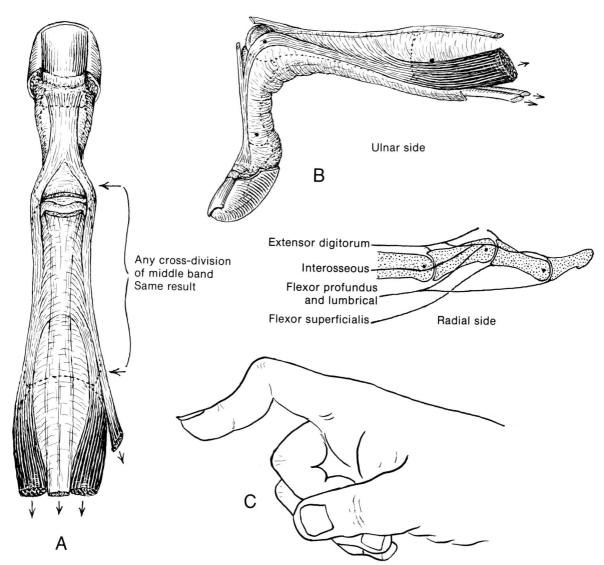

Ulnar side

B

Extensor digitorum

Interosseous

Flexor profundus
and lumbrical

Flexor superficialis

Radial side

Any cross-division
of middle band
Same result

A

C

FIG. 7–9 **A**, Experimental division of the middle band of the extensor digitorum communis from an area just proximal to the base of the middle phalanx to an area distal to the insertion of the capsule of the metacarpophalangeal joint results in a flexion deformity of the proximal interphalangeal joint and extension of the distal phalanx. In the experiment on the cadaver, simultaneous traction is applied to the interosseous, the lumbrical, the extensor digitorum communis, and the flexor sublimis and the profundus. **B**, Lateral view of such a deformity and injury. **C**, Reproduction of the deformity as seen in a living subject; this represents a deformity of the index finger of the right hand, while the diagrams represent an experiment on the middle finger of the left hand.

The deformity consists of flexion of the proximal interphalangeal joint because the balance is broken at this point in favor of the flexor superficialis. The retraction proximally of the central slip of the extensor digitorum transfers its pull to the dorsum of the metacarpophlangeal joint causing hyperextension there. The lateral bands of the interosseous-lumbrical unit, together with the lateral slips of the extensor, are shortened, transferring their pull to the distal phalanx and causing hyperextension of the distal phalanx. Constant pull of the interosseous-lumbrical bands finally induces transfer of the entire dorsal apparatus from its normal position dorsal to the transverse axis of the proximal interphalangeal joint to a position volar to the axis (Fig. 7–9).

In the living, secondary scarring and persistence of the deformity in old cases poses serious difficulties in restoration of normal function because it is necessary to overcome malposition of the lateral bands and to replace them dorsal to the axis of flexion-extension at the proximal interphalangeal joint. It is also necessary to reconstruct the insertion of the central slip of the extensor communis over the dorsum of this joint into the base of the middle phalanx to correct hyperextension of the distal phalanx.

Injury Of Entire Dorsal Apparatus. Division of the entire dorsal apparatus completely across, including its two lateral bands and the midportion of the extensor communis between the proximal interphalangeal joint and the capsule of the metacarpophalangeal joint, make extension of either the distal or the middle phalanx impossible; extension of the proximal phalanx followed. Only hyperextension of the proximal phalanx could be achieved by traction of the extensor communis; abduction and adduction were produced by traction of either one or the other interosseous acting through the insertion into the lateral aspect of the base of the proximal phalanx. Flexion at the metacarpophalangeal joint was achieved either by traction of the long flexor or simultaneous traction applied to the interossei on each side of the finger (Fig. 7–10).

Injuries of this type in patients induce serious disability and must be repaired meticulously before the retracted tendons contract and firm adhesions develop between the divided parts of the apparatus and the periosteum of the proximal phalanx. This disability can be easily differentiated from the disability caused by the division of the central slip of the extensor communis because the distal phalanx is flexed, not hyperextended.

This disability must also be differentiated from another injury that also causes flexion of the proximal interphalangeal joint and extention of the metacarpophalangeal joint. It is produced by an avulsion of the flexor profundus tendon from the volar base of the distal phalanx. In this case, the profundus tendon retracts proximally but not beyond the chiasma tendinum. It adds its flexor force to the flexor superficialis, upsetting the balance at the proximal interphalangeal joint in favor of flexion. The foreshortened dorsal apparatus still preserves its relation to the transverse axes of flexion-extension of each joint but causes hyperextension of the proximal phalanx. The distal phalanx is extended but is almost never fixed in hyperextension. Differentiation among the three types must be kept in mind because surgical repair for each case is different.

Injury Of the Extensor Digitorum Tendon. Division of the tendon of the extensor digitorum over the metacarpal produces immediate flexion of the proximal phalanx. Traction of the distal part of the extensor tendon produces hyperextension of the proximal phalanx. Because normally no traction can be transmitted through the divided tendon, no extension of the proximal phalanx was produced at all by traction of the proximal end unless the extensor communis tendons of the other fingers were pulled and the experimental division of the tendon was made proximal to the junctura tendinei. In this case, limited extension of the proximal phalanx was achieved.

Traction applied to the interossei or the lumbricals invariably produced strong flexion of

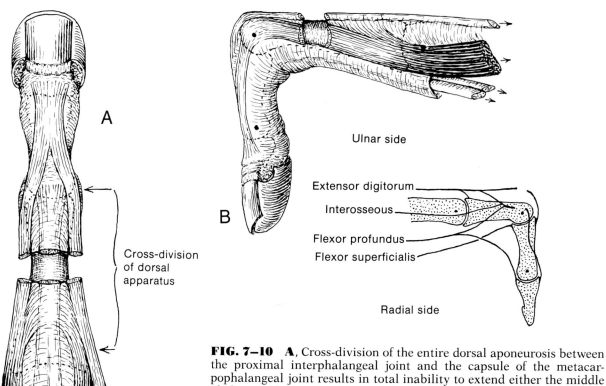

Middle Finger Left Hand

FIG. 7–10 **A,** Cross-division of the entire dorsal aponeurosis between the proximal interphalangeal joint and the capsule of the metacarpophalangeal joint results in total inability to extend either the middle phalanx at the proximal interphalangeal joint or the distal phalanx over the distal interphalangeal joint. Hypertension of the metacarpophalangeal joint can be obtained. If the action of the interossei predominates, flexion of the metacarpophalangeal joint occurs. Proximal and distal phalanges can also be flexed. When extension is attempted, the proximal phalanx is brought out of the flexed position, but the two distal phalanges remain flexed. **B,** Lateral view of same deformity; the retracted extensor digitorum communis with the lateral bands is displaced proximally with an area of interruption between the cut ends. The axis of rotation of the interphalangeal joint is still somewhat dorsal to the lateral band. With time the lateral bands displace dorsally.

the metacarpophalangeal joint and extension of the distal and proximal interphalangeal joints (Fig. 7–11).

Injury Of Dorsal Apparatus, Including Interosseous and Lumbrical. Division of the dorsal apparatus through its entire extent, including the expansion of the interosseous on each side and the tendon of the lumbrical just proximal to the metacarpophalangeal joint, produced flexion of all joints of the finger (Fig. 7–12). No extension was obtained in the distal, middle, or proximal phalanx by traction applied to the proximal parts of the extensor communis,

lumbrical, or interossei. Traction applied to the long flexors produced flexion of the distal, middle, and proximal phalanx when the wrist was in dorsiflexion or even in volar flexion because the long flexors were not restricted by the comparative shortness of the divided extensors.

• • •

In conclusion, the experiments in the cadaver indicated that the actions of the lumbrical, interossei, extensor communis, and long flexors constitute a compound unit in which

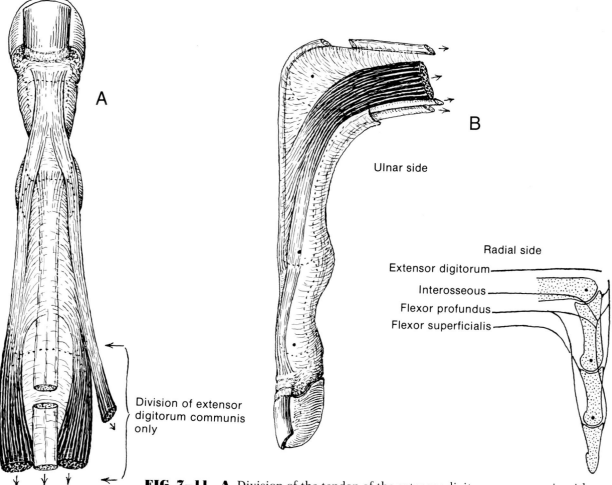

FIG. 7–11 **A**, Division of the tendon of the extensor digitorum communis without involvement of the lateral bands. The interossei and lumbricals are not opposed by the action of the extensor digitorum at the metacarpophalangeal joint. Injury to the tendon of the extensor digitorum communis anywhere between the dorsal carpal ligament and the metacarpophalangeal joint results in complete inability to extend the metacarpophalangeal joint, except for weak extension through the juncturae tendinum. An attempt to extend the metacarpophalangeal joint produces extension of the two distal phalanges and strong flexion of the metacarpophalangeal joint, similar to the position in radial nerve paralysis. Experiments on the cadaver reproduce the deformity very easily. **B**, Lateral view of this experiment with traction applied to the tendon of the extensor digitorum communis, the tendons of the flexors and the fleshy fibers of the interosseous muscle.

distinct disturbances arise when a derangement occurs in one of its components. The action of the extensor on the proximal phalanx cannot be accomplished by any other parts of this unit. The interossei and the lumbricals can substitute partly for each other in all action on the proximal, distal, and middle phalanges. The flexors profundus and superficialis can substitute imperfectly for the lumbrical and the interossei in flexion of the proximal phalanx; however, the substitution is rarely adequate.

OBSERVATIONS DURING SURGICAL PROCEDURES

The observations during surgical procedures were limited but valuable.

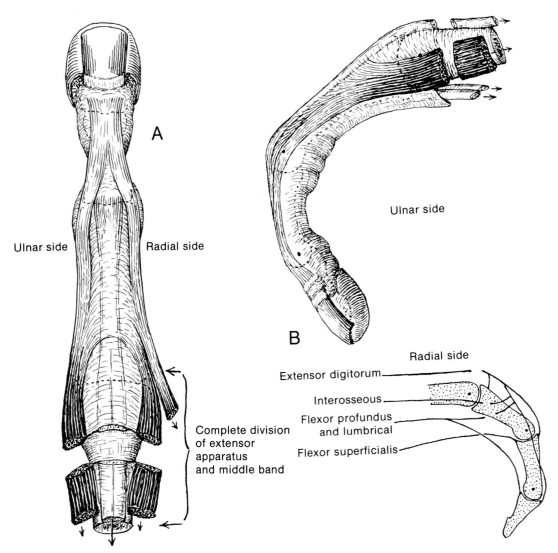

FIG. 7–12 **A,** Complete division of the extensor apparatus involving the tendon of the extensor digitorum communis, the interossei, and the lumbrical. This division, anywhere between a line just proximal to the matacarpophalangeal joint and through the neck of the metacarpal, results in a marked flexion of the distal and the middle phalanges and moderate flexion of the metacarpophalangeal joint. This results from the activity of the long flexor only, completely unopposed by the extensor units. **B,** Lateral view from the ulnar and the radial sides.

Case 1

A large lipomatous tumor was removed from the volar surface of the right hand of a woman under general anesthesia. The tumor was located between the first lumbrical and the first dorsal interosseous. After reviewing the tumor, the first lumbrical was stimulated with faradic current directly applied to the muscle body. The stimulation produced strong abduction of the index finger with slight extension of the distal and middle phalanges. Flexion of the metacarpophalangeal joint was not observed.

Stimulation of the first and second intermetacarpal spaces produced flexion of the metacarpophalangeal joints, respectively, those of the index and middle fingers with simultaneous radial deviation and strong extension of the distal and middle phalanges. Slight adduction of the index finger was noted on stimulation of the second intermetacarpal space.

Conclusions. The first lumbrical acted as a weak extensor of the distal phalanx and had no flexor action on the proximal phalanx. The first palmar interosseous (inserted into the ulnar side of the index) produced slight adduction. The first and the second dorsal interossei produced classic flexion of the proximal phalanx, radial deviation, and extension of the distal and middle phalanges.

Case 2

Four hands were examined during removal of the midpalmar aponeurosis for Dupuytren's contracture. Stimulation of the lumbricals showed very weak abduction of the index and middle fingers in most of them, irrespective of the position of the fingers; in a few fingers strong abduction was observed. However, in one of the experiments the lumbrical muscle seemed especially responsible for strong abduction of the index finger when the metacarpophalangeal joint was flexed and the index finger and thumb pressed together. In some fingers, the lumbricals produced very strong extension of the distal and middle phalanges with simultaneous flexion of the metacarpophalangeal joints.

Stimulation of the lumbricals always showed a distal displacement of the flexor profundus tendon. The displacement usually occurred when the wrist and metacarpophalangeal joint were extending, permitting the distal part of the finger to act as a fixed point. Contraction of the lumbrical then moved its origin distally, pulling the flexor profundus tendon in the same direction.

Stimulation of the interossei invariably produced radial or ulnar deviation, according to the muscle stimulated, with strong flexion of the metacarpophalangeal joint and in most cases, extension of the distal and middle phalanges of the finger. This occurred irrespective of the position of the wrist, if the patient did not attempt any action of the finger. Stimulation of the first dorsal interosseous produced very strong abduction of the index finger accompanied by simultaneous extension of the two distal phalanges. The extension of the two distal phalanges was variable. In some cases, it was very strong, and some cases showed variations in strength of extension of the distal phalanges. Only in rare cases did the stimulation produce no action on the distal phalanges. This proved that action of the first dorsal interosseous muscle on extension of the two distal phalanges does sometimes occur.

Observations were made on hands of patients under both local and general anesthesia. A mild faradic current produced by a small stimulator was applied directly to the exposed isolated lumbrical and, when possible, the interosseous muscles. When local anesthesia was used, the patient was asked to move the fingers and the wrist or to keep them still. When general anesthesia was used, isolated muscles were stimulated singly or in combinations. Generally, the results were similar, although in certain cases the normally observed responses were not seen. In flexion of the fingers there was no visible contraction of the lumbrical muscles. In voluntary extension of the distal phalanges and the metacarpophalangeal joint, strong contraction of the lumbricals could be observed, as it was in extension of the distal phalanges and simultaneous flexion of the metacarpophalangeal joint. When under local anesthesia the tendons were exposed in the hand and the patient was asked to extend the fingers slowly, while the lumbrical of one finger was stimulated, the contraction of the lumbrical was accompanied by a rapid distal advance of the flexor profundus tendon. In the surgically exposed hand, it was difficult to demonstrate any action of radial deviation with stimulation of the lumbricals. Occasionally, such action could be suspected on stimulation of the first lumbrical.

Conclusions. The lumbrical is an extensor of the two distal phalanges; it is also a flexor of the metacarpophalangeal joint. The lumbrical is not a radial deviator of the finger, except perhaps the first, which occasionally may associate its action to the first dorsal interosseous as an abductor of the index finger. The interossei act as radial and ulnar deviators of the proximal phalanx and also as flexors of the metacarpophalangeal joints. The lumbrical produces distal advancement of the flexor profundus tendon in extension of the fingers. The lumbricals are inactive in flexion of the fingers.

ANIMAL EXPERIMENTS

The left hand of an adult female rhesus monkey was dissected, and the skin was incised in the long axis of the palm and retracted. The first, second, and third lumbricals were stimulated with a faradic stimulator. On stimulation, the first lumbrical produced strong abduction of the index finger with slight flexion of the proximal phalanx. The second lumbrical produced strong flexion of the proximal phalanx of the metacarpophalangeal joint with extension of the two distal phalanges of the middle finger. The third lumbrical produced strong flexion of the ring finger at the metacarpophalangeal joint with very strong extension of the two distal phalanges. The fourth lumbrical produced moderate flexion of the metacarpophalangeal joint and extension of the two distal phalanges of the little finger.

Stimulation of the lumbrical muscles in another adult female rhesus showed that the lumbricals produced the same action as did the interossei, namely, strong flexion of the metacarpophalangeal joint and extension of the two distal phalanges in both hands. When the metacarpophalangeal joints were flexed and held in this position with the experimenter's hand, stimulation of the lumbricals produced extension of the two distal phalanges. When the proximal phalanges were held in extension, stimulation of the lumbricals also produced extension of the two distal phalanges. It was interesting that the stimulation of the flexor profundus in this specimen produced flexion at the distal, proximal interphalangeal, and metacarpophalangeal joints.

Dissection of the right hand of another female rhesus monkey showed well-developed lumbrical muscles, located similarly to those in the human. Stimulation by faradic current applied to the lumbricals showed weak action of flexion at the metacarpophalangeal joint with very slight extension of the two distal phalanges when the action of the fingers was unrestricted. Even when the fingers were held extended at the metacarpophalangeal joint, the extension of the two distal phalanges still was very weak. In contrast, stimulation of the interossei showed very strong action consisting of flexion of the metacarpophalangeal joint and extension of the two distal phalanges of the fingers corresponding to the area of stimulation. The stimulation of the lumbricals showed a distinct pull of the tendon of the flexor profundus, but in this case no lateral motion was observed.

Conclusion. Obviously, the number of experiments was very limited, but they confirmed that the lumbrical acted like the interosseous muscle with variable limited function. It also pulled the flexor profundus distally in the extension of the finger.

TESTING OF THE EXTENSORS COMMUNIS AND PROPRIUS OF THE FINGERS, THE LUMBRICALS, AND THE INTEROSSEI

Testing the extensor digitorum is simple because the tendons are easily palpated. The extension of the proximal phalanges is affected by the extensor only; all the extensor tendons become tense and can either be seen or palpated.

The extensor indicis proprius is easily observed when the extensor contracts in extension of the fingers. The tendon of the extensor proprius is palpated on the ulnar side of the tendon of the extensor digitorum of the index finger. When the extended proximal phalanx of the index finger is adducted, the proprius can be observed contracting.

It is more difficult to observe the tensing of the extensor proprius of the little finger, the most ulnar tendon of the dorsum of the hand. Nevertheless it can be observed, especially in abduction of the little finger.

Testing the interossei may be performed in several ways. Duchenne described a test for very early weakness or beginning of paralysis of the interossei. If an extended normal hand with the fingers in abduction is placed on a horizontal surface, the fingers can be adducted easily. In case of the slightest weakness of the interossei, adduction of the fingers becomes very weak or impossible.

If abduction of the fingers is impossible when the hand is placed on a horizontal surface, fairly advanced weakness of the interossei is indicated. Interosseous paralysis is further indicated when it is impossible simultaneously and actively to flex the proximal phalanx and to hyperextend the distal and middle phalanges. The characteristic position of the fingers with the proximal phalanx hyperextended and the distal and middle phalanges flexed suggests paralysis of the interossei. In old cases of complete paralysis of the interossei, the metacarpals become hypermobile in relation to each other, and the metacarpus become extremely relaxed.

The first dorsal interosseous can be palpated easily and contracts strongly in abduction of the index finger in all positions, especially on a horizontal surface. It also contracts in simultaneous flexion of the proximal phalanx and extension of the two distal phalanges.

Testing the lumbricals is also possible, especially the first and the second. To test the lumbricals, the middle and distal phalanges are strongly flexed; the proximal phalanx remains in extension. The tension of the long flexors can then be detected easily in the palm of the hand, especially if the two distal phalanges are flexed and extended several times, while the proximal phalanx is fixed in extension. Once the position of the long flexors is found, simultaneous flexion of the proximal phalanx and extension of the distal and middle phalanges permit palpation of the contraction of the lumbrical immediately radial to the long flexors.

Fixed contractures of the tendons of the extensor communis produce hyperextension of the proximal phalanges. The contracture of the flexors produces typical deformities of the fingers with flexion of either the distal or proximal interphalangeal joint, or both.

The contractures of the interossei produce typical deformities with the proximal phalanx flexed and the distal and middle phalanges extended.

Contracture of the lumbrical muscle may be overlooked. The author observed and operated on one case of isolated contracture of the second lumbrical muscle following an injury. Before the operation the patient was unable to flex the distal phalanx of the middle finger completely; the excision of the contracted lumbrical restored function.

Observation in cadavers and on a mechanical model proved that shortening the lumbrical prevented full flexion of the distal phalanx, because the contracted band between the flexor profundus and the dorsal apparatus forcibly extended the distal phalanx when traction was applied to the flexor profundus tendon.

OBSERVATIONS IN KNOWN NERVE INJURIES

Observations in known nerve injuries are of great help in estimating function in the different muscles of the hand, but they also have their limitations. Personal experience in peacetime injuries, even in special clinics, is restricted to a comparatively small number of cases.

Variations in the nerve supply are comparatively frequent and may involve the interosseous and lumbrical muscles, the extensors and flexors, and the muscles of the thenar and the hypothenar eminences, which will be considered separately.

The dissociated nerve supply may add to the difficulties, as in cases in which a separate nerve supply may be present for the extensor indicis, for the belly of the extensor of the medius, or for the flexor profundus of the index finger. In the case of the extensor indicis or the extensor communis to the medius, completely normal extensor action will be observed in the index or the medius, while all the other extensor digitorum parts may be paralyzed. In the case of the belly of the profundus, the flexor of the index finger will produce normal action and even some action in the middle finger, while all the others will be inactive owing to paralysis.

In extremely rare cases, the interosseous muscles may have an additional nerve supply from the posterior interosseous branch of the radial nerve.

There are many variations of muscular insertions. For instance, in cases in which the extensor digitorum tendon has no attachments into the capsule of the metacarpophalangeal joint, the extensor digitorum tendon will extend almost completely to the distal and middle phalanges of a finger, simulating the action of the lumbrical or interosseous muscles.

For correct analysis of the disabilities created by a nerve injury, it is imperative to test the involved muscles by all available means, including the injection of procaine around large nerve trunks, palpation of contraction, electric stimulation through the skin, surgical exposure during direct stimulation of nerves.

Experiences with nerve injuries during World Wars I and II were recorded, analyzed, and reported by a number of observers and can be found in the special literature (André-Thomas; Bunnell; Clinton; Dejerine Froment P. Marie and Meige; *Medical Department Report of the World War,* 1927; *Medical Research Council* (1942) *War Memor. #7;* Murphey, Kirklin and Finlayson: *Revue Neurologique;* Rowntree; Stookey; Sunderland; Tinel; and many others).

Isolated injuries of the median nerve just proximal to the wrist permit a study of the actions of the interossei and lumbricals with exclusion of the first and the second lumbricals, as well as of the extensors of the fingers in the presence of active long flexors. If the nerve is injured proximal to the nerve supply of the long flexors, the interossei, the third and fourth lumbrical, and the extensors can be studied with exclusion of most of the long flexors.

Isolated injuries of the ulnar nerve proximal to the deep branch with obvious paralysis of the interossei and the third and fourth lumbricals allow study of the first and the second lumbricals on the index and middle fingers and the extensor digitorum on the ring and the little fingers in the presence of the long flexors and absence of intrinsics. Isolated injury to the ulnar nerve proximal to the supply to the ulnar part of

the flexor profundus allows investigation into the action of the extensor on the ring and little fingers in the absence of the interossei, lumbricals, and flexor profundus.

Isolated injuries of the radial nerve show the action of the lumbricals and interossei when the extensor is inactive.

Combined median-ulnar nerve lesions, according to the site of the lesion, allow investigations of the action of the extensor digitorum with or without the coaction of the long flexors.

Combined median and radial nerve lesions, which would normally eliminate the extensor digitorum of all fingers and the first and second lumbricals, allow study of the action of the interossei on the index and middle fingers without the extensor and the lumbricals, and the action of the interossei and lumbricals without the extensors on the ring and little fingers. If the lesion of the median nerve is high and the long flexors are involved, isolated study of the interossei on the index finger without any other muscle becomes possible.

Combined ulnar and radial nerve lesions completely eliminate all the extensors of the ring and little fingers and the extensors and the interossei of the index and middle fingers, with action left only in the first and second lumbricals.

Limited personal experiences and review of the literature provided additional information on the mechanism of action and participation of the muscles of the hand.

Lesions of the median nerve

If the lesion occurs high in the forearm, the flexors superficialis and profundus of the index finger are completely inactive. The superficial bellies of all the fingers are inactive, but the ulnar part of the profundus, which is supplied by the ulnar nerve, may extend its supply to the profundus of the middle finger; thus, the index finger completely deprived of the flexor profundus and superficialis cannot flex the interphalangeal joints. The flexor profundus of the middle finger frequently has good flexion of the interphalangeal joints. The metacarpophalangeal joints of the index and middle fingers can flex normally in most cases, despite the expected paralysis of the first and second lumbricals. Abduction and adduction are unaffected except in cases of median supply to the first dorsal interosseous, when abduction of the index finger is impossible.

There are two good tests for paralysis of the long flexors of the index or middle fingers. In the first, the palm is placed on a table, and when asked, the patient is unable to scratch the surface of the table (Pitres and Testut). The other test consists of crossing all the fingers of both hands; the affected index finger stands out completely extended and cannot be flexed. The medius is partially flexed; complete flexion is impossible (Pitres).

In cases of injuries to the median nerve distal to the supply to the flexors, the paralysis of the lumbricals causes very little disturbance to the flexion of the metacarpophalangeal joints and extension of the two distal joints of the index and middle fingers.

The test for the first dorsal interosseous consists, as already described, in palpating the first interosseous when the index finger is abducted. The first two lumbricals can also be palpated easily, in simultaneous flexion of the proximal phalanx and extension of the distal and middle phalanges of the index and middle fingers.

Studies of paralysis of the median nerve show the following:

1. The action of the long flexors is identical with the action of these muscles established by other investigations.
2. The first and second lumbricals act similarly to the interossei, and the absence of the lumbricals does not materially affect the flexion of the metacarpophalangeal joint and extension of the two distal interphalangeal joints.

Lesions of the ulnar nerve

Lesions of the ulnar nerve must be investigated thoroughly to eliminate the possibility of the variation that carries the supply to the intrinsic muscles through the median nerve. In high lesions of the ulnar nerve the clawing of the ring and little fingers is less severe than with low lesions because the flexor profundus pull on the little finger and ring finger is lost.

With ulnar nerve lesions the proximal interphalangeal joints are hyperflexed; the metacarpophalangeal joints flex poorly or not at all. The flexor superficialis flexes the proximal interphalangeal joint; at the end of this flexion, very weak flexion of the metacarpophalangeal joint follows, but it is incomplete. The metacarpophalangeal joint hyperextends, and full extension of the distal and middle phalanges is impossible. There is no active abduction and adduction of the ring finger; the little finger remains in constant abduction owing to the action of extensor digiti minimi. With isolated injuries of the deep branch of the ulnar nerve, the general picture is the same, except that the clawing of the ring and little fingers is exaggerated by the activity of the unaffected flexor profundus.

Studies of ulnar nerve paralysis indicate the following:

1. The first and second lumbricals are not affected. With interosseous muscle paralysis, their ability to strongly extend the distal phalanges of the index and middle fingers and flexion of the proximal phalanx varies. The intact lumbricals may have some abductor action of the index and the middle fingers.
2. The extensor digitorum can completely extend the proximal phalanx. It can incompletely extend the two distal phalanges of the ring and little fingers if there is paralysis of the flexor profundus to these fingers.
3. The interossei and the lumbricals are flexors of the proximal phalanges of the ring and little fingers and can extend and hyperextend the two distal phalanges.
4. The interossei maintain the relationship of the second, third, fourth, and fifth metacarpals.

Lesions of the radial nerve

Lesions of the radial nerve affect the extensor

digitorum and completely eliminate extension or hyperextension of the proximal phalanx of the fingers. The interosseous-lumbrical unit can extend the two distal phalanges of each finger, but when this is done, the proximal interphalangeal joints flex, and the fingers can be abducted and adducted within a very limited range. When the proximal phalanges are supported in hyperextension by the examiner, the two distal phalanges extend completely, and the fingers abduct and adduct. The following conclusions are permitted:

1. The extensor digitorum is the only extensor of the proximal phalanx.
2. The interossei and the lumbricals flex the proximal phalanx and extend the distal two phalanges of the finger.
3. The interossei are abductors and adductors of the fingers in extension and also in flexion.

Lesions of the median and ulnar nerves
Combined median and ulnar nerve lesions eliminate the action of the intrinsic muscles and the long flexors and show typical clawing deformity. The extensors extend the proximal phalanx of each finger and can extend the two distal phalanges of the finger if the proximal phalanx is maintained in neutral position. The two distal phalanges can be extended actively by the extensor digitorum. The following conclusions are based on observation of these cases:

1. The extensor digitorum extends the proximal phalanx.
2. The extensor digitorum extends the two distal phalanges when hyperextension of the proximal phalanx is prevented.
3. The interosseous-lumbrical component is essential for optimal function of the extensor digitorum.

Lesions of the median and radial nerves
Combined median and radial nerve lesions indicate the following about the index and middle fingers:

1. The interossei are the principal flexors of the metacarpophalangeal joints and extend the two distal phalanges with variable power.

2. The lumbricals also perform the same function but more weakly.
3. When acting together in the ring and little fingers, the interossei and the lumbricals produce stronger action as shown in isolated paralysis of the radial nerve.

Lesions of the ulnar and radial nerves
Combined ulnar and radial nerve lesions indicate the following:

1. The power of the lumbricals varies in individuals. The first and second lumbricals, supplied by the median nerve, produce variable flexion of the metacarpophalangeal joint and extension of the two distal phalanges.
2. The distal phalanges of the index finger are slightly less flexed than the others, indicating that the lumbrical may pull the tendon of the flexor profundus distally.

CONCLUSIONS REGARDING THE MOTION OF THE FINGERS

1. Normal activity of the hand requires the participation of the flexors superficialis and profundus, the interosseous muscles, the lumbricals, the extensor digitorum, and the extensor proprius of the index and little fingers.

2. Normal activity is possible if there is additional cooperation of the extensors and the flexors of the wrist and the muscles of the thumb and hypothenar eminence, which will be considered later.

3. There is complete integration of action of all muscles, which apparently work in coordination with dominance of one or the other group, but never in single units. Whether the resulting movement is caused by actual inhibition of the subordinated group or simply a stronger impulse in the dominant group is unimportant. There is no experimental evidence that the pyramidal system has an inhibitory action on the spinal cord cells, and thus it appears probable that the theory of dominance of action is correct.

4. The relative shortness of the extensors,

which does not permit full flexion of all the joints of the fingers and wrist, and the shortness of the flexors, which does not permit full extension of the fingers and wrist, are of functional significance as mechanical factors.

5. The specific features of arrangement of the fibers of the dorsal apparatus and the variations of the insertions of the interossei and the lumbricals into the dorsal apparatus and into the sides of the base of the proximal phalanx are of mechanical significance, although the details of insertion may be of less significance than was believed.

6. The relation of the extensor digitorum tendon to the capsule of the metacarpophalangeal joint, permitting an efficient but limited range of extension and flexion without losing contact with the joint, is important.

7. There are four points of anchorage that contribute to the normal retention of the finger apparatus and its function. The retention of the tendons of the interossei in constant relation to the metacarpophalangeal joint is of paramount importance.

8. The relation of the flexors superficialis and profundus in the finger and the mechanical advantages of the chiasma tendinum are important for normal function.

9. The balance of the volar-dorsal forces over the distal interphalangeal, proximal interphalangeal, and metacarpophalangeal joints is a dynamic prerequisite for normal function.

10. Imbalance over any of these areas (item 9) causes a definite deformity that is easy to recognize.

11. The extensor digitorum is an extensor of the proximal phalanx, but it is also an extensor of the middle phalanx and indirectly, of the distal phalanx; however, the action on the middle and distal phalanges is restricted by the shortness of the long flexors and the special connection of the extensor with the capsule of the metacarpophalangeal joint. The extensor is also an abductor of the fingers in extension.

12. The flexor superficialis is the most efficient flexor of the middle phalanx, but it also has limited action on the proximal phalanx when the hand is in dorsiflexion because of its comparative shortness and actual dynamic possibility to flex the proximal phalanx after flexing the middle phalanx.

13. The flexor profundus is a flexor of the distal and proximal interphalangeal joints; under certain circumstances, it can flex the distal phalanx alone. It can also flex the metacarpophalangeal joint, like the superficialis, with the same limitations. The long flexors are adductors of the fingers in flexion.

14. The interossei are divided into two groups (dorsal and palmar) and act similarly, producing flexion of the metacarpophalangeal joint and extension of the distal and middle phalanges. They contribute to the retention of the second, third, fourth, and to a certain extent, fifth metacarpals. The dorsal interossei are abductors of the fingers in the position of extension, flexion, and most efficiently, in the flat, neutral position. The volar interossei are adductors of the fingers.

15. The lumbricals are fairly strong muscles, functionally variable in different individuals and in the hands of the same individual. They generally act similarly to the interossei, producing flexion of the metacarpophalangeal joint and extension of the two phalanges. They are important connectors between the dorsal apparatus and the flexor profundus. Apparently they contract only in extension of the finger, and in this action they pull the flexor profundus tendon toward the distal phalanx. The persistent presence of the lumbricals in different animals suggests that their function is of considerable importance. The lumbrical may be muscle adapted to relieve tension on the tendon of the flexor profundus in the usually required speed of extension as compared with the requirement of force in flexion. The special nerve supply of the lumbricals (Rabishong) and the deep structures of the hand (Stilwell) indicate their very important role as sensitive moderators balancing the action between the flexor and extensor mechanism of the fingers.

16. In normal extension of the fingers with the wrist clenched, the extensor communis acts on the middle and proximal phalanges and indirectly on the distal phalanx extending them

all. The interossei also participate in this action, but they simultaneously produce flexion of the metacarpophalangeal joint. This flexion is subordinated to the action of the extensor on the metacarpophalangeal joint, and extension of this joint ensues. The simultaneous action of these two antagonists on the metacarpophalangeal joint produces stabilization of this joint. The two distal phalanges are extended by the action of the extensor and the interossei. The lumbricals, acting in a similar manner, add their power to this motion and simultaneously pull on the tendon of the flexor profundus.

17. When the interossei contract to produce abduction with the hand flat, the extensor contracts simultaneously, predominating over the flexor component on the metacarpophalangeal joint and helping the dorsal interossei in their abduction. This also takes place in adduction of the fingers by the volar interossei.

18. The variations of the nerve supply to the intrinsic muscles must always be kept in mind, especially the median supply to the intrinsic muscles via high anastomosis in the forearm with the ulnar nerve or local branches supplying the first dorsal interosseous; the supply of the third lumbrical by the median nerve, or all the lumbricals by the ulnar nerve; the extremely rare but possible supply of the dorsal interossei by branches from the posterior interosseous of the forearm branch of the radial nerve; the possible individual supply by a branch of the posterior interosseous for the extensor indicis; the possible individual nerve supply to the flexors superficialis or the profundus.

MOTORS AND MECHANISM OF ACTION OF THE THUMB AND LITTLE FINGER

The motion of the thumb is produced by the long extrinsic and the short intrinsic muscles and is conditioned by the special structure of its metacarpocarpal joint.

The extrinsic muscles of the thumb are as follows:

Flexor pollicis longus—the flexor of the distal phalanx

Extensor pollicis longus—the extensor of the distal and proximal phalanges and the first metacarpal; the adductor of the thumb

Extensor pollicis brevis—the extensor of the proximal phalanx; the abductor of the first metacarpal; the secondary abductor of the wrist

Abductor pollicis longus—the abductor and extensor of the first metacarpal; the secondary radial abductor of the wrist.

The intrinsic muscles of the thumb are as follows:

Abductor pollicis brevis
Flexor pollicis brevis
Opponens pollicis
Adductor pollicis

The action of these muscles will be considered in relation to the specialized function of opposition of the thumb.

The extrinsic muscles of the little finger were discussed with the other extrinsic muscles of the fingers. *The intrinsic muscles of the little finger* are as follows:

Abductor digiti minimi
Opponens digiti minimi
Flexor brevis digiti minimi

Normal activity of the hand is not possible without a normal thumb and is difficult without a normally functioning hypothenar eminence. The thumb differs from the fingers because it has a movable metacarpal, permitting the special function of opposition in addition to common finger activities.

OPPOSITION OF THE THUMB

Opposition consists of a change of position of the thumb, together with its metacarpal; in this change, the thumb moves from its position of rest, lateral to the index finger, to a new location in front of all the fingers, passing forward in abduction (Fig. 7–13). When at rest or in adduction, the nail of the thumb is directed laterally or dorsally. In the new position, the nail turns anteriorly, so that the pulp of the thumb faces the pulp of the fingers and may touch each finger

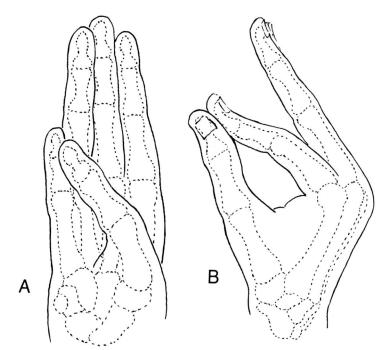

FIG. 7–13 **A**, Opposition of the thumb. **B**, Position of a pinch with tracing of the skeletal structures.

in turn. Extreme opposition, when the pulp of the thumb touches the pulp of the little finger, is accompanied by flexion of the fifth metacarpal, occurring at the metacarpohamate joint and increasing the transverse arch of the metacarpus.

Many investigators have attempted to establish whether opposition results from a rotatory or combined motion, what muscles are responsible for opposition, and whether it takes place in the metacarpocarpal joint between the trapezium and first metacarpal or whether other carpal bones are involved. Personal inquiries of the author permitted the following conclusions, based on experimentation, clinical investigation, and the findings of others:

1. Opposition of the thumb results principally from motion in the joint between the trapezium and the first metacarpal. This motion is almost never transmitted to the other bones of the carpus under normal conditions, even in extremes of opposition.
2. The motion of opposition is enhanced by lateral angulation of the proximal phalanx at the metacarpophalangeal joint, especially in opposition of the thumb to the little finger by the pull of the abductor brevis, as proved by Duchenne.
3. Opposition actually involves a rotatory motion of the first metacarpal around its longitudinal axis, but this rotation cannot be produced actively without simultaneous motion about other axes of joint.
4. The rotation of opposition is determined by several factors: the configuration of the saddle joint between the trapezium and the base of the first metacarpal (Fig. 3–1), the laxity of the capsule of this joint (Fig. 3–7), and the disposition of the small instrinsic muscles in relation to the longitudinal axis of the first metacarpal (Fig. 7–14).
5. Rotation of the first metacarpal cannot be obtained with the thumb held in any one position; it occurs only in combination with flexion of the first metacarpal from the position of extension or vice versa.
6. Abduction or adduction of the thumb is not necessarily accompanied by rotation.
7. Passive rotation of the first metacarpal can be obtained in its carpometacarpal joint in

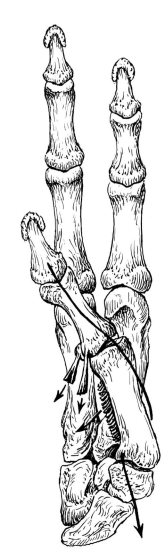

FIG. 7–14 Complete opposition of the thumb, showing traction on the radial sesamoid by the flexor brevis pollicis, on the radial base of the proximal phalanx of the thumb by the abductor brevis pollicis and by the abductor longus pollicis; the latter acts as a stabilizer and an extensor of the first metacarpal. The tendon of the extensor pollicis longus is shown without an arrow to indicate that it is not involved in this action.

flexion, extension, abduction, and adduction because of laxity of the capsule of this joint and normally does not exceed 25°.

8. Full opposition, which consists of flexion, abduction, and rotation, equals approximately 110° from full extension of the thumb to the extreme of opposition.

9. Opposition of the thumb to the little finger is enhanced by flexion of the fifth metacarpal with slight rotatory motion of the fifth metacarpal at the metacarpohamate joint.

10. The motion of flexion of the fifth metacarpal is made possible by the almost typical saddle joint between the fifth metacarpal and the ulnar half of the hamate bone and the arrangement of the hypothenar muscles.

11. Even in extremes of opposition, the first metacarpal is flexed toward the fifth metacarpal, which in turn is flexed toward the first metacarpal.

12. The thenar and the hypothenar muscles originating mostly from the volar carpal ligament have practically no effect on the carpal bones.

13. In simple, effortless opposition the abductor brevis, the opponens policis, and the flexor pollicis brevis play the dominant role.

14. In opposition requiring force, the flexor pollicis longus, the extensor pollicis longus, and the adductor pollicis play important additional roles, as do the abductor pollicis longus and the extensor pollicis brevis.

OTHER ACTIVITIES OF THE THUMB

Flexion of the distal phalanx can be achieved with the first metacarpal in extension or in flexion, showing the comparative independence of the flexor pollicis longus; however, in certain individuals flexion of the distal phalanx of the thumb is accompanied by simultaneous flexion of the distal phalanx of the index finger, showing the possible interconnection of the flexor pollicis longus and the flexor profundus indicis.

Extension of the distal and proximal phalanges and the first metacarpal is induced by the extensor pollicis longus; the extension of the proximal phalanx alone or sometimes with the distal phalanx is produced by the extensor pollicis brevis (Fig. 7–15).

Abduction is produced by the abductor brevis and opponens pollicis, which simultaneously pull the thumb forward; by the

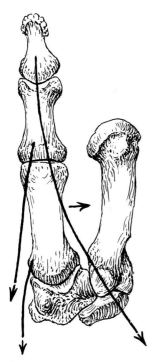

FIG. 7–15 The action of the extensor pollicis longus, which produces extension of the distal phalanx, of the proximal phalanx, and the first metacarpal with strong adduction of the first metacarpal toward the second metacarpal. The extensor pollicis brevis and the abductor pollicis longus act simultaneously as stabilizers.

flexor brevis, which is an excellent abductor; and by the abductor longus. Abduction of the thumb is accompanied by strong contraction of the extensor carpi ulnaris and sometimes by the flexor carpi ulnaris. Adduction is affected by the adductor pollicis, radial head of the first dorsal interosseous and the extensor pollicis longus. The flexor pollicis longus may also adduct the thumb.

EXPERIMENTS IN CADAVERS

Flexor Pollicis Longus. The flexor pollicis longus produced flexion of the distal phalanx when traction was applied to its tendon at the wrist. This was followed by flexion of the proximal phalanx and the first metacarpal. There is a relative shortness of the flexor pollicis longus

that, however, is not so marked as the shortness of the long flexors of the other fingers.

The experiments on the cadaver do not exactly represent the function of the flexor pollicis longus in the living because normally the flexor pollicis longus has negligible action on the proximal phalanx and practically no action on the metacarpal.

If the thumb is supported in extension with the distal phalanx hyperextended, and the distal phalanx is then released, a slight flexion of the distal phalanx is observed. Obviously, this flexion of the distal phalanx in the cadaver is caused by the tension of the comparatively short flexor pollicis longus. The same type of flexion may be observed in median nerve paralysis with involvement of the flexor pollicis longus, giving a wrong impression of activity in the paralyzed flexor pollicis longus. In complete division of the tendon of the flexor pollicis longus this phenomenon does not occur.

The flexor pollicis longus is occasionally connected with the belly of the flexor indicis profundus. In this case, flexion of the distal phalanx of the thumb produces simultaneous flexion of the two distal phalanges of the index finger.

Extensor Pollicis Longus. The extensor pollicis longus produced extension of the distal phalanx with simultaneous extension of the proximal phalanx and the first metacarpal with strong adduction of the entire thumb (Fig. 7–14). Hyperflexion of the distal phalanx and subsequent release produced slight extension of the distal phalanx on account of the relative shortness of the extensor pollicis longus. This extension did not occur if the extensor pollicis longus was divided.

The relative shortness of the long extensor also is shown when all the joints of the thumb are flexed and an attempt is made to flex the wrist. The distal phalanx cannot be maintained in flexion; it automatically extends.

Observation of the dorsal apparatus of the thumb showed that the entire apparatus becomes tense, and the tendon of the extensor pollicis longus shifts ulnarly from 4 mm to 5 mm. The shifting of the extensor longus takes place only between the metacarpophalangeal joint and Lister's tubercle. The shift permits adduction of the thumb simultaneously with extension of all its joints. If the dorsal carpal ligament is opened and the tendon of the extensor longus lifted out of its dorsal canal, traction applied to the tendon changes its normal direction and does not produce adduction simultaneously with extension of all the elements of the thumb. There is no lateral shifting of the tendon of the extensor longus over the proximal or distal phalanges of the thumb.

Extensor Pollicis Brevis.   The extensor pollicis brevis produced extension of the proximal phalanx with simultaneous strong abduction of the thumb and flexion of the distal phalanx caused by comparative shortness of the flexor pollicis longus.

It was indicated previously that there is a frequent tendinous extension of the extensor brevis into the distal phalanx. When such an extension existed, traction applied to the extension of the distal phalanx, but the extension of the distal phalanx appeared only in complete abduction of the thumb, in contrast with the extensor longus, which produced extension of the distal phalanx either in straight extension or only in adduction of the thumb (Fig. 3–20). The short extensor also produced radial inclination of the wrist after full abduction of the thumb.

Abductor Pollicis Longus.   The abductor pollicis longus acts on the first metacarpal as an abductor and extensor. After full abduction of the thumb, further traction of the long abductor proximal to its carpal retinaculum produced abduction and slight flexion of the wrist. At no time did it produce supination of the wrist (Fig. 7–14).

The experiments with the extrinsic long muscles are performed easily in the cadaver. It was more difficult to reproduce the action of the thenar and the hypothenar muscles. The following methods were used: (1) A rigid sound of small diameter was passed transversely between the muscle body under investigation and the other muscles or bone, just distal to the origin of the muscle; traction was applied to the two ends of the sound to pull the muscle near its origin. In this manner, the opponens pollicis, the opponens

digiti minimi; the abductor pollicis brevis, the flexor pollicis brevis, the adductor pollicis, the abductor digiti minimi, and the flexor digiti were investigated. (2) Traction was applied to the tendons of insertion of all intrinsic muscles.

Abductor Pollicis Brevis.   The abductor pollicis brevis produced abduction of the thumb with angulation between the proximal phalanx and the first metacarpal (Fig. 7–16). The long axis of the first metacarpal, usually continuous with the long axis of the proximal and the distal phalanges, formed an angle of about 15° to 25° at the metacarpophalangeal joint toward the radial side of the thumb with simultaneous extension of the distal phalanx (Figs. 3–22 and 7–14).

Flexor Pollicis Brevis.   The flexor pollicis brevis produced flexion of the first metacarpal and the proximal phalanx with rotation of the thumb, turning the pulp of the thumb toward the pulp of the fingers (Fig. 7–14). The flexion of the thumb was the most important motion, the rotation occurring toward the termination of the motion of flexion and taking place at the articulation between the metacarpal and the trapezium. Simultaneously, the distal phalanx extended through its tendinous expansion to the dorsal apparatus of the thumb (Fig. 3–22).

Opponens Pollicis.   The action of the opponens pollicis was difficult to observe. Traction applied to its body near the origin produced mainly flexion of the first metacarpal with very slight rotation in a few of the thumbs. The flexion was limited; the thumb barely reached the radial side of the middle finger.

Adductor Pollicis.   The adductor pollicis produced adduction of the first metacarpal and the phalanges of the thumb toward the index finger and beyond to the middle finger, moving the thumb close to the palm. Simultaneously, it extended the distal phalanx of the thumb through the fibers of connection with the dorsal apparatus (Fig. 3–22).

Duchenne stated that the adductor pollicis can move the first metacarpal in four directions. It pulls the first metacarpal into adduction, if the first metacarpal is kept (preliminary to the action of the adductor) in complete abduction by the action of the extensor brevis of the thumb. If

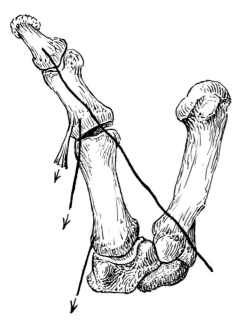

FIG. 7–16 Complete relaxation of the extensor pollicis longus, strong action of the extensor pollicis brevis, and strong action of the abductor pollicis longus and the abductor brevis, producing angulation and opposition of the proximal phalanx in relation to the first metacarpal.

the thumb is held in maximum adduction or opposition by the flexor pollicis brevis, the action of the adductor pollicis may produce abduction toward the line of origin of the adductor muscle. If the first metacarpal is kept in complete flexion at the carpometacarpal joint, the adductor pollicis may act as an extensor, bringing the thumb to the line of origin of the adductor pollicis. If the thumb is kept in complete extension by the extensor pollicis longus, the adductor may become a flexor of the first metacarpal.

Location of the motion of opposition
A special preparation was made to study the location of the motion of opposition in 15 hands. The entire hand was dissected, and all the fingers were removed, leaving only the thumb column and the distal row of the carpal bones. The triquetral and the lunate bones were removed,

but both bones of the forearm and the ligaments between these two bones and of the radio-scaphoid articulation were left intact. The volar carpal ligament was resected just ulnar to the origin of the thenar muscles. The thenar muscles were partially resected to expose the joint between the first metacarpal and the trapezium.

In imitation of opposition, traction was applied to the abductor longus and to the resected muscles between their origin and their insertion. Motion occurred only in the trapezio-metacarpal joint without the slightest transmission to any of the bones of the distal row or the scaphoid. The strongest pull on the abductor and the bands uniting the origins and insertions of the intrinsic muscles of the thumb (not shown in the illustration to demonstrate the metacarpo-multangular joint more clearly) produced no motion of the carpal bones. The relationship of the bones between the position of rest (Fig. 7–17) and complete opposition (Fig. 7–18) showed no change.

The rotatory and the flexor component of action of the flexor brevis and opponens and the abductor brevis probably arise from the pull of the muscles between the origin of these muscles and their insertions into the radial side of the proximal phalanx obliquely across the line of pull of the tendon of the flexor pollicis longus (Figs. 2–7 and 3–16).

Even with all the limitations of experiments on cadavers, and especially the removal of the volar carpal ligament, which eliminates the additional traction of the hypothenar muscles on the ulnar side of the carpus, the experiment appeared to demonstrate that motion between the carpal bones in the process of opposition is insignificant (Fig. 7–13). Incidentally, before the volar carpal ligament and the fingers were removed, the thumb was placed in complete opposition; the fifth metacarpal was placed in maximum flexion and was held in this position. The distance between the tubercle of the trapezium and the tip of the hamate hook remained the same for opposition and for neutral position of the thumb. This indicated that even in the presence of simultaneous action of the muscles of the two eminences, the probability of any motion of bones of the carpus is insignificant.

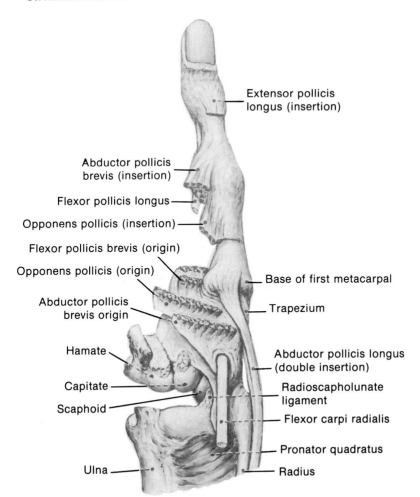

Extensor pollicis
longus (insertion)

Abductor pollicis
brevis (insertion)

Flexor pollicis longus

Opponens pollicis (insertion)

Flexor pollicis brevis (origin)

Opponens pollicis (origin)

Abductor pollicis
brevis origin

Hamate

Capitate

Scaphoid

Ulna

Base of first metacarpal

Trapezium

Abductor pollicis longus
(double insertion)

Radioscapholunate
ligament

Flexor carpi radialis

Pronator quadratus

Radius

FIG. 7–17 Figures 7–17 and 7–18 demonstrate the mechanism of opposition of the thumb. The specimen consists of the thumb, the joint between the first metacarpal and the trapezium, the joint between the trapezium and the scaphoid bone, the radioscaphoid joint, and the distal row of the carpus. The lunate, the triquetral bone, and the pisiform were removed; the distal radioulnar joint was also preserved. This preparation was made to show that opposition of the thumb does not ordinarily tansmit any motion to the bones of the carpus. To demonstrate that the joint between the first metacarpal and the trapezium was exposed by removal of the abductor brevis, the opponens, and the flexor brevis of the thumb. The double abductor longus was preserved, and the tendon of the flexor carpi radialis was left *in situ.*

Further investigation of this problem was made by roentgenographic control of the hand with the thumb in opposition and in normal attitude. The hand was placed on a flat surface, and a roentgenogram was taken with the palm facing the x-ray tube centered over the capitate bone. The thumb was placed in abduction and

extension; another roentgenogram was taken in the same position with the thumb in extreme opposition to the little finger.

The position of the hand was changed. A true lateral roentgenogram of the wrist centered over the midcarpal area through the scaphoid was taken with the thumb in opposition, and another

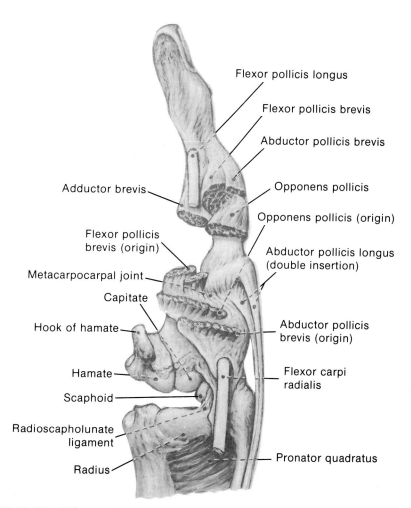

Flexor pollicis longus

Flexor pollicis brevis

Abductor pollicis brevis

Adductor brevis

Opponens pollicis

Opponens pollicis (origin)

Flexor pollicis
brevis (origin)

Abductor pollicis longus
(double insertion)

Metacarpocarpal joint

Capitate

Hook of hamate

Abductor pollicis
brevis (origin)

Hamate

Scaphoid

Flexor carpi
radialis

Radioscapholunate
ligament

Radius

Pronator quadratus

FIG. 7–18 Whereas in Figure 7–17 the thumb is in the normal position of rest, this figure shows complete forceful opposition of the thumb. The entire motion occurs in the joint between the first metacarpal and the trapezium. The relationship of the bones of the carpus does not change. The motion is not transmitted to the radioscaphoid despite the absence of the lunate and the triquetral bones and partial removal of the radiocarpal ligament. The opposition occurs in the trapeziometacarpal joint of the thumb and is possible because of the redundance of the capsule of this joint, as shown in Figure 3–7, and the configuration of the joint as shown in Figure 3–1.

roentgenogram was taken with the thumb in abduction and extension. These roentgenograms were taken in men and women of various ages and showed no significant displacement of the carpal bones from the normal position when the thumb passes into opposition. This series of roentgenograms thus confirmed the findings obtained in cadavers, namely, that the bones of

the carpus do not change their relative positions to any significant extent in opposition of the thumb.

The experiments on the muscles of the thumb indicated that for proper opposition the participation of the muscles of the thenar eminence is necessary and that the abductor longus and extensor brevis of the thumb may participate. It also showed that the distal phalanx can be extended separately in adduction and extension by the extensor pollicis longus. In abduction, the distal phalanx can be extended by the extensor brevis, which frequently inserts into the distal phalanx, in opposition, the distal phalanx extends most efficiently by action of the flexor brevis and the abductor brevis through their connection with the dorsal apparatus of the thumb and probably by the adductor pollicis, which also has connections with the dorsal apparatus (Figs. 3–13 and 3–22). The adductor also extends the distal phalanx in straight, neutral adduction.

The rotation in the trapeziometacarpal joint was observed mostly as a terminal motion of flexion and was possible because of the capsular redundance and the saddle configuration of the joint.

It is mentioned in the literature that rotation of the thumb occurs initially at the carpometacarpal joint and secondarily and *mostly* at the metacarpophalangeal joint. In multiple dissections of the thumb and in electric stimulation of the thenar muscles paired with experiments in 80 hands, it was definitely observed by the author that the entire rotation with opposition occurs principally and almost exclusively at the carpometacarpal joint. No rotation takes place at the metacarpophalangeal joint. The only movement produced at the metacarpophalangeal joint is, as mentioned previously, abduction of the proximal phalanx in extremes of opposition. In order to observe the rotatory factors of the thumb in opposition, the following experiments can be done on the living hand.

1. Pressure applied to the dorsum of the first metacarpal to flex it produces rotation of the entire thumb into full passive opposition. No rotation of the metacarpophalangeal joint is noticed. The same occurs in the cadaver.
2. Transfixion of the metacarpophalangeal joint in the cadaver by two cross-wires to prevent any motion in this joint, followed by pressure applied to the dorsum of the first metacarpal with the intent to flex the carpometacarpal joint, produces full opposition without abduction of the proximal phalanx.

3. The metacarpophalangeal joint, by arrangement of the lateral and accessory ligaments and the volar plate with the two sesamoids fixed in the plate, permits only the most insignificant rotation, not exceeding 5° to 8°.
4. Observations in cases of total ankylosis of the metacarpophalangeal joint showed no restriction of pronation. Opposition arises principally from the motion at the carpometacarpal joint under the action of the muscles, as outlined above, with addition of abduction of the proximal phalanx.

The function of the carpometacarpal joint is of major importance. It is necessary to consider the normal inclination of the articular surface of the trapezium and the first metacarpal in restoring opposition in cases of motor power loss and in pollicization procedures. This inclination can be established by roentgenographic comparison of both hands in cases of a single-hand injury or by statistical data. Terry, measuring this angle on skeletons, found that the angle varies between 44.19 and 47.06 and that there is no significant difference between the two hands.

Muscles of the hypothenar eminence
Experiments with the muscles of the hypothenar eminence showed the following:

The *abductor digiti minimi* produced slight flexion and strong abduction of the little finger by pulling the proximal phalanx into flexion and extending the two distal phalanges.
The *flexor digiti minimi brevis* produced very strong flexion of the proximal phalanx with slight adduction of the little finger and also slight flexion of the fifth metacarpal.
The *opponens digiti minimi* produced flexion of the fifth metacarpal with definite adduction of the metacarpal.

The experiments on the muscles of the hypothenar eminence, including the third palmar interosseous, indicated that their function consists of flexion and slight adduction of the fifth metacarpal to enhance opposition and also to flex the proximal phalanx and extend the two distal phalanges.

OBSERVATIONS IN NERVE INJURIES, VARIOUS PARALYSES, AND LOCAL INJURIES OF THE THUMB

Clinical observations of injuries to nerve trunks immediately after the injury and during the process of recovery and in cases of poliomyelitis and progressive muscular atrophy provide valuable means of appreciation of the action of the different muscles of the thumb.

Extensor Pollicis Longus. In the extensor pollicis longus isolated paralysis is observed rarely, but division of the tendon is common. When the tendon is interrupted proximal to the metacarpophalangeal joint, the distal phalanx rests in flexion, and the thumb is slightly abducted. Usually, there is also incomplete extension of the proximal phalanx. It is impossible in this case to adduct and extend the thumb simultaneously, but if the patient has an extensor brevis with prolongation of the insertion into the distal phalanx, complete extension of the distal phalanx is observed, but only in abduction. In opposition, the distal phalanx extends almost completely by the action of the abductor brevis and the flexor brevis, which flex, abduct, and rotate the thumb, simultaneously extending the distal phalanx. Even in neutral adduction without extension of the first metacarpal, the distal phalanx may extend actively through the expansion of the adductor into the dorsal apparatus of the thumb.

Testing the extensor pollicis longus requires full extension and simultaneous adduction of the first metacarpal. Under these circumstances, the inability to extend the distal phalanx denotes severance of the extensor pollicis longus; however, if a weak, limited range of extension of the distal phalanx is obtained after hyperflexion of the distal phalanx, this false extension results from passive tension of the tendon of the paralyzed extensor longus.

If there is absolutely no extension of the distal phalanx in adduction, abduction, or opposition, it indicates that the dorsal apparatus is interrupted completely, distal to the metacarpophalangeal joint. Paralysis of the extensor pollicis longus is not disabling, although it is quite annoying in buttoning, grasping of large objects, or the use of scissors. Often, the main disability is due to the complete extension of the proximal phalanx and the inability to elevate the adducted thumb dorsal to the plane of the hand.

Extensor Pollicis Brevis. The extensor pollicis brevis is rarely paralyzed without paralysis of the abductor longus as well. It is sometimes divided without involvement of the abductor longus. The resulting disability prevents full extension of the metacarpophalangeal joint in abduction of the thumb. In long-standing cases, the flexor pollicis brevis becomes contracted, and a peculiar deformity develops that is characterized by inability to extend the metacarpophalangeal joint and to abduct the thumb completely. The head of the first metacarpal stands out prominently, similar to a bunion of the big toe. This is observed not infrequently as a congenital deformity in some people who never have suffered paralysis of the extensor pollicis brevis or injury to this part of the hand.

The author encountered a thumb of this type in a pianist who had difficulty in stretching her hand widely because of persistent flexion of the metacarpophalangeal joint and prominence of the head of the first metacarpal.

On surgical exposure of the dorsum of the metacarpophalangeal joint, it was found that the extensor pollicis brevis was very thin and did not seem to reach its normal area of insertion at the radial side of the base of the proximal phalanx. This was considered to be caused by a variation similar to the insertion of the extensor brevis in the anthropoids, in which the tendon is either absent or fades over the dorsum of the first metacarpal.

The deformity was corrected in the following manner: The tendon of the extensor pollicis longus was split longitudinally in the middle from a point just proximal to the metacarpophalangeal joint to a point just distal to it. The split, radial half was cut across at the distal point but was left connected at the proximal end. The dorsal capsule of the joint was reefed longitudinally, and the radial half of the split-off tendon of the extensor pollicis longus was inserted securely to the radial base of the proximal phalanx where the extensor brevis inserts normally. The result was full and immediate correction of the deformity. Eight years after the operation the correction was still maintained, indicating that the absence of insertion of the extensor brevis probably was responsible for the deformity.

Abductor Pollicis Longus. The abductor pollicis longus acts in association with the extensor pollicis brevis as an abductor and extensor of the thumb by pulling the thumb out. It also acts in association with the abductor brevis when the hand and thumb are opened widely to grasp large objects.

In cases of paralysis of the abductor brevis, the thumb cannot be abducted completely despite a normal abductor pollicis longus and extensor pollicis brevis. Isolated injuries or paralysis of the abductor longus are very rare. When present, there is interference with extension of the first metacarpal.

In radial nerve paralysis when the extensor pollicis longus, extensor pollicis brevis, and abductor pollicis longus are affected simultaneously, the thumb is adducted or even pulled into the palm of the hand. The distal phalanx is sometimes flexed very slightly but can be extended by the action of the adductor pollicis, the flexor pollicis brevis, and the abductor brevis.

Strong function of the abductor pollicis longus requires the presence of a normal extensor carpi ulnaris; The flexor carpi radialis contracts secondarily.

The patient's ability to extend the proximal phalanx actively with the thumb in abduction is the usual test for the extensor pollicis brevis; first however, any contracture of the flexor pollicis brevis must be eliminated. Inability to abduct the thumb completely, despite a contracting abductor pollicis brevis, indicates a probable disability of the abductor pollicis longus, caused either by paralysis or division.

Flexor Pollicis Longus. The flexor pollicis longus is the only muscle capable of producing flexion of the distal phalanx. If the distal interphalangeal joint is moving passively but no active flexion can be produced, there is no activity in the flexor longus; however a semblance of flexion may be obtained on release of active or passive hyperextension of the distal phalanx caused by passive tension of the paralyzed muscle. It there is no motion at all, division of the tendon must be suspected.

The muscle has very insignificant action on flexion of the metacarpophalangeal joint. If there is paralysis of the thenar muscles, contraction of the flexor pollicis longus causes weak flexion of the metacarpophalangeal and carpometacarpal joints, although the distal phalanx contracts strongly.

Loss of flexion of the distal phalanx is a serious disability, especially in certain types of work (holding a needle, picking up small objects, or writing). Contractures in flexion are similar to disabilities observed in paralysis of the extensor pollicis longus but can be differentiated easily.

In high median nerve paralysis, the disorganization of the mechanism of pinch is extreme. The index finger cannot flex in any of the joints; the thumb cannot flex in any of the joints.

With contracture of the flexor pollicis longus the thumb may show strong flexion with forearm supination and be almost extended with pronation of the forearm. Lengthening the tendon may restore function and is probably a more logical operative procedure than advancement of the origin of the muscle, which may easily disturb the muscular nerve supply.

An interesting type of contracture of the flexor pollicis longus was observed by the author. A patient sustained a fracture of the two bones of the forearm just below the elbow; he was treated by immobilization, but soon after the treatment was completed he developed a functional flexion-contracture of the distal phalanx of the thumb that was evident only when the forearm was in supination. The distal phalanx would return to the normal position in pronation of the forearm. He was first seen by the author several years following the initial treatment. The peculiar behavior of the distal phalanx was explained by a probable contracture of the additional origin of the flexor pollicis longus from the ulna (muscle of Ganzer), which followed injury at the time of fracture. A simple lengthening of the tendon of the flexor pollicis longus at the wrist restored normal function of the distal phalanx, which was maintained several years later on follow-up examination.

THENAR MUSCLES

Clinical analysis of the muscles of the thenar eminence and the hypothenar eminence must consider the frequent variations in the nerve supply. The muscles are supplied by the median and the ulnar nerves.

The standard pattern of innervation, according to Rowntree, was encountered only in about a third of 226 cases. In 2% of this series, the three thenar muscles were supplied by the median nerve; in 2% of the same series, the thenar muscles and the adductor were supplied by the median nerve. In 1%, all the thenar muscles, the adductor, and the first dorsal interosseous were supplied by the median nerve. In 32%, the flexor brevis was supplied by the ulnar nerve; in 15½%, the flexor pollicis brevis had a double nerve supply; in 33%, the whole flexor brevis was supplied by the median nerve.

Of course, there are rare cases in which the entire nerve supply to the muscles of the hypothenar eminence, all the interossei, and the thenar eminence are supplied by the median nerve, as seen by the author and described by others.

It is very difficult to observe clinically the separate action of each small muscle of the thumb and the hypothenar eminence. Precise analysis of the action of each muscle, especially in the presence of variations of nerve supply, is hardly possible. There is definite evidence that dominance of one group or the other takes place in the activity of the thumb, as it takes place in the fingers and probably in all parts of the system. In cases of poliomyelitis and progressive muscular atrophy, when separate muscles may become completely paralyzed and atrophied,

studies of the remaining, relatively normal muscles bring important information.

Abductor Pollicis Brevis.   When the separate action of the abductor brevis can be observed, it produces abduction and flexion of the metacarpal and slight flexion of the proximal phalanx with simultaneous extension of the distal phalanx. Pronation of the entire thumb occurring in the carpometacarpal joint is simultaneous with the flexion of the first metacarpal. This motion is sufficient to provide normal opposition to the middle finger. The flexion and rotation of the first metacarpal become more efficient with the help of the opponens muscle, which flexes the first metacarpal and produces additional slight rotation at the carpometacarpal joint. The flexion of the first metacarpal by the opponens apparently does not go beyond the metacarpal of the index finger (Duchenne).

Flexor Pollicis Brevis.   The flexor pollicis brevis can be examined in its action in cases of progressive muscular atrophy when the abductor brevis is paralyzed. It produces extension of the distal phalanx, flexion of the proximal phalanx, and flexion with slight rotation of the first metacarpal, which occurs at the carpometacarpal joint at the termination of flexion; however, only the radial head of the flexor brevis has no abductor action. It cannot, however, pull the thumb sufficiently far forward, although it is able to flex the first metacarpal beyond the middle phalanx to the little finger. By itself it is unable to produce complete opposition to the little finger.

The *abductor brevis* is a more important muscle of opposition because it produces almost complete opposition by itself and complete opposition with the help of the opponens. It is true that this opposition does not go beyond the middle finger, but most of the activities of the hand do not require any more opposition.

Opponens Pollicis.   The opponens pollicis has never been observed to act in isolation in this author's experience. Duchenne states that

the opponens of the thumb flexes the first metacarpal with force and pulls it inward so that its head reaches the second metacarpal. It produces less opposition than the short abductor and the superficial head of the short flexor of the thumb.

Adductor Pollicis. The adductor pollicis produces strong adduction of the first metacarpal and pulls this metacarpal into close contact with the skin of the palm proximal to the middle finger. Simultaneously, it extends the distal phalanx if the flexor pollicis longus is not contracted strongly. Others have claimed that in its movement it simultaneously produces rotation of the first metacarpal and the phalanges of the thumb in reverse of opposition but the author never observed this reverse of opposition. The reverse of opposition is apparently activated by the extensor pollicis longus with the help of the adductor, which helps to overcome the action of the abductor brevis and the flexor brevis; the extensor longus overcomes the action of the abductor longus and the extensor brevis. The radial (first metacarpal) head of the first dorsal interosseous muscle assists the adductor pollicis.

Interaction of thenar muscles
The normal position of rest of the thumb is maintained by the balance of all the muscles of the thumb. When the thumb opens for a wide grasp, all the muscles participate, either as fixation muscles or actual motors. The long abductor and the short extensor pull the thumb out, the extensor longus extends the distal phalanx, but the abductor brevis, predominates over the adductor component of the extensor pollicis longus and the adductor pollicis.

When a round pinch between the thumb and the index finger is required, all the muscles of the thenar eminence are activated. The first dorsal interosseous and the adductor pollicis are in strong action; the flexor pollicis longus is in strong pull, overcoming the extensor component of the thenar muscles. The flexor profundus and the sublimis indicis overbalance the pull of the interossei. While the interossei are overcoming the pull of the extensors digitorum and the proprius of the index finger at the metacarpophalangeal joint, the abductor longus, the extensor longus, and the extensor brevis are also

active but subordinated to the action of the other muscles. Any disturbance of this balance weakens the pinch.

Some people can normally hyperextend the metacarpophalangeal joint of the thumb considerably, holding the distal phalanx extended or flexed. This is usually associated with the ability to hyperextend the proximal interphalangeal joints of all the fingers. This condition never causes complaints of disability and is probably caused by relaxation of the capsule of the metacarpophalangeal joint proximal to the sesamoids and selective extension of the extensor pollicis brevis. It is the opposite of what is observed in cases of insufficiency of the extensor pollicis brevis or contracture of the flexor pollicis brevis.

When a pinch is required with the index finger and the thumb held like pincers, the interossei of the index and first lumbrical are active, producing flexion of the metacarpophalangeal joint and extension of the distal phalanx of the index finger against the flexor sublimis. The thenar muscles are actively engaged in opposition against the action of the adductor pollicis.

Normally, complete adduction between the first and second metacarpals is produced by the adductor pollicis and the extensor pollicis longus with the aid of the first dorsal interosseous. The extensor pollicis longus acts primarily as extensor of the first metacarpal, the proximal phalanx, and the distal phalanx; then adductor action is provided. In the action of pinch between the thumb and the index finger, the adductor pollicis plays an important role of adduction, which is enhanced by the action of the first dorsal interosseous, but it also acts as an extensor of the distal phalanx of the thumb through the extension of the adductor into the dorsal expansion of the thumb.

In ulnar nerve paralysis, the pinch is extremely weak because this double action of the adductor pollicis is lost. The loss of extension of the distal phalanx of the thumb is even more pronounced by the loss of the flexor pollicis brevis (when supplied by the ulnar nerve), which also has an extension into the dorsal expansion of the thumb. Thus, in ulnar nerve paralysis an attempt to pinch between the index finger and the thumb results in strong flexion of the distal phalanx of the thumb but not enough power to hold any objects between the two. A slip of paper held between the tips of the thumb and the index finger can be pulled out easily by the examiner. This is known as *Froment's sign.* An analysis of this condition, first described by Froment, was given recently by McFarland. The forced flexion of the distal phalanx is caused by the effort of the flexor pollicis longus to overcome the absence of extension due to paralyzed adductor pollicis and flexor pollicis brevis and paralysis of the first dorsal interosseous.

In cases of atrophy or paralysis of the thenar muscles, the extensor pollicis longus predominates over the abductor longus and the extensor brevis and pulls the thumb into adduction. If only the abductor brevis is paralyzed but the flexor brevis remains active, as can be observed in certain cases of median nerve paralysis when the entire flexor brevis is supplied by the ulnar nerve, the long abductor cannot substitute for the abductor brevis to achieve true opposition.

The abductor longus, pulling the thumb completely outward, eliminates the action of the flexor pollicis brevis; however, aided by the adductor, the flexor pollicis brevis is capable of flexing the first metacarpal toward the little finger, sliding it along the palm.

When opposition is required to the index or even the middle finger, the palmaris longus usually does not participate in this motion; however, should forceful opposition be required to the little finger, the palmaris longus, when present, contracts with force. Simultaneously, the flexor digiti minimi and the opponens digiti minimi brevis contract; the fifth metacarpal flexes and adducts at the metacarpocarpal joint. Sometimes, there is slight semblance of opposition; thus, for forceful opposition between the thumb and the little finger, integrity of the hypothenar muscles is required. The abductor digiti minimi does not contract in this motion. The distance between the tip of the hamate hook and the tubercle of the trapezium does not

decrease. The palmaris longus probably contracts with the abductor pollicis brevis.

Restoration of opposition by tendon transfer and tendon grafting, developed to a high degree of proficiency by Bunnell, indicates that the substitution for the entire group of thenar muscles by one motor is sufficient for very satisfactory function with the exception, perhaps, of complete extension of the distal phalanx.

MUSCLES OF THE HYPOTHENAR EMINENCE

The Palmaris Brevis. The most mysterious muscle from a functional and developmental viewpoint, is the palmaris brevis. It is almost never absent in the human hand. (The author found it in the gorilla hand.) The muscle is embedded in the hypothenar fat pad and contracts when the abductor or the flexor digiti minimi contract, creasing the skin of the base of the hypothenar eminence. In forceful contraction of the abductor or the flexor of the little finger, the pisiform bone is displaced a few millimeters distally while the creasing occurs; however, when the flexor carpi ulnaris contracts, there is very little displacement of the pisiform, and usually there is no contraction of the palmaris brevis, if this is judged by the creasing of the skin.

Abductor Digiti Minimi. The abductor digiti minimi is a significant muscle, producing very strong abduction of the fifth finger, which is almost always accompanied by slight extension of the two distal phalanges of the little finger.

When the abductor digiti minimi is paralyzed, the extensor proprius of the little finger produces efficient abduction but no extension of the two distal phalanges.

Flexor Digiti Minimi Brevis. The flexor digiti minimi brevis is a strong flexor of the proximal phalanx with extension of the two distal phalanges. Its paralysis in ulnar nerve injuries, when the injury of the ulnar nerve is distal to the supply of the flexor profundus, shows definitely that it is the real and efficient flexor of the metacarpophalangeal joint of the little finger because flexion of this joint, despite the active flexors profundus and the sublimis, is usually inefficient. It also produces variable, active flexion of the fifth metacarpal with slight adduction. In paralysis of the hypothenar muscles, this flexion-adduction of the little finger disappears, making opposition of the thumb to the little finger more difficult.

MOTORS AND MECHANISM OF ACTION OF THE WRIST*

The movements of the wrist are closely associated with the action of the fingers and thumb. The position of the wrist is essential for normal function of the extensors or flexors and the abductors and adductors. The wrist can be flexed (volarflexed) or extended (dorsiflexed), abducted and adducted. The range of flexion and extension varies within the same age group and tends to decrease with age. Abduction or radial inclination is usually less marked than adduction or ulnar inclination. Circumduction is an uninterrupted motion through flexion, extension, abduction, and adduction. The motions of the wrist joint occur in the radiocarpal, intercarpal, and carpometacarpal joints. The proximal row of the carpal bones, excluding the pisiform, constitutes a functional unit; the distal row of the carpal bones, except for the trapezium, represents another unit. The scaphoid bone forms a functional link between the distal and proximal rows. The mechanics of the wrist joint were thoroughly investigated. At times, the approach was too mechanistic and mathematical for practical clinical purposes; at other times, it relied so much on experimental work with cadavers that the conclusions were inapplicable to the wrists of live subjects.

A combined extensive study of the mechanism of the normal wrist and the complexities of dislocations, fractures, and posttraumatic disabilities based on all available means (experimental anatomy, experimental roentgenography, anatomy, pathology) is still needed. Recent

investigations of wrist movement are based on the work of Fick.

Normally, volar flexion of the hand takes place mostly in the radiocarpal joint and secondarily in the midcarpal joint. Dorsiflexion, on the contrary, occurs mostly in the midcarpal joint and additionally in the radiocarpal joint. Radial deviation occurs mostly in the midcarpal joint, and ulnar deviation mostly in the radiocarpal articulation. The radiocarpal joint is comparatively simple and presents a concave articular surface proximally and a completely convex carpal surface distally. The articular surface of the midcarpal joint is more complicated and presents two dissimilar parts: the ulnar and the radial. The ulnar part of the midcarpal joint is formed by the ulnar side of the scaphoid, the distal side of the lunate, and the distal aspect of the triquetral in the proximal row, and the capitate and the hamate in the distal row. The radial part of the midcarpal articulation is represented by the base of the navicular and the proximal aspect of the trapezium and trapezoid.

The ulnar part of the midcarpal is similar to a mobile, diarthrodial, multiaxial joint with the center passing through the head of the capitate bone. The radial part of the midcarpal is a comparatively immobile gliding joint (Fig. 2–2). The relative positions of the carpal bones or the distal row, including the trapezium, change very little in any motion of the wrist. There is very little motion between the distal carpal row and the bases of the second and third metacarpals. The fourth has an extremely limited range of flexion and extension and is moved by the pull of the fifth metacarpal base, which has a wider range of flexion produced by the hypothenar muscles.

The articulation between the trapezium and the first metacarpal is very mobile, as mentioned earlier. The area of stability of the first metacarpal corresponding to the area of carpometacarpal stability of all the other metacarpals is transferred to the articulation between the scaphoid bone and the trapezium. This mechanism apparently developed in response to the greater mobility of the thumb.

In the author's experiments on the cadaver, roentgenographic investigations of the relative

---

* This section pertaining to the wrist contains Dr. Kaplan's unrevised material.

position of the carpal bones in opposition of the thumb and unrestricted motion of opposition in surgical fusion of the wrist joint convinced him that the opposition of the thumb does not produce any significant changes in the relative positions of the trapezium and the scaphoid bone.

It is estimated by some that 65% to 75% of volar flexion and 55% to 60% of ulnar deviations occur in the radiocarpal articulation, and that 75% to 85% of dorsal flexion and 60% to 65% of radial deviation take place in the midcarpal articulation.

The carpal bones of the proximal row change their relation in the movements of the wrist because of the special position of the scaphoid bone, which belongs to the distal and proximal rows. Some free motion definitely occurs between the scaphoid and the lunate and the lunate and the triquetral in volar flexion, although the range of this motion is decidedly variable. In certain fresh specimens, it appears to be practically nonexistent, while in others it is quite marked. It is possible that individuals who have a wider range of mobility of the carpal bones of the proximal row are more susceptible to dislocations of the lunate bone. The wedgelike form of the lunate with its volar aspect wider than the dorsal in relation to the scaphoid and the triquetral makes its position relatively insecure in dorsiflexion of the wrist. The scaphoid, the lunate, and the triquetral appear to be closer together in dorsiflexion.

In specially dissected wrists with the collateral ligaments preserved (Figs. 4-5 and, 4-13*A*) the proximal row of bones of the carpus show motion between each other in volar and dorsiflexion of the wrist. In dorsiflexion, the posterior margin of the radius appears to push the lunate volad from behind, thus contributing to its possible dislocation in sudden and forceful dorsiflexion of the wrist.

Motion in the radiocarpal, midcarpal, and between the carpal bones of the proximal row occurs continuously and smoothly, passing from one stage to the other without interruption, either in dorsal or volar flexion, radial and ulnar deviation, or circumduction.

Roentgenographic investigations of the motion of the carpal bones show the following:

1. In hyperflexion, the lunate turns its distal articular surface anteriorly; the capitate turns and becomes almost vertical; the head of the capitate is barely palpable from the dorsal aspect of the wrist. The lunate is almost horizontal, oriented such that its proximal articular surface is dorsal, instead of being in contact with the articular surface of the radius. The proximal end of the scaphoid follows the lunate in its dorsal rotation, while the distal end of the scaphoid follows the base of the capitate. The scaphoid becomes more or less vertical under these circumstances (Fig. 7–19).

2. In extension and hyperextension, the lunate turns its distal articular surface dorsally; the capitate turns and becomes vertical with its base oriented dorsally (if the forearm is held horizontally); the head of the capitate is completely unpalpable because it is placed completely volad in contact with the distal articular surface of the lunate. The neck of the capitate abuts the posterior lip of the radius. The proximal end of the scaphoid follows the lunate, but the distal part of the scaphoid follows the capitate only partially, straining the scaphotrapezial articulation. The scaphoid bone forms an angle with the capitate, open dorsally (Fig. 7–19).

3. In radial inclination, the entire proximal surface of the scaphoid is in contact with the articular surface of the radius; the styloid process of the radius touches the trapezium; the lunate moves under the triangular cartilage; the capitate is almost vertical. The range of radial inclination is not as marked as the range of ulnar inclination (Fig. 7–20).

4. In ulnar inclination, the lunate moves nearer to the radial styloid process; the capitate deflects slightly to the ulnar side of the hand. The center of rotation in the midcarpal joint passes through the head of the capitate in radial and ulnar deviations.

Interesting results were obtained by the author in limited experiments on which movement in cadavers with well-preserved movable joints, transfixed by wires through the skin in various combinations to observe by the roentgenograms how transfixion influences the various movements of the wrist. In the first experiment, the two bones of the forearm were

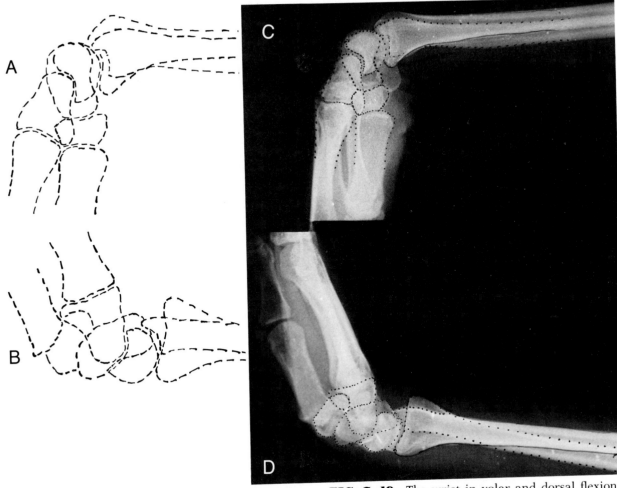

FIG. 7–19 The wrist in volar and dorsal flexions. **A**, Volar flexion with outlines of the capitate, lunate, scaphoid, and trapezium. **B**, The wrist in dorsiflexion (extension) with the same bones in changed relationship. **C**, In volar flexion, most of the proximal articular surface of the lunate can be palpated dorsally. The capitate is almost vertical with the base downward; the scaphoid tends to become almost parallel with the capitate. **D**, In dorsiflexion, the lunate recedes almost completely under the radius; the capitate is vertical with the base upward; the scaphoid forms an angle with the capitate of almost 90 degrees.

transfixed by a horizontal wire proximal to the distal radioulnar joint; this prevented supination and pronation but did not appreciably alter flexion and extension, as well as abduction and adduction of the wrist. Transfixion of the scaphoid and the lunate bones did not change radial or ulnar deviation, or flexion and extension of the wrist. Transfixion of the scaphoid and the lunate from the radial side and the lunate and the triquetral from the ulnar side did not appear to influence abduction, adduction, flexion, or extension of the wrist. This experiment indicated that the proximal row of the carpal bones apparently acts as a single unit between the radius and the triangular ligament; however, this experiment will have to be amplified by various combinations of carpal bone transfix-

ions. It is obvious that accurate studies of the relationship of the movement between the distal and proximal rows of bones will have to be continued.

A study of the various curves of the carpal bones in relation to the movement of the wrist was made by VanLamoen. It showed that the

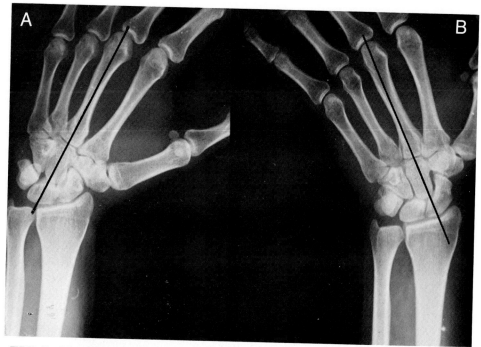

FIG. 7—20 Roentgenogram of the hand in ulnar and radial deviations, showing the movement of the axis of the third metacarpal and the capitate in relation to the lunate and the scaphoid. **A**, The combined axis of the third metacarpal and the capitate passes through the middle of the lunate and intersects the distal radioulnar joint in radial deviation. **B**, The combined axis of the third metacarpal and the capitate passes through the proximal part of the scaphoid in ulnar deviation.

movements of the individual carpal bones are more complex than the ordinary x-ray films usually indicate and are conditioned by the irregularities of the surfaces of the capitate, lunate, and scaphoid bones. MacConaill's studies of the mechanics of wrist joint movement are also significant.

MUSCLES OF THE WRIST

All of the muscles of the wrist are attached to the metacarpals, except the flexor carpi ulnaris. Motion is transmitted through the fixed carpometacarpal articulations to the midcarpal and the radiocarpal joints. Additional attachments to the carpal bones occasionally occur. All these muscles work conjointly. For descriptive and analytic purposes, they are separated into the following groups:

Flexors:
  Flexor carpi radialis
  Flexor carpi ulnaris
  Palmaris longus
  Long flexors of the fingers
  Abductor pollicis longus
Extensors:
  Extensor carpi radialis longus and brevis
  Extensor carpi ulnaris
  Extensors digitorum communis and proprius of the little and index fingers
  Extensor pollicis longus
Radial Deviators:
  Abductor pollicis longus
  Extensor carpi radialis longus
  Flexor carpi radialis
Ulnar Deviators:
  Extensor carpi ulnaris
  Flexor carpi ulnaris

Flexor Carpi Radialis. The flexor carpi radialis is inserted into the volar aspect of the base of the second metacarpal and not infrequently into the base of the third metacarpal as well; it also has frequent insertions into the trapezium. It acts as a strong flexor of the wrist, transmitting its pull to the midcarpal articulation, mostly on the radial side of the hand. In conjunction with the extensor carpi radialis longus, it produces radial inclination of the hand. The flexor carpi radialis contracts strongly when the finger extensors are in action. This action is apparently synergistic with the contraction of the extensors of the fingers. When the common extensors are paralyzed, an attempt to extend the fingers results in flexion of the wrist. Very strong contraction of the flexor carpi radialis produces some pronation of the forearm after complete flexion of the wrist.

Flexor Carpi Ulnaris. Isolated contraction of the flexor carpi ulnaris induces flexion of the wrist over the ulnar side of the hand. In strong contraction, it actually produces slight supination of the ulnar border of the hand.

Duchenne denied its action as an ulnar deviator, basing his conclusions on absence of ulnar deviation when the muscle was stimulated separately by faradic current. He also thought that in the neutral position of the forearm, strong flexion of the wrist eliminated any ulnar deviation of the wrist because of the close contact of the joint surfaces.

The following can be observed by palpation:

In extension, ulnar deviation of the wrist is not accompanied by simultaneous contraction of the flexor carpi ulnaris.

In flexion, the flexor carpi ulnaris contracts strongly when ulnar deviation is attempted against resistance.

In the neutral position, between supination and pronation of the forearm, the flexor carpi ulnaris contracts strongly with the extensor carpi ulnaris, if ulnar deviation is resisted. If there is no resistance to ulnar deviation, there is remarkably little contraction of the flexor carpi ulnaris.

When abduction of the thumb is attempted in a normal hand, the flexor carpi ulnaris does not contract, while the extensor carpi ulnaris contracts very strongly. This shows that the ulnar fixation of the wrist necessary for adequate abduction of the thumb is not produced by the flexor carpi ulnaris, as would be expected were this muscle an important ulnar deviator.

Palmaris Longus. The action of the palmaris longus is not always very clear. The relation of the tendon of insertion of the muscle to the volar carpal ligament conditions its action.

The palmaris longus is considered to be a flexor of the wrist. Frequently, flexion of the wrist is achieved in the cadaver and during surgical procedures by traction applied to the tendon, but sometimes flexion is not achieved in the same type of experiments. The absence of flexor action on the wrist is easily explained in these cases by the continuation of the tendon into the midpalmar aponeurosis without firm connections with the volar carpal ligament, or by the insertion of the tendon proximal to the volar carpal ligament.

The muscle is considered to be a synergist in thumb opposition; it contracts strongly, and its tendon becomes very tense when opposition of the thumb is attempted or maintained. The contraction was thought to produce synergistic tension of the volar carpal ligament to provide better fixation at the origins of the thenar muscles.

Frequently, the tendon is inserted into the abductor pollicis brevis (Fig. 2–30) or the hypothenar muscles and apparently acts directly on these muscles in opposition. Tensing of the volar carpal ligament was not observed either on surgical exposure or in the experiments on the cadaver and is problematic; however, direct contraction of the palmaris longus with tension of its tendon is frequently observed in abduction of the thumb and is probably caused by the relation of the tendon to the abductor pollicis brevis.

The palmaris longus is an unimportant flexor of the wrist and a strong synergist of abduction of the thumb and through abduction, with opposition of the thumb. In paralysis of other flexors of the wrist, it may become a fairly important flexor if it is firmly connected to the volar carpal ligament or with the bones of the carpus.

Long Flexors of the Fingers. The long flexors, as was indicated previously, normally have very insignificant flexor action on the wrist. The comparative shortness of the extensors of the fingers does not permit flexion of the wrist when the fingers are flexed. In normal hands, strong flexion by the long flexors of the fingers produces a synergistic contraction of the extensors of the wrist. The regulation of this synergy is so nearly perfect that the slightest contraction of the long flexors of the fingers produces a proportionate contraction of the extensors of the wrist. Thus, the long flexors of the fingers, paradoxically, should be considered extensors of the wrist, instead of flexors of the wrist when the fingers are flexed.

In the cadaver, traction of the long flexors of the fingers produces flexion of the wrist. If the fingers are prevented from flexion in the distal and proximal interphalangeal joints, either by extension contracture of these joints or by outside resistance, the long flexors of the fingers may become flexors of the wrist.

Abductor Pollicis Longus. Contractions of the abductor pollicis longus produce abduction and flexion of the thumb through traction of the first metacarpal. When abduction and flexion of the first metacarpal are at a maximum by the action of this muscle, further contraction produces flexion and radial deviation of the hand; however, this action is effective only with the synergistic coaction of the abductor pollicis brevis and the extensor carpi ulnaris. In a case of paralysis of either or both of these muscles, the thumb cannot be abducted effectively despite the presence of an active abductor pollicis longus. Naturally, the wrist flexion that follows the normal abduction and flexion of the thumb cannot be executed by the abductor pollicis longus in the presence of paralysis of the abductor brevis and the extensor carpi ulnaris.

Extensors Carpi Radialis Longus and Brevis and the Extensor Carpi Ulnaris. Contraction of the extensors transmits their action to the radiocarpal and midcarpal joints. The long radial extensor extends the wrist with radial deviation. The short radial extensor is an almost straight dorsal extensor. When the two act together the extension of the wrist is very strong, with marked radial deviation. In very strong dorsiflexion against resistance, the two radial extensors act together with the extensor carpi ulnaris.

The radial extensors and the extensor carpi ulnaris act together as synergists of the long flexors of the fingers. Whenever the long flexors of the fingers contract, the two radial extensors and the extensor carpi ulnaris contract simultaneously and directly in proportion to the force used by the flexors of the fingers. Patients with paralysis of the long flexors (profundus and superficialis) dorsiflex their wrists whenever they are asked to flex the fingers.

The extensor carpi ulnaris contracts strongly when abduction of the thumb is attempted and maintained. In ulnar deviation, the extensor carpi ulnaris contracts with the flexor carpi ulnaris; the stronger contraction is felt in the extensor carpi ulnaris. In radial deviation, the extensor carpi radialis longus contracts simultaneously with the abductor pollicis longus. However, in this case, slight action of the abductor pollicis prevents the thumb from abduction and permits comparatively free motion of the thumb in radial deviation of the wrist. Isolated paralysis or division of the radial extensors produces a continuous pull of the hand toward the ulna. This can be very disabling.

The Common and Proper Extensors. The common and proper extensors of the fingers participate in the motion of the wrist in a complex manner. It has been stated previously and is well established that the strong extension of the fingers in the interphalangeal and metacarpophalangeal joints produces synergistic and simultaneous contraction of the flexor carpi radialis and the flexor carpi ulnaris. The extension of the interphalangeal joints with extension of the metacarpophalangeal joint of a finger is caused by simultaneous action of the intrinsic muscles and the long digital extensors. The intrinsic muscles extend the interphalangeal joints and simultaneously flex the metacarpophalangeal joint.

The extensor communis overcomes the flexor element of the intrinsic muscle on the metacarpophalangeal joint and extends this joint; it also extends the middle phalanx. Only the extension of all the joints of the fingers produces synergistic action of the flexors of the wrist (the flexor carpi radialis and ulnaris), and full extension is produced by the extensor communis and the intrinsic muscles together. Under these circumstances, the extensor communis does not produce any extensor action on the wrist.

If the fingers are relaxed in flexion and the wrist is extended against resistance, the extensor communis contracts and brings a few degrees of additional extension with simultaneous, slight extension of the metacarpophalangeal joints without contraction of the flexor carpi radialis and ulnaris but with further contraction of the finger flexors in the interphalangeal joints. If the extended fingers are pushed into flexion while the wrist is extended, the flexor carpi radialis and the carpi ulnaris relax greatly.

In one case of fusion of the interphalangeal joints of the four fingers, the extensor communis produced a slight additional extension of the wrist, simultaneously extending the metacar-pophalangeal joints. In one case observed by the author of complete division of the long flexors of all the fingers, hyperextension of the metacarpophalangeal joints did not produce additional extension of the wrist. Further observations of such cases are necessary for more definite information concerning extension of the wrist by the common and proper extensors.

In summary, the extensor communis and the extensor proprius, under certain exceptional conditions, may have slight extensor action on the wrist.

Extensor Pollicis Longus. The extensor pollicis longus is apparently capable of producing limited extension of the wrist in exceptional cases, as a terminal phase after extending the distal and proximal phalanges and the first metacarpal.

The variations of the muscles and their insertions, the state of the ligaments of the joints, the vagaries of nerve supply, and the peculiarities of certain afflictions of the nervous or muscular systems may present problems difficult to interpret and analyze, requiring meticulous and thorough observations of groups of muscles and motion as a whole.

Important Muscular Variations of the Hand and Forearm

Emanuel B. Kaplan
Morton Spinner

Variations in general and especially muscular variations are important to the surgeon. The description of variations and their relationship to comparative anatomy preoccupied the anatomists of the 19th century, but gradually the interest faded, and now only occasionally is description found in the special surgical literature.

In the description of muscles given earlier, some of the variations are mentioned. The variations observed by the authors during surgical procedures and personal dissections were supplemented with observations collected during anatomic dissections by medical students. Only muscles having direct action on the hand and wrist will be described.

EXTRINSIC MUSCLES

Flexor Carpi Radialis. The flexor carpi radialis varies at the site of insertion. Occasionally, an insertion is found to the trapezium either in the tunnel of passage or outside to the ridge of this bone, or an insertion may be found into the scaphoid tubercle anteriorly. Once the tendon passes into the hand, the insertion runs toward the base of the second metacarpal and may extend toward the third and fourth metacarpals. A tendinous extension occasionally may run toward the abductor pollicis brevis.

Palmaris Longus. The palmaris longus is one of the most variable muscles. Its use in hand surgery as a source of tendon material for free tendon grafts makes its variations important.

The palmaris longus may present the following arrangement in the forearm. It may consist of a tendon only from the origin to insertion or consist of a muscle body only. The structure may be reversed, presenting a tendinous origin and a fleshy insertion into the palmar fascia or a fleshy body in the middle and a tendinous origin and insertion (Fig. 7–21). At times, there are two muscles running from the origin to insertion as two independent parallel structures with variations of origin or insertion patterns (Fig. 9–21). A variation was even reported in which the muscle consisted of three distinct muscles. The variations of origin are numerous. The muscle may come from almost any muscle of the ulnar side of the forearm or from the coronoid process of the ulna. Its insertions also are variable. It may be absent or may stop at the antebrachial fascia, or scaphoid or pisiform, or the abductor pollicis brevis.

Although most of the variations were described by LeDouble, Testut, and English anatomists, the authors observed a case of a double palmaris longus, in which one head arose from the common origin of muscles on the medial epicondyle and the other from the fascia covering the flexor superficialis. The epicondylar muscle became tendinous at the junction of the upper and middle third of the forearm and inserted into the transverse carpal ligament; the second fascially originating head ran parallel with and radial to the epicondylar head of the muscle. This tendon reached the transverse carpal ligament, crossed it, and continued into the midpalmar fascia of the hand (Fig. 7–21C).

In two other instances, the flexor superficialis to the little finger was absent. The palmaris longus tendon crossed the transverse carpal ligament and joined the abductor pollicis brevis. At the point of insertion of the palmaris longus tendon to the abductor pollicis brevis, a musculotendinous branch came off and supplied a structure running into the flexor tunnel of the little finger.

A case was observed in which the palmaris

Variation—reversed
palmaris longus

A

H. Thomas

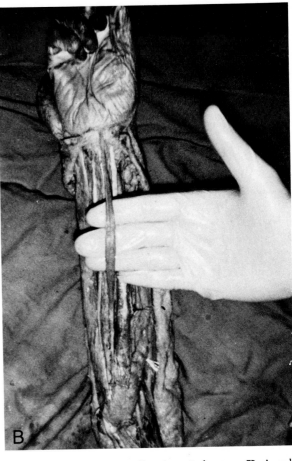

B

FIG. 7–21   **A**, Reversed palmaris longus. **B**, A palmaris longus muscular from origin to insertion. **C**, Variant palmaris longus arising from the fascia of the flexor digitorum superficialis.

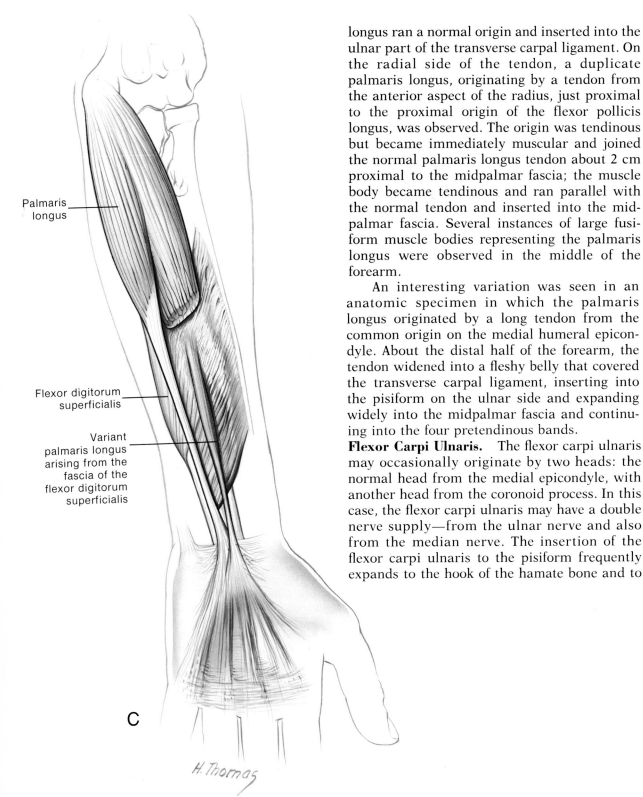

Palmaris longus

Flexor digitorum superficialis

Variant palmaris longus arising from the fascia of the flexor digitorum superficialis

C

H. Thomas

longus ran a normal origin and inserted into the ulnar part of the transverse carpal ligament. On the radial side of the tendon, a duplicate palmaris longus, originating by a tendon from the anterior aspect of the radius, just proximal to the proximal origin of the flexor pollicis longus, was observed. The origin was tendinous but became immediately muscular and joined the normal palmaris longus tendon about 2 cm proximal to the midpalmar fascia; the muscle body became tendinous and ran parallel with the normal tendon and inserted into the midpalmar fascia. Several instances of large fusiform muscle bodies representing the palmaris longus were observed in the middle of the forearm.

An interesting variation was seen in an anatomic specimen in which the palmaris longus originated by a long tendon from the common origin on the medial humeral epicondyle. About the distal half of the forearm, the tendon widened into a fleshy belly that covered the transverse carpal ligament, inserting into the pisiform on the ulnar side and expanding widely into the midpalmar fascia and continuing into the four pretendinous bands.

Flexor Carpi Ulnaris.   The flexor carpi ulnaris may occasionally originate by two heads: the normal head from the medial epicondyle, with another head from the coronoid process. In this case, the flexor carpi ulnaris may have a double nerve supply—from the ulnar nerve and also from the median nerve. The insertion of the flexor carpi ulnaris to the pisiform frequently expands to the hook of the hamate bone and to to the fifth and sometimes the fourth metacarpal bases. A definite muscle expansion is frequently continued between the pisiform and the hook of the hamate; this muscle is the uncipisiform muscle. The tendon of insertion into the pisiform not infrequently continues directly into the abductor digiti minimi.

Flexor Superficialis. The flexor superficialis frequently varies in origin as well as in insertion. The muscle may have an additional origin from the coronoid process with insertions to the flexor profundus or the flexor pollicis longus. Occasionally, the muscle body is separated into four distinct units for each finger. Not infrequently, a flexor superficialis to the little finger may be completely absent; at times, this absent flexor superficialis may be substituted by a muscle from the palmaris longus as described above, from the transverse carpal ligament, or even from a lumbrical. Quain mentions rare cases in which the medial and lateral tendons are absent and replaced by a sheet of muscle representing an additional superficial flexor. LeDouble mentions a case described by Turner in which a slip of the flexor superficialis crossed to the palmaris longus and joined the lower part of the brachioradialis.

Flexor Digitorum Profundus. The connections between the flexor digitorum profundus and the flexor superficialis may assume various forms. A connection of the flexor profundus with the flexor pollicis longus through a slip connecting the flexor profundus of the index finger with the flexor pollicis longus is not infrequent. This is important because the flexor profundus to the index finger may form an independent part of the flexor profundus, assuring a varying degree of free movement of the index finger. An extension of the flexor profundus may be found originating proximal to the pronator teres from the radius, crossing the pronator teres, and joining the main body of the flexor profundus. The connection of the flexor profundus with the part of the flexor profundus to the index finger may assume various forms. In two cases observed by the author, a muscle slip emerged just proximal to the tendinous portion of the flexor pollicis longus. Running parallel with the normal tendon of the flexor pollicis longus, it entered the carpal canal, passing between the tendon of the flexor pollicis longus and the tendon of the profundus indicis. Before coming out of the carpal canal the accessory tendon split into two parts— one part joining the flexor profundus indicis tendon and another lateral part joining the first lumbrical muscle. In one case, the flexor profundus to the little finger was absent; instead, the flexor superficialis to the little finger just proximal to the transverse carpal ligament divided into a posterior and an anterior tendon. The anterior tendon represented a normal flexor superficialis; the posterior tendon ran as a normal flexor profundus. The lumbrical muscle to the little finger did not originate from the variant flexor profundus tendon but from the flexor profundus tendon of the ring finger together with its lumbrical to the ring finger. The flexor digitorum profundus of the little finger can send a slip to the flexor superficialis of the ring finger (Fig. 7–22, *insert*).

Flexor Pollicis Longus. Most of the variations of the flexor pollicis longus were given in the description of normal muscles; however, variations of special interest are presented here. An accessory muscle orginating from the coronoid process is very frequent. It inserts in three ways: most often the muscle fibers attach to the muscular portion of the proximal flexor pollicis longus, another may join the flexor digitorum profundus, and the third may join the flexor superficialis. The accessory muscle originating from the coronoid process forming a special slip for the flexor profundus was described by Gantzer as the *accessorius ad flexorum profundum digitorum*. Gantzer also described the accessory slip from the coronoid process to the flexor pollicis longus, which he named *musculus accessorius ad pollicem*, as mentioned in the description of the normal flexor pollicis longus; thus, Gantzer described the musculus accessorius ad flexorum profundum digitorum (accessory to the flexor profundus) and also the musculus accessorius ad pollicem (accessory to the flexor pollicis longus). These two accessory muscles should not be confused. This anomalous accessory head of origin of the flexor pollicis

FIG. 7–22 Gantzer's muscle, an accessory head of the flexor pollicis longus, here arising from the medial epicondyle is seen penetrating the median nerve in the proximal forearm. In the arm the median nerve was found to course posterior to the brachial artery. *(Insert)*, the flexor digitorum profundus of the little finger is seen sending a slip to the flexor superficialis of the ring finger. The flexor superficialis of the little finger is absent.

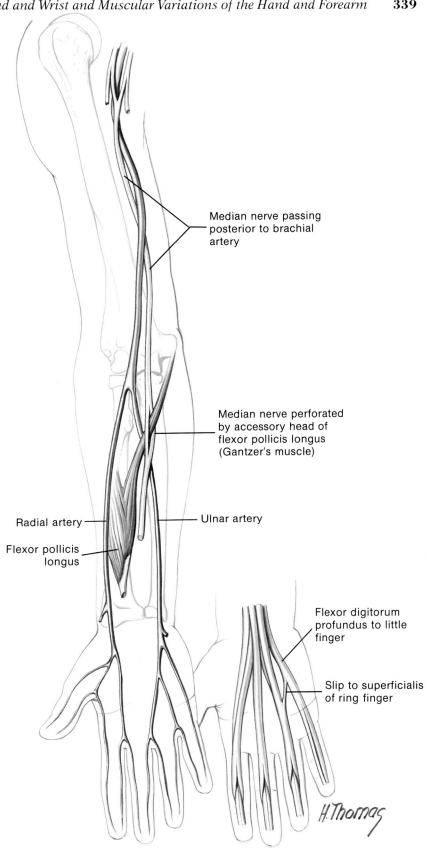

Median nerve passing posterior to brachial artery

Median nerve perforated by accessory head of flexor pollicis longus (Gantzer's muscle)

Radial artery

Flexor pollicis longus

Ulnar artery

Flexor digitorum profundus to little finger

Slip to superficialis of ring finger

H. Thomas

longus has been seen penetrating the median nerve in the proximal forearm (Fig. 7–22). LeDouble states that the accessory to the flexor pollicis longus was described before Gantzer by Albinus and other anatomists.

Macalister, as mentioned by LeDouble, described several interesting flexor pollicis longus variations: (1) a muscle origin from the coronoid process forming the origin of the pronator teres and the accessory to the flexor pollicis longus sent a few slips to the flexor superficialis; (2) a slip from the coronoid divided into three parts: for the flexor pollicis longus, the flexor profundus digitorum, and the flexor superficialis; (3) the coronoid slip divided into two parts: for the pronator teres and the flexor profundus digitorum; and (4) a coronoid process origin that replaced the head of the pronator teres and passing dorsal to the ulnar artery, joined entirely the flexor pollicis longus after some connection with the flexor superficialis.

The author observed three cases in which an accessory of the flexor pollicis longus formed a separate tendon in the midforearm, parallel with the main tendon of the flexor pollicis longus and ending in the first lumbrical muscle, which joined the flexor profundus indicis tendon in the palm. Besides the accessory coronoid process muscle, a muscular origin to the flexor pollicis longus arises from the medial epicondylar region of the humerus. It is important to realize that the accessory origins of the flexor pollicis longus are found in more than one third of human forearms, as observed by early anatomists and by Mangini.

Brachioradialis.   The brachioradialis is now used frequently in transplantation for other paralyzed muscles. The muscle presents certain variations that may make it unsuitable or only partly useful for transplantations. The variations may be observed in origin as well as insertion.

The origin of the brachioradialis may ascend into the area of the deltoid muscle. The insertion of the muscle may be found at times just distal to the pronator quadratus without reaching the styloid process, or sometimes it may not go beyond the insertion of the pronator teres, as seen by Testut. On the other hand, the brachioradialis

has been observed to extend its insertion distal to the styloid process of the radius and attach to the scaphoid and also to the trapezium. The muscle is sometimes divided into two parts of which one, situated deeper, is inserted 3 cm proximal to the styloid and the other, more superficial, is attached to the radial styloid.

The muscle is absent in cases of congenital absence of the radius. At times, there is intimate connection of the brachioradialis with the radial extensors of the wrist and with the abductor pollicis longus. LeDouble cites a case of Wood's in which the terminal tendon divided into three branches: one inferior, inserting into the styloid radial process; another middle, inserted proximal to the pronator quadratus on the anterior surface of the radial shaft; and the third superior, as the middle of the lateral surface of the radial shaft. The superficial radial nerve passed between the superior and the middle parts of the variant brachioradialis insertion.

Extensors Carpi Radialis Longus and Brevis. The extensors carpi radialis longus and brevis are reasonably considered together in comparative anatomy. In some of the mammals, the two muscles are represented by one muscle; in human anatomy, the absence of the extensor carpi radialis brevis is not uncommon and was observed by a number of anatomists. The absence of the extensor carpi radialis brevis was observed by Kaplan in three separate cadavers. In two specimens, the absence was noted in both forearms. The absence of the extensor brevis was also observed in two surgical patients.

In cases of absence of the extensor carpi radialis brevis, the extensor carpi radialis longus usually inserts into the second and third metacarpal bases. A rare additional muscle is mentioned by Quain—the extensor carpi radialis intermedius, which originates independently from the humeral epicondyle between the two radial carpal extensors and inserts into the bases of the second and third metacarpals (Fig. 7–23). Another additional muscle—the extensor carpi radialis accessorius—originates in the region of the extensor carpi radialis longus and runs distally for insertion into the base of the first metacarpal bone. The insertion may vary considerably and extend to the proximal phalanx or to the abductor pollicis brevis. The insertions of the normal extensors longus and brevis may extend to two or three metacarpal bases each.

Extensor Digitorum. Most variations of the extensor digitorum involve the number of tendons. The most common is either an increase or decrease in the number of tendons; at times, this is accompanied by an increase of separate muscular bellies. The author observed several cases of separate muscular bellies for the middle finger with a separate tendon running below the other extensor tendons and joining the common extensor to the middle finger slightly on the ulnar side of the metacarpophalangeal joint, similar to the extensor indicis proprius insertion to the index finger. The number of tendons may be double; all the tendons may be united in one continuous layer over the dorsum of the hand with separate, very short extension into each finger at the metacarpophalangeal joint. One of the important and frequent arrangements is an absence of a common extensor to the little finger. Instead of this, a short junctura tendinum is extended from the common extensor of the ring finger near the metacarpophalangeal joint of the little finger to the extensor expansion of this finger. The extensor proprius of the little finger is almost always double, as reported by Schenk. In use of this tendon of the extensor of the little finger for surgical transplantation, it must be remembered that the two most ulnar tendons of the little finger belong to the extensor proprius of the little finger.

An additional tendon from the muscular belly or the tendon of the extensor proprius of the index finger may be found rather frequently running to the extensor pollicis longus at the level of the first metacarpal either through the tunnel of the extensor pollicis longus or with the extensor indicis. The author observed several cases of this type on surgical intervention and anatomic dissections. A division of the muscle body of the extensor digitorum into four separate heads may occasionally be observed. This is usually connected with marked independence of extension of each finger, despite the presence of the juncturae tendinum. Apparently, the juncturae themselves do not restrict the independent action of each finger.

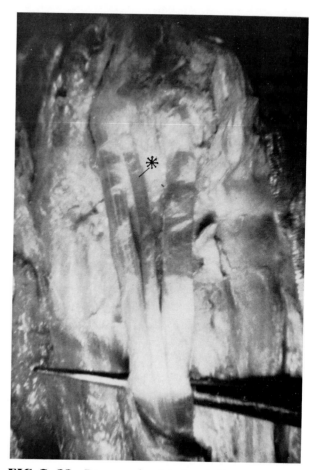

FIG. 7–23 Dorsum of a right hand dissection; note an extensor carpi radialis intermedius (✶) inserting onto the medial side of the base of the second metacarpal. The extensor carpi radialis longus is seen attaching to the dorsoradial side of the base of the second metacarpal, while the extensor carpi radialis brevis attaches to the base of the third metacarpal.

Extensor Digiti Minimi. The extensor digiti minimi normally has two tendons; but it may occasionally have more than two tendons (Fig. 7–24). Rarely, the extensor of the little finger may be completely absent and may be substituted by an extensor either from the common extensor of the ring finger or from the extensor carpi ulnaris.

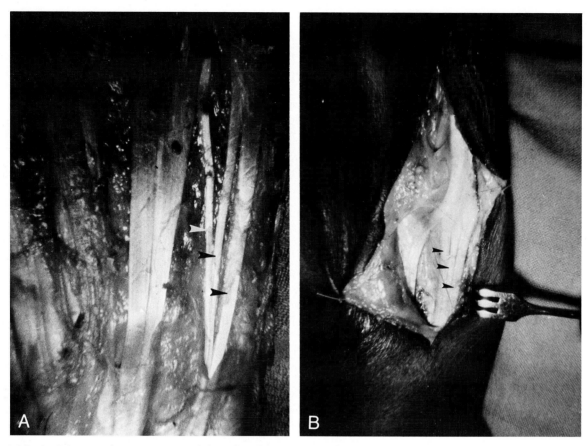

FIG. 7–24   A cadaver specimen (**A**) and operative case (**B**) with a three-tendoned extensor digiti minimi (*arrows*).

Extensor Indicis.   The extensor indicis may rarely be completely absent or very thin and functionally insignificant. At times, the tendon does not reach the base of the proximal phalanx but stops at the dorsum of the second metacarpal. The tendon may be found to be double (Fig. 7–25). The authors have observed a case in which the extensor indicis sends an additional tendon to the common extension of the middle finger. Extensor proprius tendons to the middle and ring fingers have been reported in the literature. Connections of the extensor indicis with the extensor pollicis longus are occasionally seen.

Extensor Carpi Ulnaris.   The extensor carpi ulnaris normally has a single origin from the epicondyle, the intermuscular septum, and the fascia of the forearm; however, the muscle is sometimes double, and rarely it has an additional origin from the lower dorsal surface of the ulna. The additional muscle is inserted into the base of the proximal phalanx of the little finger and is known as the *ulnaris digiti minimi* (Wood). A tendinous extension from the lower part of the tendon of the extensor carpi ulnaris was observed several times by Kaplan. The extension runs toward the proximal phalanx of the little finger (Fig. 7–26). At times, it may replace the extensor digiti minimi and then may run to the base of the middle phalanx. The extensor carpi ulnaris is sometimes connected with the extensor of the little finger in the forearm. Extensions of the tendon may be traced to the abductor and to the opponens of the little finger. Connections with the pisiform also are occasionally present.

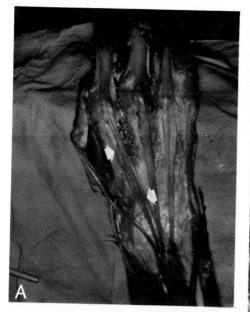

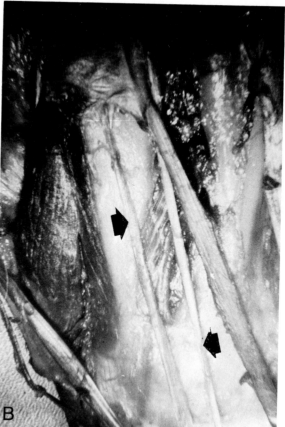

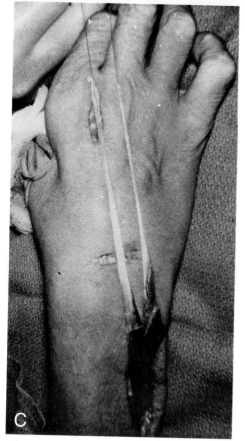

FIG. 7–25 **A**, Right hand anatomic specimen with a double extensor indicis (*arrows*). **B**, Close-up of specimen in **A**; the extensor digitorum communis to the index finger has been retracted; the two tendons of the extensor indicis are seen (*arrows*) attaching to the extensor expansion radial and ulnar to the attachment of the communis. **C**, An operative case where a double extensor indicis was found and used as a tendon transfer to restore opposition to the thumb.

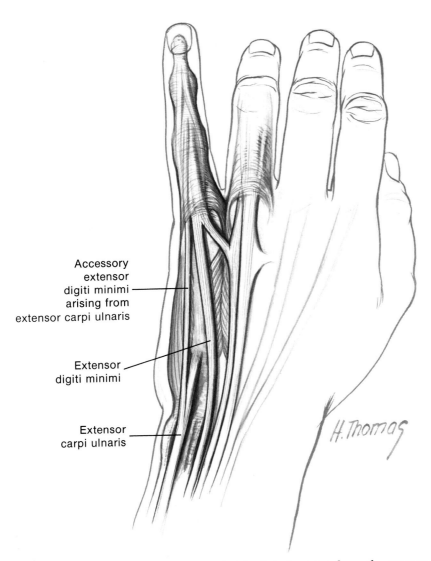

Accessory
extensor
digiti minimi
arising from
extensor carpi ulnaris

Extensor
digiti minimi

Extensor
carpi ulnaris

H. Thomas

FIG. 7—26   An accessory extensor digiti minimi arising from the extensor
carpi ulnaris.

Extensor Pollicis Brevis, Abductor Pollicis Longus, and Extensor Pollicis Longus.   The extensor pollicis brevis, abductor pollicis longus, and extensor pollicis longus present many variations. The three are considered together because in most variations all may be involved. The most frequent variation of the extensor pollicis brevis is its insertion into the base of the distal phalanx. This was observed by the author on many occasions on surgical exposure of the thumb and in anatomic specimens. In some instances the abductor pollicis longus and the extensor pollicis brevis form a single muscle body with separate tendons running to the base of the first metacarpal, and an additional tendon running toward the base of the proximal phalanx. Most frequently, the tendon of the abductor longus divides into several tendinous slips running toward the thenar muscles, the transverse carpal ligament, the trapezium, and the scaphoid. The extensor pollicis brevis may also divide into several slips running in the same tunnel with the tendon of the abductor longus or in a separate tunnel. The extensor pollicis longus often may replace the absent extensor pollicis brevis; when the extensor pollicis brevis is absent, the abductor pollicis longus is usually present. The abductor pollicis longus may be completely absent; in this case, the extensor pollicis brevis has tendinous extensions into the base of the first metacarpal.

The extensor pollicis longus is rarely, if ever, absent. It may have a double muscle head with a duplication of the tendon of insertion. In addition to the insertion into the terminal phalanx, the extensor pollicis longus is almost always inserted into the base of the proximal phalanx. The tendon of the extensor longus is at times connected with the extensor indicis, the extensor digitorum, or the abductor longus. It is necessary to add a rare variety representing a muscle between the extensor indicis and the extensor pollicis longus with an insertion into the index and thumb. It may replace either the extensor pollicis longus or the extensor indicis.

INTRINSIC MUSCLES

The intrinsic muscles of the hand present variations that are explained by their evolutionary development. Humphry, McMurrich, LeDouble, Macalister, and others have developed views explaining the existing variations. The present concern is the practical application of the variations. The intrinsic muscles of the thenar eminence and the thumb will be considered first; followed by the intrinsic muscles of the hypothenar eminence and the interossei and the lumbricals and concluded with the short extensors of the hand.

The thenar eminence

The abductor pollicis brevis seldom varies significantly. Most of the variations consist of a more extensive origin from the transverse carpal ligament, the trapezium, and the scaphoid. The muscle may be divided into two separate bodies, of which one is connected with an addi-

tional tendon that comes from the abductor pollicis longus or other muscles in this region. The absence of the abductor pollicis brevis is mentioned in the literature, and the authors have observed it. Some anatomists have observed a cutaneous thenar muscle 3 cm to 4 cm long and a few millimeters wide. This muscle inserts into the lateral base of the proximal phalanx and runs into the skin of the thenar eminence; it is separated from the abductor brevis by the thenar fascia.

The flexor brevis is described in a recent study by Napier that clarifies its significance and its division into the superficial and deep heads. The division of the thenar muscles into the abductor brevis, the opponens, and the flexor brevis is known; however, separation of the opponens from the flexor brevis is somewhat arbitrary. Cruveilhier attempted to divide the thenar muscles according to their relationship to the radial and the ulnar sesamoids:

My consideration of these small muscles is based on their distal insertions, because their origins are overlapping, so that their separation is somewhat arbitrary. I am dividing these muscles of the thumb into two groups: muscles directed from the carpus to the first metacarpal and to the radial side of the proximal phalanx, and muscles which are directed from the carpus to the ulnar side of the proximal phalanx. The first which could be considered as a single and same muscle comprising the abductor brevis, opponens and short flexor, the second consisting of the adductor pollicis, which I regard as the first palmar interosseous.*

It is often difficult to separate this muscle from the opponens and even from the abductor brevis; however, the deep part of the flexor brevis is almost always present and runs posterior to the flexor pollicis longus tendon from the common origin with the adductor pollicis to the radial sesamoid. The opponens muscle is difficult at times to separate from the flexor brevis.

Variations of the adductor pollicis muscle

---

*Cruveilhier J: Traité d'Anatomie Descriptive, 2nd ed, vol 2, p 298 1843.

are not common. One variation consists of a wide separation between the transverse and oblique heads. As mentioned previously, it is also known that a separate small head of the adductor pollicis may be observed almost constantly, which may be considered as the first palmar interosseous.

The hypothenar eminence

The muscles of the hypothenar eminence present more variations than are usually observed in the thenar eminence. The palmaris brevis is very seldom absent; however, its extent from the ulnar to the radial side of the hand may vary considerably. LeDouble mentioned that the fibers of the palmaris brevis may be followed under the palmar aponeurosis to the scaphoid and even the trapezium, as fibrous extensions of this muscle. It may also occasionally extend to the pisiform and receive fibers of reinforcement from the flexor carpi ulnaris.

The abductor digiti minimi may be absent. It originates either from the pisiform only or from the pisiform and the flexor carpi ulnaris. It may be found to be double, and it is sometimes difficult to separate the muscle from the flexor digiti minimi brevis. It is sometimes reinforced by additional small muscles from the volar carpal ligament, from the antebrachial fascia, and from the palmaris longus. In one case reported by Wood, the abductor of the little finger was covered by a muscle mass coming off the antebrachial fascia over the flexor carpi ulnaris and the palmaris longus. This mass was much larger than the abductor. The author observed an aberrant muscle in which one part derived from the palmaris longus at its junction with the palmar aponeurosis, and the other part originated from the antebrachial fascia over the flexor carpi ulnaris in the distal third of the forearm. The two parts joined at the pisiform and extended toward the abductor digiti minimi. The ulnar artery passed on top of the first muscle. The ulnar nerve passed on top of the first muscle in the forearm but on reaching the pisiform penetrated under the second part of the muscle into the abductor digiti minimi.

The flexor digiti minimi brevis varies in size and additional muscle bodies, which may come off the antebrachial fascia, sometimes proximal to the pisiform. Mangini described an anomalous muscle of the flexor brevis of the little finger arising from the antebrachial fascia with absence of the opponens and fusion of the flexor brevis and the abductor of the little finger. The palmaris longus also was absent. The variant muscle often simulates tumors or tenosynovitis and must be considered in diagnosis.

Lumbricals

The lumbrical muscles frequently vary in the number of the muscles, their origin and course, and relation to other muscles. LeDouble estimated the incidence of variation as about one in eight individuals. Four lumbricals are considered normal; however, the number may increase to five. Although the normal origin of the lumbrical is from the tendon of the flexor profundus, the muscle may arise not from the flexor profundus tendon in the palm but from other tendons located in the forearm or even from other structures. In personal observations the lumbrical was found originating from an accessory flexor pollicis longus, from a profundus tendon of the index finger in the forearm. An accessory lumbrical of the index finger has been seen arising from the proximal portion of the flexor pollicis longus (Fig. 7–24C). A muscle slip from the sheath of the median nerve was seen in one case, coming off just proximal to the transverse carpal ligament and joining the first lumbrical, which originated from the flexor profundus of the index finger.

The first lumbrical may be completely absent without any influence on the function of the distal phalanx. The first lumbrical may originate from the flexor superficialis of the index finger or from the flexor pollicis longus. The first lumbrical was seen originating from the flexor superficialis near the coronoid process (Figs. 7–27A and B). Additional lumbricals also are observed. LeDouble cites Froment, who found a supernumerary lumbrical for the index finger coming off the first metacarpal and the

FIG. 7–27 **A**, An anomalous lumbrical arising from the flexor digitorum superficialis in the proximal forearm. **B**, An accessory first lumbrical arising in the forearm. **C**, An accessory lumbrical arising from the flexor pollicis longus. (From Dr. Emanuel B. Kaplan's anatomical sketches, circa 1924–1928)

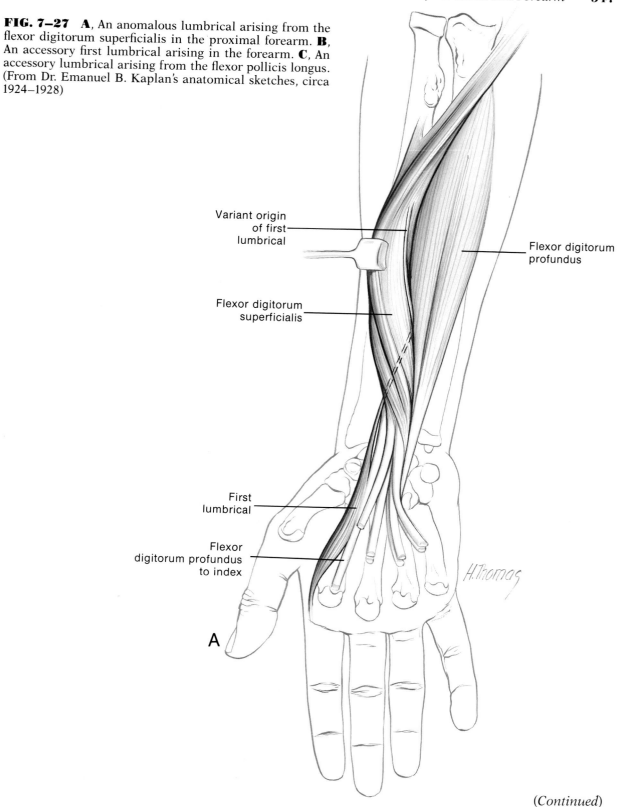

Variant origin of first lumbrical

Flexor digitorum profundus

Flexor digitorum superficialis

First lumbrical

Flexor digitorum profundus to index

H.Thomas

A

(Continued)

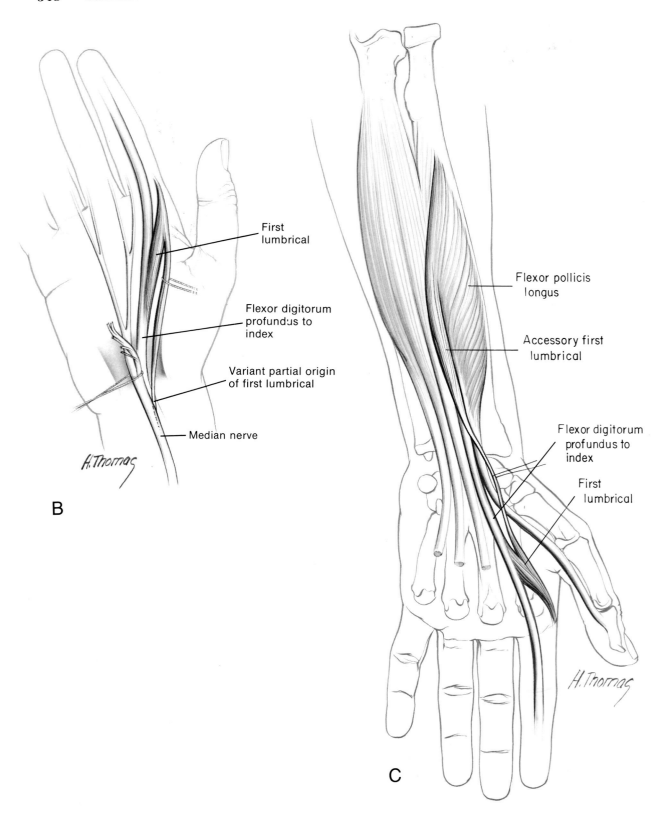

First
lumbrical

Flexor digitorum
profundus to
index

Variant partial origin
of first lumbrical

Median nerve

H.Thomas

B

Flexor pollicis
longus

Accessory first
lumbrical

Flexor digitorum
profundus to
index

First
lumbrical

H.Thomas

C

opponens pollicis in one hand and from the long abductor and the short extensor of the thumb in the other hand. The second lumbrical also may be absent; it may be double, inserting into the radial side of the middle finger and the ulnar side of the index finger. The third lumbrical also may be absent, even if all the others are present. The third lumbrical may be inserted on the ulnar side of the middle finger instead of the radial side of the ring finger. Some anatomists observed two lumbricals to the ring finger with simultaneous absence of the lumbrical to the little finger. The third and fourth lumbricals are the most variable; the fourth lumbrical frequently is absent or has two insertions.

Interossei

The interossei and their variations were described in the section on the Muscles of the Fingers. It is important to repeat that the insertions of the interossei extend toward the proximal phalanges, that the volar as well as the dorsal interossei may extend their action to the dorsal expansion, and that the first dorsal interosseous frequently extends its action to the distal and middle phalanges.

It is not correct to state that the first dorsal interosseous never extends its action through the dorsal expansion to the distal and middle phalanges. The variations of the interossei consist in the different insertions of the volar and dorsal interossei to the lateral bases of the phalanges and to the dorsal expansion. The first volar interosseous may be considered the separate head of the oblique portion of the adductor pollicis, which originates between the bases of the first and second metacarpals and runs toward the ulnar sesamoid with the other parts of the adductor pollicis. A similar narrow head originates in the same area, but instead of running on the ulnar side of the flexor pollicis longus tendon, it crosses the flexor pollicis longus tendon on its dorsal side and emerges on the radial side of this tendon to insert into the radial sesamoid with the flexor brevis pollicis (superficial part).

Extensor Brevis Manus

The extensor brevis manus is a variable muscle that does not occur frequently, but its presence is important because unsuspected, it may give an impression of a swelling or tumor on the dorsum of the hand. It is similar to the short extensor of the foot; it usually originates from the dorsum of the lunate, capitate, or triquetrum or from the ligaments uniting these bones. It may originate from the extensor retinaculum or from the distal margin of the radius. It represents a muscle belly that terminates in tendinous expansions joining the long extensor tendons at the metacarpophalangeal joints. There are usually only one or two tendons to the index and middle fingers. Although as many as three and even four tendons may be found, this is probably exceedingly rare. The authors observed this muscle in 22 cases, mostly on surgical exposure, but never saw more than one tendon to the index finger and one to the middle finger in the same hand. It is innervated most often by terminal branches of the posterior interosseous nerve.

Part Three
Surgical Anatomy

8
Surface Anatomy of the Hand and the Wrist

Daniel C. Riordan
Emanuel B. Kaplan

The relationship of the deep structures of the hand to its surface creases and bony prominences should be known to all emergency room physicians, upper extremity surgeons of all specialties, and anatomy students.

THE VOLAR ASPECT

On the palmar surface of the normal hand, the distal and proximal palmar flexion creases and the thenar crease, in addition to the pisiform and trapezial tubercle, are the constant landmarks. Kaplan defined the cardinal line of the hand as a line drawn from the apex of the interdigital fold between the thumb and index finger toward the ulnar side of the hand, parallel with the proximal palmar crease (Fig. 8–1) and passing about 4 mm to 5 mm distal to the pisiform bone. With this line the relationships between many important deep structures of the hand can be established.

A second line, drawn as a continuation of the ulnar line of the ring finger in a proximal direction toward the wrist, transects the cardinal line of the hand at a point slightly radial and distal to the pisiform (Fig. 8–2). The point of intersection of these two lines corresponds almost exactly with the tip of the hook of the hamate bone. This point of intersection defines the locations of the ulnar artery and veins and the volar sensory branches of the ulnar nerve, which pass directly over the hook of the hamate. A point halfway between the hook of the hamate and the pisiform is the point of

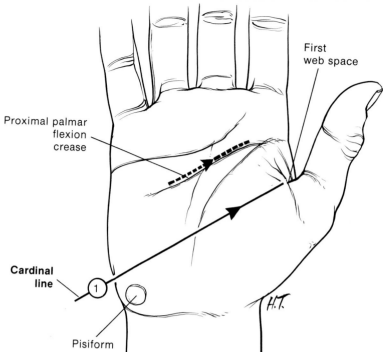

FIG. 8–1   The cardinal line (1) is located by drawing a line from the apex of the first web space parallel to the proximal palmar crease.

FIG. 8–2   A line (2) drawn proximally as a continuation of the ulnar side of the ring finger intersects the cardinal line (1) at the hook of the hamate. A line drawn from this point to the ulnar side of the fifth metacarpal traces the course of the ulnar digital nerve of the little finger. The surface representation of the deep branch of the ulnar nerve, the common digital nerve to the radial side of the little finger and ulnar side of the ring finger, the ulnar artery, and vein are easily mapped out with the help of these lines. *(Insert)*, The hook of the hamate is an excellent point of reference to the articulation between the base of the fourth and fifth metacarpals.

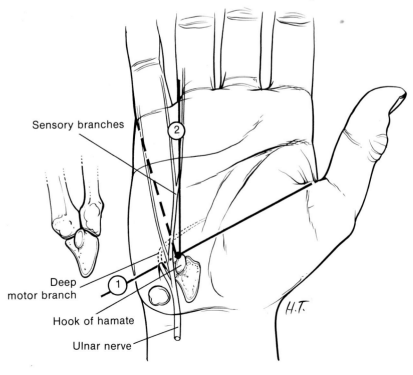

penetration of the deep branch of the ulnar nerve into the deep, retrotendinous part of the hand.

The line uniting the tip of the hamate hook (as identified by the intersection of the cardinal line and the ulnar line of the ring finger with the ulnar side of the metacarpophalangeal joint of the fifth finger) traces the precise course of the ulnar digital nerve of the fifth finger. The nerve is covered by a thin fascia in the distal part of the palm and by the ulnar palmar fat pad and the palmaris brevis muscle around the hook of the hamate bone.

The intersection of the thenar crease with the cardinal line corresponds to the emergence of the motor branch of the median nerve (Fig. 8–3). A third line can be drawn by continuing the radial side of the middle finger in a proximal direction until it intersects the cardinal line, which locates the point of penetration of the

motor branch of the median nerve into the thenar muscles. The recurrent branch of the median nerve is occasionally found slightly higher on the cardinal line. In these cases, instead of crossing at the thenar line as one branch, the median nerve is divided into several smaller branches as it enters the thenar muscles.

A fourth line can be drawn from the flexion crease on the palmar surface of the second metacarpal head to the flexion crease on the palmar surface of the fifth metacarpal head (Fig. 8–4). A trapezoidal area is thus formed by the lines drawn from the radial border of the middle finger to the cardinal line, from the ulnar border of the ring finger to the cardinal line, the cardinal line itself, and the line from the second to the fifth metacarpal heads. This trapezoid indicates the locations of the vascular arches of the hand. The deep palmer arch is located slightly proximal to the cardinal line, and proximal to the

FIG. 8–3   The intersection of the cardinal line (1) and thenar crease corresponds to the emergence of the motor branch of the median nerve (x). The intersection of line (3), which is a proximal continuation of the radial side of the long finger and the cardinal line, locates the point of penetration of this motor branch of the median nerve into the thenar muscles.

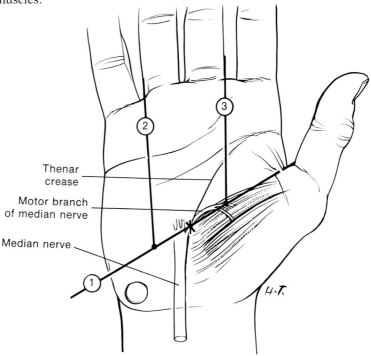

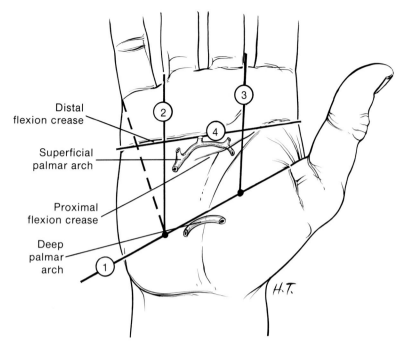

FIG. 8—4 When line 4 is drawn from the palmar flexion crease of the index finger to the palmar flexion crease of the little finger, a trapezoidal area is formed by it and the cardinal line (1), line 2, and line 3. The vascular arches are located in relation to this trapezoid.

FIG. 8—5 A line drawn from the intersection of line 3 and the cardinal line (1) to the radial side of the palmodigital crease of the index finger outlines the course of the digital nerve to the radial side of this digit. Similarly, the course of the digital nerve to the ulnar side of the little finger follows a line drawn from the intersection of line 2 and the cardinal line and the ulnar side of the palmodigital crease of the little finger.

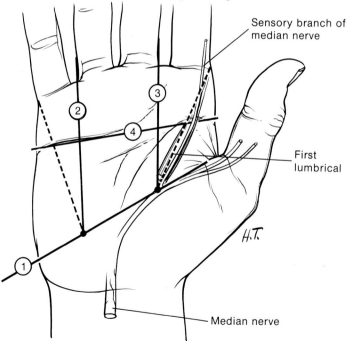

distal transverse line the distal convexity of the superficial palmar arch is found. In some cases this arch will not quite reach the transverse line, but it will usually be within 3 mm to 5 mm of this line. A line drawn from the point of intersection of the cardinal line and the radial line of the middle finger to the radial side of the palmodigital crease of the index finger outlines the course of the digital nerve to the radial side of the index finger. The nerve is a satellite of the first lumbrical muscle, as it is located parallel with and on the radial side of the muscle (Fig. 8–5).

The point of intersection of the thenar line with the cardinal line represents an important area (Fig. 8–3). A penetrating wound at this point will injure the motor branch of the thenar muscles; if the injury is deep, the nerve to the first dorsal interosseous, the nerve to the first lumbrical, and the nerve to the adductor pollicis may be divided, with paralysis of the corresponding muscles. Such a wound may also divide the cutaneous digital nerves to the thumb and index finger.

The identification of the tip of the hook of the hamate bone permits recognition of other important relationships (Fig. 8–2, *insert*). The distal point of the ridge of the hamate hook corresponds almost exactly to the articular interline between the bases of the fourth and fifth metacarpals. The ulnar side of the hook corresponds to the metacarpohamate joint of the fifth finger.

The radial side of the wrist joint proximal to the thenar eminence displays a bony prominence that can be palpated even in obese people. The prominence corresponds to the proximal end of the ridge of the trapezium and is known as the tubercle of the trapezium. Immediately proximal to the tubercle, the tendon of the flexor carpi radialis can be palpated; this tendon then disappears under the tubercle. The tubercle continues distally as a ridge that is 10 mm to 12 mm long and can be palpated along its entire length. The ridge forms the radial wall of the canal for the tendon of the flexor carpi radialis (Figs. 2–7, 2–63, and 8–6). The trapezial ridge has an oblique course toward the distal part of the hand. The continuation of the line of the ridge

distally intersects the ulnar side of the head of the third metacarpal. The distal end of the ridge stops at the articular line of the saddle joint between the trapezium and the first metacarpal. The articular line of the trapezium and first metacarpal saddle joint is directed obliquely toward the distal ulnar side of the hand; its continuation would cross the neck of the fifth metacarpal (Fig. 8–6).

The volar branch of the radial artery courses over the oblique articular line of the trapeziometacarpal joint about 2 mm distal to the joint line.

The tubercle of the scaphoid bone can be palpated just radial to the flexor carpi radialis and can be felt easily if the wrist is slightly flexed against resistance. The distal volar crease of the wrist is represented by a line drawn between the proximal edge of the pisiform and the proximal edge of the tubercle of the trapezium. This crease corresponds to the articular line between the trapezium and the scaphoid bone on the radial side and the cleft between the triquetrum and the lunate on the ulnar side (Fig. 8–6). It passes in front of the neck of the capitate, just distal to the articular edge of the head of the capitate. The lunate is normally proximal to this line (Fig. 2–3). The proximal volar crease of the wrist corresponds approximately to the radiocarpal joint.

THE DORSAL ASPECT

On the dorsal surface of the hand are a few easily discernible landmarks. One of the most important is the tubercle of Lister, which terminates at the posterior border of the radius (Fig. 8–7). It can be palpated as a prominence just proximal to the radiocarpal joint over the dorsum of the radius almost halfway between the radial styloid process and the radioulnar joint (Fig. 3–14). This key point leads to many structures of the wrist.

On the ulnar side of the tubercle runs the tendon of the extensor pollicis longus; parallel to the radial side of the tubercle is the tendon of the extensor carpi radialis brevis. The two ten-

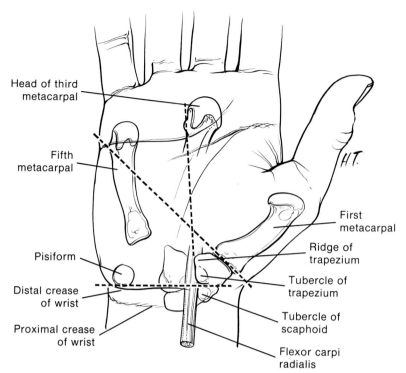

Head of third
metacarpal

Fifth
metacarpal

Pisiform

Distal crease
of wrist

Proximal crease
of wrist

H.T.

First
metacarpal

Ridge of
trapezium

Tubercle of
trapezium

Tubercle of
scaphoid

Flexor carpi
radialis

FIG. 8–6 A line continuing the oblique course of the trapezial ridge distally intersects the ulnar side of the head of the third metacarpal. A line continuing the articular surface of the trapeziometacarpal joint ulnad intersects the neck of the fifth metacarpal. A line drawn between the proximal edge of the tubercle of the trapezium and the proximal edge of the pisiform overlies the distal volar flexion crease of the wrist.

dons cross immediately distal to the tubercle and form for it a tendinous cradle; the tendon of the extensor pollicis longus runs more superficially than the tendon of the extensor carpi radialis brevis (Fig. 3–14). The tip of the tubercle is just proximal to the radiocarpal joint and corresponds to the line of articulation between the scaphoid and lunate bones.

The position of the lunate bone in relation to Lister's tubercle and the long axis of the third metacarpal changes in radial and ulnar deviations of the wrist. In the neutral position, the long axis of the third metacarpal passes through the long axis of the capitate and through the lunate, such that the lunate is mostly on the ulnar side of the axis of the third metacarpal. In radial deviation, the relationship with the axis of the third metacarpal is maintained, although the axis shifts slightly to the

radial side of the lunate and continues into the radioulnar joint (Fig. 7–20A). In ulnar deviation, the axis of the third metacarpal passes through the capitate but shifts completely out of the limits of the lunate and passes either between the scapholunar articulation or slightly more radially, through the scaphoid bone (Fig. 7–20B).

When the wrist is in the neutral position, palpation of the dorsum of the hand in the second intermetacarpal space between the bases of the second and third metacarpals reveals a slight prominence similar to Lister's tubercle. The prominence is formed by the styloid process of the base of the third metacarpal and the process of the second metacarpal. A line uniting the prominence of the second and third metacarpal bases with Lister's tubercle corresponds roughly to the articular line between the capitate on the ulnar side and the trapezoid and the scaphoid bones on the radial side (Fig. 8–7). The styloid process of the radius is palpated on the radial side of the wrist. The ulnar styloid process is palpated on the posteroulnar side of the wrist and is higher (more proximal) than the radial process. The styloid process of the radius contributes to the formation of the anatomic snuff-box, which is located on the radial aspect of the wrist.

The snuff-box consists of a depression with borders formed by the tendon of the extensor pollicis brevis on the radial side and by the tendon of the extensor pollicis longus on the ulnar side. The distal border on the snuff-box is formed by the prominent edge of the base of the first metacarpal, and the proximal border is formed by the styloid process of the radius. The skin overlying the snuff-box is movable and contains within its fascia one or several large veins. The snuff-box also serves as a passage for a few terminal branches of the musculocutaneous nerve and for the radial nerve as it passes to the ulnar side of the thumb. The floor of the snuff-box is formed by the dorsal tubercle of the trapezium and is crossed by the radial artery in its course toward the apex of the angle formed by the first and second metacarpals. A part of the floor is formed by the dorsal surface of the scaphoid tubercle, which can be felt under the tip of the styloid process of the radius. The small part of the osseous floor of the snuff-box, which may still be felt, is part of the dorsal surface of the trapezium (Figs. 3–1 and 7–15).

When the wrist is in neutral position, the snuff-box is 10 mm to 12 mm wide and 16 mm to 20 mm long. The width and height of the snuff-box varies with wrist position. Its height decreases in hyperextension of the thumb and decreases considerably in radial deviation of the wrist; its height increases in adduction of the thumb and increases considerably in ulnar deviation of the wrist.

Although the variations are less obvious than that in height, the snuff-box also changes slightly in width during abduction and adduction of the thumb, especially if combined with extension of the distal phalanx of the thumb.

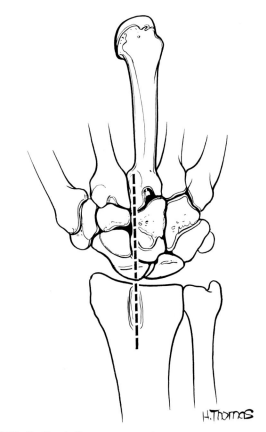

FIG. 8–7 A line uniting the prominence between the second and third metacarpal bases and Lister's tubercle passes between the trapezoid and capitate joint.

This change in width results from the slight lateral motion of the tendon on the extensor pollicis longus over the dorsum of the first metacarpal when the thumb moves from abduction into adduction and vice versa; this motion, as mentioned earlier, is 4 mm to 5 mm. Any surgical or fibrous fixation of the tendon of the extensor pollicis longus with elimination of the lateral motion would interfere with abduction and adduction of the thumb.

When the wrist is completely extended, the following may be observed by palpation:

Immediately proximal to the base of the second metacarpal is a depression that corresponds to the trapezoid and is covered by the strong tendons of the radial extensors of the wrist. The scaphoid bone is almost completely impalpable because it is hidden under the distal end of the radius.

Immediately proximal to the base of the third metacarpal is a deeper depression that corresponds to a small surface of the dorsum of the body of the capitate bone. The lunate bone is impalpable because it is hidden by the distal end of the radius.

Immediately proximal to the fourth and fifth metacarpal bases, the dorsal aspect of the hamate bone is palpable.

When flexion is begun from the position of extreme extension, the first prominence that appears to creep from under the posterior edge of the distal end of the radius corresponds to the ulnar end of the scaphoid and the radial end of the lunate, which form one unit. These two bones are intimately united by their interosseous ligament and are covered by cartilage so smoothly that it is sometimes difficult to find their line of articulation. These two bones, especially the lunate, are increasingly palpable as flexion of the wrist increases. In complete flexion of the wrist, the prominence found on palpation corresponds to the lunate. The capitate is palpable on full flexion and remains in a small depression distal to the lunate bone. In persons who can flex the wrist beyond 90 degrees, the proximal head of the capitate can be palpated as a second bony prominence just distal to the prominence of the dorsal surface of the lunate. The entire dorsal aspect of the trapezoid is palpable through the thickness of the radial extensors of the wrist when the wrist is fully flexed. The hamate bone remains palpable proximal to the fifth metacarpal, and the triquetrum can be palpated immediately distal to the ulna.

The metacarpophalangeal and the interphalangeal articular lines are easy to identify. These interarticular lines are always located distal to the highest bony point of each joint. At the metacarpophalangeal joint of each finger, the distance between the highest point and the articular line is 10 mm to 12 mm. At the metacarpophalangeal joint of the thumb and the proximal interphalangeal joint of each finger, this distance does not normally exceed 4 mm to 5 mm. At the distal interphalangeal joints of the fingers and thumb, the distance ranges from 1 mm to 3 mm.

Other lines and points of reference, when marked, make further identification of structures comparatively easy. The distal palmar crease over the ulnar side of the hand crosses the neck of the fifth metacarpal and runs to the ulnar edge of the hand. This point of the distal crease of the palm is marked. The tubercle of the trapezium is palpated, and a mark is placed exactly 1 cm distal to its most prominent point. These two marks are then connected with a line, which crosses the thenar crease before reaching the mark over the trapezium. The line is continued to the tendon of the abductor pollicis longus. The part of this line between the thenar crease and the tendon of the abductor pollicis longus represents a direct approach to the volar aspect of the carpometacarpal joint of the thumb (Fig. 8-6). The line can be continued posteriorly in the same curved position to the same joint or curved up along the radial edge of the first metacarpal; this line, confined either to the area between the thenar crease and the abductor pollicis longus or extended posteriorly in the same line, is an excellent approach for Bennett's fractures, removal of the trapezium, or any other procedure requiring exposure of this area.

9
Surgical
Approaches

Lee W. Milford
Emanuel B. Kaplan

Surgery of the hand requires carefully considered surgical approaches. The principles of a good surgical approach are as follows:

1. Adequate exposure, providing ease of surgical procedures
2. Avoidance of injury to important structures
3. Option of extension of exposure if the need arises
4. Placement of the skin incision correctly to avoid disabling scars and interference with critical sensory nerves

It was felt at one time that skin incisions should be made near or parallel to major skin creases; however, in fact, skin incisions may be made almost anywhere in the hand, as long as they adhere to certain basic principles. The basic linear incision is always later converted into a mobile, oval or elliptical opening by undermining the skin and fat as the underlying fascia is exposed. The line of the skin incision does not dictate the orientation of further dissection. In other words, a skin incision may be in one direction, and the underlying dissection may be at 90 degrees to this. An S-shaped incision always has two basic flaps created by the undermining of the skin and its underlying fat. Care should be taken in certain instances that these flaps thus created have adequate blood supply for healing.

The skin incisions are placed according to Langer lines whenever possible. In 1861, Langer described lines of cleavage of the skin caused by the disposition of the subcutaneous, longitudinal elastic fibers. The fibers are located mostly parallel with the lines of Langer. Because of tension of these fibers, circular punctures in the skin tend to become elliptical. Investigations concerning contractures of the skin appear to produce evidence that skin incisions parallel with Langer lines are not always productive of good scars. Any scar running across a joint is subject to greater tension and may eventually become contracted. A scar running parallel with a joint axis will not be subject to tension and will not have a tendency to contract.

Several years ago, Min-Chyang Ju investigated the mechanism of contractures in experiments that explain satisfactorily the reasons for some of the contractures on the basis of differences of the tensions of normal and healing skin based on the differences in physical proper-

ties of the normal skin and the scars. The importance of skin creases was amplified by further observations.

Circular scars show a great tendency to contract. The reason for contractures of circular scars, irrespective of their relation to Langer's lines, resides in the continuity of the circle of scar tissue without interposition of normal skin. Such scars cannot be relieved by circular excision of the contracting band. Only a Z-plasty may be effective in treatment of these constricting bands. On the other hand, semicircular or U-shaped scars placed parallel with Langer's lines produce less contracture than if placed across Langer's lines.

The skin incisions of the hand and the fingers present special problems. Most of the

FIG. 9–1 Dorsal and palmar lines of the hand. The dorsal lines are transverse and slightly curved, parallel with the articular creases of the interphalangeal joints. The skin lines of the dorsum of the hand are mostly transverse; the skin lines of the wrist also are transverse. The volar lines are mostly longitudinal and parallel to the long axes of the fingers, except for those volar creases associated with the joints. The lines to the thumb fan out from the metacarpophalangeal crease toward the thenar line of the palm.

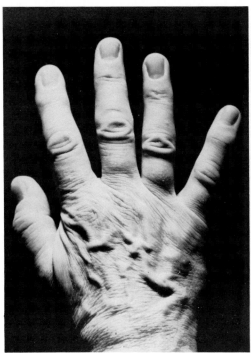 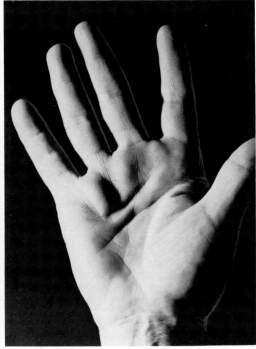

skin lines of the dorsal aspect of the hand are transverse. Over the phalanges, the lines are parallel with the dorsal creases of the interphalangeal joints; they are transverse over the distal part of the metacarpophalangeal line; and they become oblique toward the proximal parts of the metacarpophalangeal joints. Farther proximally, the lines become transverse over the dorsum of the hand and over the wrist.

On the volar surface of the hand, the line creases are directed differently. They are parallel with the long axes of the fingers except across the transverse lines of the interphalangeal and metacarpophalangeal lines. Over the thenar eminence, the skin lines run obliquely from the thenar crease toward the metacarpophalangeal line of the thumb on the ulnar side of the thenar eminence. On the radial side of the thenar eminence and the first metacarpal, the skin line becomes parallel with the metacarpophalangeal crease of the thumb (Fig. 9–1).

INCISIONS OVER FINGERS

Incisions over the fingers may be made volar, lateral, or dorsal (Figs. 9–2 and 9–3). If made volar, the incision may be zigzag; if made midline, it should be converted to a Z-plasty or should not extend more than one phalanx in order not to cross a flexor crease at a right angle.

LATERAL INCISIONS

The lateral incision opens the finger like an envelope, and the neurovascular bundle may be brought with the volar flap or left dorsally attached to its original bed. This incision permits exposure of the flexor tendon and its sheath and digital nerves and vessels over the palmar aspect. The opposite digital nerve and vessel can also be exposed. Extension of the lateral incision proximally is limited, especially in the middle and ring fingers because at the finger web, the vessels and nerves become deep and cannot be continually mobilized with the volar flap. The finger webs should be preserved and the natatory

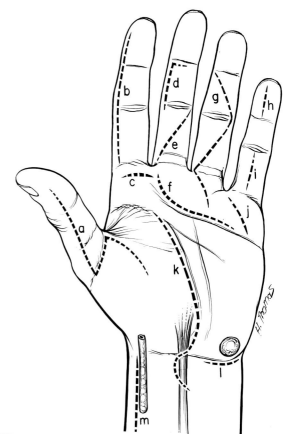

FIG. 9–2 Useful incisions on palmar side of hand: (a) Incision to expose entire flexor surface of thumb. (b) Lateral approach to digit, see also Fig 9-4. (c) Transverse incision to expose proximal portion of flexor tendon sheath. (d) Limited incision for flexor tendon sheath at middle phalanx. (e) Oblique incision to lateral flexor tendon sheath proximal phalanx. (f) Transverse incision for distal palmar approach. (g) Utility incision for entire flexor tendon sheath. (h) Midline incision of distal pulp for drainage of abscess. (i) Vertical incision for limited exposure of flexor sheath. (j) Oblique incision to expose underlying flexor tendon sheath. (k) Utility incision for exposing entire palm. (l) Transverse incision for limited exposure to flexor carpi ulnaris tendon. (m) Incision to expose radial artery at distal forearm.

ligaments protected to eliminate contracting scars.

On making a lateral incision, the surgeon should note that the incision is truly lateral and that the skin entry is slightly dorsal to the dorsal

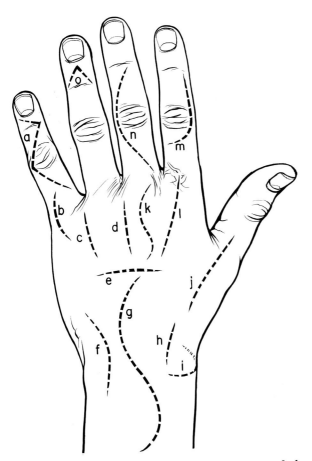

FIG. 9-3 Useful incisions on the dorsum of the hand: (a) extensive exposure of dorsum of finger. (b) Limited exposure of underlying extensor tendon MP joint. (c) and (d) Limited exposures for drainage of infection or extensor tendon injury. (e) Transverse incision for exposing mid-dorsum of hand. (f) Limited exposure to ulnar aspect of wrist. (g) Extensive exposure midwrist area. (h) Limited exposure to extensor of thumb. (i) Exposure of the underlying abductor pollicis longus tendon. (j) Exposure of the extensor tendon to the metacarpophalangeal area. (k) Exposure of metacarpal joint area. (l) Exposure of extensor tendon of index. (m) Exposure of dorsum of the PIP joint. (n) Extensive exposure of the dorsum of PIP joint and extensor mechansim. (o) Utility incision for exposure of DIP joint and extensor tendon insertion.

margin of the flexor creases at the distal and proximal interphalangeal joints, as is seen while flexing these two joints and noting the dorsal extent of the crease. The incision may begin distally at the lateral nail margin and may extend proximally just dorsal to the finger web. After the skin incision is completed, the incision is dissected in a plane slightly volad but maintaining the digital vessels and nerve in the volar flap. This volar direction is important, especially at the level of the distal and proximal interphalangeal joints in order to skirt these joints and avoid entering them because they have very little fat over their lateral margins. The ligament of Cleland is cut because it lies dorsal to the neurovascular bundles, enabling the digital neurovascular bundles to be brought volad with the mobilized volar flap (Fig. 9-4).

The flexor tendon sheath is left bare as the plane of dissection is developed. The opposite digital nerve and vessel can also be dissected (if necessary for repair) through this incision. It is more practical to make the incision on the side of the lacerated nerve; the incision can be extended slightly into and across the palm from the ulnar side of the little finger and from the radial side of the index finger because no finger webs limit the extension. This extension is achieved by continuing the incision at a right angle, at the level of the metacarpophalangeal joints of the middle phalanx and little fingers. This can also be fashioned at a point just distal to the web of the middle and ring fingers when the digital nerve and vessels have already been divided by trauma at the level of the proximal finger crease.

The lateral approach has been for many years the preferred approach for repair of the flexor tendons and digital nerves within the finger. Many surgeons leave the digital nerve and vessels attached at their original locations in the dorsal aspect of the incision; it has the advantage of being extendable into the palm from any finger, but has the theoretical if not actual disadvantage of voiding a part of the volar flap of its sensibility because the small fibers of the digital nerve feeding the flap are cut on one side. This approach is also technically more difficult to do correctly. By leaving the digital nerve and vessels behind on the dorsal flap, the distal end of the incision may be extended across the finger at the level of the pulp to expose the insertion of the flexor digitorum profundus tendon. Care should be taken not to cut the terminal branches of the digital nerve in this critical area of sensibility.

Lateral finger incisions can be placed on either the radial or ulnar side of the finger, but it is advisable to avoid placing the incision on the radial side of the index finger in particular, as well as the middle and ring fingers to preserve normal touch contact with the thumb. This principle also applies to the ulnar side of the little finger; however, in most cases expediency requires placing the incision on the radial side of the other fingers; this can be done with awareness of the dorsal branch of the digital nerve, especially of the index finger, which should be avoided.

FIG. 9–4 **A**, Transverse section illustrates the need of entering a digit midlaterally and then disecting a bit volarly in order to enter the flexor tendon sheath. **B**, The dotted line indicates the need to place the incision well dorsal to transverse creases of the joints. These creases normally extend dorsally beyond the midline. **C**, The ligaments of Cleland have been sectioned. This sectioning exposes the underlying neurovascular bundles that lie palmarward of the flexor tendon sheath.

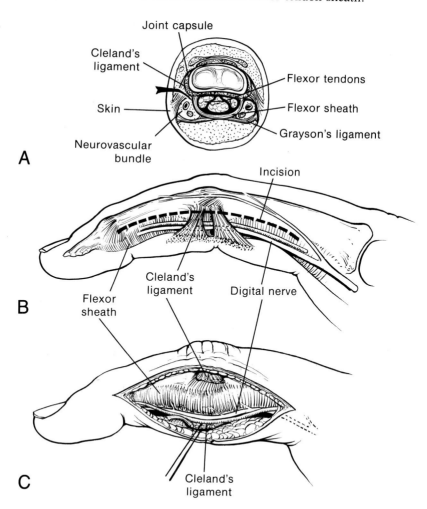

VOLAR INCISION

Most recently, the volar zigzag incision has been increasingly used. This incision provides a direct approach to the flexor tendon; it may be extended into the palm with ease because it does not mobilize either neurovascular bundle (Fig. 9-5). It may use three flaps within each finger or five flaps; the five-flap zigzag incision requires a sharper angle flap and is usually not used because of preference for the three-flap incision. In either type of incision, it is essential to protect the digital nerves and vessels on each side. These vital structures lie just under the point of the flap, and there the point should be dissected only skin deep to assure no damage to the underlying vessels and nerves. In the unlikely event that the digital artery is nicked on each side of the finger, a necrosis of the fingertip may well develop. Care must be taken during closure to avoid the needle's entry into the digital artery. In cases where

there is a tightness of the volar skin, the zigzag incision tends to migrate toward the midline, and a Z-plasty should be fashioned.

In cases such as tumors or infections where there is a need for exposure of the midpulp, a straight-line incision may be made over the exact middle of the distal phalanx beginning just proximal to the nail and extending just proximal to the distal finger crease. This straight incision avoids the major branches of the digital nerves, invades few terminal branches, and is generally a nontender, healed incision. It provides a direct approach to a bone felon or a tumor that otherwise would be difficult to dissect.

A fishmouth incision is mentioned only to condemn it for the morbidity it may cause. L-shaped or S-shaped incisions at the base of the fingers may be used for certain tumors requiring limited exposure. These do not cross flexor creases and do not invade digital nerves because

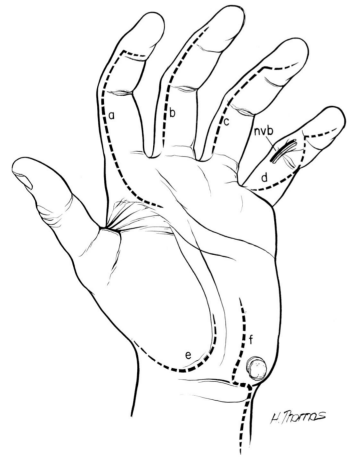

FIG. 9—5 (a) Approach to the flexor tendons of the index finger with extension into the palm through a flap incision according to Rank and Wakefield. (b and c) Regular incision of the flexor of the middle finger through a lateral incision, dorsal to the neurovascular bundle. (d) Zigzag exposure of the flexor sheath and to its contents along with the neurovascular bundles. (e) Approach for removal of the trapezium through an incision, the anterior part of which is useful in the open treatment of Bennett's fractures, according to Gedda. (f) Exposure of the hypothenar eminence and in particular the ulnar nerve and its branches.

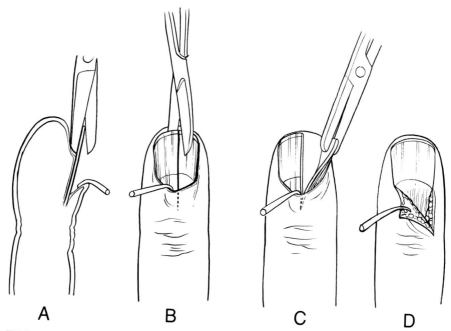

FIG. 9–6 Incision for removal of glomus tumor from the subungual area and for drainage of subungual abscesses or osteomyelitis of the distal phalanx.

the incision is confined to one segment of the finger.

The surgical approach to the nail bed of the finger is very simple. In cases of glomus tumors or infections around or deep in the nail bed, the nail is removed by longitudinal splitting from the tip to the base and by using a spiral twist and avulsion of each half of the nail. The nail bed is incised longitudinally and treated according to the affliction (Fig. 9–6).

DORSAL INCISIONS

Incisions on the dorsum of the fingers need not be as exacting as those placed on the volar aspect because the skin is more mobile, there are fewer vital structures (*i.e.*, digital nerves), and the skin creases do not cause problems of scar hypertrophy (Fig. 9–3); however, under certain circumstances oblique incisions over the dorsum of the joint creases may be useful. Oblique incisions over the dorsum of the phalanges permit adequate exposure of the dorsum of the middle

and the proximal phalanges. On exposure of the extensor apparatus over the proximal phalanx, a longitudinal incision through the midband of the extensor apparatus may be extended to the proximal interphalangeal joint without producing a disinsertion of the midtendon from the base of the middle phalanx (Fig. 9–7).

Incisions to expose the dorsal surface of the distal interphalangeal joint must avoid entering the nail matrix to avoid eventual deformity after future growth of this nail. They should also avoid unintentional cutting of the extensor tendon. An inverted-V incision permits exposure of the insertion area of the extensor tendon, gives minimal danger to the nail matrix, and does not impair the terminal branches of the dorsal digital nerve to the margin of the nails. An inverted V-shaped incision is made with its point distally placed between the most distal crease of the distal interphalangeal joint and the cuticle of the nail. The legs of this incision extend down to the dorsal lateral aspect of the finger near the distal interphalangeal joint. This dorsal flap has the advantage of being vascularized proximally; it

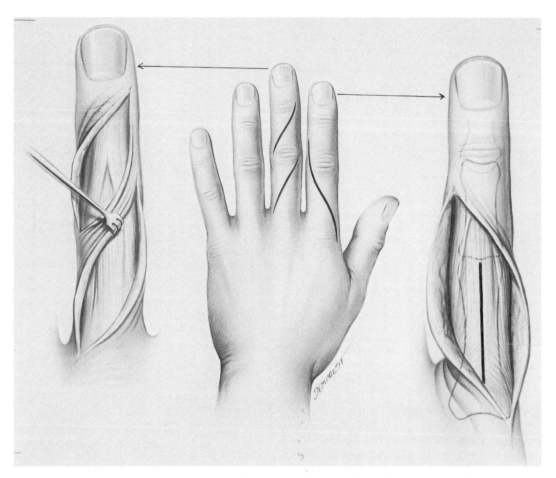

FIG. 9–7 Oblique incisions over the dorsum of the middle and the proximal phalanges of the middle finger. These can be used to explore the entire dorsal expansions of the finger. An oblique incision bypassing the proximal interphalangeal joint can be used for the same purpose. Skin retraction permits exposure of the expansion. A longitudinal incision in the dorsal expansion permits exploration of the proximal interphalangeal joint. The incision is not extended to the middle phalanx; however, if necessary, it may be extended to the middle phalanx, if the midtendon is not detached from the point of insertion.

permits exposure of the extensor tendon and the distal interphalangeal joint. The extensor tendon may be either severed and resutured or 1 mm of each lateral margin may be excised and, by alternate retraction to one side and the other, the joint may be adequately exposed for synovectomy and other procedures. It also has the advantage of causing minimal scarring, and healing usually is quite rapid.

The distal interphalangeal joint may also be approached by the J-shaped incision (Fig. 9–8).

It has the disadvantage of causing three sides of the skin margins to lack entry of blood. The nail itself takes up one side, and the two sides where the incision is made sever its blood supply, leaving only one lateral side of the flap. This is usually adequate but under conditions that have already caused crushing of this skin, slow healing may result. When the J incision is used, veins should be salvaged where possible. A straight transverse or vertical incision over the distal interphalangeal joint permits very limited exposure.

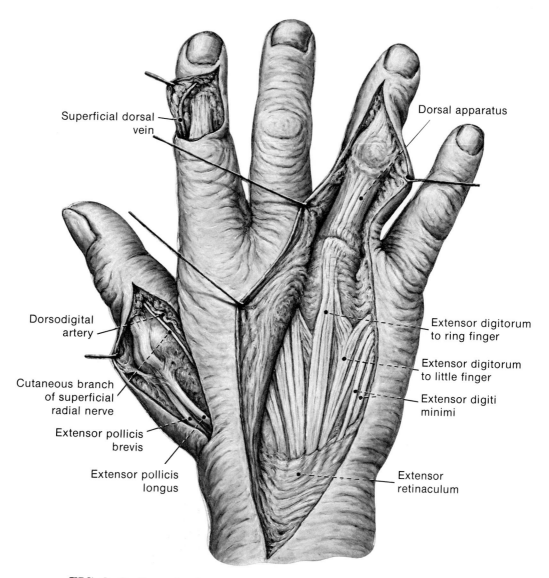

FIG. 9–8 Extensive incision for simultaneous exposure of the extensor digitorum communis tendons and tendon to one finger. This incision can be started on any finger, can be restricted to the dorsum of the hand and the wrist only, or to the dorsum of the finger only. Incision placed for repair of the dorsal apparatus over the middle phalanx of the index finger. Through this incision, any tear of the dorsal extensor apparatus can be repaired. Exposure for approach to the dorsoulnar side of the thumb or to the posterior aspect of the thumb.

For exposure of the entire dorsal apparatus, an extended, curved incision from the area distal to the distal interphalangeal joint reaching the metacarpophalangeal joint may be used (Fig. 9–3, incision). This incision can be extended easily into the dorsum of the hand (Fig. 9–8).

Through the long incision of the finger, the joints of the finger can be approached for various reconstruction procedures, excisions, arthrodesis, and others. After the skin incision is made and the dorsal apparatus is exposed, a lateral incision on the dorsal apparatus can be made and the entire structure reflected, permitting exposure of the underlying connections of the apparatus with the phalangeal joints (Fig. 2–60).

For exposure of the metacarpophalangeal joint of the index finger from the dorsum, a curved incision over the radial side of the index permits excellent exposure. After the skin is incised, the dorsal apparatus is incised between the tendon of the extensor communis indicis and the first dorsal interosseous to the point of insertion of the lumbrical muscle (Fig. 9–9). Proximal extension of this incision permits a total approach to the entire metacarpal.

For exposure of the metacarpophalangeal joint of the middle or ring finger, a straight incision is placed over the dorsum of the hand between these two fingers. For exposure of the joint, the same principle is followed by dividing the structures between the corresponding extensor tendon and the belly and the tendon of the interosseous muscle to the point of insertion of the lumbrical muscle. The metacarpophalangeal joints of the ring and little fingers may be approached through a vertical incision between the ring and little fingers. Extension of these incisions into the dorsum of the hand gives full access to the corresponding metacarpals.

In the various approaches to the metacarpophalangeal joint, curved or straight incisions permitting access to one or two joints may be used for resection of the heads of the metacarpals. After the skin is incised the most proximal part of the dorsal apparatus is separated from the interosseous muscle. The origin of the interosseous muscle is separated subperiosteally from the bone. The extensor digitorum tendon is retracted to the corresponding finger.

In reduction of untreated or unsuccessfully reduced metacarpophalangeal dislocations of the fingers, the joint may be approached through the dorsum as described above; however, certain dislocations cannot be reduced by an approach through the dorsum. Dislocations of the metacarpophalangeal joint of the index present characteristics requiring a different approach.

In a typical case, the proximal phalanx is hyperextended at the metacarpophalangeal joint and sits on the dorsum of the second metacarpal,

the phalanx is deviated toward the middle finger overlapping it on the radial side, and the distal and the proximal phalanges of the finger are flexed slightly. The head of the corresponding metacarpal can be felt in the palm of the hand between the thumb and the third metacarpal (Fig. 9–10A). In cases of this type of dislocation, the fibrocartilaginous plate of the metacarpophalangeal joint is torn from the neck of the metacarpal, the flexor tendons displace to the ulnar side of the metacarpal head and the lumbrical muscle to the radial side. The pretendinous band of the midpalmar fascia remains on the ulnar side of the metacarpal head, the volar cartilaginous plate follows the proximal phalanx and lands on the dorsum of the neck of the metacarpal, the lateral collateral ligaments lock the phalanx in the abnormal position. The natatory ligament distally and the superficial transverse metacarpal ligament proximally lock the head in a quadrangle.

To reduce dislocations of this type, the incision is placed in the proximal crease of the palm over the metacarpophalangeal joint of the index finger and if necessary, extended over the radial side of the proximal phalanx of the finger. The natatory band and the superficial transverse fibers then can be divided and the dislocation reduced (Figs. 9–10B and C).

Becton and others have described a dorsal incision to reduce the complex dislocation of the metacarpophalangeal of the index finger. This incision gives full exposure of the fibrocartilaginous volar plate, which is, of course, the structure that blocks reduction. It also permits ample protection to the digital nerves and permits observation of the joint for possible osteochondral fractures of the metacarpal head.

A dorsal incision is made over the index metacarpophalangeal joint in a 4-cm straight line, exposing the extensor tendon, which is split along its axis, as well as the joint capsule. The volar plate then is noted and cut longitudinally (this should not be confused with the metacarpal head). The wrist is flexed, thus releasing tension on the flexor tendon, which is then allowed to slip around the metacarpal head as reduction is accomplished by flexing the finger. An

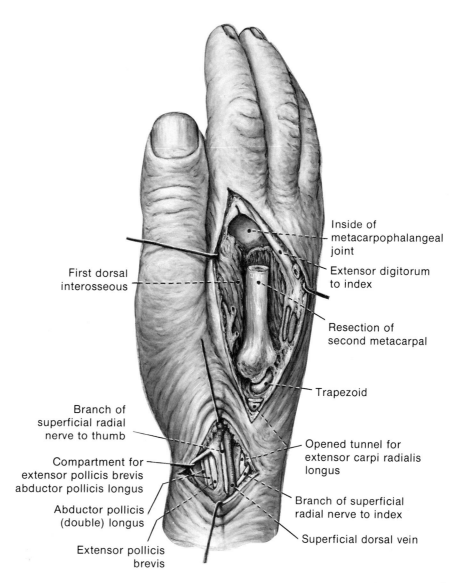

First dorsal interosseous

Inside of metacarpophalangeal joint

Extensor digitorum to index

Resection of second metacarpal

Trapezoid

Branch of superficial radial nerve to thumb

Compartment for extensor pollicis brevis abductor pollicis longus

Abductor pollicis (double) longus

Extensor pollicis brevis

Opened tunnel for extensor carpi radialis longus

Branch of superficial radial nerve to index

Superficial dorsal vein

FIG. 9–9 Incision for resection of a part or the whole second metacarpal and incision for DeQuervain's disease. Through a curved incision with the convexity directed toward the ulnar side of the hand, running from the lower third of the dorsum of the proximal phalanx of the index toward the base of the second metacarpal, the second metacarpal can be approached easily. The capsule and the interosseous muscles are detached subperiosteally. The forked base of the second metacarpal is easy to identify and can be disarticulated, if necessary, after disinsertion of the tendon of the extensor carpi radialis longus. For DeQuervain's disease, a transverse or curved incision about 4 cm long is placed over the radial styloid. Blunt dissection uncovers the superficial branches of the radial nerve and the dorsal vein. The tendons of the abductor pollicis longus and the extensor pollicis brevis are located easily in the tunnel, which is incised longitudinally. The incision must be very superficial until the branches of the radial nerve are exposed. It should not be extended too far to the ulnar side because it is easy to get into the tunnel of the extensor carpi radialis longus.

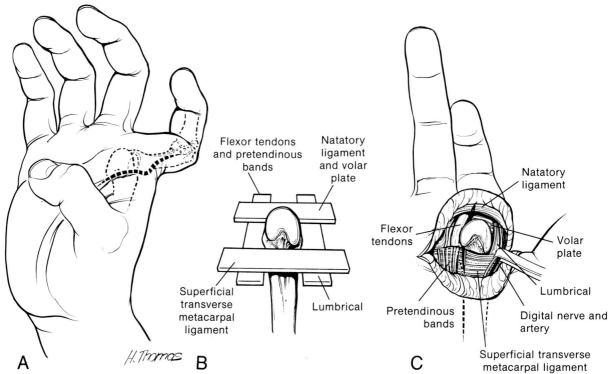

FIG. 9–10 **A**, Position of the index finger in metacarpophalangeal dislocation viewed from the lateral aspect of the hand. Incision for approach to the area of dislocation. **B** and **C**, Anatomy of the dislocation of the metacarpophalangeal joint of the index and mechanism to locking of the metacarpal head.

osteochondral fracture of the metacarpal head may be noted and either excised, or if a major portion of a ligament is attached to it, appropriately repaired. The joint capsule, tendon, and skin are each sutured. It is not necessary to transfix the joint with a pin. Splinting is usually sufficient and maintained for approximately 3 weeks before motion is started.

INCISIONS OVER THE THUMB

The exposures for various surgical procedures involving the thumb must be placed correctly and with precision (Figs. 9–2, 9–3, and 9–11). Over the volar surface of the distal and the proximal phalanges, the incisions are similar to the incisions of the other fingers. The distal phalanx can be incised over the radial or ulnar

aspect or midline of the pulp for drainage of infections of the closed space or removal of a sequestrum of the distal phalanx. Fishmouth incisions are not advised.

Lateral incisions over the radial side of the thumb to expose the digital nerve or artery or approach the tendon of the flexor pollicis longus. This incision can be extended into the metacarpophalangeal crease and even into the hand, as will be described later.

The transverse incision in the crease of the metacarpophalangeal joint of the thumb is very useful for treatment of stenosing tendovaginitis of the sheath of the flexor pollicis longus (Fig. 9–11, incision *a*). Certain precautions must be taken when this incision is used. The incision must be made just through the dermis, especially over its radial part, because the digital nerve and artery to the radial side of the thumb are very superficial and have a surprisingly anterior course between the skin and the radial sesamoid. The skin incision can and should be extended more toward the ulnar side but should not divide the interdigital web between the thumb and index finger (Fig. 9–12).

The relationship of the digital nerves of the thumb to the sesamoids should be well understood (Figs. 3–3 and 3–12). The approach to the tunnel of the flexor pollicis longus is made by careful, blunt exposure between the radial and ulnar digital nerves of the thumb. The incision does not permit much space. The tendon sheath can be split blindly by introducing the scissors between the tendon and the tendon sheath and slitting the sheath distally; this procedure is wrought with danger if done proximally. The blind splitting of the tendon sheath in a proximal direction may reach the bifurcation of the branch of the median nerve to the thumb and may inadvertently divide either one or the other branch (Figs. 5–14 and 9–13) to the thumb.

The exposure of the greater length of the flexor pollicis longus requires a special incision that can be combined easily with the radial incision over the thumb and the transverse incision over the metacarpophalangeal joint of the thumb (Fig. 9–2). The additional incision starts near the ulnar end of the metacarpophalangeal crease and runs toward the thenar crease of the palm in a curved line. It crosses the thenar line to the ulnar side and running parallel with this line for about 5 mm to 6 mm to its ulnar side, it reaches the midline of the wrist ulnar to the tendon of the palmaris longus (Fig. 9–13).

Extending the incision into the depth on the ulnar side of the tendon of the palmaris longus, the transverse carpal ligament is incised, and the median nerve is identified. The median nerve is approached from its ulnar side and is retracted toward the thumb without exposing the motor thenar branch, which supplies the thenar muscles from the radial side of the nerve. Retraction of the median nerve toward the thumb permits rapid localization of the tendon of the flexor pollicis longus, which can be identified in the radial bursa as the

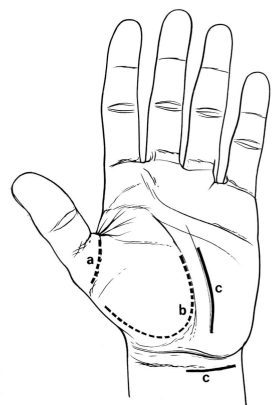

FIG. 9–11 (a) Useful transverse incision for release of trigger thumb. (b) Incision utilizing retrograde flap to expose underlying thenar eminence. (c) and (d) Double skin incisions for a carpal tunnel release. The scars are located in skin creases.

deepest and most radially placed tendon in the carpal canal. The entire length of the flexor pollicis longus tendon can be exposed in the palm with the proper retraction of the digital branches of the median nerve to the thumb, index, and middle fingers (Fig. 9–13). This incision permits good exposure of all the digital nerves of the median nerve and the thenar motor branch of the thenar muscles if this is necessary.

Similar to the above incision is one that uses the same two distal limbs, namely the lateral approach to the thumb from the radial aspect, extending across the metacarpophalangeal joint to the ulnar aspect, but instead of proceeding to a point beyond the thenar crease, a more radial

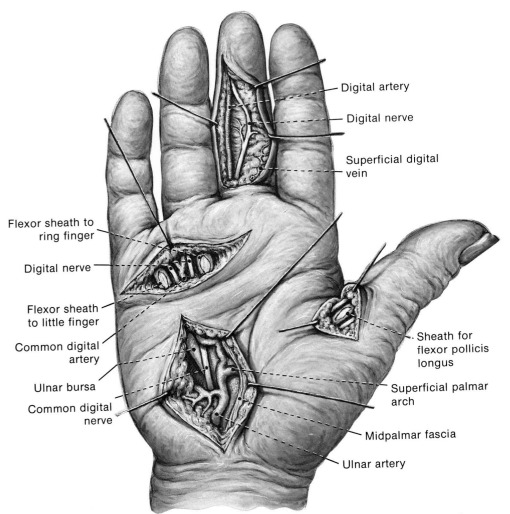

FIG. 9–12 Incisions for approach to the digital nerve and the digital artery of a finger. There are no venae comitantes; the nerve exhibits articular branches. Incision for a trigger thumb; note proximity of the digital nerve to the radial side of the incision. Incision for approach to the snapping ring and the little fingers and also to the midpalmar space, distal to the distal crease. Incision for exposure of the ulnar bursa; approach to one of the branches of the ulnar nerve and to the superficial volar arch.

alignment of the incision is made by going proximal but parallel on the radial aspect of the thenar crease. This more proximal limb of the incision is about 1/2 cm on the radial aspect of the thenar crease and is therefore more directly over the area of the flexor tendon of the thumb. Great care must be taken not to sever the recurrent branch of the median nerve. This does not permit an adequate exposure to the median nerve, but does permit a more direct approach to the flexor pollicis longus tendon, which is frequently found when severed and is seated between the muscle bellies of the abductor pollicis brevis and the flexor pollicis brevis.

A special approach to the volar aspect of the metacarpocarpal joint of the thumb is

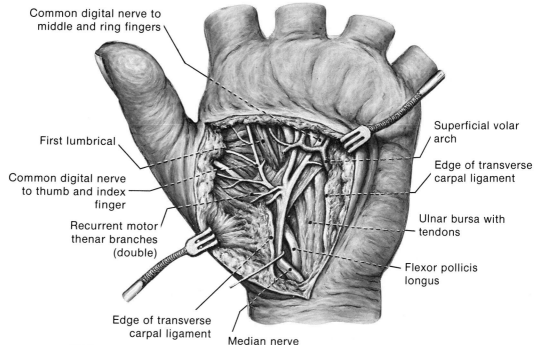

Common digital nerve to middle and ring fingers

First lumbrical

Common digital nerve to thumb and index finger

Recurrent motor thenar branches (double)

Edge of transverse carpal ligament

Median nerve

Superficial volar arch

Edge of transverse carpal ligament

Ulnar bursa with tendons

Flexor pollicis longus

FIG. 9–13 Incision for approach to the median nerve in the hand and to the flexor pollicis longus. Through this incision to the ulnar side of the thenar crease, the palmaris longus and the median nerve are approached transversely. The carpal ligament is divided for exposure of the median nerve; the median nerve is then retracted toward the radial side of the wrist. Retraction of the nerve permits exposure of the radial bursa, which is incised, and the flexor pollicis is exposed. Through this incision, the distal part of the flexor pollicis longus can also be exposed safely.

sometimes required. The author used a special approach in cases of old subluxation and dislocation of the thumb for treatment of this condition. In dislocations of this joint, the volar part of the capsule becomes distended or tears. The posterior dorsal part of the capsule, which is reinforced by the tendons of the extensors pollicis longus and brevis, does not tear as easily as the volar part covered by the origin of the abductor brevis and the opponens pollicis.

The volar aspect of the trapeziometacarpal joint of the thumb is approached in the following manner: an incision is made starting about 1 cm proximal to the cardinal line (Figs. 8–4 and 9–5) along the proximal part of the thenar crease, then following the proximal curve of the thenar eminence distal to the tubercle of the trapezium. The incision is extended radially to the insertion

of the tendon of the abductor pollicis longus. The origins of the abductor pollicis brevis and opponens pollicis are elevated from the volar carpal ligament distal to the ridge of the trapezium and radial to the tunnel of the tendon of the flexor carpi radialis. The surgical repair of the exposed joint consists of reefing and plication of the capsule (Figs. 2–7, 2–63, and 3–16). After this is done the muscles of the thenar eminence are repositioned and secured with a few sutures to the transverse carpal ligament.

The trapezium also can be excised through this approach, but the trapeziometacarpal joint can also be approached from a longitudinal curved or a horizontal incision made through the anatomic snuff-box and then longitudinally between the tendons of the extensors pollicis longus and brevis. With the wrist in ulnar deviation, the trapezium may be approached safely and excised carefully; however, this approach is not as adequate as the approach described for the exposure of the volar aspect of the trapeziometacarpal joint, which does not endanger the flexor carpi radialis tendon when the trapezium is separated from the volar structures in the process of removal.

In fractures, dislocations of the base of the thumb metacarpal, known as Bennett's fractures, it is necessary to overcome the dorsal and radial subluxation of the metacarpal and to reduce the fracture of the ulnar base of the proximal phalanx. Although closed reduction with the first metacarpal firmly held in place with plaster only may give satisfactory results, an open reduction or percutaneous pinning with transfixion of the metacarpal and the fragment in place is a more dependable procedure.

Milford and others have advocated percutaneous pinning of the first metacarpal to the second metacarpal or carpus to maintain adequate reduction of the Bennett fracture. Traction is placed on the thumb with the wrist in flexion while holding the thumb in abduction. The first metacarpal is brought into alignment with the fragment on the ulnar aspect. Two Kirschner wires are introduced through the metacarpal across the joint or into the second metacarpal or to the carpal bones to stabilize the first metacarpal in the reduced position. Accurate reduction can then be determined by x-ray without details being obscured by a cast; however, a cast is applied once adequate reduction is obtained. This method avoids open reduction of the fracture, but if accurate reduction is not obtained, open reduction can still be done. This is more easily done through a volar approach at the base of the thumb. Gedda and Moberg have also made a thorough study of the subject that resulted in the clearest understanding of the mechanism and treatment of this condition. The approach to the metacarpophalangeal joint is simplified and made more precise by the following method.

The ulnar end of the distal crease of the palm is marked as a point. Another point is marked 1 cm proximal to the prominent tubercle of the trapezium on the thenar eminence; the two points are united by a line. This line on the base of the thenar eminence corresponds exactly to the carpometacarpal articular interspace. An incision over this line at the base of the thenar eminence, extending slightly distally along the thenar eminence, gives the most direct approach to the joint.

For an approach to the trapezium, this line can be extended posteriorly along the same curve, first crossing the tendons of the extensor pollicis brevis and the abductor pollicis longus and then the tendons of the extensor pollicis longus. This permits an exposure of the anterior and posterior aspects of the trapezium (Fig. 9–5A[e]).

Irreducible dislocations of the metacarpophalangeal joint of the thumb require a special surgical approach. The pathology of the dislocation is conditioned by the anatomic relationship of the sesamoids connected with the volar plate of this joint and the connection of the thenar muscles with the sesamoids. There is practically no capsule over the base of the proximal phalanx; instead of the capsule there is the volar fibrocartilaginous plate with the sesamoids. Over the head and the neck of the metacarpal, the capsule is intimately connected with the tendons of the thenar muscles (Figs. 3–3, 3–12, and 3–16).

To treat intelligently dislocations of the thumb through an appropriate approach, the pathology of the dislocation must be understood. In these dislocations, the metacarpal head usually tears through the flexor brevis muscle and dislocates forward and radially. The base of the proximal phalanx dislocates dorsally and becomes displaced on the dorsoulnar side of the neck of the first metacarpal, carrying with it the entire intersesamoid ligament, which is actually the glenoid ligament, with the tunnel of the flexor pollicis longus and the two sesamoids. In the dislocations, the tunnel of the flexor pollicis longus usually is displaced toward the ulnar side, crossing the ulnar neck of the first metacarpal. The two sesamoids completely clear the head of the first metacarpal and move toward the dorsum of the neck of the first metacarpal, together with the base of the proximal phalanx. The radial and ulnar digital nerves become com-

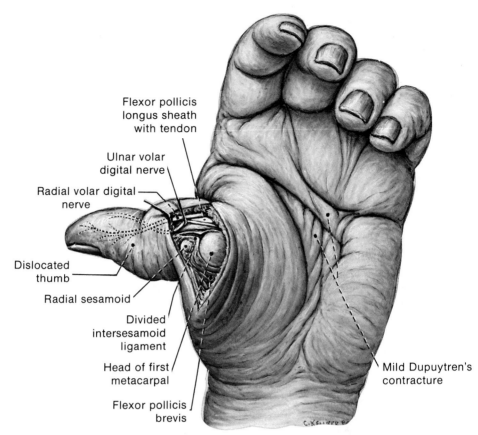

Flexor pollicis
longus sheath
with tendon

Ulnar volar
digital nerve

Radial volar digital
nerve

Dislocated
thumb

Radial sesamoid

Divided
intersesamoid
ligament

Head of first
metacarpal

Flexor pollicis
brevis

Mild Dupuytren's
contracture

FIG. 9–14 Approach for reduction of dislocated thumb, irreducible by the closed method. Dislocation of the thumb in a hand afflicted with a mild Dupuytren's contracture. The incision is made at the ulnar end of the metacarpophalangeal crease of the thumb, running parallel with this crease toward its radial end, then deflecting toward the dorsum of the first metacarpal. The head of the first metacarpal is located easily when torn through the flexor pollicis brevis. The nerves and the vessels run together with the flexor pollicis longus on the ulnar side of the neck of the first metacarpal. The intersesamoid ligament (volar plate) is freely divided longitudinally, permitting a complete reduction of the dislocation. The digital nerve of the radial side of the thumb loses its relation to the radial sesamoid and is displaced notably toward the ulnar side of the thumb, making it comparatively easy to divide the intersesamoid ligament just ulnad to the radial sesamoid.

pletely displaced and move to the ulnar side of the head of the first metacarpal. The radial digital nerve of the thumb loses its constant relationship with the radial sesamoid (Fig. 9–14).

Occasionally, the dislocation may occur through the adductor pollicis. Then, the head of the first metacarpal is dislocated anteroulnarly; the tunnel of the flexor pollicis longus with the tendon is displaced radially and rests on the radial side of the neck of the first metacarpal.

The pathology of the dislocation makes the procedure and the incision obvious in cases where closed reduction is difficult or impossible. The incision is started at the ulnar end of the metacarpophalangeal crease of the thumb and is carried parallel with this crease toward the radial end of the crease. It then turns in line with this crease toward the dorsum of the thumb, crossing the dorsum of the first metacarpal. Through this long incision, the intersesamoid ligament, the volar plate, or the glenoid ligament are approached and in accordance with the type of dislocation, is divided to separate the two sesamoids. This division permits release of the stranglehold the glenoid ligament forms over the dorsal neck of the first metacarpal and permits the reduction of the phalanx with restoration of the flexor pollicis longus tunnel to its normal position (Fig. 9–14).

The anterior part of the metacarpophalangeal joint of the thumb, as has been mentioned, has practically no capsule. The dense glenoid ligament represents the volar aspect of the capsule. The distal and the proximal movements of this glenoid ligament, together with the sesamoids in their restored position, permit flexion and extension of this joint.

In the operative approach to a dislocated thumb in which the head of the metacarpal protrudes toward the radiovolar side of the metacarpophalangeal joint, the head of the metacarpal is covered with dense fibrous tissue that results from the tear and fibrous healing of the flexor pollicis brevis on the radial side or of the adductor pollicis on the ulnar side. In old cases it is therefore necessary to excise this dense, fibrous tissue to free the head of the metacarpal from the surrounding fibrous tissue.

It is also possible to divide the glenoid ligament from the posterior aspect to free the flexor tunnel and the two sesamoids. The displacement of the volar plate with the sesamoids to the neck of the metacarpal in dislocations of the thumb makes it accessible from the dorsal aspect of the joint. If, for some reason, an approach of this type is decided on, a curved dorsal incision either on the radial or the ulnar side of the metacarpophalangeal joint may be used (Fig. 9–8). The capsule is incised between the extensors pollicis longus and brevis; however, this approach is somewhat restricted because the displaced thumb frequently forms a 90-degree angle with the first metacarpal.

Some injuries of the metacarpophalangeal joints of the thumb do not produce dorsal dislocations of the proximal phalanx but produce subluxations, mostly radial, with instability of the joint. These injuries are of two types: acute injuries, which produce a total disruption of the ulnar capsular structures, including the ulnar lateral ligament of the metacarpophalangeal joint (Aldred, Moberg, and Stener); and gradual subluxations, which result in radial deviations of the proximal phalanx with instability and weakness of adduction. In both types of subluxation, in addition to the displacement of the proximal phalanx the tendon of the extensor pollicis longus is displaced to the radial side of the metacarpal head, and the ulnar sesamoid with the adductor pollicis is displaced toward the volar side of the joint. The displacement of the extensor pollicis becomes permanent and increases the deformity when an attempt is made to extend the thumb.

Extensive experience with acute injuries and observations in late results after acute injuries by Stener showed that the subluxations are caused by the disruptions of the ulnar collateral ligament, and on occasion, the dorsal adductor expansion is torn (Fig. 9–15). Kaplan was able to produce experimentally in cadavers subluxations of the metacarpal head without disruption of the ulnar collateral ligament but with rupture of the extensor expansion of the adductor muscle. The mechanism proposed was rotation of the thumb with disruption and deflection of the extensor pollicis longus tendon. In acute cases of rupture of the ligament, primary repair of the ligament is the best treatment. In cases of radial subluxation of the proximal phalanx and displacement of the tendon of the extensor pollicis longus, in which there is no history of acute injury, transplantation of the tendon of the extensor indicis into the extensor pollicis longus gave satisfactory results. Others have recommended ligamentous reconstruction with a free tendon graft (Curtis, Smith); Nevaiser recommends adductor pollicis advancement.

The incision over the metacarpophalangeal joint may be as indicated in Figure 9–16; In other instances, an oblique incision over the dorsum of the metacarpophalangeal joint, running from the ulnar side of the middle of the proximal

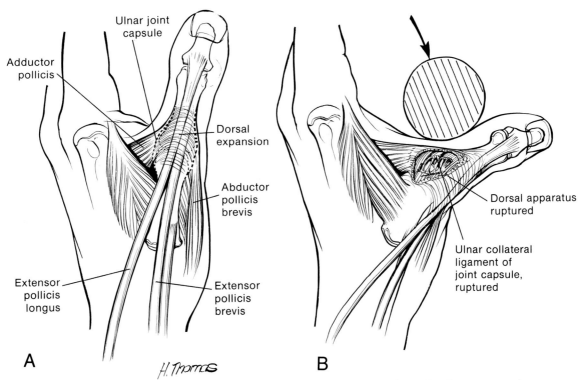

FIG. 9–15 **A**, Anatomy of normal thumb as seen from the dorsum. **B**, When excessive pressure is exerted at proximal phalanx, a tear may occur at ulnar aspect of metacarpophalangeal joint, stretching or tearing the joint and dorsal apparatus and the ulnar collateral ligament.

phalanx to the neck of the first metacarpal, gives a better view of all the structures involved. The volar approach for dislocations of the metacarpophalangeal joint also has an advantage; it can be used for resection of the metacarpal head if correction of the dislocation cannot be obtained after division of the volar plate between the two sesamoids and if the resection becomes necessary.

Several dorsal incisions may be used for exposure of the region over the metacarpophalangeal joint of the thumb for tendon work. When placed on the dorsoradial side of the joint, the tendon of insertion of the abductor pollicis brevis is exposed and can be used for implantation of transplanted tendons, for instance in a case of loss of opposition. When placed on the dorsoulnar aspect, the incision can be used for tendon surgery of the extensor

pollicis brevis or longus (Fig. 9–8). If this incision is extended proximally (Fig. 9–3), it permits exposure of the entire length of the tendon of the extensor pollicis longus.

The incision starts on the ulnar side of the dorsum of the proximal phalanx of the thumb and runs parallel with the ulnar side of a line connecting the ulnar tubercle of the base of the first metacarpal to Lister's tubercle of the radius (Fig. 9–3). The identification of the tendon is easy, even if the tendon retracts in cases of its traumatic division or attrition. The tendon of the extensor pollicis longus is superficial to the two radial extensors of the wrist. Immediately distal to the tubercle of Lister, the tendon crosses, in the form of a X, the tendon of the extensor carpi radialis brevis. The extensor pollicis longus is more superficial than the tendon of the extensor carpi radialis brevis.

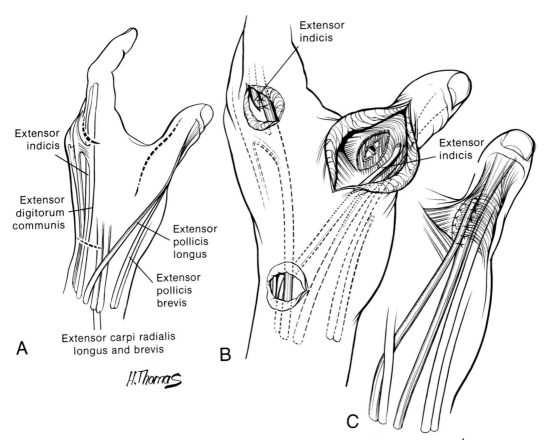

FIG. 9–16 Kaplan's method of repairing radial subluxation of the metacarpophalangeal joint of the thumb.

The extensor pollicis longus is hidden in an osteofibrous tunnel formed by Lister's tubercle and the dorsal carpal ligament. In its course through this short tunnel, the extensor pollicis longus changes its tendinous structure into the bipennate muscular form of its belly (Fig. 3–14). To locate the extensor pollicis longus when it retracts, it is necessary to incise the tunnel longitudinally and look for the bipennate muscle belly.

SURGICAL APPROACHES TO THE PALM OF THE HAND

Incisions within the palm are frequently in addition to or are extensions of finger or wrist incisions. The need for this possible finger or wrist extension should be anticipated; drawing out the incision with a sterile skin pencil is helpful to accurately coordinate these possible extensions if needed or when old scars or recent traumatic incisions must be correlated with new incisions. Use of already committed openings challenges the surgeon's ingenuity because he or she must avoid too narrow a distally based flap or parallel incisions that are too close together. When scars are used as a part of a new incision, heavy collagen tissue may encompass or distort the underlying nerves, vessels, and tendons, making it difficult not to damage these. To avoid damage, the area proximal and distal to the scar should be dissected first, slowly identifying the vital structures lying within the scar. These may be already severed or partially severed, but further damage should be meticulously avoided.

Any incision made in the palm can actually be carried immediately to the depth of the palmar fascia with safety (an exception is the area of the recurrent branch of the median nerve and at the distal palmar fat pad, where there is no palmar fascia). Once the fascia is encountered, fat and skin are dissected off the fascia, converting the linear opening into an oval shape for better exposure. The exposed fascia may then be spread or excised, thus exposing the underlying structures. The palmar skin is less mobile than the dorsal skin because it must provide a stable, padded, fixed surface during grasping and pinching. This skin fixation causes a problem when skin rotation may be desirable, such as in Z-plasties within the palm. The thumb and finger webs are an entirely different problem because the web height can be lowered to accommodate for the extra skin needed. Owing to the tight fixation of the palmar skin and its underlying fat, soft tissue tumors such as lipomas and ganglia are difficult to palpate until they reach considerable size. Symptoms of pressure may be the presenting complaint rather than a mass. For the same reason, swelling from infection can frequently be seen more easily and earlier when located in the dorsum of the hand. This dorsal swelling is also caused by the venous and lymphatic dorsal drainage. Tenderness in an area of the suspected abscess may be a more dependable sign of its extent than attempting palpation of its ill-defined borders.

Specific incisions for specific problems will be described later; traditionally, most incisions in the palm have been transverse in nature, paralleling the flexor creases. These have generally served well for excision of tumors, drainage of infection, and repair of tendons with an additional but separate incision in the fingers when necessary. The exploration needed for reconstruction of proximal flexor tendon pulleys, synovectomy of the finger, palm, and wrist, rheumatoid disease, and decompression

for high-pressure injection injuries is more efficiently done with one continuous incision that is more vertical in nature within the palm; however, the incision still adheres to the principles of not crossing flexor creases at near right angles. Incisions are zigzag in the digits with extension into the palm and wrist (Fig. 9–2, incisions *g* and *k*). This type of incision is not quite the same as a general utility incision described many years ago by Bunnell. It is a more direct approach to the pathology involved and elevates less skin as flaps.

In principle, when draining an abscess within the palm the procedure should be done using an arm tourniquet but by eliminating most of the blood before elevation of the tourniquet pressure by a 2-minute elevation of the entire extremity instead of wrapping the arm to exsanguinate the area. Once the incision is made and the area of abscess is identified, it is safer to proceed to the area by blunt dissection, instead of using the usual sharp knife or scissor. Structures may be distorted by the swelling and nerves and arteries drawn tight over the area of abnormal appearing anatomy. Pushing the blunt scissors or hemostat into the abscess, gently spreading it, provides the drainage to the sometimes necrotic or rather badly distorted area.

SURGICAL APPROACHES AND ANATOMY OF DUPUYTREN'S CONTRACTURE

Treatment of the hand with intact skin may present special problems such as the treatment of Dupuytren's contracture (Fig. 9–17). The history, etiology, and pathology of this affliction have been described extensively; the treatment is a matter of meticulous work. The author believes that a thorough excision of the contracted fascia, properly executed, produces satisfactory functional results. Surgical treatment requires knowledge of the usual relationship of the contracted fascia bands to the nerves and vessels of the hand and fingers. The exci-

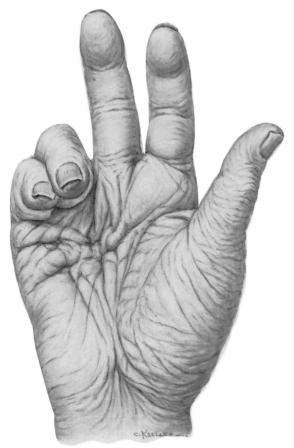

FIG. 9–17 Dupuytren's contracture. The dissection of this hand is shown in Figures 9–18 and 9–19.

sion of the contracted bands must be accomplished without injury to the digital nerves and arteries.

The material available in most anatomic laboratories presents frequent opportunities for dissection of the hand afflicted with Dupuytren's contracture. Study of these hands permits more extensive observations than is possible during surgical procedures (Fig. 9–18).

One of the constant impressions obtained by the author was concerned with the relationship of the contracted bands to the digital nerve and vessels. Constantly, the pretendinous contracted bands of the midpalmar aponeurosis appeared to be running deeply to the digital nerve and artery of the fingers. If a branch of a

pretendinous band formed an additional bridge to the next finger, the additional bridge ran deeply to the digital nerve and artery (Figs. 9–19 and 9–20). Resection of a part of the nerve and the artery in the illustrated specimen over the radial side of the contracted ring finger and the ulnar side of the contracted little finger shows the pretendinous contracted band of the fifth finger and a branch running from the contracted band to the next finger deeply to the nerve and the artery.

In the palm of the hand, the nerves and the vessels are located deeper than the contracted aponeurosis. The superficial transverse ligament is always superficial to the nerves and the vessels in contrast with the pretendinous bands in the fingers. The tendon of the palmaris longus muscle is frequently missing. When present, the tendon and the palmaris longus muscle are not involved in the contracture.

The varied configurations of deformity secondary to the proliferating fibroblasts in Dupuytren's contracture provoke the surgeon's ingenuity and imagination to develop appropriate incisions needed for correction of these deformities. These individualized incisions may be of three general types, while still adhering to the basic principles of incisions about the hand: an incision may be needed to remove only the palmar portion of disease and is usually transverse (Figs. 9–2, incision *f*, and 9–12); an incision may be needed on the volar side of the finger to permit excision of the underlying pathology and to obtain extension of the joints (Figs. 9–2, incision *g*, and 9–20); and an incision may be needed to not only provide exposure of the underlying pathology but to provide a means of transferring skin in an effort to relieve the skin contracture (Z-plasty, or Y-to-V advancement techniques are recommended).

Transverse Incision. The transverse incision may be made at almost any level of the palm with the exception of an incision that directly crosses the thenar crease as it connects the radial and ulnar sides of the palm. Paralleling the distal two palmar creases at any level may be carried out to expose the underlying nodules

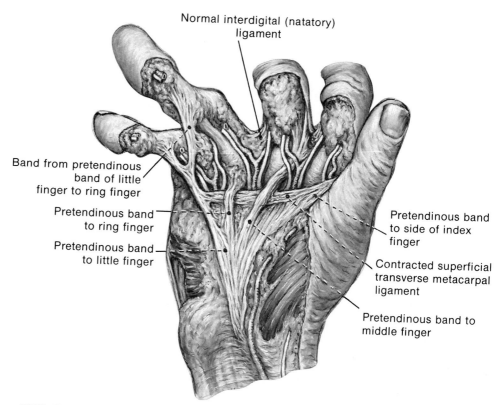

Normal interdigital (natatory)
ligament

Band from pretendinous
band of little
finger to ring finger

Pretendinous band
to ring finger

Pretendinous band
to little finger

Pretendinous band
to side of index
finger

Contracted superficial
transverse metacarpal
ligament

Pretendinous band to
middle finger

FIG. 9–18 Dupuytren's contracture, right hand (the left hand of the same cadaver also afflicted with Dupuytren's contracture is shown in Figure 9–14). The pretendinous band to the little finger is very contracted and sends an additional contracting branch to the ring finger. The contracture extends to the middle phalanx of the little and the ring fingers. The artery and the nerve are volar to the contracting bands. The pretendinous bands to the ring finger are attached to the tunnel of the flexor tendon in the region of the metacarpal head. The pretendinous band to the middle finger forms dense adhesions with the radial side of the proximal phalanx of this finger. The superficial transverse ligament is extremely dense, forming a cordlike structure from the pretendinous band of the little finger to the radial side of the index finger. This specimen had no palmaris longus tendon.

FIG. 9–19 Detail of the ulnar side of the contracted little and ring fingers of the hand shown in Figure 9–18.

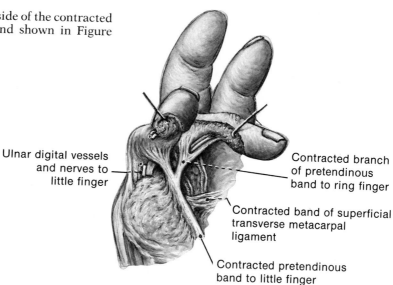

Ulnar digital vessels
and nerves to
little finger

Contracted branch
of pretendinous
band to ring finger

Contracted band of superficial
transverse metacarpal
ligament

Contracted pretendinous
band to little finger

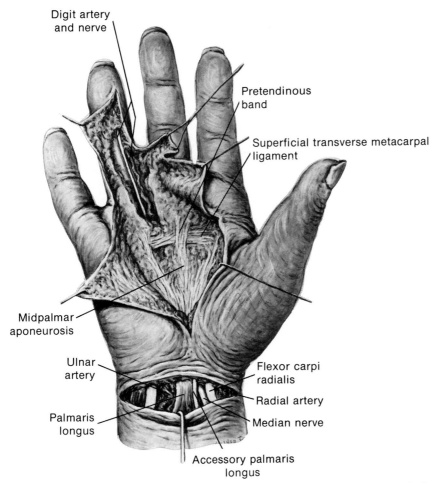

Digit artery
and nerve

Pretendinous
band

Superficial transverse metacarpal
ligament

Midpalmar
aponeurosis

Ulnar
artery

Flexor carpi
radialis

Radial artery

Palmaris
longus

Median nerve

Accessory palmaris
longus

FIG. 9—20   The principle of direct extended exposure of the offending underlying
fascia by an incision continuous from the palm into the fingers is shown here.

or fascial contractures; however, after the initial incision is carried completely through the skin, the skin should be undermined immediately to avoid the underlying neurovascular bundles that may be distorted, especially in Dupuytren's disease. By undermining, the incision is then converted into a oval-shaped exposure, providing ample visualization of the underlying fascia for safe excision. Closure of this incision should be loose and drained frequently with ample splinting of the hand and wrist. Forty-eight hours of elevation of the hand immediately postoperatively helps to prevent pernicious hematoma.

Zigzag Incision.   When skin contracture is not a major problem, a zigzag incision may be made through the mid- and distal palm and extended into the volar aspect of the fingers. This can be a stretched-out, multiple Z-shaped incision or in combination with a separate transverse palmar incision. This has the disadvantage of leaving an undermined bridge of skin at the distal palm. This direct Z-shaped approach to the underlying contracting bands maintains ample blood supply to the flaps, and prompt healing is expected. This incision may later migrate toward the midline in some instances, but this is generally not a serious disadvantage. The points of the incision should be made with care because they overlie the digital nerves. The incision should be closed with loosely placed sutures to permit drainage.

Z-Plasties. The third type of incision is that in which a single or multiple Z-plasties are fashioned to provide exposure and to convert a vertical incision into a zigzag closure. This approach is advantageous for removal of skin areas that are pitted or very thin. By planning the incision and outlining it with a skin pencil, the surgeon can envision how certain areas of the skin may be eliminated when closing the flaps. This direct approach to the underlying pathology makes it much easier to envision and protect the frequently distorted path of the digital nerves. Digital nerves may be looping the lateral deforming fascial bands and are frequently embedded in the fibrous tissue, especially proximal to and at the level of the proximal interphalangeal joint. The Z-plastic flaps should be created such that the transverse central segment of the "Z" will lie within or at least parallel to the normal creases of the fingers.

INCISIONS FOR RELEASE OF CARPAL TUNNEL SYNDROME

Carpal tunnel syndrome in the majority of cases is caused by a nonspecific synovitis that results in pressure on the median nerve. This pressure frequently causes the patient to awaken at night with burning or numbness in the hand that may be relieved by exercises. Tinel's sign may be demonstrated in patients at the wrist level. Atrophy of the thenar muscle, innervated by the median nerve, may also be present. This syndrome may be caused by other space-occupying lesions, such as tumors, malalignment of the carpal canal as in a distal radial fracture, dislocation of the lunate, and other carpal bone dislocations. Aberrant muscles are another (but rare) cause of median nerve compression, and thrombosis of a patent median artery has also been reported.

An incision parallel to the thenar crease beginning at the level of the base of the thumb web and extending parallel with the thenar crease to the carpal volar wrist crease and then gently curving ulnad is a safe incision through which the underlying fat and the more proximal antebrachial fascia are dissected. The transverse carpal ligament lies distal to the transverse volar wrist creases, but it can be more safely approached, proximal to distal, by first isolating the nerve at the level of the flexor volar crease and opening the overlying structures from this point distally. It is important to realize that the palmar branch of the median nerve usually lies between flexor carpi radialis tendon and the palmaris longus and may be sectioned should the incision extend too far radially, causing a very painful postoperative neuroma. It should therefore be protected.

Nerve of more vital importance is the recurrent branch of the median nerve, which (it must be realized) can arise from the ulnar aspect or the volar aspect of the nerve trunk. Location of this branch can generally be made by Kaplan's cardinal lines (see Fig. 8–3). Following complete release of the median nerve by being certain that the distal margin of the transverse metacarpal ligament is cut, the wound may be closed by placing deep interrupted vertical sutures. Subcutaneous sutures are not necessarily needed. Care should be taken to make the skin closure level. Postoperatively, a rubber drain is frequently helpful; a volar splint is helpful for 10 days to 2 weeks postoperatively to avoid wrist flexion and possible herniation of the tendons. Finger motion is encouraged.

INCISIONS FOR TRIGGER FINGER

Incision for the triggering finger that occurs in adults (usually after 40 years of age) may be associated with collagen diseases. It is more common in the middle finger and may be diagnosed by a palpable fusiform swelling or nodule over the flexor tendon just proximal to the true tendon sheath at the distal palm. Pressure on this nodule will accentuate the triggering effect of the finger. Sectioning of this sheath may be indicated if other conservative measures have been inadequate. Incisions may be either transverse or vertical over the sheath, but again adhering to the principle of not crossing a crease of the palm at right angles. A transverse incision is generally adequate just distal to the distal palmar crease (Fig. 9–12).

After making the incision and converting it to an oval shape, the distinct proximal margin of the tendon sheath should be located by blunt dissection. At this point, a small primary opening of the sheath should be carried out with a knife to allow visualization of the underlying tendon; insertion of slightly opened scissors pushed gently distally, opens the sheath from this point to the level just beyond the proximal finger crease. Undermining the skin and fat above the sheath will make this easier. Elevation of the tendons from their bed will confirm that there is no nodule on the tendons and that they are free to move and that an adequate release has been carried out. Single interrupted sutures to close the wound are adequate without subcutaneous sutures, and a compression dressing can be applied, elevating the hand immediately postoperatively. This permits early motion within 24 hours.

INCISIONS INTO THE DORSUM OF THE HAND

The dorsum of the hand presents problems of approach to the metacarpals and the extensor tendons of the fingers. These incisions can be placed in a manner that permits their extension into the wrist and even the forearm if necessary. The incision along the dorsoulnar or the dorsoradial side of the finger can be extended easily in a curved line with the apex toward the ulnar side of the hand. Such an incision gives a wide exposure of the extensor tendons of the dorsum of the hand (Fig. 9–8). This incision placed between the superficial branches of the radial cutaneous nerve and the cutaneous branches of the ulnar nerve permits unhampered access to the extensor tendons.

A straight-line incision over the dorsoradial side of the second metacarpal permits excellent access to the second metacarpal, including the head and the base of this metacarpal. After the skin incision is made, the first dorsal interosseous muscle is stripped away with a sharp periosteal elevator toward the palm of the hand; the tendon of this interosseous is separated and also displaced toward the palm of the hand. The metacarpal can be freed from the muscles of the second intermetacarpal space in the same manner, and any part of the metacarpal can be isolated completely. The superficial veins are ligated or retracted. The cutaneous branches of the radial nerve are carefully avoided when the skin incision is made (Fig. 9–9).

A straight-line incision along the dorsoulnar side of the fifth metacarpal permits an adequate exposure of the fifth metacarpal, which can be completely stripped of its muscles.
A longitudinal incision between the fourth and third metacarpals permits an approach to the second contiguous metacarpals. As mentioned previously, the second and fifth metacarpals can be approached from the dorsoradial side of the second or dorsoulnar side of the fifth, respectively; however, if the second and third have to be approached simultaneously, an incision is made between the second and third metacarpals. For a similar approach to the fourth and fifth metacarpals an incision is made between the fourth and fifth. The extensors digitorum and the proprius tendons are retracted after incision of the fascial planes. The cutaneous branches of the ulnar or radial nerves should be retracted.

SURGICAL APPROACHES TO THE WRIST

In principle, the best approach to the wrist joint from either the volar or dorsal aspect while minimizing postoperative scars should be made through transverse incisions. The important deep structures of the wrist and distal forearm run a longitudinal course; therefore, the transverse incisions are frequently insufficient to permit exposure in the more complicated procedures.

When the surgical requirements are confined to limited areas, transverse incisions are satisfactory. When large exposures are necessary, the incisions must be placed across the wrist in curved and oblique lines to meet both the requirements of extensive exposures and the properties of the skin.

APPROACHES TO THE VOLAR ASPECT OF THE WRIST

The most useful transverse incision is placed near the proximal crease of the wrist, but the incision must be made parallel with and proximal to a line uniting the proximal pole of the pisiform with the proximal part of the tubercle of the multangulum major. The ulnar and radial ends of the incision must be placed at a distance from the pisiform and the tubercle of the multangulum major because the scar placed too near the insertion of the flexor carpi ulnaris or near the entrance of the flexor carpi radialis into its canal tends to contract in these areas. The incision is made from the radial to the ulnar side of the wrist (Fig. 9–20). If the transverse incision is not sufficient for the required surgical procedure, the incision can be extended on the radial or ulnar side of the distal forearm. For certain exposures, especially in the more distal part of the wrist, the incision may have to be curved across the wrist (Fig. 9–2).

The incision is made superficially, and the superficial veins and the cutaneous nerves are treated adequately. The tendon of the palmaris longus can be palpated and is visible, running longitudinally in the most superficial fascia in the midline of the wrist. The tendon is ensheathed in its own fascial cover, separated from the deeper structures by the antebrachial fascia.

All the important structures of the wrist retain a constant relationship, making it comparatively easy to identify them, unless the wrist is severely mutilated. The few variations that occur in this region are not confusing, if known.

Upon the location of the tendon of the palmaris longus, the tendon of the flexor carpi radialis is normally located on the radial side of the wrist covered by the antebrachial fascia, which completely encloses the tendon and is quite dense near the entrance of the tendon into the channel formed by the ridge of the trapezium. The tendon of the flexor carpi ulnaris is found on the ulnar side of the exposed wrist. This tendon is also covered by the antebrachial fascia, which adheres firmly to the tendon near its insertion into the pisiform bone.

The tendon of the palmaris longus, when present and not involved in a variation, can be considered the key to the structures of the wrist in the carpal canal. The tendon of the flexor carpi radialis and the tendon of the flexor carpi ulnaris are completely outside of the carpal canal.

Immediately under the tendon of the palmaris longus, but separated from this tendon by the antebrachial fascia and the volar carpal ligament, is found the median nerve. Immediately under the trunk of the median nerve is found the tendon of the flexor superficialis to the index finger; deeper and toward the tendon of the flexor indicis superficialis is found the tendon of the flexor indicis profundus. Not infrequently, the flexor indicis superficialis shifts its position to the ulnar side of the wrist. In this case, immediately under the trunk of the median nerve lies the tendon of the flexor indicis profundus.

In the same horizontal plane as the trunk of the median nerve but to the ulnar side of the trunk is found the thickest tendon of the wrist, the flexor superficialis to the middle finger. On the ulnar side of the flexor superficialis to the middle finger is found the superficialis tendon to the ring finger. These two tendons are sometimes separated by a synovial fold; the most ulnar superficial tendon, to the ulnar side of the ring finger, is the thin tendon of the flexorsuperficialis to the little finger. Deep to the tendons of the flexor superficialis of the ring and the little fingers are found the flexor profundus tendons of the middle, ring, and little fingers.

The most radial deep corner of the carpal canal is occupied by the tendon of the flexor pollicis longus (Fig. 2–31). In the incisions of the volar aspect of the wrist, as soon as the fascia under the tendon of the palmaris longus is divided and retracted, the largest structure encountered is the tendon of the flexor sublimis of the middle finger. The tendon is joined by oblique muscular fibers on the radial side, the lowermost part of the belly of the flexor sublimis to the middle finger, which runs in a distal ulnar direction to this tendon forming an arched proximal curtain from under which emerges the trunk of the median nerve (Fig. 2–30).

The ulnar nerve and artery are found on the ulnar side of the wrist under the antebrachial fascia between the tendon of the flexor carpi ulnaris and the carpal canal, completely outside the carpal canal. The radial artery is completely radial to the tendon of the flexor carpi radialis and the carpal canal (Fig. 2–7 and 2–31).

The exposure of the carpal bones through a volar incision is not easy through a transverse incision. A curved or an extended transverse incision may be required. The approach depends on which bone requires exposure.

The lunate bone can be approached with comparative ease because it is located proximal to the line uniting the tubercle of the trapezium and the proximal pole of the pisiform bone immediately under the anterior lip of the lower end of the radius, ulnar to the long axis of the middle finger and its metacarpal (Figs. 2–2, 2–3, and 2–63). With the hand placed in strong dorsiflexion, the lunate is in good position for enucleation or other procedures. Although the positions of the skeletal parts are convenient, the dissection of the soft tissues is extensive. The incision must be extended deeply between the flexor tendons contained in the ulnar bursa and the median nerve on one side and the flexor carpi radialis on the other or between the flexor tendons in the bursa. The tendons must be dislocated after incision of the volar carpal ligament. The deep volar fat pad (Fig. 6–13) must be removed or retracted distally into the palm, and the vessels of the anterior aspect of the carpus must be properly controlled to prevent bleeding after the temporary hemostatis is discontinued.

The capitate bone may be approached from the volar aspect, if necessary, through the same incision as the lunate, if the head of the capitate requires a special procedure; otherwise, it is easier to approach the capitate from the dorsal aspect of the wrist.

The scaphoid bone may be approached from the anterior and lateral aspects. It is not an easy approach but with proper precautions may give sufficient exposure for extensive procedures. A transverse incision is made from the tendon of the palmaris longus over the anterior radial aspect of the wrist and across the anatomic snuff-box to the tendon of the extensor pollicis longus. The tunnel of the flexor carpi radialis is opened, and the tendon is reflected in an ulnar direction. The common retinaculum of the abductor pollicis and extensor pollicis brevis is opened, and the tendons are reflected outwardly. This provides sufficient room for exposure of the bone and the procedures over the volar aspect of it.

A further step, consisting of retraction of the abductor pollicis longus and extensor pollicis brevis in one direction and the extensor pollicis longus in the opposite direction toward the ulnar side of the hand with the hand in ulnar deviation provides additional exposure of the scaphoid bone from the lateral aspect.

Otto Russe has advised a volar longitudinal incision to the carpal scaphoid for bony non-union. This, he feels, avoids damage to the blood supply of the scaphoid, which has been shown to have major vessels entering dorsally. The incision is also cosmetically acceptable and gives ample exposure to the fracture site. Under appropriate operating room conditions, the longitudinal incision, 3 cm to 4 cm in length, is made just radial to the flexor carpi radialis tendon beginning at the proximal crease of the wrist or at about the radial styloid. The flexor carpi radialis tendon is retracted toward the ulnar side, and the capsule is entered at the same section alignment as the skin incision. The radial artery is protected on the radial aspect.

After entering the capsule, the non-union of the carpal scaphoid can be noted. If there is any doubt about the site, an x-ray in the operating room will confirm. A cavity is formed by using a small gouge at the sclerotic bone ends. From the opposite iliac crest, an oblong piece of cancellous bone is taken to form a peg, which is

FIG. 9–21 Variation of the anterior structures of the wrist and the distal part of the forearm revealed by further dissection of the skin of Figure 9–20.

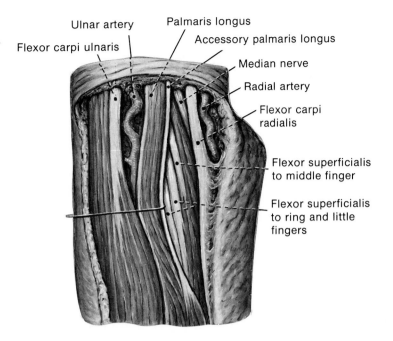

Ulnar artery
Flexor carpi ulnaris
Palmaris longus
Accessory palmaris longus
Median nerve
Radial artery
Flexor carpi radialis
Flexor superficialis to middle finger
Flexor superficialis to ring and little fingers

Proximal

placed in the center of the cavity with multiple small chips placed about it, thus completely obliterating the cavity. This procedure may be similar to filling the cavity in the tooth; x-rays determine the degree of excavation and filling of the cavity. The tourniquet should be removed before closure, especially if there is doubt concerning damage to the radial artery.

The approach to the trapezium from the volar surface was described with the procedures for the thumb.

The triquetral, hamate, and the trapezoid are fairly inaccessible from the volar aspect of the wrist. The pisiform is superficial and can be approached with care if the location and proximity of the ulnar nerve and artery are kept in mind constantly. The hook of the hamate may also be approached in cases of necessity, keeping in mind its relation to the ulnar nerve and its deep branches.

In the approaches to the wrist certain occasional variations must be kept in mind. The palmaris longus is the most accessible, palpable, and visible superficially and is also the most variable. About 12% of hands have no palmaris

longus; the absence is usually bilateral but may be found in only one hand of the same individual. The palmaris longus may deflect to the radial or the ulnar side of the hand (Fig. 2–30, see variations).

Instead of the tendon, a muscle belly may be found which may completely confuse the uninitiated (Figs. 9–20 and 9–21). In an illustrative case in a cadaver, a transverse incision showed, instead of a normal tendon of the palmaris longus, a wide muscular band with a thin tendinous band on one side of the muscular band. Further dissection disclosed that the muscular band covered completely the normal flexor tendon underneath it and that the band presented a variation of the palmaris longus with an additional thin, almost independent palmaris longus. Reflection of the palmaris longus complex revealed the normal flexor tendons of the fingers and the median nerve.

The median nerve may be found to consist of two trunks instead of one, each of smaller diameter than the single trunk; however, when this variation occurs, both trunks retain their relation to the tendon of the palmaris longus and to the fleshy fibers of the tendon of the flexor sublimis of the middle finger.

The tendon of the flexor carpi radialis varies in its additional insertions into the carpal bones or the volar carpal ligament, presenting no surgical difficulties.

The flexors of the fingers vary in number. Some of the tendons fuse together; some other tendons split in two of three separate parts. The flexor superficialis to the little finger or to the index may be absent; the tendons of the flexors profundus or superficialis may fuse together, especially in the ring and little fingers. Additional tendons deriving from additional muscle bellies are occasionally found (see variations).

In rare instances, the flexor pollicis longus tendon is absent. In some other instances, the tendon may be intimately connected with the tendon of the flexor profundus of the index finger.

Sometimes, the flexor carpi ulnaris is found to be double; in rare instances, the tendon is fused proximally with the flexor tendons of the fingers.

APPROACHES TO THE RADIAL ASPECT OF THE WRIST

The approach to the radial aspect of the wrist in the region of the snuff-box and to the radial styloid process can be accomplished through a transverse incision (Fig. 9–3, incision *i*) or through a Z-shaped incision. The transverse incision starts about 5 mm radial to the flexor carpi radialis tendon, extends across the radial aspect of the wrist just proximal to the radial styloid process, and ends slightly ulnar to the tendon of the extensor pollicis longus (Fig. 9–9). By then dissecting the underlying soft tissues, veins, and nerves longitudinally, the incision is then converted into an oval shape for better and safer exposure. The transverse incision heals well without contractures, but the tendons of the region cannot always be exposed widely. It again should be emphasized that damage to the underlying superficial radial nerve may result in a disabling, painful neuroma.

longitudinal incision is convenient, but it contracts in healing and forms a long, irregular, and sometimes widened, sensitive scar. To avoid the disadvantages of a longitudinal incision and enlarge the necessary exposure, Z-shaped incisions may be used. The longitudinal branch of the incision, about 5 cm long, is placed over the anatomic snuff-box, the distal branch of the Z is extended over the dorsum of the wrist, and the proximal branch of the Z is extended over the volar surface of the distal forearm.

The skin of the transverse or Z approach must be incised superficially to avoid injury to the superficial branches of the radial nerve and the dorsal veins. The veins are superficial to the nerve. When the branches are identified they are retracted gently; the fibers of the extensor retinaculum, which form the tunnel for the abductor pollicis longus and the extensor pollicis brevis, are exposed.

The approach to this region is comparatively simple. The tunnel for the passage of the tendons is opened through a longitudinal splitting of the dense fibrous cover (Fig. 9–9). The tendon of the abductor pollicis longus very frequently splits into two separate tendons and sometimes into three separate units; occasionally, the tendon of the extensor pollicis brevis is split into two tendons. The split tendons are of unequal size. The most common type consists of three separate tendons, one for the extensor pollicis brevis and two for the abductor pollicis longus, as can be seen in a cross-section (Fig. 2–31). The floor of the tunnel for these tendons is formed by the extension of the insertion of the tendon of the brachioradialis muscle (Fig. 3–19). The tendon of the brachioradialis itself is frequently split into two tendons (Fig. 9–22) before its insertion into the radial styloid.

INCISION FOR STENOSING TENOSYNOVITIS OF THE ABDUCTOR POLLICIS LONGUS AND EXTENSOR POLLICIS BREVIS (DeQUERVAIN'S DISEASE)

Women are affected with DeQuervain's disease about ten times more frequently than are men. Like carpal tunnel compression of the median nerve, it is usually caused by an idiopathic synovitis. It is commonly associated with rheumatoid arthritis. The thickening of the synovium causes a stenosing effect on the tendons passing through it. Sharp ulnar deviation of the wrist with the patient's thumb held in adduction (Finkelstein's test) is probably the most pathognomonic sign. Exquisite local tenderness at the radial styloid over the tendon sheath is also a common finding. Anatomic variations of the insertion of the tendon of the abductor pollicis longus are frequent, as mentioned above. It may be considered normal, however, for a portion of the abductor pollicis longus to insert into the trapezium and for another portion to insert to the base of the first metacarpal.

The extensor pollicis brevis lying ulnar to this larger tendon may be enclosed in a separate sheath; therefore, it is imperative to observe at the time of surgery that both sheaths, if present, are opened. A transverse incision just proximal to the radial styloid is carried down to the superficial veins. The incision is converted into an oval-shaped incision, and the continuation of the dissection is now in a vertical orientation. This helps protect the small branches of the superficial radial nerve and provides exposure to the underlying tendon sheath, which must be incised vertically.

Incision of the sheath should be carried through its entire extent over the ulnar aspect (Fig. 9–9), thus helping to eliminate the possibility of subluxation of the abductor pollicis longus tendon radially on wrist flexion in the immediate postoperative period. It is extremely important to avoid cutting a portion of the superficial radial nerve; neuromas following severance of this nerve are frequently disabling to the entire hand and are refractory to treatment. A longitudinal skin incision at this site causes hypertrophy of scar. An alternate incision might be a vertical incision converted to a Z-plasty, but this may be more than is necessary to release the sheath.

When the transverse incision is used for an approach to the scaphoid, it must be placed more distally, halfway between the base of the

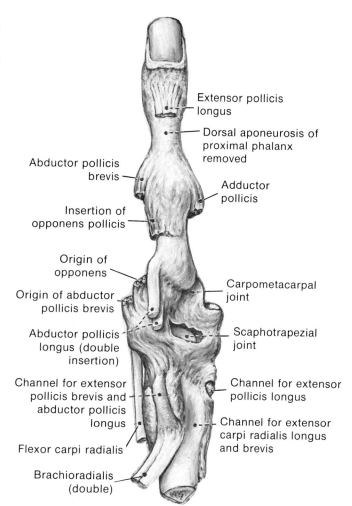

FIG. 9–22 Dorsum of the right thumb and lateral surface of the radius and carpus. The tendon of the extensor pollicis is resected. Double insertion of the abductor pollicis longus is shown. A window is opened into the scaphoidotrapezial joint. The tendon of the brachioradialis, which is double in this illustration, forms the floor for the tunnel of the extensor pollicis brevis and the abductor pollicis longus. Over the front of the radius the tendon of the flexor carpi radialis entering the tunnel under the crest of the trapezium is crossed by the origin of the abductor brevis, the opponens, and the flexor brevis of the thumb.

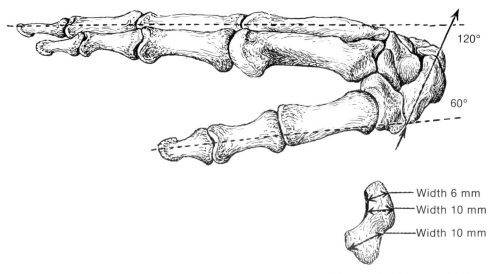

FIG. 9–23 Illustration of the direction of the long axis of the scaphoid bone, which is about 60 degrees to the horizontal in a dorsal and proximal direction. This line intersects the long axis of the middle finger at an angle of about 120 degrees. It is also about 60 degrees to the lower end of the radius. The scaphoid is about 10 mm at its widest part and about 6 mm at its narrowest part.

first metacarpal and the styloid process of the radius instead of the incision passing near the end of the styloid process. After incision of the skin, the cutaneous branches of the radial nerve are exposed and retracted. The radial artery is located in the anatomic snuff-box between the tendons of the extensor pollicis brevis and the extensor pollicis longus. The hand is placed in strong ulnar deviation in a horizontal position (neutral position between dorsiflexion and volar flexion). This brings out the scaphoid bone from under the radius (Fig. 7–20B).

The direction of the long axis of the scaphoid bone is easily determined. The proximal half of the floor of the anatomic snuff-box between the radial styloid and the base of the first metacarpal is occupied by the lateral portion of the scaphoid; the distal half of the floor of the anatomic snuff-box is occupied by the trapezium. The long axis of the scaphoid bone forms an angle of 60 degrees with the horizontal plane in a dorsal and proximal direction. The long axis of the scaphoid also forms an angle of 60 degrees with the long axis of the radius (Fig. 9–23).

The trapezium in its dorsal aspect may be exposed through the same incision if necessary, but the exposure will be quite limited.

A long longitudinal incision over the radiovolar aspect of the distal part of the forearm may be used for drainage of the space of Parona, if a prudent collection develops there spontaneously or through rupture of the flexor radial bursa (containing the flexor pollicis longus) or the flexor ulnar bursa (containing all the flexor tendons with the exclusion of the flexor pollicis longus). The skin incision, about 7.5 cm long, runs along the radius, starting from the styloid process proximally, and is extended between the flexor carpi radialis and the brachioradialis toward the anterior aspect of the pronator quadratus. The radial artery must be protected carefully (Fig. 2–29). This incision is used for counterdrainage in conjunction with the incision for drainage of the flexor sheath of the flexor pollicis longus in the hand.

A lateral incision placed in a curved line over the dorsum of the first metacarpal and curving slightly anteriorly toward the volar aspect of the wrist, then posteriorly to the lateral surface of the radius, can be made and extended between the extensor pollicis brevis and the abductor pollicis longus on one side and the extensor pollicis longus on the ulnar side. Some branches of the radial artery, the dorsal radial carpal artery, and the dorsal first intermetacarpal artery may be ligated because they produce bleeding. This incision may be continued on the lateral surface of the radius up to the fleshy fibers of the extensor pollicis brevis. Subperiosteally, the ulnar part of the incision may be widened, lifting up the extensors carpi radialis longus and brevis; the tendon and the fleshy fibers of the extensor pollicis brevis and the abductor pollicis longus can be retracted, exposing the entire lower third of the radius.

A radiolateral incision for wrist arthrodesis

Riordan and Haddad have described a technique of arthrodesis of the wrist by an approach from the radiolateral aspect. This technique has certain advantages in that it does not disturb the extensor tendons or their beds, nor does it disturb the flexor surface of the wrist. The danger of course is in damaging the superficial branch of the radial nerve and possibly the radial artery. An extremely high rate of fusions have been accomplished through this method of arthrodesis.

A J-shaped incision is made beginning 1 inch proximal to the radial styloid in the middle lateral aspect of the forearm extending distally and then curving dorsally over the base of the second metacarpal. The superficial branch of the radial nerve is identified and retracted. The volar aspect of the radius is approached at an interval between the extensor carpi radialis longus and the abductor pollicis longus and extensor pollicis brevis. The abductor pollicis longus is mobilized by subperiosteal dissection as is the extensor pollicis brevis. The wrist and finger extensors are retracted to the opposite side of the incision. The extensor carpi radialis longus tendon is divided just proximal to its insertion at the base of the second metacarpal and can be sutured later to the remaining stump. The capsule of the radiocarpal joint and the second carpometacarpal joint are exposed. The

dorsal branch of the radial artery to the dorsal carpal arch is ligated. The radiocarpal joint and the articular surface are denuded. An iliac crest bone-graft is taken from the inner aspect measuring 1½ inch by 1 inch in length. A slot is then cut in the lateral aspect of the radius, including the distal end of the radius, the carpal bones, and the base of the second and third metacarpals. The medial aspect of the radius is preserved, as is the integrity of the distal radioulnar joint. Into this slot the graft is inserted with the wrist in neutral or slightly dorsiflexed position. Kirschner wires may be added to the graft if it is unstable; the wires are cut off under the skin. A volar plaster splint is applied after the wound is closed. Two weeks later, the volar splint is converted into a solid gauntlet cast with the thumb included, having had the sutures removed and the wound observed as healing.

APPROACHES TO THE ULNAR SIDE OF THE WRIST

The ulnar side of the wrist can be approached for extensive or limited procedures for drainage of the space of Parona, resection of the distal end of the ulna, or resection or arthrodesis of the carpal and the radiocarpal joints.

Drainage of the space of Parona is effected through an incision of from about 5 cm to 7.5 cm between the pisiform bone, along and parallel with the ulna. The incision extends between the ulna and the flexor carpi ulnaris under direct view, safe-guarding the ulnar nerve and its dorsal branch and artery.

An ulnar incision for approach to the distal end of the ulna and to the carpal bones on the ulnar aspect was devised by Darrach and Smith-Petersen. The Darrach incision consists of exposure of the ulna between the extensor carpi ulnaris and the flexor carpi ulnaris with preservation of the styloid process and excision of a segment of the distal end of the ulna. In the Smith-Petersen incision (Fig. 9–24), the skin line is placed over the ulnar side of the fifth metacarpal and is then extended over the dorsum of the carpus and the lower end of the ulna. Through this incision, the metacarpal is approached, the

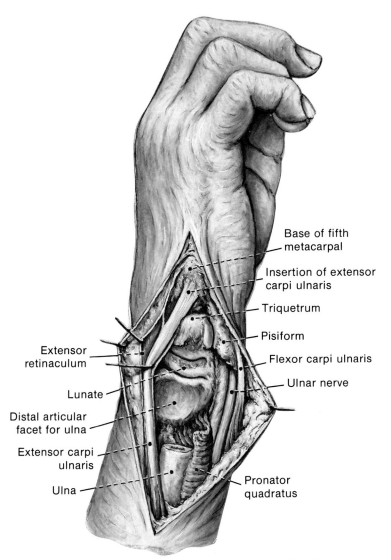

Base of fifth
metacarpal

Insertion of extensor
carpi ulnaris

Triquetrum

Pisiform

Flexor carpi ulnaris

Ulnar nerve

Extensor
retinaculum

Lunate

Distal articular
facet for ulna

Extensor carpi
ulnaris

Ulna

Pronator
quadratus

FIG. 9–24   The Smith–Petersen incision begins in the middle of the dorsum of the fifth metacarpal, continues to the lateral aspect of the wrist, and further extends proximally to the lateral aspect of the ulna. Through this incision the distal end of the ulna can be approached and completely resected just proximal to its articulation to the radius, permitting a wide exposure of the bones of the carpus. Several important considerations should be kept in mind. The extensor carpi ulnaris, which is inserted into the base of the fifth metacarpal, extends much more distally than does the flexor carpi ulnaris, which is inserted into the pisiform. The flexor carpi ulnaris tendon is located much more radially. The ulnar nerve is exposed very easily and conceals the ulnar artery immediately underneath. The pronator quadratus descends low on the radius. The articular facet for the ulna, which is exposed on the medial side of the radius after resection of the ulna, is frequently distorted and enlarged and irregular. The freeing of the extensor carpi ulnaris is easy after complete division of the extensor retinaculum.

extensor carpi ulnaris is located, and the dorsal carpal ligament is incised longitudinally, freeing this tendon. A subperiosteal separation between the tendon of the extensor carpi ulnaris and the flexor carpi ulnaris is done. In this subperiosteal separation, the fibers of the pronator quadratus are involved.

The flexor carpi ulnaris is placed quite anteriorly; therefore, great care must be exercised to avoid injury not only to the dorsal branch of the ulnar nerve, but to the ulnar nerve itself and to the ulnar artery, which lies right in front of the nerve. Retraction in this area must be done cautiously. The lower end of the ulna is resected completely, including the ulnar collateral ligament. The fibrocartilage between the ulna and the triquetral bone is removed, and the ulnar articular facet of the radius is exposed.

In older people, the ulnar articular facet of the radius frequently changes its shape and is widened, making the recognition of this facet somewhat difficult. The tendons of the extensor carpi radialis and the flexor carpi radialis after fusion of the wrist may be excised, tenodesed, or fixed in any manner desirable.

APPROACHES TO THE DORSUM OF THE WRIST

Curved incision continued in a curved line from the dorsum of the fingers is very useful. The synovial sheath of the extensor digitorum communis involved in various processes requires this type of excision (Figs. 9–8 and 9–25). In average cases the cutaneous nerves are easily preserved in this location, and the scar resulting from this type of curved incision is satisfactory. In patients with rheumatoid arthritis, this incision should be straight or nearly straight to avoid developing lateral flaps that frequently are delayed in healing.

If deeper structures must be approached, transverse incisions may be used for excision of separate carpal bones or for other procedures on these bones. The scaphoid bone can be approached if the hand is placed in a horizontal position and a deep exposure made between the extensor pollicis longus, which is retracted radially, and the extensor carpi radialis longus, which is retracted ulnarly.

An incision between the tendon of the extensor digitorum along a line uniting the tubercle of Lister with the hook of the base of the third metacarpal gives access to the joint between the lunate located on the ulnar side of this line and the scaphoid located on the radial side of the same line. More distally, the line separates the capitate on the ulnar side of this line from the trapezoid on the radial side.

The lunate bone is easily exposed, when the hand is in volar flexion, immediately distal to the base of the lower end of the radius, ulnar to the long axis of the third metacarpal and the middle finger. The triquetral and the hamate bones are approached between the extensor carpi ulnaris and the extensor proprius of the fifth finger.

In the approach to all carpal bones, the previously described ligaments with their blood supplies must be preserved. Hemostasis must be obtained to prevent bleeding from the rich network of blood vessels formed by the dorsal transverse arteries and veins derived from the radial, ulnar, and interosseous arteries and veins of the forearm. To avoid interference with the blood supplies of these bones, it is better to approach them through longitudinal incisions in the ligaments, then through transverse incisions.

For extensive exposures of the carpus, when resection of the wrist is required or arthrodesing operations are indicated, more appropriate incisions must be used mostly through the dorsum or the dorsoulnar aspect of the carpus.

The incision described long ago by Ollier is probably the precursor of the most appropriate approaches. It starts approximately over the middle of the dorsum of the second metacarpal on the radial side of the extensor communis digitorum indicis, following this line toward the wrist, approximately to the middle between the radial and ulnar styloids. The incision is extended proximally for about 6 cm to 7 cm.

Upon exposure of the extensor digitorum indicis communis, a deeper incision is made slightly radial to this tendon down to the second metacarpal. The dorsal carpal ligament is then incised between the extensor indicis communis and the extensor pollicis longus. The extensor

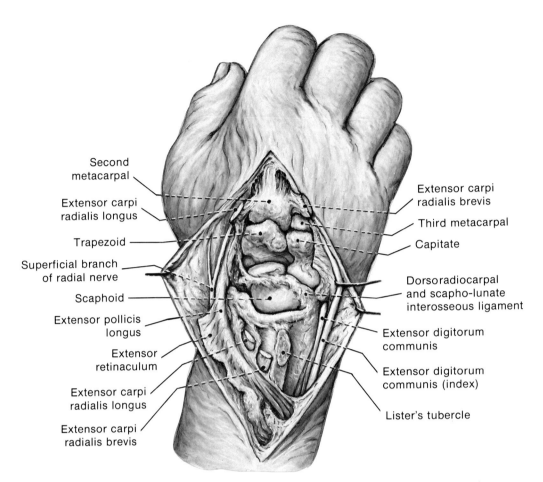

Second metacarpal

Extensor carpi radialis longus

Trapezoid

Superficial branch of radial nerve

Scaphoid

Extensor pollicis longus

Extensor retinaculum

Extensor carpi radialis longus

Extensor carpi radialis brevis

Extensor carpi radialis brevis

Third metacarpal

Capitate

Dorsoradiocarpal and scapho-lunate interosseous ligament

Extensor digitorum communis

Extensor digitorum communis (index)

Lister's tubercle

FIG. 9–25 Approach to the dorsum of the wrist joint, exposing the second metacarpal, the trapezoid, the capitate, the scaphoid, and the distal end of the radius. The incision is placed between the extensor pollicis longus and the extensor digitorum communis to the index. The extensors longus and brevis of the wrist are divided, the extensors pollicis longus and digitorum are retracted, and the capsule is excised for fusions of the wrist joint or excision of the carpal bones.

communis tendons are retracted in an ulnar direction, and the extensor pollicis longus is retracted in a radial direction. The long and the short radial extensors of the wrist are separated subperiosteally from the radius and also retracted in a radial direction.

This incision was used by Ollier mostly for partial resection of the bones of the carpus; for complete excision of the bones Ollier supplemented this incision by an ulnar incision which was placed in the following manner: The additional skin incision started approximately 3 cm proximal to the styloid process of the ulna and

extended about 2 cm distal to the base of the fifth metacarpal. The incision extended volar to the tendon of the extensor carpi ulnaris, carefully avoiding the dorsal branch of the ulnar nerve, which was retracted dorsally. Ollier used this incision mostly for complete excision of the bones of the carpus, trying to preserve, after complete resection of the carpal bones, the radial and the ulnar extensors of the wrist.

The extensor pollicis longus is preserved carefully in its sheath and retracted radially. The extensor digitorum communis tendons and the proper extensor tendons, together with the tendon of the extensor carpi ulnaris, are retracted ulnad. All these tendons are replaced before the wound is closed to preserve the function of the fingers.

At present, the double incision of Ollier is not in general use. The fusion of the wrist may be performed through one skin incision (Fig. 9–25), although sometimes it is necessary to incise the dorsal carpal ligament on the radial and ulnar sides of the extensor digitorum communis and retract the tendons either to the radial or ulnar side for better and complete exposure of the carpal bones. Modern orthopedic surgical procedures seldom require resection of all the carpal bones.

The approach for fusion of the wrist joint may be made through an incision proposed by Abbott and his associates. Through a straight or curved incision over the dorsum of the wrist, passing over Lister's tubercle, the extensor pollicis longus and the extensor digitorum communis tendons are exposed. An incision is made into the dorsal carpal ligament between the extensor pollicis longus, together with the radial extensors, which are separated from the radius and retracted radially, and the tendons of the extensor digitorum communis, which are separated from the radius and retracted ulnarly. The radiocarpal joint is exposed, and the ligaments uniting the two are divided transversely. After appropriate treatment of the radiocarpal joint consisting of removal of the cartilage from the radius and the proximal aspect of the carpus, an osteoligamentous flap is raised from the dorsal aspect of all the carpal bones in adults and is sutured to the radial periosteum. In children, the intercarpal joints are denuded of cartilage and are filled with bone chips. The subsequent fusion, if successful, eliminates motion between the bones of the carpus but permits some motion in the carpometacarpal joints.

The preservation of the radial extensors of the wrist in Abbott's procedure is apparently intended for the postoperative motion in the carpometacarpal joints, which are not fused and compensate for the loss of motion in the radiocarpal joint.

Through Abbott's incision, as well as other dorsal incisions, bone grafts can be placed, bridging the bones of the wrist with the metacarpus or with the bones of the forearm. The distal radioulnar joint is not fused to preserve supination and pronation.

Kocher described an ulnar-dorsal approach. The incision in this approach is placed over the dorsum of the fifth metacarpal, extending over the middle of the wrist joint proximally into the lower end of the forearm. After division of the dorsal carpal ligament between the extensors to the fifth finger and the extensor carpi ulnaris, the triangular fibrocartilage is approached and, if necessary, excised. The triquetral bone is excised; the hamate bone is excised, leaving the hamate hook. The flexor tendons are then visualized and lifted up; the flexor carpi radialis is preserved. The extensors are then carefully separated from the dorsum of the radius, the thumb is deviated forcibly to the lateral side, and the carpal bones can be removed.

It is obvious that Kocher's incision was devised mostly for resection of the carpal bones with attempts to preserve carefully the radial extensors of the wrist. In cases where such a procedure is indicated, the Kocher incision might be chosen instead of the Ollier incision or the others.

When the carpal bones are exposed, it is comparatively simple to recognize each individual bone, its shape and relation to the surrounding bones. The forked appearance of the base of the second metacarpal and the hook of the radial aspect of the base of the third metacarpal represents significant landmarks. The trapezoid is articulated with the fork of the second metacarpal (Fig. 9–25). The articular base of the third metacarpal is joined to the base of the capitate. These four bones (second and third metacarpals, capitate, and the trapezoid) meet in the form of an almost perfect cross (Fig. 2–2), simplifying their identification. The operative handling of all the carpal bones requires gentleness to avoid crushing them and care to avoid injury to their volar ligaments and other important structures (Figs. 2–31 and 2–63).

10
Amputations in the Hand: Concepts and Treatment

Alfred B. Swanson
Genevieve deGroot Swanson
Emanuel B. Kaplan

In congenital or acquired hand amputations the capacity for infinite patterns of action may be lost, but some basic prehensile potential may be retained as long as the hand still has sensation and is pain-free. The tenets of all hand surgery—maintaining a system with good architectural structure, mobile joints, balance between extrinsic and intrinsic musculature, and a durable, flexible skin cover with good sensibility—are paramount in surgery of an amputated hand. The patient with partial hand amputation has usually lost only structured parts or their arrangement. The control apparatus is usually intact; therefore, the usefulness of the reconstructed partial hand and the effectiveness of its substitutionary functional adaptations and re-acquired prehensile skills will largely depend on the mobility of the system. The amazing prehensile skills seen in the congenitally malformed partial hand demonstrate the substitutionary patterns that can be attained in the pain-free, mobile hand. Knowledge of the normal structure and function of the hand and its response to the abnormal is essential for proper management of a patient with amputation of the fingers or hand.

Ideal restoration of function provides a strong grasp with good sensation. The importance of *function* rather than cosmetic appearance should be emphasized. There is a great tendency for concern with the appearance of the hand rather than with what the hand can do. The decision regarding the treatment to be given to a particular patient should be based on evaluation of the patient's capacity for function, his needs as they relate to the anatomic defect, and his capacity for training.

PRINCIPLES OF TREATMENT

The main goal in the initial management of a severely mutilated hand is to preserve as much viable tissue and length as possible. The surgeon responsible for initial management of the case should consider potential reconstruction and save tissues such as bone, tendon, nerve, and skin flaps presenting good viability and sensitivity that can be a use in reconstructive surgery.

Primary treatment of major amputations requires use of the main operating room and preferably general anesthesia, although block anesthesia can be used to advantage. A preoperative evaluation of motion and sensation with the patient awake is helpful to determine the viability of structures and degree of involvement. Initial operative cleansing of the damaged part is time consuming. The skin is thoroughly scrubbed with soap and water; Iodine (Betadine) soap is preferred. All antiseptics should be kept out of the wound, and it should be copiously irrigated with saline or Ringer's solution. A pneumatic tourniquet is almost always applied to allow proper visualization of the deep structures; it should be released for evaluation of vascular supply to the digitis and skin flaps.

Minor finger tip amputations involving soft tissues alone can be resurfaced with a split or a full-thickness skin graft, according to the size of the defect. If skin loss is so extensive that secondary contraction would not provide full-thickness coverage, a full-thickness skin graft is preferred. Loss of digital pulp should be restored with tissue that provides adequate padding, sensibility, and pseudomotor function. According to the situation, cross-finger flaps, island pedicle flaps, or adjacent pedicle flaps such as an advancement flap can be used. Distal phalangeal finger amputations or pulp losses can be resurfaced with local triangular advancement flaps, providing that the volar tissue loss is not greater than the dorsal loss. Such flaps were originally described by Kutler, Atosoy, and Kleinert. Loss of less than half of the distal pulp surface in very young children will often heal primarily without surgical intervention.

When amputation of a finger occurs at the level of the cuticle, the germinal matrix is preserved and can produce a fingernail. Primary replacement of the soft tissue is necessary to avoid clawlike growth of the nail over the stump. When the fingernail cannot be salvaged, minor shortening of the digit may allow direct wound closure without tension and can be warranted for the middle and ring fingers. Amputations of the distal phalanx require a longer volar flap. The preservation of the distal phalanx (even a few millimeters) can be very important. Bone length should be preserved whenever possible; spicules or irregularities should be neatly trimmed. In digital disarticulations, the condyles should be tapered to prevent a bulbous tip. Good soft tissue cover must be provided over cartilage to avoid chronic chondritis.

Unstable fractures should be reduced and fixed with small Kirschner wires. Internal fixation can be maintained with cross-wires or a transverse wire through the metacarpal heads; a vertical wire in the intramedullary canal can be used to prevent angulation. Metacarpal bone length should be maintained, and Kirschner wires can be used as spacers by bending them appropriately to maintain the necessary length; this simplifies subsequent bone grafting and reconstructive procedures. Phalangeal fractures can be treated by multiple small Kirschner wire fixation. Bone should not be removed unless it is completely detached from all soft tissues.

The digital nerve and artery to the unsalvageable part are individually identified. A neuroma will always form at the distal amputated nerve end. To help avoid troublesome dysesthesia and pain, the nerve ends should be placed in healthy tissues that will be free of scar. In amputations the nerves, when sacrificed, are pulled into the wound, cut clearly across, and allowed to retract into healthy tissues. Digital arteries and subcutaneous veins are ligated separately.

In digital amputations, the extensor and flexor tendons are pulled down, cut, and allowed to retract. In amputation through the middle phalanx, the flexor profundus does not retract beyond the proximal phalanx because it is held by vincula; the flexor superficialis remains attached to the stump of the middle phalanx unless too much of the middle phalanx is removed; even then, however, the tendon does not retract beyond the proximal phalanx. Suturing the extensor apparatus to the flexor tendons over the stump of the amputated middle phalanx interferes with the motion of the stump, causing incomplete extension of the stump and incomplete flexion of the adjacent digit. In amputations through the proximal phalanx, the flexors superficialis and profundus tendons retract beyond the metacarpophalangeal joint because the chiasma of Camper is transected in the division through the volar surface of the finger, and frequently, the vinculum to the flexor profundus is located near the base of the proximal phalanx. The resulting stump is effective and has a full range of motion. The extensor digitorum tendon retains all the elements for extension of the proximal phalanx through its insertion into the dorsal base or capsule of the metacarpophalangeal joint. The connections of the interossei tendons with the extensor apparatus of the fingers and with the sides of the base of the proximal phalanx affect flexion of the proximal phalanx. The flexor profundus re-attaches into the volar surface of the proximal phalanx and acts as a flexor of this phalanx; however, in amputation of the ring and little fingers at the level of the metacarpophalangeal joint, the extrinsic tendons are attached to the distal end of the bone to provide increased motion of the palmar arch.

Adequate skin cover is essential to obtain primary wound healing. Secondary healing in the hand results in scarring and fixation, which is disastrous to function. Skin debridement should be minimal; even small tags of viable skin may be useful. Metacarpals should not be resected merely for skin closure. If a digit is considered unsalvageable, its skin can be filleted and used as a local flap for additional skin coverage. If closure is inadequate, a primary skin flap may be used. Such a flap may be local, from a cross finger or island pedicle, or distant, from the thorax, abdomen or contralateral arm. These flaps can be designed as random flaps, arterial flaps, or free flaps, as necessary and feasible. Split-thickness skin grafts can be readily applied and are usually preferred during primary treatment.

Small silicone rubber drains are placed in the wound, and a voluminous conforming dressing including a plaster splint is applied. Prevention of swelling through continuous elevation and early motion of joints is of paramount importance for eventual restoration of function. Wrist splinting in dorsiflexion, allowing the metacarpophalangeal joints to be in flexion and the interphalangeal joints to be in extension, is of great importance. Frequent active exercises for the entire extremity should be prescribed. An aggressive effort at this stage may prevent excessive swelling and the development of a causalgic syndrome. Proper operative and postoperative care to avoid secondary problems of drainage and swelling and the institution of early mobilization may make the difference between a stiff and secondarily deformed hand and a useful, prehensile mechanism capable of substitutionary prehensile functions.

CONCEPTS OF SINGLE DIGIT AMPUTATION

The concepts of treatment of single-digit and multiple-digit injuries are different and will be discussed separately.

The Thumb
The thumb represents 40% of the functional value of the entire hand. It serves as the opposing pole for prehension; its effectiveness is in direct proportion to its length, mobility, and placement. Obviously, the integrity of its skele-

tal structure and motor balance, especially at its carpometacarpal joint, are important. The thumb web space provides freedom of action and also a cleft for the grasping space. The fingernail is essential for fingernail pinch.

The short thumb can be a very functional digit as long as the other digits can reach it and the cleft is deep enough; however, there should be no sacrifice of length to gain primary coverage. Primary split-thickness coverage in the multiple-digit injury is indicated. In isolated distal thumb injuries, closure can be obtained with local flaps, cross-finger flaps from the radial side of the index or middle finger or island flaps, or distant pedicles from the thorax, abdomen, or contralateral arm. Retention of the base of the distal phalanx may be important to function as long as there is a tactile pad covering. A neurovascular skin pedicle may be used for restoring critical sensibility to the thumb with a scarred, anesthetic tip. The use of this island pedicle for restoration of sensation may also make worthwhile other skin pedicle and bone reconstructions.

Amputation through the proximal portion of the proximal phalanx is disabling. Function can be markedly improved if the cleft is deepened by local tissue flaps, grafts, or distant pedicles. Amputation at the metacarpophalangeal joint is considered to be complete loss of the thumb; deepening of the web space or pollicization of a digit may be considered as secondary procedures (Figs. 10–1 and 10–2). In trapeziometacarpal disarticulation, the nerve stumps are treated with great circumspection because of the proximity of the median nerve and its terminal branches and the possible development of causalgic manifestations. The deep branch of the radial artery passing between the two metacarpals may easily be injured in this process.

The Index Finger

The index finger represents 20% of the functional value of the hand. Its most important function is to provide an opposing pole for grasping and pinching. It provides spread for grasp, opposition to the thumb for palmar pinch, fingertip pinch, and lateral (key) pinch; it is important in percussion adaptations of the hand. Maintenance of length is of great importance in this finger, and the index finger is the only digit other than the thumb that needs to have its length maintained by cross-finger or thenar skin pedicle coverage. When amputation occurs proximal to the distal interphalangeal joint, pinch is usually transferred to the middle finger. When amputation occurs at or proximal to the proximal interphalangeal joint (*i.e.*, proximal to the insertion of the superficialis tendon), the stump has no great functional value and acts mainly in widening the palm. However, some lateral pinch can still occur and may be of functional importance, especially in the absence of the middle or ring fingers. In amputations distal to the insertion of the superficialis tendon, all salvageable length must be preserved. In amputations proximal to the insertion of the superficialis tendon, the bone may be slightly shortened to facilitate primary closure.

Amputation at or proximal to the metacarpophalangeal joint destroys function. If other fingers are present, the unsightly and nonfunctional short index stump or the protruding metacarpal head are preferably resected more proximally. Two different methods have been proposed. The first method is an oblique amputation through the metacarpal neck with preservation of the attachment of the deep transverse metacarpal ligament of the palm to maintain the breadth and stability of grasp; the first dorsal interosseous is elevated subperiosteally from the metacarpal and transferred to the base of the proximal phalanx of the middle finger. In the second method, a resection of the second ray is carried out through a racquet incision, with care taken to place the suture lines away from the web space and the palm. The proximal half of the metacarpal is exposed, and an angulated osteotomy through its proximal quarter is performed to prevent protrusion of the bone stump into the web space and to preserve the attachment of the extensor carpi radialis longus (Fig. 10–3*A* and *B*). The extensor digitorum communis is cut short and allowed to retract. The extensor indicis is transferred to the

Fig. 10–1 Common incisions for elective finger amputation; metacarpal or ray resection; Z-plasty for deepening thumb web space.

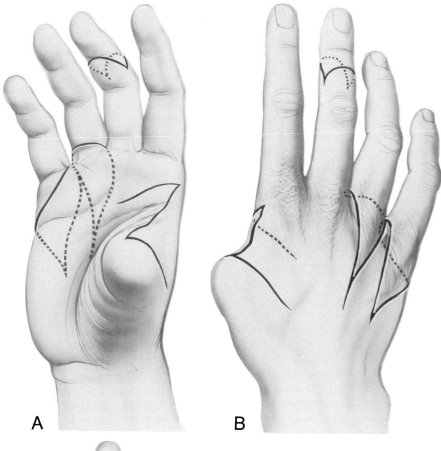

FIG. 10–2 Pollicization of the index finger to replace thumb loss can provide necessary opposing pole for pinch and grasp functions. Nerves, tendons, and vessels are moved along with finger as a pedicle, thus supplying sensation, nutrition, and motion.

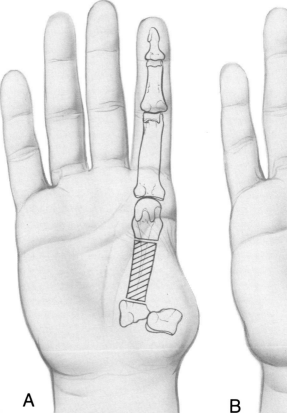

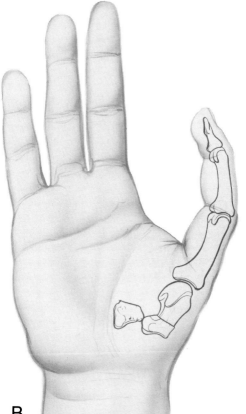

A   B

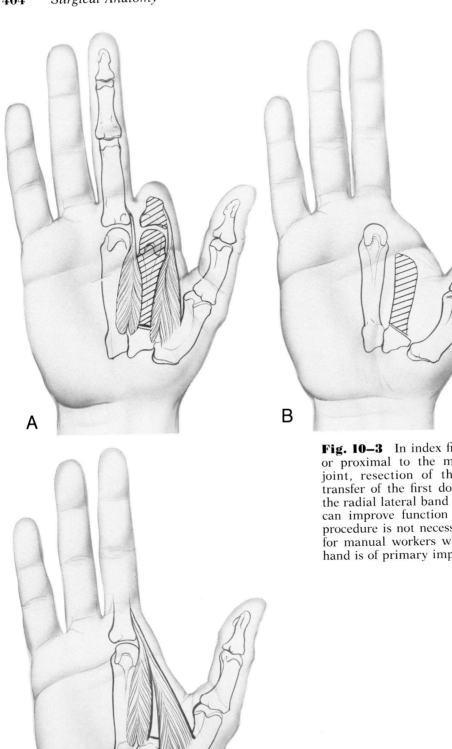

A

B

C

Fig. 10–3 In index finger amputation at or proximal to the metacarpophalangeal joint, resection of the second ray and transfer of the first dorsal interosseous to the radial lateral band of the middle finger can improve function and cosmesis; this procedure is not necessarily recommended for manual workers where breadth of the hand is of primary importance.

extensor mechanism of the middle finger to increase its independent extension. Both flexor tendons are cut short and allowed to retract. The digital arteries are ligated and the nerves are placed in healthy tissues. The first dorsal interosseous is sectioned at its insertion and transferred to the radial lateral band of the middle finger to augment abduction of this finger in pinching (Fig. 10–3C). If the first dorsal interosseous is attached to the extensor mechanism of the middle digit, a swan-neck or intrinsic-plus deformity will result. This procedure opens up the thumb web space and improves the functional relationship between the thumb and middle finger.

The Middle Finger

The middle finger represents 20% of the functional value of the hand and contributes to strong grasp, pinch, hook, and percussion actions. It reinforces the index finger's action and may substitute for it completely. In single-digit amputation, the critical amputation level is proximal to the proximal interphalangeal joint, resulting in loss of cup or scoop action of the hand; small objects fall through the closed hand. More proximal amputation through the metacarpal further results in loss of the stabilizing effect of the transverse metacarpal ligament, and the adjacent fingers roll away from the missing finger. The third metacarpal also provides an origin for the strong adductor pollicis muscle.

In amputations proximal to the proximal interphalangeal joint that result in an incompetent palmar cup or objectionable cosmetic effect, the space may be closed by metacarpal amputation alone or preferably by transfer of the adjacent second ray to the base of the amputated metacarpal to prevent malrotation of the ulnar digits (Fig. 10–4A). In transferring the index

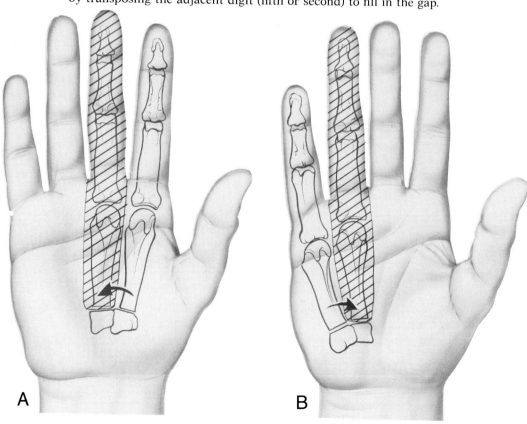

Fig. 10–4 In amputation of the third or fourth digit proximal to the proximal interphalangeal joint, incompetence of the palmar cup and cosmesis can be improved by transposing the adjacent digit (fifth or second) to fill in the gap.

A   B

metacarpal to the third metacarpal, it is important to place the osteotomies at the junction of the proximal and the middle third of the metacarpals; cut the flexor and extensor tendons of the middle digit short and allow them to retract; ligate the blood vessels and place the long nerve stump in a protracted area; preserve the transverse intermetacarpal ligaments and firmly resuture them to help stabilize the ring finger; excise either one or both the second or third dorsal interosseous, if they are too bulky; and provide excellent fusion by use of an intramedullary bone peg, appropriate Kirschner-wire fixation, and plaster immobilization. Following this procedure, when indicated, both the cosmetic appearance and function of the hand can be greatly improved.

The ring finger

The ring finger fills in the finger span and represents 10% of the hand's functional value. Along with the little finger, it provides the palmar arch with mobility. As for the middle finger, the critical amputation level is proximal to the proximal interphalangeal joint, and loss of the metacarpal head results in rotary deviation of adjacent fingers. Subperiosteal resection of the distal two thirds of the fourth ray, with or without transfer of the little finger to the base of the fourth ray, can be considered to correct an incompetent palmar cup or an objectionable cosmetic effect. The principles of the procedure are similar to those described for the transfer of the index finger (Fig. 10–4B). Attention should be given to proper rotation of the metacarpal in the transfer and to sufficient lengthening of the digit without causing excessive tightness of the digital motors.

The little finger

The little finger represents 10% of the hand's functional value. It adds to the width and strength of the grasp. Its presence is especially important in loss of the other fingers. It is frequently spared in multiple finger loss and its importance in function because of its polar situation is obvious. Because it is the least important digit functionally, single-digit amputation is best managed by ray amputation, if the residual stump is too short (proximal to the proximal interphalangeal joint) to contribute to hand function or if it is cosmetically unacceptable.

This is carried out obliquely through the base of the fifth metacarpal to avoid a cosmetically and functionally deterring hump on the ulnar side of the hand (Fig. 10–5). The incisions should be planned on the dorsal or palmar aspect of the hand, away from the ulnar aspect. It is important to preserve the dorsal branch of the ulnar nerve and its branches to the ring finger to avoid anesthesia to the new ulnar side of the hand. The abductor digiti minimi is elevated subperiosteally from the metacarpal. After oblique amputation through the base of the metacarpal, it is brought over the cut bone, and its tendon is sutured to the ulnar lateral band of the ring finger: The muscle belly of the abductor digiti minimi is sutured to that of the fourth dorsal interosseous at the end of the procedure to avoid dead spaces. This technique offers good soft tissue coverage and protects the nerves. The extensor digiti minimi tendons are cut short and allowed to retract. The extensor digitorum slip to the little finger often passes from the extensor to the ring finger just proximal to the metacarpophalangeal joint. Care must be taken not to injure the extensor tendon to the ring finger in sectioning this slip. The flexor tendons are cut short and allowed to retract. The digital vessels are ligated and cut short, but the nerves are left long and placed deep in the interosseous space to avoid neuromata problems.

CONCEPTS OF MULTIPLE DIGIT AMPUTATION

When amputation of more than one finger or major portions of the hand occurs, the problem of functional rehabilitation of the injured hand becomes increasingly complex. Creation of prehension with sensation is the main objective of surgical rehabilitation of such a hand. The manner in which the functions of the hand are achieved depends upon the severity of loss (Fig.

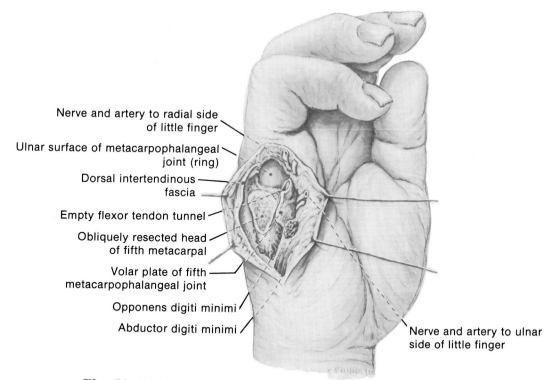

Nerve and artery to radial side
of little finger

Ulnar surface of metacarpophalangeal
joint (ring)

Dorsal intertendinous
fascia

Empty flexor tendon tunnel

Obliquely resected head
of fifth metacarpal

Volar plate of fifth
metacarpophalangeal joint

Opponens digiti minimi

Abductor digiti minimi

Nerve and artery to ulnar
side of little finger

Fig. 10–5 Amputation disarticulation of the little finger, showing an oblique section through the head and the neck of the fifth metacarpal. The preservation of the volar plate of the metacarpophalangeal joint is essential to safeguard the continuity of the intermetacarpal retention apparatus. In little finger amputation proximal to the proximal interphalangeal joint, partial resection of the fifth metacarpal can improve function and appearance; however, on occasion, maintenance of the breadth of the palm could be of more importance.

10–6). Some partial hands could require a transplanted toe or toes, a surgical post, a partial prosthesis, or an activated prosthesis. The management is individualized (Fig. 10–7). A prosthetic thumb and index and middle fingers can be activated; the activated fingers are cable-controlled to an axillary loop similar to a standard prosthesis; the prosthesis is then covered with a cosmetic glove.

In wrist disarticulation, the styloid processes should be trimmed off only slightly to preserve a wedge-shaped stump to facilitate snug fitting of the prosthesis unless a Krukenberg forceps is done. In children, after disarticulation at the carpometacarpal joint, some useful wrist motion may be gained if a total prosthesis is not used. At operation, the wrist tendons should be attached to the carpus, and a wrist disarticulation type of prosthesis should be prescribed.

With a transmetacarpal amputation at this level, a prosthetic device may be fitted to provide a surface against which the hand stump can be opposed, thus providing prehension. After amputation at this level, a partial prosthesis will provide prehension, or phalangization of the metacarpals may be performed. The hand has great compensatory ability to substitute function, and many of its grosser functions may be accomplished despite severe tissue loss.

The main objective in surgery of the severely disabled hand is to salvage all remaining digits

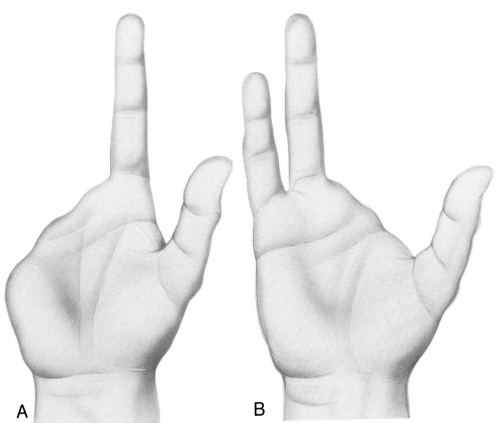

Fig. 10–6   Example of partial hands that can function satisfactorily.

and digital remnants, to save as much length as possible to preserve the palm, and to provide a functional thumb and an opposing pole for pinch and grasp. Skin grafts and atypical flap closures to cover fingertips assume greater importance, and resection of much bone to obtain smooth stump closure should be avoided. When all fingers are lost, as much metacarpal length as possible should be saved. In the primary procedures, the resulting remnants may be insufficient for necessary function, and secondary reconstructive procedures will be in order. The importance of having adequate tissues to work with in reconstruction cannot be stressed too much.

In amputations of all four fingers proximal to the proximal interphalangeal joint with preservation of good thumb function, some useful hand function is usually preserved (Fig. 10–8). When all three central digits are absent, a rotation osteotomy through the base of the first and fifth metacarpals will improve opposition of the radial and ulnar sides of the hand (Figs. 10–9 and 10–10). In metacarpophalangeal disarticulations and distal transmetacarpal amputations of all fingers with preservation of the thumb, phalangization of the first metacarpal can improve opposition. The use of a surgical post in selected cases (*e.g.,* transfer of a second toe) or use of a partial prosthesis can improve function. In absence of all digits and amputation of the thumb at the metacarpophalangeal level, flexion and opposition can be improved by flexion-rotation osteotomies of the mobile fourth and fifth metacarpals; the first metacarpal can be phalangized and the thumb web deepened by release procedures and a Z-plasty (Fig. 10–11). Resection of the second metacarpal will further open the space. The principle of formation of a cleft between two opposing poles, which adduct parallel to each other or which are rotated to diametrically oppose each other, should be used to obtain a good grasping mechanism. This can be achieved by osteotomy and tendon transfer.

Transmetacarpal and Transcarpal Amputation

In transmetacarpal amputations through half or more than half of the metacarpal length of all digits or in transcarpal amputations, some function can be obtained if there is active flexion and extension of the radiocarpal joint. Especially in children, the hook action of a flexible wrist can be of real assistance. In transcarpal amputations, the wrist extensor and flexor tendons should be attached distally. A partial prosthesis can be fitted to provide a surface against which the hand stump can be opposed. An open-end socket can be used with an attached palmar post to provide prehension with sensation between the post and distal stump. A hook can be attached to the socket to allow more strength and versatility.

Fig. 10–7 Partial prosthesis provides a post for pinch and grasp. This patient was rehabilitated to useful function of this extremity.

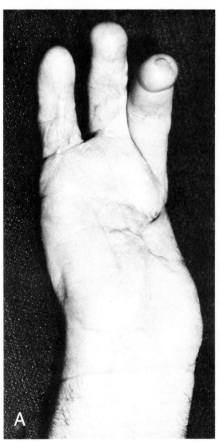
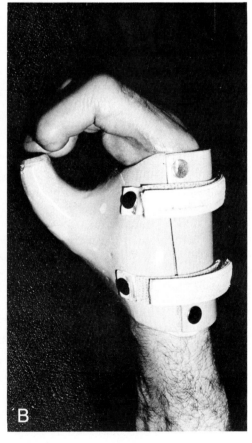

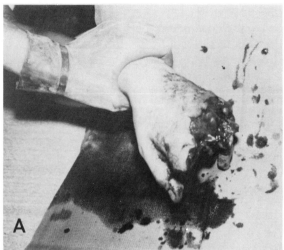

A

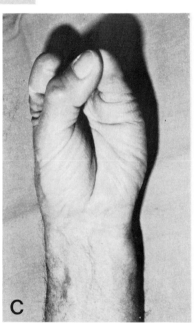

Fig. 10–8 A, Gunshot wound of the hand with severe loss of tissue; the initial surgery included careful evaluation of potential parts for reconstruction, debridement, and cleansing. The patient had a secondary closure and achieved primary healing. **B**, **C**, and **D**, A soft pliable and supple hand with good stability, pinch and grasp, and sensibility. The breadth of the grasp allows three-point fixation for holding larger objects. The mobility allows for good pinch strength and the two poles for pinching which are available to the thumb by the index and little finger stump, providing a variety of pinch adaptations. This patient eventually became a medical student and a successful general surgeon.

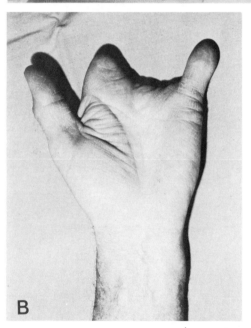

B

C

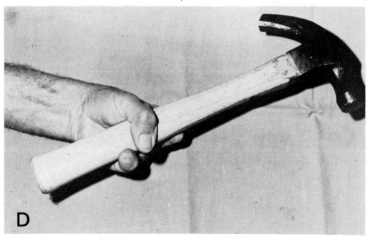

D

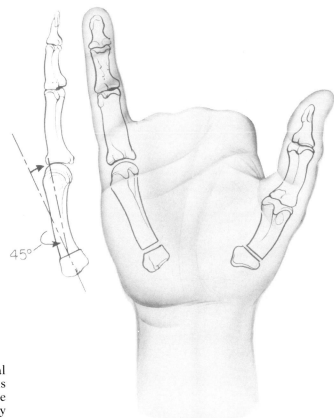

Fig. 10—9 In amputation of all three central digits, osteotomy of the first and fifth metacarpals aids in opposing the radial and ulnar sides of the hand so that the pulp of the little finger can easily oppose to the pulp of the thumb.

WRIST DISARTICULATION

In wrist disarticulation, the radial and ulnar styloids should be trimmed only slightly, because the wedge-shaped stump can be fitted satisfactorily and helps pronate and supinate the prosthesis. This is preferable to a distal forearm amputation, in which the distal radioulnar articulation is lost.

BILATERAL HAND LOSS— THE KRUKENBERG PROCEDURE

The patient with bilateral hand loss presents a great rehabilitation challenge because he lacks tactile gnosis where he wears his artificial limbs.

The Krukenberg procedure splits the forearm stump into a prehensile forceps with sensation. This procedure is indicated for the blind patient with bilateral hand loss, whether congenital or posttraumatic, and for patients living in areas where prosthetic devices are unavailable. It can be considered for any patient with bilateral hand loss if approximately three fifths of the forearm is present with reasonably normal skin coverage of the stump. The advantage of readily available prehension with sensation is significant, especially in dressing, bathing, eating, and toilet activities. An artificial limb is usually recommended for the opposite extremity as an assistive hand (Fig. 10–12). If the patient desires to wear an artificial limb over the Krukenberg stump, a standard prosthesis can be easily fitted

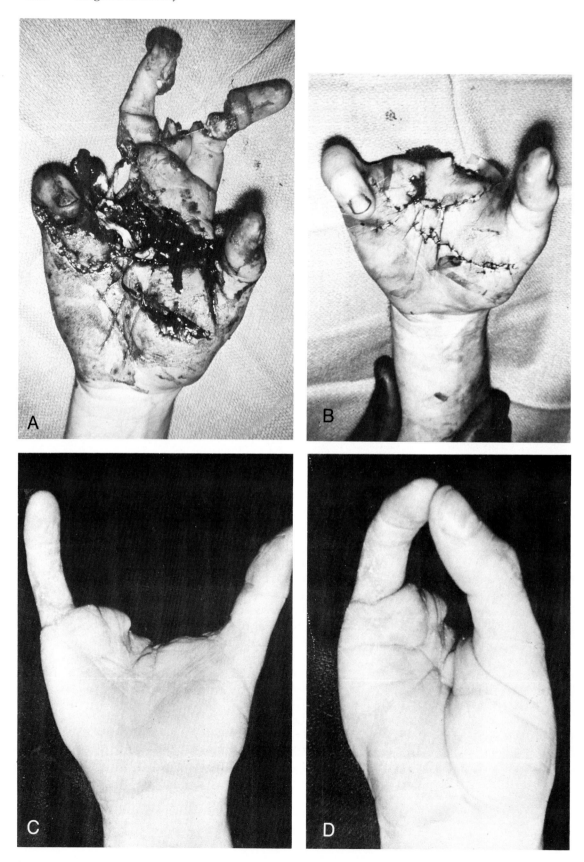

Fig. 10–10 **A**, Severe lacerating avulsing wound of the hand in a young male; careful evaluation of the viability and reconstructive potential of the remaining parts is important. **B**, A careful surgical debridement and cleansing with stabilization of the remaining digits in a functional position; loose closure of the skin flaps over drains was possible in this relatively tidy wound. **C**, This patient's result demonstrated a good grasping mechanism. **D**, The patient has good pinch with good stability and sensibility.

Fig. 10–11 In amputation of all the digits and the thumb, excision of the second metacarpal and phalangization of the first metacarpal provide a grasping mechanism. Flexion-rotation osteotomy of the first, fourth, and fifth metacarpals aids opposition.

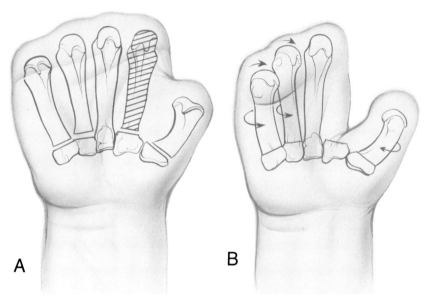

A   B

and the patient will still have the advantages of the Krukenberg stump for home activities. Using the simple mechanical principle of chopsticks, these patients can function with amazing dexterity. In children the procedure should be done as soon as feasible, usually in the second year of life. The functional pattern of adaptations are rapidly developed, and the epiphyses are not disturbed if the procedure is carefully done.

The goal of the Krukenberg procedure is to convert the forearm into a strong active forceps with the radial ray opposing the ulnar ray. Tactile sensation should be present between the tips of the forceps, and therefore the distal skin should be full thickness with good nerve and blood supply. Digits, if present, are left undisturbed, including their vessels and tendons. The forceps should spread wide enough to accommodate ordinary objects, such as a drinking glass, and should be strong enough to hold the objects securely. If the forceps is too long, it may lack strength; if it is to short, it may lack distal spread. The forceps length depends on the length of the radius and ulna distal to the pronator teres radii muscle, which limits the depth of the forceps proximally.

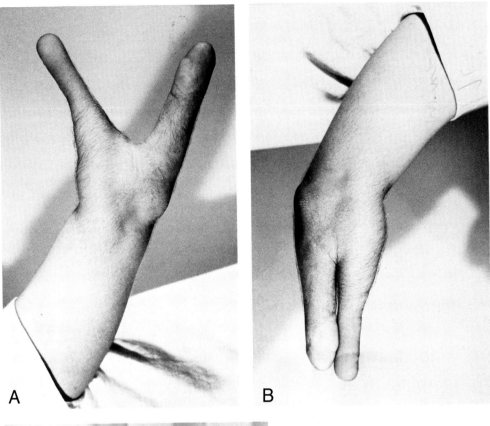

A

B

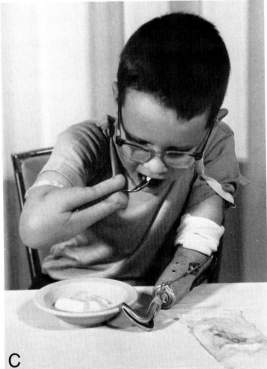

C

Fig. 10–12 A and **B**, Opening and closing of the radial and ulnar ray; note the strong muscle development. This boy was born with left upper transverse arrest (short below-elbow type) and a right transverse arrest (wrist disarticulation type), a transverse arrest of the left lower extremity with absence of the foot and a right transverse lower extremity of the below-knee type. Since childhood he has used the Krukenberg stump as his dominant hand with strong prehension and sensation. **C**, Patient with bilateral hand loss rehabilitated with Krukenberg's procedure in right arm and shoulder prosthesis with two-fingered hook for left arm.

Separation of the two rays and the design of their skin coverage is similar to the technique described by Bunnell for separation of finger syndactylism. The incision on the flexor aspect of the forearm is placed slightly radially and the dorsal incision slightly ulnad. The ulnar nerve is directed with the ulnar ray, and the median nerve with the radial ray as the forearm is divided. The muscles and tendons are divided between the radial and ulnar rays as shown in Figure 10–13. The interosseous membrane is divided along its ulnar periosteal attachment, avoiding the interosseous vessel and nerve. The distal ends of the tendons of the restrained muscles in each ray are sutured to the periosteum and capsular structures of the distal end of the radius or ulna. The pronator quadratus, the flexor digitorum profundus, the flexor and abductor pollicis longus, and extensor pollicis brevis may be resected if they do not activate a single digit or if they make the stump too bulky and prevent easy closure. The pronator teres should not be disturbed because it will serve as one of the strongest adductors of the radius.

The distal portions of the rays are resurfaced with local skin flaps placing the scarline away from the tips and opposing surfaces. The skin flaps should be closed without tension, and excess fat, fibrous tissue, or muscle substance should be removed. If severe scarring of the distal end of the stump is present after traumatic amputation in the adult, some shortening of the radius and ulna may be necessary to obtain good rotation and closure of the skin to provide tactile sensation between the forceps tips. In juvenile patients the distal ulnar and radial epiphyseal plates are carefully preserved. The secondary V flap is rotated in the axilla of the forceps, and any residual defect on the proximal volar surface of the radial ray is resurfaced with a split-thickness skin graft. The skin over the distal radius and ulna may be anchored by suturing the superficial fascia to the periosteum to provide stability during grasp. The opposing ends of each ray should touch for best function. A secondary osteotomy can be done to correct any angulation of the radius that would prevent good opposition to the ulnar ray.

A training program is started within 2 to 3 weeks after the operation, and patients rapidly learn to grasp and release naturally (Fig. 10–12). Pronation and supination are strong, normal movements; abduction and adduction of the rays, however, are important to learn for maximum benefit. The motion occurs at the radiohumeral and proximal radioulnar joints. The major adduction-abduction motion of the Krukenberg stump is accomplished by moving the radius toward or away from the relatively fixed ulna. In strong gripping, however, ulnar adduction is also important. The abductors of the radius are the brachioradialis, the extensors carpi radialis longus and brevis, the radial portion of the extensor digitorum communis, and the biceps. The adductors of the radius are the pronator teres, supinator, flexor carpi radialis, the radial aspect of the flexor digitorum profundus, and the palmaris longus. The abductors of the ulna are the extensor carpi ulnaris, the ulnar part of the extensor digitorum communis, and the triceps. The adductors of the ulnar ray are the flexor carpi ulnaris, the ulnar part of the flexor digitorum profundus, the brachialis, and the anconeus.

The therapist is invaluable in training patients to use standard implements and to adapt to a normal environment. Two-handed activity is encouraged, using the hook on the opposite side. Patients become increasingly adept at using the Krukenberg forceps, and the prehension and sensibility it affords significantly improve the quality of life. The procedure should be used more extensively in patients with bilateral hand loss.

PROSTHESES

Providing the disabled hand with sensation and functional prehension by reconstructive surgery is superior to use of a prosthesis; however, if the hand remnant has too much hand function to warrant total amputation but too little to make

(Text continues on page 418)

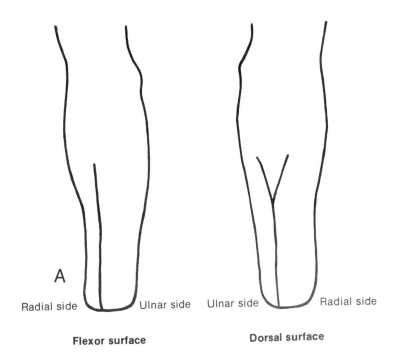

Radial side   Ulnar side   Ulnar side   Radial side

Flexor surface   **Dorsal surface**

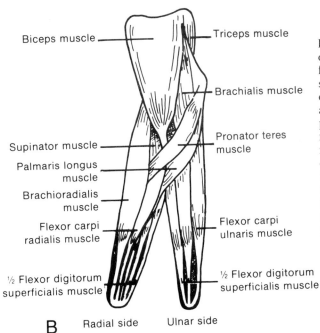

Biceps muscle ⎯⎯⎯⎯⎯⎯   ⎯⎯⎯ Triceps muscle

⎯⎯⎯ Brachialis muscle

Supinator muscle ⎯⎯⎯⎯   Pronator teres
                                         muscle
Palmaris longus
muscle

Brachioradialis
muscle

Flexor carpi   Flexor carpi
radialis muscle   ulnaris muscle

½ Flexor digitorum   ½ Flexor digitorum
superficialis muscle   superficialis muscle

B   Radial side   Ulnar side

Flexor surface

Fig. 10–13 **A**, Skin incision on dorsal surface of forearm is slightly to the ulnar side and on flexor aspect slightly on the radial side. V-shaped, secondary incision is made at the time of skin closure to determine its proper size more accurately. **B**, Division of muscles on flexor aspect into radial and ulnar rays. **C**, Muscles separated into two moieties for the radial and ulnar rays on the dorsal aspect. **D**, Skin closure on dorsal surface shows the suture lines away from the contact surface. The secondary skin flap is rotated into the axilla of the wound. The skin folded over the end of the ray is noted. Skin closure on flexor aspect of forearm shows split graft needed for closure on the radial ray.

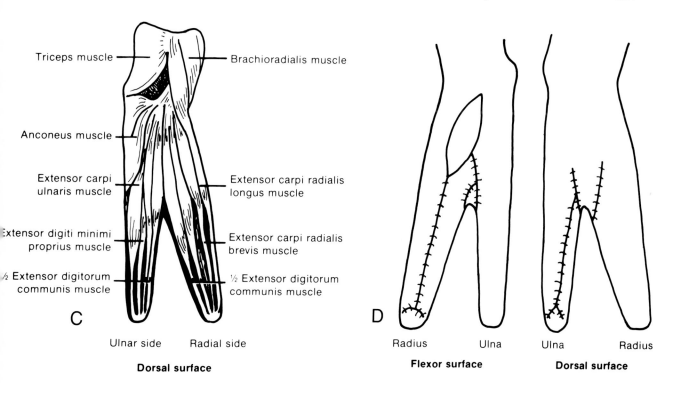

Triceps muscle

Brachioradialis muscle

Anconeus muscle

Extensor carpi ulnaris muscle

Extensor carpi radialis longus muscle

Extensor digiti minimi proprius muscle

Extensor carpi radialis brevis muscle

½ Extensor digitorum communis muscle

½ Extensor digitorum communis muscle

C

Ulnar side   Radial side

Dorsal surface

D

Radius   Ulna   Ulna   Radius

Flexor surface   **Dorsal surface**

Fig. 10–14 Partial prostheses can provide function for a partial hand, allowing use of tactile sensation and providing an opposing pole for a strong partial hand segment.

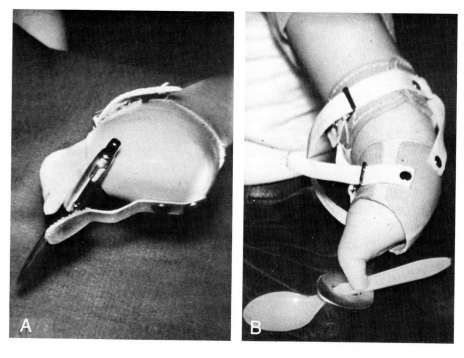

restoration of hand function possible without prosthetic assistance, a partial prosthesis can be of real value (Figs. 10–7 and 10–14). It may act as an opposing pole for prehension and may be designed to enable the patient to perform some specific work. It may also be prescribed for covering with a cosmetic glove, although this defeats the principle of allowing tactile skin to be exposed. The surgeon's first responsibility should be to restore function. Rehabilitation should emphasize the functional aspect, and if it is successful, most patients will accept the greater importance of function over beauty. A partial prosthesis will prove its value to the patient in direct proportion to the part that sensation plays in hand function. If the patient benefits from the available sensation and if grasp is strong and efficient, the partial prosthesis will be important in the patient's rehabilitation. If the prosthesis is comfortable, well-fitting, and efficient, it will be accepted.

If a reasonable partial prosthesis cannot be fitted, total prosthetic replacement can be very satisfactory. Amputation should be performed as a last resort in an upper extremity in which functional prehension with sensation cannot be restored by surgical reconstruction or by a partial prosthesis. Amputation is preferred, in fact, to multiple fruitless surgery on a stiff, anesthetic, or painful hand remnant. Most patients are fitted with a voluntarily opening hook for most activities and later may be fitted with a body-powered mechanical hand.

Classic Bibliography

Since the appearance of the Second Edition, many studies have been made on the morphology, function, and surgery of the hand. The expansion of literature did not obscure the fundamental and precise knowledge of the classical anatomists. Many new references were added to the present list. It must be mentioned again that a bibliography of this type cannot be all-inclusive. So much was written on the hand that doubtless many very important articles were omitted. This has not been done intentionally. As mentioned in the Introduction, this book is not encyclopedic. A large part of the material is based on personal investigation.

Very short commentaries on the significance of a few references are given to draw the reader's attention to some specific factor. Although it is known that very pertinent and "modern" material can be found in the writings of classical authors, it is surprising how much can actually be added to our modern knowledge and how much improvement can be introduced into our methods of analysis and treatment by reading some of the very old texts. A few of the classical references were given with this particular purpose in view.

DESCRIPTIVE AND FUNCTIONAL ANATOMY

Albinus, Bernard Sigfried: Historia musculorum hominis, Leidae Batavorum, pp 479, 639 and others. 1724
Excellent descriptive anatomy of the muscular system with important considerations on muscular physiology, with exquisite illustrations and line drawings of the muscles of the hand. Illustrated by Jan Wandelaer. Albinus understood the action of the intrinsic muscles of the hand. He described first the scalenus minimus, now rightfully called the muscle of Albinus.

Alcott WA: The Structure, Uses and Abuses of the Human Hand, Boston, MA, Sabbath School Society, 1856

Anson BJ: An Atlas of Human Anatomy, 2nd ed., Philadelphia, WB Saunders, 1963
Valuable addition to anatomic literature re-emphasizing precision and importance of variations. Excellently illustrated.

Ashby BS: Hypertrophy of the palmaris longus muscle. J Bone Joint Surg **46-B**:230, 1964

Basmajian JV: Muscles Alive. Their Function Revealed by Electromyography, Baltimore, Williams & Wilkins, 1962

Baumann JA: Value, variations and equivalences of extensor inteross., adductor and abductor muscles in man, Acta Anat **4**:10, 1947

Baumann JA: Anatomie, fonctions et chirurgie de l'ensemble tendineux extenseur au dos des doigts (main et pied), Rev Orthop **34**:25, 1948

Bell, Sir Charles: The Hand—Its Mechanism and Vital Endowments as Evincing Design. London, William Pickering, 1833
Written by a great British anatomist and surgeon of the 19th century. The English is delightful, the factual material very interesting and instructive. The illustrations reflect the author's genius as a scientific illustrator.

Bibliography on the worker's hand: Ciba Symposia, vol 4, no. 4, July 1942

Birch-Jensen A: Congenital Deformities of the Upper Extremities. Copenhagen, Munksgaard, 1949

Blunt, MJ: The vascular anatomy of the median nerve in the forearm and hand. J Anat **93**:1, 1959

Borchardt M, Wjasmbenski: Der nervus medianus. Beitr Klin Chir **107**:553, 1917

Borchardt M: Der nervus radialis. Beitr Klin Chir **170**:475, 1919

Borchardt M: Anatomy and function of extensor complex. Br J Plast Surg **2**:175, 1949

Bourgery JM: Traité complet de l'anatomie de l'homme comprenant la médecine opératoire, Parts I-VIII. Paris, CA Delauney, 1832-1854

Braitwaite F, Charnell GD, Moore FT, Willis J: The applied anatomy of the lumbrical and interosseous muscles of the hand. Guy's Hosp Rep **97**:185, 1948

Brand PW, Beach RB, Thompson DE: Relative tension and potential excursion of muscles in the forearm and hand. J Hand Surg **6**:209–219, 1981

Braus H: Anatomie des menschen. Dritte Auflage, vol. 1. Berlin, Springer Verlag, 1954
A modern German anatomy reflecting the functional viewpoint.

Bryce TH: Quain's Elements of Anatomy, 11th ed. vol. 4, part 2. London, Longmans, Green 1923

Burman M: Kinetic disabilities of the hand and their classification. Am J Surg **61**:167, 1943

Camper Petri: Demonstrationum anatomico-pathologicarum liber primus. Continens brachii humani fabricum et morbos. Amstelaedami, 4, 19, 1760, Tab. 1, Fig. II.
Excellent atlas of anatomic drawings with precise anatomic descriptions. Not mentioned frequently. Detailed description of the insertion of the flexor superficialis tendon is given with credit to Albinus. For the first time, this insertion is called Chiasma Tendinum. This is not generally known.

Cauldwell EW, Anson BJ, Wright RR: Q Bull N U Med S **17**:267, 1943

Cleland J: On the cutaneous ligaments of the phalanges, J Anat Physiol **12**:526, 1878.

Clifton EE: Unusual innervation of intrinsic muscles by median and ulnar nerve. Surgery **23**:12, 1948

Cockshott P: Carpal fusions. Am J Roentgenol **89**:1260, 1963

Coleman SS, Anson BJ: Arterial patterns in the hand based upon a study of 650 specimens. Surg Gynecol Obstet **113**:409, 1961

Cornacchia M: Considerazioni sulla meccanica articolare del pollice. Chir Organi Mov **33**:137, 1949

Cruveilhier J: Traité d'anatomie Descriptive. 2nd ed. Paris, Labe, 1843
A great anatomy text written in the tradition of the 19th century French anatomists, replete with original research, understanding of medicine and great respect for precise description of anatomic structures.

Day MH, Napier JR: The two heads of flexor pollicis brevis. J Anat **95**:123, part 1, 1961

DeLeeuw B: The Stratigraphy of the Dorsal Wrist Region as Basis for an Investigation of the Position of the M. Extensor Carpi Ulnaris in Pronation and Supination of the Forearm. (De Stratigrafie van het dorsale Polsgebied als uitgangspunt voor een Onderzoek naar de Positie van de m. extensor carpi ulnaris Tijdens het Proneren en Supineren van de Onderarm) Thesis. Leiden, Luctor et Emergo, 1962

Dolgo-Saburow BA: Innervation der Venen. Berlin, Veb Verlag Volk und Gesundheit, 1963

Destot Étienne: Traumatismes du Poignet. Paris, Masson, 1923
Thorough pioneer work on the mechanism of the normal and injured wrist by roentgenography. Very important contribution on the subject, rapidly joining the long list of important but forgotten books.

Dubreuil-Chambardel, L: Des muscles fléchisseurs et extenseurs sur un pouce à trois phalanges. Bull Soc Anat Paris, 1919

Dubreuil-Chambardel, L: Traité des variations du système artériel. Variations des artères du membre supérieur. Paris, Masson, 1926
The only known treatise on the variation of the arterial system of the upper extremity.

Duchenne GB: Physiology of Motion, Demonstrated by Means of Electrical Stimulation and Clinical Observation and Applied to the Study of Paralysis and Deformities. Philadelphia, JB Lippincott, 1949. Translated and edited by Emanuel B. Kaplan
The most valuable contribution in the world literature on the activity and the kinesiology of the muscles of the human body. The most comprehensive study on the physiology of a normal and abnormal hand by one of the great neurologists of the 19th century.

Duensing F: Über die Wirkungsweise des Extensor digitorum communis (mit Untersuchungen über die Entstehung der Krallenhand bei den Ulnaris-lähmungen). Deutsch Z Nervenheilk **156**:141, 1944

Dwight T: Variations of the Bones of the Hands and Feet. Philadelphia, JB Lippincott, 1907
Roentgenographic study of the skeletal variations of the hand. Based on the material in the Warren Museum, Boston.

Elze C: Bewegungsapparat, *In* Braus-Anatomie des Menschen, 3rd ed, vol. 1, Berlin, Springer Verlag, 1954

Emmel VE: The BNA Arranged as an Outline of Regional and Systematic Anatomy, 2nd ed, Philadelphia, Wistar Institute, 1927

Eyclesheimer AC: Anatomic Names, Especially the Basle Nomina Anatomica (BNA), p 118. Wood, 1917
Very informative text combining important historical data with signficance and development of anatomic names.

Eyeler DL, Markee JE: The anatomy and function of the intrinsic musculature of the fingers. J Bone Joint Surg **36-A**:1, 1954

Fick R: Bemerkungen über die Schnappgelenke. Morph J **66**:1, 1931

Forster A: Die Mm. contrahentes und Interossei Manus in der Säugetierreihe und beim Menschen Arch Anat Physiol p 101, 1916

Forster A: Considérations sur l'os central du carpe de l'homme dans l'espèce humaine. Arch Anat (Strasb) **37**:385, 1933-34

Franklin KJ: A Monograph on Veins. Springfield, Charles C Thomas, 1937

Froment J: Paralysie des muslces de la main et troubles de la préhension, J Méd. Lyon, 1920
Interesting study by a master neurologist based on the experiences of World War I.

Galen: Oeuvres anatomiques, physiologiques et médicales, translated by Dr. Ch. Daremberg, Paris, Baillière, 1854. V. de l'Utilité des Parties du Corps Humain. Livre Premier de la Main.

Gambier R, Asvazadurian A, Venturini G: Recherches sur la vascularisation des tendons. Rev Chir Orthop **48**:225, 1962

Goldner JL, Irwin CE: An analysis of paralytic thumb deformities. J Bone Joint Surg **32-A**:627, 1950

Grayson J: The cutaneous ligaments of the digits. J Anat **75**:164, 1941

Greulich WW, and Pyle SI: Radiographic Atlas of Skeletal Development of the Hand and Wrist, 2nd ed. Stanford, Stanford University Press, 1959
The book is a continuation of a study, initiated by T. Wingate Todd, on important material investigating long-term changes of human growth. Important contribution.

Grodinsky M, Holyoke EA: The fasciae and fascial spaces of the palm. Anat Rec **79**:435, 1941

Gruber W: Über den Anomalie verlauf des Nervus ulnaris vor dem Epitrochleus. Arch Anat p 560, 1867

Gruber W: Über die Verbindung des Nervus medianus mit dem Nervus ulnaris am Unterarme des Mensche unter der Saugethiere, Arch Anat p 501, 1870

Haines RW: The mechanism of the metatarsals and spread foot. Chiropodist **2**:197, 1947

Haines RW: The flexor muscles of the forearm and hand in lizards and mammals, J Anat **84**:13, 1950.

Haines RW: The extensor apparatus of the finger. J Anat **85**:251, 1951
Study of the extensor apparatus confirming the viewpoints of Landsmeer.

Harris H, Joseph J: Variations in extension of the metacarpo-phalangeal and interphalangeal joints of the thumb. J Bone Joint Surg **31-B**:547, 1949

Henle J: Handbuch der Systematischen anatomie den Menschen, Braunschweig, Von Friedrich Vieweg und Sohn, 1868
Fundamental anatomic textbook based on original research by a master anatomist.

Hovelaque A: Anatomie des nerfs craniens et rachidiens et du système grand sympathique, Paris, Doin, 1927
Excellent, complete descriptive anatomy of the peripheral nervous system. When in quest of some obscure or unknown detail on the peripheral nervous system, the answer may be found here.

Huber CG: Piersol's Human Anatomy, 9th ed. Philadelphia, JB Lippincott, 1930

Hughes, HV, Dransfield JW: McFadyeans Osteology and Arthrology of the Domesticated Animals, 4th ed. London, Baillière, Tindall and Cox, 1953

Humphry GM: Observations in Myology. Cambridge—London, Macmillan, 1872
Remarkable collection of observations of great interest and importance on the significance of muscular variations.

Hyrtl J: Handbuch der topographischen Anatomie, bd. 2. Vienna, 1882
A great German topographic anatomy of the brilliant period of the development of anatomy.

International Federation of Societies for Surgery of the Hand: Terminology for Hand Surgery, 1970

Kaplan EB: Extension deformities of the proximal interphalangeal joints of the fingers. J Bone Joint Surg **18**:781, 1936

Kaplan EB: The palmar fascia in connection with Dupuytren's contracture. Surgery **4**:415, 1938

Kaplan EB: Device for measuring length of tendon graft in flexor tendon surgery of the hand. Bull Hosp Joint Dis **3**:97, 1942

Kaplan EB: Functional significance of the insertions of the extensor digitorum communis in man. Anat Rec **92**:293, 1945

Kaplan EB: The relation of the extensor digitorum communis tendon to the metacarpo-phalangeal joint. Bull Hosp Joint Dis **6**:149, 1945

Kaplan EB: Notes on the upper extremity of the gorilla. Bull Hosp Joint Dis **7**:129, 1946

Kaplan EB: Embryological development of the tendinous apparatus of the finger. J Bone Joint Surg **32-A**:820, 1950

Kaplan EB: Anatomical problems of opposition of thumb. Bull Hosp Joint Dis **15**:56, 1954

Kaplan EB: Notes on the surgical anatomy of the hand. J St. Barnabas Med Center **2**:3–6, 1964

Kaplan EB: Variation of the ulnar nerve at the wrist. Bull Hosp Joint Dis **24**:85, 1963

Kendall HO, Florence P: Muscles. Testing and Function. Baltimore, Williams & Wilkins, 1949

Kessler I, Silberman Z: An experimental study of the radiocarpal joint by arthrography. Surg Gynecol Obstet **112**:33, 1961

King RB: Anomalous innervation of the hand muscles. J Neurosurg **8**:528, 1951

Kopsch Fr: Die Nomina anatomica des Jahres 1895 (BNA) nach der Buchstabenreihe geordnet und gegenübergestellt den Nomina anatomica des Jahres 1935 (INA), Leipzig, Thieme, 1937

Krogman WM: The anthropology of the hand, Ciba Symposia, vol 4, no 4, 1942

Lacey TII, Goldstein LA, Tobin CE: Anatomical and clinical study of the variations in the insertions of the abductor pollicis longus tendon, associated with stenosing tendovaginitis. J Bone Joint Surg **33-A**:347, 1951

Lamoen: In Matricali EAM: Een Ontleekundig-Functioneel Onderzoik Van het Polsgewricht. Norduijn en Zoon, 1961

Landsmeer JMF: The anatomy of the dorsal aponeurosis of the human finger and its functional significance. Anat Rec **104**:31, 1949
Thorough study of the dorsal apparatus.

Landsmeer JMF: Anatomical and functional investigations on the articulation of the human fingers. Acta Anat Suppl 24, **25**:1 1955

Lanz Von, T, Wachsmuth W: Prartische Anatomie. Erster Band, Driter Teil. Arm. Berlin, Springer-Verlag, 1935

Laurent E: Lexicum medicum polyglottum. Paris, Maloine, 1906

Lazortes, G: Le système neurovasculaire. Étude anatomique, physiologique, pathologique et chirurgicale. Paris, Masson, 1949

LeDouble AF: Traité des variations du système musculaire de l'homme et de leur signification au point de vue de l'anthropologie zoologique. Paris, Schleicher Frères, 1897
Most complete and valuable contribution on the variations of muscles of the human body with excellent comparative anatomic and bibliographic notes on the subject.

Legueu MMF, Juvara E: Des aponévroses de la paume de la main. Bull Soc Anat Paris, p. 393, May, 1892
One of the initial original studies of the aponeurosis of the hand still referred to in the descriptions of the aponeurosis found in the French textbooks of anatomy, including the latest publications.

Littler JW: The hand and wrist. In Howorth MB: A Textbook of Orthopedics. Philadelphia, WB Saunders, 1952
A most contributive series of articles on principles of reconstruction and understanding of hand mechanisms by a master surgeon and artist.

Littler JW: The physiology and dynamic function of the hand. Surg Clin North Am **40**:259, 1960

Loomis LK: Variations of stenosing tenosynovitis at the radial styloid process. J Bone Joint Surg **33-A**:340, 1951

Lubotsky DN: Priority of N. I. Pirogoff in problems of surgical anatomy of the extremities, Khirurgia (Russian), no. 12, p. 11, 1950

MacConaill MA: The mechanical anatomy of the carpus and its bearings on some surgical problems. J Anat **75**:166, 1940–41

Mackenzie Sir Colin: The Action of Muscles. London, Lewis, 1930
A frequently mentioned text. Some of the observations and conclusions of this book can be seriously questioned.

Mangini U: Os styloideum carpi. Arch Putti Chir Organi Mov, vol. 9, 1957

Mangini U, Boni V: Gli Elementi accessori delle ossa del carpo. Arch Putti Chir Organi Mov, vol. 12, Florence, 1959

Mangini U: Illustrazione di una rara variazione della muscolatura ipothenar. Arch Putti Chir Organi Mov, vol. 7, 1956

Mangini U: Flexor pollicis longus muscle. Its morphology and clinical significance. J Bone Joint Surg **42-A**:467, 1960

Mannerfelt L: Studies on the hand in ulnar nerve paralysis. A clinical-experimental investigation in normal and anomalous innervation. Acta Scand Orthop Suppl. 87, 1966

Marie P, Foix Ch: Atrophie isolée de l'éminence thénar d'origine névritique. Rôle du ligament annulaire antérieur du carpe dans la pathogénie de la lésion. Rev Neurol **26**:647, 1913

Mason ML: Rupture of tendons of the hand, with study of extensor tendon insertions in fingers. Surg Gynecol Obstet **50**:611, 1930

Mierzecki H: Symbolism and pathognomy of the hand. Ciba Symposia, vol. 4, no. 4, 1942

Miller RA: Evolution of the pectoral girdle and forelimb in the primates. Am J Phys Anthropol **17**:1, 1932

Mittelmeier H: Experimentelle Untersuchungen zur Pathologie und Verhutung der posttraumatischen Sehnenverwachsung. Berlin, Springer, 1963

Moberg E: Examination of sensory loss by the Ninhydrin printing test in Volkman's contracture. Bull Hosp Joint Dis **21**:296, 1960

Montagu MFA: An Introduction to Physical Anthropology, 2nd ed. Springfield, Charles C Thomas, 1951
Important textbook on physical anthropology. Its wide and human approach to the subject of study of man makes it valuable for the surgeon and the anatomist.

Montant R, Baumann A: Recherches anatomiques sur le système tendineux extenseur des doigts de la main. Ann Anat Pathol Paris **14**:311, 1937

Murphey F, Kirklin JW, Finlayson AI: Anomalous innervation of the intrinsic muscles of the hand. Surg Gynecol Obstet **83**:15, 1946

McCormack LJ, Cauldwell EW, Anson BJ: Brachial and antebrachial arterial patterns. A study of 750 extremities. Surg Gynecol Obstet **96**:43, 1953

McFarlane RM: Observations on the functional anatomy of the intrinsic muscles of the thumb. J Bone Joint Surg **44-A**:1073, 1962

McMurrich JP: The phylogeny of the forearm flexors. Am J Anat **2**:177, 1902

Napier JR: The form and function of the carpometacarpal joint of the thumb. J Anat **89**:3, 1955

Napier JB: Studies of the hands of living primates. Proc Zool Soc (London) **134**:647, 1960

Napier JB: Functional aspects of the anatomy of the hand. Physiological Memorandum #12 P.O., London, Research Station, Registered Case #20412

Noback CR, Robertson GG: Sequences of appearance of ossification centers in the human skeleton during the first five prenatal months. Am J Anat **89**:1, 1951

Nomina Anatomica Tokyo, 4th ed. Amsterdam-Oxford, Excerpta Medica, 1977

O'Rahilly R: Morphological patterns in limb deficiencies and duplications. Am J Anat **89**:135, 1951

O'Rahilly R: A survey of carpal and tarsal anomalies. J Bone Joint Surg **35-A**:626, 1953

O'Rahilly R: The developmental anatomy of the extensor assembly. Acta Anat **47**:363, 1961

Parona F: Dell' oncotomia negli accessi profundi diffusi dell' avambracchio. Annali Universali di Medicina e Chirurgia, Milan, 1876. (Abstracted in Jahresbericht über die Leistungen und Fortschritte in der gesamten Medizin, 1877.)

Paturet G: Membres supérieurs et inférieurs. In Traité d'Anatomie Humaine. Tome II, Paris, Masson, 1951

Pirogoff NI: Complete course of applied anatomy of the human body. (Polnii coorse pricladnoi anatomii chelovecheskavo tiela.)

Pitres JA, Vaillard M: Maladies des nerfs periphériques et du sympathique. Paris, Baillière, 1924
Fundamental important studies on the afflictions of the peripheral nervous and autonomic systems. Many important details and facts connected with recognition of the most obscure cases of nerve injuries are described lucidly.

Pitres JA, Testut L: Les nerfs en schémas. Paris, Doin, 1925
A most useful contribution to the anatomy and the physiology of the peripheral nerve system. The diagrams are masterpieces of lucidity; they are widely imitated in modern textbooks, either directly or with "modifications."

Poirier P, Charpy A: Traité d'anatomie humaine, new ed. (A. Nicolas, ed) Paris, Masson, 1926

Primrose A: The anatomy of the orangoutang. University of Toronto Studies, Anatomical Studies, no. 1, 94 pages, 1900

Rabishong P: L'innervation proprioceptive des muscles lombricaux de la main chez l'homme. Rev Chir Orthop **48**:234, 1963

Raven HC: Comparative anatomy of the sole of the foot. American Museum Novitates, no. 871, July, 1936
A delightful study of the subject. Short, informative, useful.

Raven HC: The anatomy of the gorilla, The Henry Cushier Memorial volume. The studies of H. C. Raven and contributors arranged and edited by W. K. Gregory. New York, Columbia University Press, 1950
Valuable, but incomplete as far as the hand is concerned.

Reininger W: The hand in art. Ciba Symposia, vol. 4, no. 4, 1942

Riordan DC: Congenital absence of the radius. J Bone Joint Surg **37-A**:1129, 1955

Rosen G: The worker's hand. Ciba Symposia, vol. 4, no. 4, 1942

Rouvière H: Anatomie des Lymphatiques de l'Homme. Paris Masson, 1932
Collective anatomy of the lymphatic system.

Rowntree T: Anomalous Innervation of the hand muscles. J Bone Joint Surg **31-B**:505, 1949

Rushfort AF: A congenital abnormality of the trapezium and first metacarpal bone. J Bone Joint Surg **31-B**:543, 1949

Salmon M, Dor J: Les artères des muscles des membres et du tronc. Paris, Masson, 1933

Salisbury: The interosseous muscle of the hand. J Anat **71**:395, 1936-1937
Important investigation on the subject.

Sappey PhC: Traité d'Anatomie. Paris, Delahaye et Lecrosnier, 1888
A 19th century treatise of anatomy which can be considered contemporary now on account of the original contributions of the author. The descriptions are excellent; the illustrations are not numerous but very valuable and precise. Some of these illustrations are reproduced in the most modern books (as for instance, the lymphatic system).

Schenck R: Variations of the extensor tendons of the fingers. Surgical significance. J Bone Joint Surg **46A**:103, 1964

Shevkunenko VN: Atlas of the peripheral and venous Systems, State Edition of Medical Literature. Leningrad, 1943 (Russian)

Spinner M: Injuries to Major Branches of Peripheral Nerves of the Forearm, 2nd ed. Philadelphia, WB Saunders, 1978

Stack HG: Muscle function in the fingers. J Bone Joint Surg **44-B**:899, 1962

Stein AH: Variations of the tendons of the abductor pollicis longus and the extensor pollicis brevis. Anat Rec **110**:49, 1950

Steindler A: Mechanics of Normal and Pathological Locomotion in Man. Springfield, Charles C Thomas, 1935

Stilwell DL, Jr: The innervation of tendons and aponeuroses. Am J Anat **100**:289, 1957

Stilwell DL, Jr: Regional variations in the innervation in the deep fasciae and aponeuroses. Anat Rec **127**:635, 1957

Stilwell DL, Jr: The innervation of the deep structures of the hand. Am J Anat **101**:75, 1957

Stopford JSB: The nerve supply of the interphalangeal and metacarpo-phalangeal joints. J Anat, vol. 56, 1921-1922
Thorough investigation of the subject.

Straus WL: The phylogeny of the human forearm extensors. Human Biol **13**, no 1: 23-50; **13**, no. 2: 203-238, 1941
Important contribution to the understanding of the pattern of development of the muscles of the forearm and hand.

Straus WL: The homologies of the forearm flexors: urodeles, lizards, mammals. Am J Anat **70**:281, 1942

Straus WL: Rudimentary digits in primates. Q Rev Biol **17**:228, 1942

Straus WL: Significance of hypothenar elevation in movements of opposition of the thumb. Aust NZ J Surg **13**:155, 1944

Straus WL: Blood supply of the nerves of the upper extremity. Arch Neurol Psychiatr **53**:91, 1945

Straus WL: The actions of the extensor digitorum communis, interosseous and lumbrical muscles. Am J Anat **77**:189, 1945

Valuable contribution to the understanding of finger motion and hand action based on excellent analysis of clinical material.

Straus WL: Blood supply of peripheral nerves. Arch Neurol Psychiat **54**:180, 1945

Sunderland S: Flexion of distal phalanx of the thumb in lesions of median nerve. Aust NZ J Surg **13**:157, 1944

Sutton JB: Ligaments: Their Nature and Morphology. London, Lewis, 1887

Terry RJ: The inclination of the saddle surface of the trapezium with respect to the angle between the thumb and wrist. Am J Phys Anthrop **1**:No. 2, 1943

Testut L: Les anomalies musculaires chez l'homme expliquée par l'anatomie comparée. Leur importance en anthropologie. Paris, Masson, 1884
Thorough, extensive study of the subject. Source of valuable information based on personal extensive investigations and specialized literature.

Testut L, Latarget A: Traité d'anatomie humaine, 8th ed. vol. 1. Paris, Doin, 1928
A monumental, thorough, informative, complete anatomy, probably unsurpassed in any language.

Thompson A: Third annual report of the committee of collective investigation of the anatomical society of Great Britain and Ireland for 1891 and 1892. J Anat Physiol **27**:183, 1892-93

Todd TW: Atlas of Skeletal Maturation. St. Louis, Mosby, 1937
Todd began a long-term investigation of human growth in 1929 in Cleveland, Ohio. The material contained in this atlas is of great value in determining standards of growth in children.

Toldt C: An Atlas of Human Anatomy (Adapted to English and American and international terminology by M. Eden Paul), vols. 1 and 2. New York, Macmillan, 1928

Trarieux J: La préhension. Son mechanisme et ses modes. Thèse presentée à la Faculté de Médecine et de Pharmacie de Lyon, 1921

Travaglini F: Arterial circulation of the carpal bones. Bull Hosp Joint Dis **20**:No. 1, 1959

Tubiana R, Valentin P: L'extension des doigts. Rev Chir Orthop **49**:543, 1963

Vallois HV: Arthrology. *In* Poirier and Charpy: Traité d'anatomie humaine, 4th ed. (A. Nicolas, ed.), vol. 1. Paris, Masson, 1926

Vaschide N: Essai sur la psychologie de la main. Paris, Marcel Rivière, 1909

Von Lanz WW: Praktische Anatomie. Berlin, Springer, 1935
A masterpiece of illustrative anatomy, modern in trend of combining function with description of structures; complete; precise; instructive.

Walsh JF: The Anatomy and Functions of the Hand and of the Extensor Tendons of the Thumb. Philadelphia, Charles H. Walsh, 1897

Most contributive personal investigation of the motors of the hand, based on anatomic studies and critical review of literature.

Waugh RL, Sullivan RF: Anomalies of the carpus. J Bone Joint Surg **32-A**:682, 1950

Weitbrecht J: Syndesmologia sive historia ligamentorum corporis humani, quam secundum observationes anatomicas concinnavit, et figuris and objecta recentia adumbratis illustravit. Petropoli, ex typographia academiae scientiarum, 1742
A delightful large volume with an excellent description of the ligaments of the human body. Weitbrecht first described the oblique radio-ulnar ligament, bearing his name.

Wetherington RK: A note on the fusion of the lunate and triquetral centers. Am J Phys Anthropol new series 19. no **3**:251, 1961

Willan R: The action of the extensor, lumbrical and interosseous muscles in the hand and foot. Anat Anz **11**:145, 1912

Winslow JB: The usage of the muscles of the hand. Exposition anatomique de la structure du corps humain, 2nd ed. p 349. Amsterdam, 1752
One of the early, thorough anatomic texts explaining the motions of muscles. It can be compared favorably with some of the most modern speculations on muscle action.

Wood-Jones F: Man's Place Among the Mammals. London, Arnold, 1929

Wood-Jones F: The principles of anatomy, 2nd ed. Baltimore, Williams & Wilkins, 1942
An important serious study on many aspects of the anatomy of the hand. All phases connected with the hand are treated interestingly and lucidly by the learned anatomist.

Wright WG: Muscle Function. New York, Hoeber, 1928

Yerkes RM: Almost Human. New York, Century, 1925

Yerkes RM, Ada W: The Great Apes. New Haven, Yale University Press, 1929

Zeren Z: Les passages fibro-tendineux annexes aux muscles chez l'homme comptes rendus, XLII-Reunion. Paris, July 25-30, 1955

Zeren Z: A propos les arcades et tunnels annexés aux muscles. Acta Anat (Switz.) 1957

SURGICAL ANATOMY

Adams W: Observations on Contraction of the Fingers (Dupuytren's Contraction). London, Churchill, 1879
A most interesting study of Dupuytren's contracture, treated with understanding of the fundamental principles involved in the causation of this entity.

Barsky AJ: Congenital anomalies of the hand. J Bone Joint Surg **33-A**:35, 1951

Bateman JE: Trauma to Nerves in Limbs. Philadelphia, WB Saunders, 1962

Bolton H, Fowler PJ, Jepson RP: Natural history and treatment of pulp space infection and osteomyelitis of the terminal phalanx. J Bone Joint Surg **31-B**:499, 1949

Borges AF, Alexander JE: Relaxed skin tension lines, Z-plastics on scars, and fusiform excision of lesions. Br J Plastic Surg **15**:242, 1962

Boyes JH: Flexor tendon grafts in the fingers and thumb. J Bone Joint Surg **32-A**:489, 1950

Boyes JH: Bunnell's Surgery of the Hand, 5th ed. Philadelphia, JB Lippincott, 1970
Current 4th edition revised by Joseph H. Boyes—a master surgeon who added invaluable new material and advanced information on function and structure of the hand.

Brand PW: Paralytic claw hand. J Bone Joint Surg **40-B**:618, 1959

Brickel ACJ: Surgical Treatment of Hand and Forearm Infections. St. Louis, Mosby, 1939
Useful textbook on surgery of infections, reflecting personal experiences and investigations of the subject.

Brooks DM: Inter-metacarpal bone graft for thenar paralysis. J Bone Joint Surg **31-B**:511, 1949

Bruner JM: Incisions for plastic and reconstructive (non-septic) surgery of the hand. Br J Plastic Surg **4**:48, 1951

Bruner JM: The selective treatment of Dupuytren's contacture with special reference to complications and indications for treatment. Trans Int Soc Plastic Surg 244, 1960

Bunnell S: Surgery of the Hand, 2nd ed. Philadelphia, JB Lippincott, 1948
An important edition of a text on surgery of the hand, covering the subject in its entirety. When first appeared, it was responsible for the creation of a whole generation of surgeons with an unsurpassed devotion to the reconstruction of the injured and disabled human hand.

Bunnell S: Discussion of spontaneous compression of the median nerve at the wrist by G. S. Phalen. JAMA **145**:1132, 1951

Bunnell S: Ischaemic contracture, local in the hand. J Bone Joint Surg **35-A**:88, 1953

Byrne JJ: The Hand. Its Anatomy and Diseases. Springfield, Charles C Thomas, 1959

Cadenat FM: Les voies de pénétration des membres. 2nd ed. Paris, Doin, 1948
A complete informative study of surgical approaches to the extremities. Very useful, well illustrated, based on fruitful personal investigations.

Camey M: Un cas d'ablation complète du flechisseur commun superficiel des doigts. Rev Orthop **37**:196, 1951

Cornacchia M: Indirizzi terapeutici nella perdita della funzione di opposizione del pollice. Chir Organi Mov **33**:201, 1949

Curtis RM: Capsulectomy of the interphalangeal joints of the fingers. J Bone Joint Surg **36-A**:1219, 1954

Cutler CW: The Hand: Its Disabilities and Diseases. Philadelphia, WB Saunders, 1942

Dionis: A Course of Chirurgical Operations, Demonstrated at the Royal Garden at Paris, p 392. London, Jacob Tonson, 1710
An early 18th century surgery which was translated into several languages and was very popular throughout Europe of that period. The surgical methods and techniques, including tendon sutures, could be interpreted as quite modern.

Dornan, A: The results of treatment in Kienböck's disease. J Bone Joint Surg **31-B**:518, 1949

Dwyer FC: Excision of the carpal scaphoid for ununited fracture. J Bone Joint Surg **31-B**:572, 1949

Ender J, Krotcscheck H, Simon Weidner R: Die Chirurgie der Handverletzungen. Vienna, Springer-Verlag, 1956

Farabeuf LH: Précis de manuel opératoire, new edition. Paris, Masson, 1889
One of the greatest surgical anatomies written by a French anatomist of the 19th century who left an indelible imprint on the development of French surgery and surgical technique.

Flynn JE: Surgical significance of the middle palmar septum of the hand. Surgery **14**:134, 1943

Gedda KO: Studies on Bennett's fracture. Acta Chir Scand Suppl 193, Goteborg, 1954

Gedda KO, Moberg E: Open reduction and osteosynthesis of the so called Bennett's fracture in the carpometacarpal joint of the thumb. Acta Orthop Scand **12**, No. **3**:249, 1953

Grant JCB: A Method of Anatomy, 4th ed. Baltimore, Williams & Wilkins, 1948

Harris C, Riordan DC: Intrinsic contracture in the hand and its surgical treatment. J Bone Joint Surg **36-A**:10, 1954

Harvey GW: Excision of the trapezium for osteoarthritis of the trapezio-metacarpal joint. J Bone Joint Surg **31-B**:537, 1949

Hilgenfeldt O: Operativer Daumenersatz und Beseitigung von greifstörungen bei Fingerverlusten. Stuttgart, Enke, 1950
Thorough, important contribution to reconstructive surgery of the hand, reflecting original thoughts, ingenuity and mastery of the subject.

Iselin M, Gosse L, Boussard S, Benoist D: Atlas de Technique Opératoire. Chirurgie de la Main Flammarion. Paris, 1958

James JIP: A case of rupture of flexor tendons secondary to Kieböck's disease. J Bone Joint Surg **31-B**:521, 1949

Jamieson JG: The fascial spaces of the palm. With special references to their significance in infections of the hand. Br J Surg vol. 38, July, 1950-April, 1951

Jones T, Shepard WC: A Manual of Surgical Anatomy. Philadelphia, WB Saunders, 1945

Kanavel A: Infections of the Hand, 6th ed. Philadelphia, Lea & Febiger, 1933
One of the great books on the hand, which inspired a large

number of surgeons and initiated interest and serious scientific search in the methods of prevention of disabilities of the hand and understanding of the finer structures of the hand.

Kaplan EB: Pathology and operative correction of finger deformities due to injuries and contractures of the extensor digitorum tendon. Surgery **6**:35, 1939

Kaplan EB: Mallet or baseball finger. Surgery **7**:784, 1940

Kaplan EB: Correction of a disabling flexion contracture of the thumb. Bull Hosp Joint Dis **3**:51, 1942

Kaplan EB: Surgical anatomy of the flexor tendons of the wrist. J Bone Joint Surg **27**:368, 1945

Kaplan EB: Dorsal dislocation of the metacarpophalangeal joint of the index finger. J Bone Joint Surg **39-A**:1081, 1957

Kaplan EB: Anatomy, injuries and treatment of the extensor apparatus of the hand and the digits. Clin Orthop **13**:24, 1959

Kaplan EB: Lateral subluxation of the metacarpophalangeal joint of the thumb: experimental study. Bull Hosp Joint Dis **21**:200, 1960

Kaplan EB: The pathology and treatment of radial subluxation of the thumb with ulnar displacement of the head of the first metacarpal. J Bone Joint Surg **43-A**:541, 1961

Kaplan EB: Surgical treatment of spastic hyperextension of the proximal interphalangeal joints of the fingers, accompanied by flexion of the distal phalanges (case report). J Hosp Joint Dis **23**;35, 1962

Koch SL: Division of flexor tendons within digital sheath. Surg Gynecol Obstet **78**:9, 1944

Kocher Th: Chirurgische Operationslehre, 5th ed. Jena, Fischer, 1907
Well-known and great operative surgery apparently being mentioned less and less, forgotten more and more. Curiously enough, a number of most modern operative approaches can be found in this text under earlier names.

Lampe EW: Surgical anatomy of the hand. Ciba Clinical Symposia, vol. 3, no. 8, 1951

Lapidus P, Fenton R: Stenosing tendovaginitis at the wrist and fingers (Report of 423 cases in 369 patients with 354 operations). Arch Surg **64**:475, 1952

Lasserre Ch, Pauzat D, Derenes R: Osteoarthritis of the trapezio-metacarpal joint. J Bone Joint Surg **31-B**:534, 1949

Lecen P: Chirurgie des os des articulations des membres. Paris, Masson, 1929

Littler JW: Metacarpal reconstruction. J Bone Joint Surg **29**:723, 1947

Littler JW: Free tendon grafts in secondary flexor tendon repair. Am J Surg **74**:315, 1947

Littler JW: Tendon transfers and arthrodeses in combined median and ulnar nerve paralysis. J Bone Joint Surg **31-A**:225, 1949

Littler JW: The neurovascular pedicle method of digital transposition for reconstruction of the thumb. Plastic Reconstr Surg **12**:303, 1953

Littler JW: Principles of reconstructive surgery of the hand. Am J **92**:88, 1956

Littler JW: The prevention and the correction of adduction contracture of the thumb. Clin Orthop **13**:182, 1959

Littler JW: The severed flexor tendon. Surg Clin North Am **39**:435, 1959

Littler JW: Basic principles of reconstructive surgery of the hand. Surg Clin North Am **40**:383, 1960

Luck JV: Dupuytren's contracture. J Bone Joint Surg **41-A**:4, 1959

Maisonnet J, Coudane R: Anatomie clinique et opératoire, vol. 1 Paris, Doin, 1950
A truly clinical and surgical anatomy with numerous excellent illustrations covering the entire field of anatomy, in 3 volumes. Very valuable contribution indicating the proper method of approach to anatomy.

Mangini U, Laus S: La compressione del nervo median al polso o sindrome del canale del carpo. Arch Putti Chir Organi Mov **9**:9, 1957

Marcer E: Chirurgia reparatrice della mano, Relazione al XXXIII Congresso della Societa Italiana di Ortopedia e Traumatologia. Bologna, Ottobre, 1948
Excellent review of surgery of the hand.

Milford L: Hand surgery. In Grenshaw AH (ed): Campbell's Operative Orthopedics, 6th ed. St. Louis, Mosby, 1980

Min-Chyang Ju, D: The physical basis of scar contraction. Plastic Reconstr Surg **1**:343, 1951

Moberg E: Surgery of the hand. Transactions of the Northern Surgical Association, Copenhagen, 1951

Moberg E, Stenner B: Injuries to the ligaments of the thumb and fingers. Diagnosis, treatment, and prognosis. Acta Chir Scand **106**:166, 1953

Moersch FP: Median thenar neuritis. Proc Mayo Clin **13**:220, 1938

Montant R, Baumann A: Rupture-luxation de l'appareil extenseur des doigts au niveau de la première articulation phalangienne. Rev Orthop **25**:4, 1938

Müller GM: Arthrodesis of the trapeziometacarpal joint for osteoarthritis. J Bone Joint Surg **31-B**:540, 1949

Nichols, HM: Repair of extensor-tendon insertions in the fingers. J Bone Joint Surg **33-A**:836, 1951

Nicola T: Atlas of Surgical Approaches to Bones and Joints. New York, Macmillan, 1945

Ollier L: Traité des résections et des opérations conservatrices, vol 2. Paris, Masson, 1888
A rich source of descriptions of surgical approaches which sometimes bear new names in the newest surgical literature.

Phalen GS: Spontaneous compression of the median nerve at the wrist. JAMA **145**:1128, 1951

Potenza D: Clinical evaluation of flexor tendon healing and adhesion formation within artificial digital sheaths. An experimental study. J Bone Joint Surg **45-A**:217, 1963

Pulvertaft RG: Contractures of the Hand. Modern Trends in Orthopaedics (second series), 1972

Rank BK, Wakefield AR: Surgery of Repair As Applied to Hand Injuries. London, Livingstone, 1953

Riordan DC: Tendon transplantations in median-nerve and ulnar-nerve paralysis. J Bone Joint Surg **35-A**:312, 1953

Riordan DC: Fractures about the hand. Southern M J **50**:637, 1957

Riordan DC: Surgery of the paralytic hand. Am Acad Orthop Surg Instructional Course Lectures, **16**:79, 1959

Riordan DC: The hand in leprosy (a seven-year clinical study). Part 1. General aspects of leprosy. Part 2. Orthopaedic aspects of leprosy. J Bone Joint Surg **42-A**: 661, 1960

Robbins H: Anatomical study of the median nerve in the carpel tunnel and etiologies of the carpal tunnel syndrome. J Bone Joint Surg **45-A**: 1963

Russell TB: Intercarpal dislocations and fracture dislocations. J Bone Joint Surg **31-B**:524, 1949

Slocum DB: An Atlas of Amputations. St. Louis, Mosby, 1949

Slocum DB: Amputations. In Grenshaw AH (ed): Campbell's Operative Orthopaedics, 4th ed. St. Louis, Mosby, 1963

Spak I: Tenodesis of the distal finger joint—A method of repair for loss of the flexor profundus function. Acta Chir Scand **110**:338, 1955/56

Steindler A: The traumatic deformities and disabilities of the upper extremity. Springfield, Charles Chomas, 1946

Stenner B: Displacement of the ruptured ulnar collateral ligament of the metacarpophalangeal joint of the thumb. A clinical and anatomical study. J Bone Joint Surg **44-B**:869, 1962

Stookey B: Surgical and mechanical treatment of peripheral nerves. Philadelphia, WB Saunders, 1922

Strandell G: Total rupture of the ulnar collateral ligament of the metacarpophalangeal joint of the thumb. Result of surgery in 35 cases. Acta Chir Scand **118**:72, 1959

Tanzer RC, Littler WJ: Reconstruction of the thumb, by transposition of an adjacent digit. Plastic Reconstr Surg **3**:533, 1948

Tinel J: Les Blessures des Nerfs. Paris, Masson, 1916
An important contribution to the physiopathology of nerve injuries. One of the greatest books of our times which added to better understanding of disabilities of injured peripheral nerves. Originator of Tinel sign of nerve regeneration.

Tubiana R: Greffes des tendons fléchisseurs des doigts et du pouce. Rev Chir Orthop **46**:191, 1960

Vasconcelos E: Modern Methods of Amputation. Philosophical Library of New York, Dept. of War Medicine, 1945

Vaughan-Jackson OJ: A case of recurrent subluxation of the carpal scaphoid. J Bone Joint Surg **31-B**:532, 1949

Verdan C: Chirurgie réparatrice et fonctionelle des tendons de la main. Expansion Scientific Française, Impz. Wallon-Vichy, 1951

Verdan C, Michon J: Le traitement des plaies de tendons fléchisseurs des doigts. Rev Chir Orthop **47**:285, 1961

Watson-Jones R: Leri's pleonosteosis, carpal tunnel compression of the median nerves and Morton's metarsalgia. J Bone Joint Surg **31-B**:560, 1949

White, WL: Restoration of function and balance of the wrist and hand by tendon transfer. Surg Clin North Am **40**:427, 1960

Zachary RB: Thenar palsy due to compression of the median nerve in the carpal tunnel. Surg Gynecol Obstet **81**:213, 1945

Current Bibliography

FINGERS

Bowers WH, Wolf JW, Jr, Nehil JL, Bittinger S: Proximal interphalangeal joint volar plate. I. Anatomical and biomechanical study **5**:79–88, 1980

Bowers WH: Proximal interphalangeal joint volar plate. II. Clinical study of hyperextension injury **6**:77–81, 1981

Moss SH, Schwartz, KS, Von Drasek-Ascher G, Ogden LL, Wheeler CS, Lister GD: Digital venous system. (Submitted to J Anat)

Milford LW: Retaining Ligaments of the Digits of the Hand. WB Saunders, Philadelphia, 1968

Schultz RJ, Krishnamusthy S, Johnson L: A gross anatomical and histologic study of the innervation of the proximal interphalangeal joint of the hand. Read at 38th annual meeting, American Society for Surgery of the Hand. March 7, 1983, Anaheim, Calif.

TENDONS

Beckman C, Greenlee TK, Jr.: Chick vincula: elastic structures with a check-rein mechanism. J Anat **119**:295–308, 1975

Boyes JH, Stark HH: Flexor-tendon grafts in the fingers and thumb. J Bone and Joint Surg **53-A**:1332–1342, 1971

Brockis JG: The blood supply of the flexor and extensor tendons of the fingers in man. J Bone and Joint Surg **35-B**:131–138, 1963

Caplan HS, Hunter JM, Merklin RJ: Intrinsic vascularization of flexor tendons. In symposium on tendon surgery in the hand. A.A.O.S. CV Mosby Co, St. Louis, 48–58, 1975

Duran RJ, Houser RG: Controlled passive motion following flexor tendon repair in zones 2 and 3. In symposium on tendon surgery in the hand. A.A.O.S. CV Mosby Co, St. Louis, 105–114, 1975

Edwards DAW: The blood supply and lymphatic drainage of tendons, J Anat **80**:147–152, 1964

Edwards EA: Organization of the small arteries of the hand and digits. Am J Surg **99**:837–846, 1960

Leffert RD, Weiss C, Sthanasoulis CA: The vincula with particular references to their vessels and nerves. J Bone and Joint Surg **56-A**:1191–1198, 1974

Lindsay WK, Thompson HG: Digital flexor tendons: An experimental study, Part 1. The significance of each component of the flexor mechanism in tendon healing. Br J Plast Surg **12**:289–316, 1960

Lister GD, Kleinert HE, Kutz JE, Atasoy E: Primary flexor tendon repair followed by immediate controlled mobilization. J Hand Surg **2**:441–451, 1977

Lundborg G, Myrhage R, Rydevik B: The vascularization of human flexor tendons within the digital synovial sheath region-structional and functional aspects. J hand Surg **2**:417–427, 1977

Lundborg G, Rank F: Experimental intrinsic healing of flexor tendons based upon synovial fluid nutrition. J Hand Surg **3**:21–31, 1978

Matsui T, Merlin RJ, Hunter JM: A microvascular study of the human flexor tendons in the digital fibrois sheath—normal blood vessel arrangement of tendons and the effects of injuries to tendons and vincula on distribution of tendons blood vessels. Journal of the Japanese Orthopedic Association **53**:307–320, 1979

Matthews P, Richards H: The repair potential of digit flexor tendons. J Bone and Joint Surg **56-B**:618–625, 1974

Matthews P: The fate of isolated segments of flexor tendons within the digital sheath—a study of synovial nutrition. Brit J. Plast Surg **29**:216–224, 1976

Mayer L: The physiological method of tendon transplantation. 1. Historical anatomy and physiology of tendons. Surg Gynecol Obstet **182**:182–197, 1916

McDowell CL, Snyder DH: Tendon healing: An experimental model in the dog. J Hand Surg **2**:122–126, 1977

Nichols HM, Lehman WL, Meek EC: Alteration of the blood supply of flexor tendons following injury. Am J Surg **87**:379–383, 1954

Ochiai N, Matsui T, Miyaji N, Merlin RJ, Hunter JM: Vascular anatomy of flexor tendons, I. Vincular system and blood supply of the profundus tendon in the digital sheath. J Hand Surg **4**:321–330, 1979

Peacock EE, Jr.: A study of the circulation in normal tendons and healing grafts. Ann Surg **149**:415–428, 1959

Potenza AD: Tendon healing within flexor digital sheath in dog. J Bone and Joint Surg **44-A**:49–64, 1962

Potenza AD: Concepts of tendon healing and repair. In symposiun of tendon surgery of the hand. A.A.O.S. CV Mosby Co, St. Louis, 18–47, 1975

Smith JW: Blood supply of tendons. Am J Surg **109**:272–276, 1965

Tsuge K, Ikuta Y, Matsuishi Y: Repair of flexor tendons by intratendinous tendon suture. J Hand Surg **2**:436–440, 1977

Verdan CE: Half a century of flexor-tendon surgery, J Bone and Joint Surg **54-A**:472-491, 1972

Young L, Weeks PM: Profundus tendon blood supply within the digital sheath. Surgery Forum **21**:504–506, 1971

THUMB

Ahstrom JP, Jr: Pollicization in congenital absence of the thumb. In Ahstrom, JP, (ed): Current Practice in Orthopaedic Surgery 5. CV Mosby Co, St. Louis, 1973

Buck-Gramcko D: Pollicization of the Index Finger: Method and Results in Aplasia and Hypoplasia of the Thumb. J Bone Joint Surg **53**:1605–1617, 1971

Bunnell S: Physiological Reconstruction of the Thumb after Total Loss, Surg Gynecol Obstet **52**:245–248, 1931

Iselin M: Chirugie de la Main, 10th ed. Paris, 1955

Linburg RM, Comstock BE: Anomalous tendon slips from the flexor pollicis longais to the flexor digitorum profundus. J Hand Surg 79–83, 1979

Littler JW: The Neurovascular Pedicle Method of Digital Transposition for Reconstruction of the Thumb, Plastic, and Reconstructive Surgery, **12**:303–319, 1953

Littler JW: Subtotal reconstruction of the thumb. Plastic and Reconstructive Surgery **10**:215, 1952

Riordan DC: Pollicization for congenital absence of the thumb. Campbell's Operative Orthopaedics. 6th ed. CV Mosby, St. Louis, 1982

WRIST

Bryce TH: On certain points in the anatomy and mechanism of the wrist joint reviewed in the light of a series of roentgen ray photographs of the living hand. Journal of Anatomy and Physiology **31**:59, 1896

Capener N: The hand in surgery. J Bone Joint Surg (Br) **38**:128, 1956

Cyriax EF: On the rotatory movements of the wrist. J Anat **60**:199, 1926

Destot E: Injuries of the Wrist. A radiological study. London, Ernest Benn Limited, 1925

Fisk GF: Carpal instability and the fractured scaphoid. Ann R Coll Surg Eng. 46–63, 1970

Ghia C: Contributo allo studio della articolazione della mano. Chir degli Organi di Movimento. **24**:344, 1939

Gilford WW, Bolton RH, Lambrinudi C: The mechanism of the wrist joint with special reference to fractures of the scaphoid, Guy's Hosp. Rep. 92–52, 1943

Johnston HM: Varying positions of the carpal bones in the different movements at the wrist. Part I. Extension, ulnar and radial flexion. J Anat Physiol **41**:109, 1907

Kauer, JMG: The interdependence of carpal articulation chains. Acta Anat **88**:481, 1974

Kauer JMG: The articular disc of the hand. Acta Anat **93**:590, 1975

Kauer JMG: The relation of the ulnar styloid process—triangular disc in the gibbon. Acta Morphol Neerl Scand **15**:328, 1977

Kauer JMG: Functional anatomy of the wrist. Clin Orthop **149**:9, 1980

Kessler I, Silberman Z: An experimental study of the radiocarpal joint by arthrography. Surg Gynecol Obstet 112–33, 1961

Kirk JA, Ansell BM, Bywaters EGL: The hypermobility syndrome. Ann Rheum Dis **26**:419, 1967

Lewis OJ, Hamshere RJ, Bucknill TM: The anatomy of the wrist joint. J Anat **106**:539, 1970

Lichtman DM, Swafford AR, Scneider JR: Midcarpal subluxation. Presented at the Members Day Program, Am Soc Surg Hand Atlanta, GA, February 3, 1980

Linscheid RL, Dobyns JH, Beabout JW, Bryn RS: Traumatic instability of the wrist. J Bone Joint Surg (Am) **54**:1612, 1972

Mayfield JK, Johnson RP, Kilcoyne RK: Carpal dislocations: pathomechanics and progressive perilunar instability. J Hand Surg **5**:226, 1980

Navarro A: Anales del instituto de clinica quirurgica y cirugia experimental, Montevideo. Imprenta Artistica de Dornaleche Hnos, 1935

Palmer AK, Werner FW: Triangular fibrocartilage of the wrist, anatomy and function. J Hand Surg **6**:153, 1981

Sutro CJ: Hypermobility of bones due to "overlengthened" capsular and ligamentous tissues, Surgery **21**:67, 1947

Taleisnik J: The ligaments of the wrist, J Hand Surg **1**:110, 1976

Taleisnik J: Wrist: Anatomy, function and injury. Amer Acad Orthop Surg Instructional Course Lectures **27**:6, 1978

Testut L, Laterjet A: Tratado de anatomia humana, Vol 1, 9th ed, Rev., Buenos Aires, 1951, Salvat Editores

Weber ER: Biomedical implications of scaphoid waist fractures. Clin Ortho 149:83, 1980

Wright RD: A detailed study of movement of the wrist joint. J Anat **70**:137, 1935

SURGERY

Curtis RM: Joints of the hand. In Flynn JE (ed) Hand Surgery. 3d ed, pp 335–353, Williams & Wilkins, Baltimore, 1982

Smith RJ: Post-traumatic inotability of the thumb. J Bone Joint Surg **59-A**:17–21, 1977

Swanson AB: The treatment of war wounds of the hand. Clin Plast Surg **2**:615–626, 1975

Swanson AB: Severe congenital malformations of the upper limb: Considerations for classifications and treatment. Ann Clin **29**:433–462, 1975

Swanson AB: Multiple finger amputations: Concepts of treatment. Journal of the Michigan State Medical School **61**:316–320, 1962

Swanson AB: Restoration of hand function by the use of partial or total prosthetic replacement, Part I. The use of partial prostheses. J Bone Joint Surg **45-A**:276–283, 1963

Swanson AB: The Krukenberg procedure in the juvenile amputee. J Bone Joint Surg **461-A**:1540–1549, 1964

Swanson AB, Swanson G, deGrott: The Krukenberg procedure in the juvenile amputee. Clin Orthop **148**:55–61, 1980

Emanuel B. Kaplan Bibliography

1932

Kaplan EB: Early signs of tuberculous spondylitis by Dr. S. Kofman, U.S.S.R. translated from the German. J Bone Joint Surg 14:143–144, 1932

1934

Kaplan EB: Treatment of ganglion. Am J Surg 24:151, 1934
Kaplan EB: Multiple fractures associated with blue sclera. J Bone Joint Surg 16:625–630, 1934

1938

Kaplan EB: The palmar fascia in connection with Dupuytren's contracture. Surgery 4:415–422, 1938

1939

Kaplan EB: Operation for Dupuytren's contracture (in Russian). Russian Med Soc NY Fifteenth Anniversary Bulletin, 78–82, September 1939

1940

Kaplan EB: Mallet or baseball finger. Surgery 7:784–791, 1940

1941

Kaplan EB: Surgical approach to the proximal end of the radius and its use in fractures of the head and neck of the radius. J Bone Joint Surg 23:86–92, 1941

1942

Kaplan EB; Nelson LS: Hallux valgus. Bull Hosp Joint Dis 3:17–25, 1942
Kaplan EB: Correction of a disabling flexion contracture of the thumb. Bull Hosp Joint Dis 3:51–54, 1942
Kaplan EB: Device for measuring length of tendon graft in flexor tendon surgery of the hand. Bull Hosp Joint Dis 3:97–99, 1942

1943

Kaplan EB: The coraco-humeral ligament of the human shoulder. Bull Hosp Joint Dis 4:62–65, 1943

1944

Kaplan EB: Treatment of fractures of metacarpals and proximal phalanx by skeletal traction. Bull Hosp Joint Dis 5:99–109, 1944

1945

Kaplan EB: The surgical and anatomic significance of the mammillary tubercle of the last thoracic vertebra. Surgery 17:78–92, 1945
Kaplan EB: Functional significance of the insertions of the extensor communis digitorum in man. Anat Rec 92:293–303, 1945
Kaplan EB: Surgical anatomy of the flexor tendons of the wrist. J Bone Joint Surg 27:368–372, 1945
Kaplan EB: The relation of the exterior digitorum communis tendon to the metacarpophalangeal joint. Bull Hosp Joint Dis 6:149–154, 1945
Kaplan EB: Surgical anatomy. Langer's muscle of the axilla. Bull Hosp Joint Dis 6:78–79, 1945

1946

Kaplan EB: The illiotibial band. Bull Hosp Joint Dis 7:84–86, 1946
Kaplan EB: The place of anatomy in the training of resident orthopaedic surgeons in a hospital not affiliated with a medical school. Bull Hosp Joint Dis 7:4–10, 1946
Kaplan EB: The blood vessels of the gluteal region. Bull Hosp Joint Dis 7:165–168, 1946
Kaplan EB: Notes on the upper extremity of the gorilla: Clinical application. Bull Hosp Joint Dis 7:129–136, 1946

1947

Kaplan EB: Variations of the subclavian vessels in the region of the scalenus anterior muscle. Bull Hosp Joint Dis 8:217–281, 1947

1948

Kaplan EB: Duchenne of Boulogne and the physiologie des movements. Victor Robinson Memorial Volume. Essays on Historical Medicine, pp 1–16, 1948
Kaplan EB: Resection of the obturator nerve for relief of pain in arthritis of the hip joint. J Bone Joint Surg 30A:213–216, 1948

Kaplan EB: Obturator nerve avulsion in the treatment of painful hip joints. Surg Clin North Am, pp 473–480, 1948

Kaplan EB: Variations in length of the nerve to the extensor hallucis longus. Bull Hosp Joint Dis 9:88–90, 1948

1949

Kaplan EB: Hemangiopericytoma of the hand. Bull Hosp Joint Dis 10:69–74, 1949

Kaplan EB: The ligamentum teres femoris in relation to the position of the femur. Bull Hosp Joint Dis 10:112–117, 1949

Kaplan EB: Basic sciences in the training of residents in orthopaedic surgery. Bull Hosp Joint Dis 10:269–276, 1949

1950

Kaplan EB: Surgical approach to the planter digital nerves. Bull Hosp Joint Dis 11:96–97, 1950

Kaplan EB: Transverse dorsal approach for triple anthrodesis of the foot. Bull Hosp Joint Dis 11:48–52, 1950

Kaplan EB: Embryological development of the tendinous apparatus of the fingers. J Bone Joint Surg 32A:820–826, 1950

1951

Kaplan EB: Circular hand saw for cutting small bones. J Bone Joint Surg 33A:270–274, 1951

Kaplan EB: Duchenne's sign. Bull Hosp Joint Dis 12:273–277, 1951

1953

Kaplan EB: Reference points in surgery of the vertebral column. Bull Hosp Joint Dis 14:292–303, 1953

Kaplan EB: Functional and Surgical Anatomy of the Hand. Philadelphia, JB Lippincott, 1953

1954

Kaplan EB: Anatomical problems of opposition of the thumb. Bull Hosp Joint Dis 15:56–59, 1954

Kaplan EB: Anatomical pitfalls in the surgical treatment of torticollis. Bull Hosp Joint Dis 15:154–161, 1954

1955

Kaplan EB: The tibialis posterior muscle in relation to hallux valgus. Bull Hosp Joint Dis 16:88–93, 1955

Kaplan EB: The embryology of the menisci of the knee joint. Bull Hosp Joint Dis 16:111–124, 1955

1956

Kaplan EB: Reflections on orthopaedic terminology. Chairman's Address Before Orthopaedic Section on the 150th Annual Meeting of the New York State Medical Society, May 10, 1956

Kaplan EB: The lateral menisco-femoral ligament of the knee joint. Bull Hosp Joint Dis 17:176–182, 1956

Kaplan EB: Peter Camper, 1722–1739. Bull Hosp Joint Dis 17:371–385, 1956

1957

Kaplan EB: Discoid lateral meniscus of the knee joint. J Bone Joint Surg 39A:77–87, 1957

Kaplan EB: Factors responsible for the stability of the knee joint. Bull Hosp Joint Dis 18:51–59, 1957

Kaplan EB: Dorsal dislocation of the metacarpophalangeal joint of the index finger. J Bone Joint Surg 39A:1081-1086, 1957

1958

Kaplan EB: Tendon passer for hand surgery. Bull Hosp Joint Dis 19:109–110, 1958

Kaplan EB: Comparative anatomy of the extensor digitorum longus in relation to the knee joint. Anat Rec 131:129–149, 1958

Kaplan EB: The iliotibial tract. J Bone Joint Surg 40A:817–832, 1958

Kaplan EB: The genesis of an eponym. Bull History Med 32:451–455, 1958

1959

Kaplan EB: Injuries and afflictions of the menisci of the knee. Am Acad Orthop Surg Instr Course Lectures 16:153–160, 1959

Kaplan EB: Treatment of tennis elbow (epicondylitis) by denervation. J Bone Joint Surg 41:147–151, 1959

Kaplan EB: Morphology and function of the muscle quadratus plantae. Bull Hosp Joint Dis 20:84–95, 1959

Kaplan EB: Personal observations of effects of spinal anesthesia for operation on the lower extremity. Bull Hosp Joint Dis 20:112–116, 1959

Kaplan EB: Anatomy, injuries and treatment of the extensor apparatus of the hand and the digits. Clin Orthop 13:24–41, 1959

Kaplan EB: Duchenne's Physiology of Motion (translation). Philadelphia, WB Saunders, 1959

1960

Kaplan EB: Lateral subluxation of the metacarpophalangeal joint of the thumb: Experimental study. Bull Hosp Joint Dis 21:200–205, 1960

1961

Kaplan EB: The fabellofibular and short lateral ligaments of the knee joint. J Bone Joint Surg 43A:169–179, 1961

Kaplan EB: Cyst (ganglion) connected with the proximal tibofibular joint. Bull Hosp Joint Dis 22:105–107, 1961

Kaplan EB: The pathology and treatment of radial subluxation of the thumb with ulnar displacement of the head of the first metacarpal. J Bone Joint Surg 43A:541–546, 1961

1962

Kaplan EB: Some aspects of functional anatomy of the human knee joint. Clin Orthop 23:18–29, 1962

Kaplan EB: Surgical treatment of spastic hyperextension of

the proximal interphalangeal joints of the fingers, accompanied by flexion of the distal phalanges (case report). J Hosp Joint Dis 23:35–39, 1962

Kaplan EB: Intraneural neurofibroma of the posterior tibial nerve. Bull Hosp Joint Dis 23:153–157, 1962

1963

Kaplan EB: Variation of the ulnar nerve at the wrist. Bull Hosp Joint Dis 24:85–88, 1963

Kaplan EB: Avulsion fracture of proximal tibial epiphysis. Bull Hosp Joint Dis 24:119–122, 1963

1964

Kaplan EB: Some principles of anatomy and kinesiology in stabilization operations of the foot. Clin Orthop 34:7–13, 1964

Kaplan EB: The quadrate ligament of the radio-ulnar joint of the elbow. Bull Hosp Joint Dis 25:126–130, 1964

Kaplan EB: Notes on surgical anatomy of the hand. J Saint Barnabas Medical Center 2:3–6, 1964

1965

Kaplan EB: Arteritis involving the arteries of the hand. Bull Hosp Joint Dis 26:52–55, 1965

Kaplan EB: Functional and surgical anatomy of the hand, 2nd ed. Philadelphia, JB Lippincott, 1965

1966

Kaplan EB: Development of tendon surgery in the past 50 years. Clin Orthop pp 65–72, 1966

Kaplan EB: The participation of the metacarpophalangeal joint of the thumb in the act of opposition. Bull Hosp Joint Dis 27:39–45, 1966

Kaplan EB: Replacement of an amputated middle metacarpal and finger by transposition of the index finger. Bull Hosp Joint Dis 27:103–108, 1966

Kaplan EB: Anatomy and kinesiology of the hand. In Flynn JE (ed): Hand Surgery, pp 11–28. Baltimore, Williams & Wilkins, 1966

Kaplan EB: Surgical Approaches to the Neck, Cervical Spine and Upper Extremity. Philadelphia, WB Saunders, 1966

1967

Kaplan EB: Smith RJ: Rheumatoid deformities at the metacarpophalangeal joints of the fingers. A correlative study of anatomy and pathology. J Bone Joint Surg 49A :31–47, 1967

Kaplan EB: Intratruncular tumor of the posterior tibial nerve. Bull Hosp Joint Dis 28:26–29, 1967

1968

Kaplan EB, Smith RJ: Camptodactyly and similar atraumatic flexion deformities of the proximal interphalangeal joints of the fingers. J Bone Joint Surg 50A:1187–1204, 1968

Kaplan EB: Guide lines to deep structures and dynamics of intrinsic muscles of the hand. Surg Clin North Am 48:993–1002, 1968

1969

Kaplan EB: Muscular and tendinous variations of the flexor superficialis of the fifth finger of the hand. Bull Hosp Joint Dis 30:59–67, 1969

Kaplan EB, Nathan P: Accessory extensor pollicis longus. Bull Hosp Joint Dis 30:202–207, 1969

Kaplan EB: Anatomical dissertation on muscular variations. Gantzer's muscle (translation from the Latin). Bull Hosp Joint Dis 30:191–198, 1969

Kaplan EB: Weitbrecht's Syndesmology (translation). Philadelphia, WB Saunders, 1969

1970

Kaplan EB: Anterior surgical approach for resection of the trapezium. Bull Hosp Joint Dis 31:178–187, 1970

Kaplan EB: Antero-posterior width of the vertebral bodies. Bull Hosp Joint Dis 31:197–198, 1970

Kaplan EB, Spinner M: The quadrate ligament of the elbow—Its relationship to the stability of the proximal radio-ulnar joint. Acta Orthop Scand 41:632–647, 1970

Kaplan EB, Spinner M: The extensor carpi ulnaris and its relationship to the distal radio-ulnar joint disability. Clin Orthop 68:124–129, 1970

1971

Kaplan EB: Intraosseous ganglion of the scaphoid bone of the wrist. Bull Hosp Joint Dis 32:50–53, 1971

1972

Kaplan EB, Zeide MS: Aneurysm of the ulnar artery. Bull Hosp Joint Dis 33:197–199, 1972

Kaplan EB: The tingling sign in peripheral nerve lesions by J. Tinel. In Spinner M (ed): Injuries to major branches of nerves of the forearm. Philadelphia, WB Saunders, 1972

1973

Kaplan EB, Kane E, Spinner M: Observations on the course of the ulnar nerve in the arm. Ann Chir 27:487–496, 1973

1975

Kaplan EB: Anatomy and kinesiology of the hand. In Flynn JB (ed): Hand Surgery, 2nd ed. Baltimore, Williams & Wilkins, 1975

1976

Kaplan EB, Spinner M: The relationship of the ulnar nerve to the medial intermuscular septum in the arm and its clinical significance. Hand 8:239–242, 1976

1980

Kaplan EB, Spinner M: Normal and anomalous innervation patterns in the upper extremity. In Omer G, Spinner M (ed): Management of Peripheral Nerve Problems. Philadelphia, WB Saunders, 1980

1978

Kaplan EB: The "tingling" sign in peripheral nerve lesions by J. Tinel. In Spinner M (ed): Injuries to Major Branches of Peripheral Nerves of the Forearm, 2nd ed. Philadelphia, WB Saunders, 1978

1981

Kaplan EB: Forward. In Tubiana R (ed): The Hand, vol 1. Philadelphia, WB Saunders, 1981

1982

Kaplan EB: Anatomy and kinesiology of the hand. In Flynn JE (ed): Hand Surgery, 3rd ed. Baltimore, Williams & Wilkins, 1982

Index

An *f* following a page number indicates a figure; a *t* represents tabular material.